Advances in Nanomaterials in Biomedicine

Advances in Nanomaterials in Biomedicine

Editor

Elena I. Ryabchikova

MDPI • Basel • Beijing • Wuhan • Barcelona • Belgrade • Manchester • Tokyo • Cluj • Tianjin

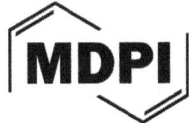

Editor
Elena I. Ryabchikova
Institute of Chemical Biology and Fundamental Medicine,
Siberian Branch of the Russian Academy of Sciences (ICBFM SB RAS)
Russia

Editorial Office
MDPI
St. Alban-Anlage 66
4052 Basel, Switzerland

This is a reprint of articles from the Special Issue published online in the open access journal *Nanomaterials* (ISSN 2079-4991) (available at: https://www.mdpi.com/journal/nanomaterials/special_issues/Biomedicine_Nanomaterials).

For citation purposes, cite each article independently as indicated on the article page online and as indicated below:

LastName, A.A.; LastName, B.B.; LastName, C.C. Article Title. *Journal Name* **Year**, *Volume Number*, Page Range.

ISBN 978-3-0365-0868-9 (Hbk)
ISBN 978-3-0365-0869-6 (PDF)

© 2021 by the authors. Articles in this book are Open Access and distributed under the Creative Commons Attribution (CC BY) license, which allows users to download, copy and build upon published articles, as long as the author and publisher are properly credited, which ensures maximum dissemination and a wider impact of our publications.

The book as a whole is distributed by MDPI under the terms and conditions of the Creative Commons license CC BY-NC-ND.

Contents

About the Editor vii

Elena Ryabchikova
Advances in Nanomaterials in Biomedicine
Reprinted from: *Nanomaterials* **2021**, *11*, 118, doi:10.3390/nano11010118 1

Vanessa Acebes-Fernández, Alicia Landeira-Viñuela, Pablo Juanes-Velasco, Angela-Patricia Hernández, Andrea Otazo-Perez, Raúl Manzano-Román, Rafael Gongora and Manuel Fuentes
Nanomedicine and Onco-Immunotherapy: From the Bench to Bedside to Biomarkers
Reprinted from: *Nanomaterials* **2020**, *10*, 1274, doi:10.3390/nano10071274 7

Kyle Bromma and Devika B. Chithrani
Advances in Gold Nanoparticle-Based Combined Cancer Therapy
Reprinted from: *Nanomaterials* **2020**, *10*, 1671, doi:10.3390/nano10091671 79

Boris Chelobanov, Julia Poletaeva, Anna Epanchintseva, Anastasiya Tupitsyna, Inna Pyshnaya and Elena Ryabchikova
Ultrastructural Features of Gold Nanoparticles Interaction with HepG2 and HEK293 Cells in Monolayer and Spheroids
Reprinted from: *Nanomaterials* **2020**, *10*, 2040, doi:10.3390/nano10102040 105

Antoine D'Hollander, Greetje Vande Velde, Hilde Jans, Bram Vanspauwen, Elien Vermeersch, Jithin Jose, Tom Struys, Tim Stakenborg, Liesbet Lagae and Uwe Himmelreich
Assessment of the Theranostic Potential of Gold Nanostars—A Multimodal Imaging and Photothermal Treatment Study
Reprinted from: *Nanomaterials* **2020**, *10*, 2112, doi:10.3390/nano10112112 129

Sérgio R. S. Veloso, Raquel G. D. Andrade, Beatriz C. Ribeiro, André V. F. Fernandes, A. Rita O. Rodrigues, J. A. Martins, Paula M. T. Ferreira, Paulo J. G. Coutinho and Elisabete M. S. Castanheira
Magnetoliposomes Incorporated in Peptide-Based Hydrogels: Towards Development of Magnetolipogels
Reprinted from: *Nanomaterials* **2020**, *10*, 1702, doi:10.3390/nano10091702 147

Tao Luo, Jinliang Gao, Na Lin and Jinke Wang
Effects of Two Kinds of Iron Nanoparticles as Reactive Oxygen Species Inducer and Scavenger on the Transcriptomic Profiles of Two Human Leukemia Cells with Different Stemness
Reprinted from: *Nanomaterials* **2020**, *10*, 1951, doi:10.3390/nano10101951 161

Harsh Kumar, Kanchan Bhardwaj, Eugenie Nepovimova, Kamil Kuča, Daljeet Singh Dhanjal, Sonali Bhardwaj, Shashi Kant Bhatia, Rachna Verma and Dinesh Kumar
Antioxidant Functionalized Nanoparticles: A Combat against Oxidative Stress
Reprinted from: *Nanomaterials* **2020**, *10*, 1334, doi:10.3390/nano10071334 181

Xue Bai, Gaoxing Su and Shumei Zhai
Recent Advances in Nanomedicine for the Diagnosis and Therapy of Liver Fibrosis
Reprinted from: *Nanomaterials* **2020**, *10*, 1945, doi:10.3390/nano10101945 207

Gurbet Köse, Milita Darguzyte and Fabian Kiessling
Molecular Ultrasound Imaging
Reprinted from: *Nanomaterials* **2020**, *10*, 1935, doi:10.3390/nano10101935 225

Wan Khaima Azira Wan Mat Khalir, Kamyar Shameli, Seyed Davoud Jazayeri, Nor Azizi Othman, Nurfatehah Wahyuny Che Jusoh and Norazian Mohd Hassan
In-Situ Biofabrication of Silver Nanoparticles in *Ceiba pentandra* Natural Fiber Using *Entada spiralis* Extract with Their Antibacterial and Catalytic Dye Reduction Properties
Reprinted from: *Nanomaterials* **2020**, *10*, 1104, doi:10.3390/nano10061104 253

Martin Škrátek, Andrej Dvurečenskij, Michal Kluknavský, Andrej Barta, Peter Bališ, Andrea Mičurová, Alexander Cigáň, Anita Eckstein-Andicsová, Ján Maňka and Iveta Bernátová
Sensitive SQUID Bio-Magnetometry for Determination and Differentiation of Biogenic Iron and Iron Oxide Nanoparticles in the Biological Samples
Reprinted from: *Nanomaterials* **2020**, *10*, 1993, doi:10.3390/nano10101993 279

Pawan Kumar, Meenu Saini, Brijnandan S. Dehiya, Anil Sindhu, Vinod Kumar, Ravinder Kumar, Luciano Lamberti, Catalin I. Pruncu and Rajesh Thakur
Comprehensive Survey on Nanobiomaterials for Bone Tissue Engineering Applications
Reprinted from: *Nanomaterials* **2020**, *10*, 2019, doi:10.3390/nano10102019 299

Humaira Idrees, Syed Zohaib Javaid Zaidi, Aneela Sabir, Rafi Ullah Khan, Xunli Zhang and Sammer-ul Hassan
A Review of Biodegradable Natural Polymer-Based Nanoparticles for Drug Delivery Applications
Reprinted from: *Nanomaterials* **2020**, *10*, 1970, doi:10.3390/nano10101970 359

Weikun Meng, Ana Rey-Rico, Mickaël Claudel, Gertrud Schmitt, Susanne Speicher-Mentges, Françoise Pons, Luc Lebeau, Jagadeesh K. Venkatesan and Magali Cucchiarini
rAAV-Mediated Overexpression of SOX9 and TGF-β via Carbon Dot-Guided Vector Delivery Enhances the Biological Activities in Human Bone Marrow-Derived Mesenchymal Stromal Cells
Reprinted from: *Nanomaterials* **2020**, *10*, 855, doi:10.3390/nano10050855 381

Jonas Urich, Magali Cucchiarini and Ana Rey-Rico
Therapeutic Delivery of rAAV *sox9* via Polymeric Micelles Counteracts the Effects of Osteoarthritis- Associated Inflammatory Cytokines in Human Articular Chondrocytes
Reprinted from: *Nanomaterials* **2020**, *10*, 1238, doi:10.3390/nano10061238 397

Anna S. Pavlova, Ilya S. Dovydenko, Maxim S. Kupryushkin, Alina E. Grigor'eva, Inna A. Pyshnaya and Dmitrii V. Pyshnyi
Amphiphilic "Like-A-Brush" Oligonucleotide Conjugates with Three Dodecyl Chains: Self-Assembly Features of Novel Scaffold Compounds for Nucleic Acids Delivery
Reprinted from: *Nanomaterials* **2020**, *10*, 1948, doi:10.3390/nano10101948 411

Sandra Noske, Michael Karimov, Achim Aigner and Alexander Ewe
Tyrosine-Modification of Polypropylenimine (PPI) and Polyethylenimine (PEI) Strongly Improves Efficacy of siRNA-Mediated Gene Knockdown
Reprinted from: *Nanomaterials* **2020**, *10*, 1809, doi:10.3390/nano10091809 431

Evgeny Apartsin, Nadezhda Knauer, Valeria Arkhipova, Ekaterina Pashkina, Alina Aktanova, Julia Poletaeva, Javier Sánchez-Nieves, Francisco Javier de la Mata and Rafael Gómez
pH-Sensitive Dendrimersomes of Hybrid Triazine-Carbosilane Dendritic Amphiphiles-Smart Vehicles for Drug Delivery
Reprinted from: *Nanomaterials* **2020**, *10*, 1899, doi:10.3390/nano10101899 447

About the Editor

Elena I. Ryabchikova graduated from Novosibirsk State University where she learned different microscopic methods and their application in various studies. She obtained her PhD degree in Anatomy, Histology and Embryology from Moscow State University (1980), and in 1982, she joined the State Research Center of Virology and Biotechnology "Vector" in Koltsovo, Novosibirsk region. She successfully used electron microscopy in studies of natural nano-objects—viruses, their structure and interaction with host cells. Her studies of biological properties and pathogenesis of Ebola and Marburg filoviruses were published in leading virological journals and were highly valued by the scientific community. She obtained a Doctor of Biological Sciences degree in 1998 for studies of filoviral pathogenesis. In 2009, Elena Ryabchikova moved to the Institute of Chemical Biology and Fundamental Medicine of the Siberian Branch of the Russian Academy of Sciences in Novosibirsk and started to work with artificial nano-objects. She applied her experience in virus investigations to understanding nanoparticle–cell interactions. A group led by Elena Ryabchikova obtained and published new data on gold, silica and palladium nanoparticles' interaction with a cell, which showed new facets in nanoparticle biology. In her publications, Elena Ryabchikova shows the need for a deep understanding of the mechanisms of interaction of nanoparticles with cells for the successful and safe development of nanobiotechnologies.

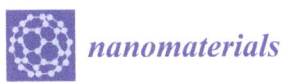

Editorial

Advances in Nanomaterials in Biomedicine

Elena Ryabchikova

Institute of Chemical Biology and Fundamental Medicine, Siberian Branch of Russian Academy of Science, 8 Lavrentiev Ave., 630090 Novosibirsk, Russia; lenryab@yandex.ru

Received: 25 November 2020; Accepted: 5 January 2021; Published: 7 January 2021

Keywords: nanotechnology; nanomedicine; biocompatible nanomaterials; diagnostics; nanocarriers; targeted drug delivery; tissue engineering

---

Biomedicine is actively developing a methodological network that brings together biological research and its medical applications. Biomedicine, in fact, is at the front flank of the creation of the latest technologies for various fields in medicine, and, obviously, nanotechnologies occupy an important place at this flank. Based on the well-known breadth of the concept of "Biomedicine", the boundaries of the Special Issue "Advances in Nanomaterials in Biomedicine" were not limited, and authors could present their work from various fields of nanotechnology, as well as new methods and nanomaterials intended for medical applications. This approach made it possible to make public not only specific developments, but also served as a kind of mirror reflecting the most active interest of researchers in a particular field of application of nanotechnology in biomedicine. The Special Issue brought together more than 110 authors from different countries, who submitted 11 original research articles and 7 reviews, and conveyed their vision of the problems of nanomaterials in biomedicine to the readers.

A detailed and well-illustrated review on the main problems of nanomedicine in onco-immunotherapy was presented by Acebes-Fernández and co-authors [1]. It should be noted that the review is not limited to onco-immunotherapy, and gives a complete understanding of nanomedicine in general, which is useful for those new to this field. The review is well structured, and clear schemes help the reader to follow complicated problems of cancer diagnostics and treatment using nanomedicine approaches.

The review authored by Bromma and Chithrani [2] critically discusses the state of the art problems and prospects for using AuNPs (gold nanoparticles) in combined cancer therapy. The authors presented variants of nanoplatforms based on AuNPs and the role of their physicochemical characteristics in determining the pathways of interaction with cells, and they draw attention to the problem of NPs biocompatibility for their successful application. This review analyzes the use of AuNPs as radiosensitizers and in chemoradiotherapy, highlighting problems and outlining prospects for the development of existing applications. The use of multicellular spheroids as adequate experimental tumor models is mentioned in this review, and the article presented by Chelobanov and co-authors [3] provides new data on spheroids formed by human hepatoma cells (Hep-G2) and human kidney cells (HEK293). The authors show the preservation of organ specificity in the structure of HepG2 spheroids, whose cells form bile capillaries and "pseudosinusoids". For researchers working with spheroids, it will be interesting to know that the outer surface of the spheroids, which is in contact with the nutrient medium, is formed by the basal regions of cells. This work also reported the inability of HepG2 cells to internalize "naked" AuNPs in both monolayer and spheroids, in contrast with active uptake of the same AuNPs covered with polyethylenimine (PEI) or bovine serum albumin (BSA). The HEK293 cells were devoid of this "selectivity" and internalized all types of AuNPs.

AuNPs possess many unique physico-chemical properties and are widely used in various biomedicine studies, mostly in spherical form, which can be easily synthesized and functionalized. D'Hollander and co-authors [4] reported obtaining and characterizing gold nanostars, and their high potential as agents of theranostics. This paper presents the successful use of gold nanostars that were coated with a polyethyleneglycol-maleimide for in vitro and in vivo photoacoustic imaging, computed tomography, as well as photothermal therapy of cancer cells and tumor masses. The work was carried out using a wide range of methods; however, an understandable presentation of experiments will allow other researchers to reproduce the obtaining of nanostars and conduct studies with them. The experiments performed by the authors convincingly demonstrate the high potential of the nanostars they obtained for theranostics and clinical use.

Iron NPs are another widely used object in biomedicine, and the Special Issue has combined their research in a variety of areas, reflecting the interest of a broad audience in this object. Thus, Veloso and co-authors [5] shared their experience in obtaining a new nanoform, representing a combination of solid and aqueous magnetoliposomes with supramolecular peptide-based hydrogels. Such complex constructions are primarily intended for the safe and targeted delivery of toxic drugs that are used in cancer therapy, and the authors provided evidence for their architecture and spatial organization.

Luo and co-authors [6] presented a new level of iron NPs application. Using RNA sequencing, the ability of Fe_3O_4 NPs coated with 2,3-Dimercaptosuccinic acid (DMSA) to induce the production of reactive oxygen species (ROS), as well as the ability of Prussian blue NPs to be ROS scavengers, was shown on two leukemia cell lines (KG1a and HL60). This research is part of a promising new approach to the treatment of leukemia—the development of nanomedical drugs as inducers of ferroptosis in cancer cells. The authors applied modern methods of transcriptome analysis and showed that two types of iron NPs differently regulate many genes expression. Surprisingly, it turned out that NP treatment of cells could affect the expression of many important genes, including those associated with antioxidant effects, lipid metabolism, vesicle movement, innate immune system, and the cytoskeleton. The importance of this work lies not only in its elucidation of iron NPs' cytotoxicity mechanisms for leukemic cells, but also in demonstration that NPs could affect the molecular mechanisms of cell metabolism. Obviously, the time has come to study the effects of NPs on cells and the organism at the molecular level, not limited to standard cytotoxicity tests.

Thus, the effect of NPs can lead to the disruption of cellular intermolecular interactions, in particular, to enhance the processes of peroxidation, which play an important role in stress development. However, it is well known that a poison can be a medicine, and vice versa, and Kumar with co-authors in their paper [7] reviewed the possibility of using various nanomaterials as anti-stress agents. Having shown the role of peroxide reactions in the development of various diseases, the authors move on to the analysis of antioxidants and the possible use of NPs, including metallic, to combat oxidative stress. They present information on the antioxidant properties of a number of NPs, as well as on the use of NPs as carriers of antioxidants and on the functionalization of NPs with antioxidants. The use of nanomaterials as antioxidants is a new direction in nanomedicine, and this review gives a comprehensive understanding of the state of research in this area. The text provides detailed characteristics of nanomaterials that have shown antioxidant properties and discusses the problems of their implementation into practice.

The Special Issue includes a review on the use of nanomedicines in the diagnosis and treatment of liver fibrosis [8], which remains among the difficult-to-diagnose and poorly treatable diseases. Xue Bai and co-authors inform readers about the crucial role of hepatic stellate cells in pathogenesis of liver fibrosis and briefly summarize routine approaches for the treatment and diagnostics of this severe disease. Then, data on use of magnetic NPs in magnetic resonance imaging for fibrosis diagnostics are presented. Analyzing the application of different nanomaterials for the treatment of liver fibrosis, the authors pay attention to the positive therapeutic effects of metallic NPs, drug delivery by various NPs and the use of targeted ligands to improve drug delivery. To complete the review, the authors show the advantages and disadvantages of using nanomedicines for liver fibrosis treatment and diagnosis, and express their confidence that all the imperfections of nanomedicine could be overcome by the design and fabrication of nanosystems based on knowledge about their properties.

The paper submitted by Köse and co-authors [9] presents molecular ultrasound imaging basing on nanoconstructions, such as microbubbles, nanobubbles, and nanodroplets, which are able to significantly improve standard ultrasound examinations. This paper demonstrates the advantages of new imaging systems in the visualization of blood vessels in particular, which is an important task for many clinical examinations. The authors emphasize that the presented means of molecular ultrasound diagnostics have been tested in laboratory models and, in fact, are at the level of preclinical studies. They focus on the "painful" problem of translating new developments into the clinic, which requires appropriate funding. This issue has also been noted in other articles in the Special Issue, and it is hoped that this podium will better demonstrate the potential of new developments in nanomedicine and attract the attention of potential investors.

The Special Issue "Advances in Nanomaterials in Biomedicine", among others, announced the topic "New Effective Antimicrobials". Khalir and co-authors [10] presented a process of preparing Ag-NPs on alkali-treated C. pentandra fibers as supporting material, and also provided detailed characteristics of the resulting products. The C. pentandra/Ag-NPs showed catalytic activity towards the Rhodamine B and methylene blue dyes, and good antibacterial activity towards both Gram-positive and Gram-negative bacteria S. aureus, E. faecalis, E. coli and P. vulgaris. Thus, C. pentandra/Ag-NPs could be evaluated as a promising nanomaterial for biomedical applications such as wound healing and the coating of biomaterials, wastewater treatment, food packaging, etc.

The growing use of nanomaterials is a cause for concern, as many of them have negative effects on living organisms. The assessment of this effect is often complicated by the presence of one or another element in biogenic forms in the body, which raises the problem of distinguishing between a biogenic and an element originating from nanomaterials. The article by Škrátek and co-authors [11] shows how it is possible to detect and differentiate iron, which comes from nanomaterials, and iron, which is naturally present in living organisms. To this end, the authors improved the SQUID magnetometric method, and showed that the developed method makes it possible to detect "artificial" iron in solid and liquid samples of animal tissues, and to distinguish it from biogenic iron naturally present in tissues and blood.

The creation of ever new nanomaterials and the study of the possibility of their application in biomedicine gave rise to the need for the analysis of published data in accordance with individual branches of medicine. The review presented by Kumar and co-authors [12] summarizes the data on prospects for the use of nanomaterials in the field of solid tissue engineering and analyzes the types of nanomaterials suitable for this particular area. The main tasks that can be solved using nanomaterials are shown, including the construction of scaffolds that mimic the extracellular matrix; regeneration of bones and cartilage; fighting infection through the properties of nanomaterials

The problems of using nanomaterials for drug delivery attract the attention of many researchers, and it is not surprising that five original articles and one review in the Special Issue are devoted to the development of delivery vehicles, based on various types of nanomaterials. A review by Idrees and co-authors [13] critically examines the use of naturally occurring biodegradable polymers in drug delivery systems for local or targeted and controlled release of drugs. The authors dwell in detail on the most used biodegradable and biocompatible substances, such as chitosan, alginate, albumin, hyaluronic acid and hydroxyapatite, giving not only their main characteristics, but also analyzing their advantages and disadvantages. This review will be useful to novice researchers, who can gain comprehensive information on the state of art in the field of drug delivery using biodegradable delivery vehicles.

Meng and co-authors [14] demonstrated a new approach to the treatment of articular cartilage injuries using a nanoconstruct based on selected carbon dots coupled to a recombinant adeno-associated virus (rAAV) vector for the delivery of highly chondroreparative cartilage-specific sex-determining region Y-type high-mobility group 9 (SOX9) transcription factor or transforming growth factor beta to human bone marrow-derived mesenchymal stromal cells. All experiments are detailed in this article, and the data presented convincingly demonstrates that the selected carbon dots are systems for efficient gene transfer through rAAV. Many people suffer from osteoarthritis, which is associated with irreversible degradation of key components of the articular extracellular cartilage matrix (ECM) (proteoglycans, type II collagen), with the critical involvement of pro-inflammatory cytokines (interleukin 1 beta and tumor necrosis factor alpha). Urich and co-authors [15] reported effective, micelle-guided rAAV SOX9 overexpression, which enhanced the deposition of ECM components and the level of cell survival. In other words, the operation of this rAAV vector system provided the neutralization of negatively acting cartilage cytokines, and polymer micelles, in turn, provided its controlled delivery, thereby evidencing the significance of appropriate nanomaterial development.

The efficient delivery of therapeutic nucleic acids into cells is one of the most important problems, and numerous and diverse nanoconstructions are being created to solve it. In the Special Issue, in addition to carbon dots and polymer micelles, two more types of carriers are presented: dodecyl-containing oligonucleotides [16] and nanosystems based on tyrosine-modified polypropylenimine (PPI) and polyethylenimine (PEI) [17]. In the first, Pavlova and co-authors [16] showed the formation of micellar nanostructures by the self-assembly of amphiphilic "like-a-brush" oligonucleotide conjugates, and their penetration into HepG2 cells. This is the first report on the self-assembly of "like-a-brush" triple chains-contained dodecyl-bearing oligonucleotides and their ability to enter the cells; thereby, this work widened a set of means for nucleic acids delivery. The authors of the second article exploit chemical modification to improve siRNA delivery with well-known cationic polymers, namely polyethylenimine (PEI) and polypropylenimine (PPI). Noske and co-authors [17] for the first time modified PPI, including dendrimer form, by tyrosine and showed that this modification significantly improved the siRNA complexation, complex stability, siRNA delivery, knockdown efficacy and biocompatibility. It should be noted that analysis of the effect of corresponding siRNAs on cytokines TNF-α and INF-γ was carried out in mice, which makes conclusions about the effect of tyrosine modification more convincing. As a whole, this work demonstrated that tyrosine-modified PPIs or PEIs are promising polymeric systems for siRNA formulation and delivery.

An example of the self-assembly of nanoconstructions for drug delivery has been given in the paper by Apartsin and co-authors [18], who designed a new class of dendritic amphiphiles self-assembling into vesicle-like supramolecular associates (dendrimersomes). The rationally designed molecular topology of dendrons permits us to use simple procedures to yield monodisperse pH-sensitive NPs. As a proof-of-concept study, anti-cancer drugs doxorubicin and methotrexate were encapsulated into dendrimersomes and delivered into human leukemia cells. Drug-loaded dendrimersomes efficiently penetrate into cells and induce cell death.

Author Contributions: E.R. solely contributed to the editorial. The author has read and agreed to the published version of the manuscript.

Funding: This research received no external funding.

Acknowledgments: We are grateful to all the authors who contributed to this Special Issue. We also express our acknowledgments to the referees for reviewing the manuscripts.

Conflicts of Interest: The author declares no conflict of interest.

References

1. Acebes-Fernández, V.; Landeira-Viñuela, A.; Juanes-Velasco, P.; Hernández, A.-P.; Otazo-Perez, A.; Manzano-Román, R.; Gongora, R.; Fuentes, M. Nanomedicine and Onco-Immunotherapy: From the Bench to Bedside to Biomarkers. *Nanomaterials* **2020**, *10*, 1274. [CrossRef]
2. Bromma, K.; Chithrani, D.B. Advances in Gold Nanoparticle-Based Combined Cancer Therapy. *Nanomaterials* **2020**, *10*, 1671. [CrossRef] [PubMed]
3. Chelobanov, B.; Poletaeva, J.; Epanchintseva, A.; Tupitsyna, A.; Pyshnaya, I.; Ryabchikova, E. Ultrastructural Features of Gold Nanoparticles Interaction with HepG2 and HEK293 Cells in Monolayer and Spheroids. *Nanomaterials* **2020**, *10*, 2040. [CrossRef] [PubMed]
4. D'Hollander, A.; Velde, G.V.; Jans, H.; Vanspauwen, B.; Vermeersch, E.; Jose, J.; Struys, T.; Stakenborg, T.; Lagae, L.; Himmelreich, U. Assessment of the Theranostic Potential of Gold Nanostars—A Multimodal Imaging and Photothermal Treatment Study. *Nanomaterials* **2020**, *10*, 2112. [CrossRef]
5. Veloso, S.R.S.; Andrade, R.G.D.; Ribeiro, B.C.; Fernandes, A.V.F.; Rodrigues, A.R.O.; Martins, J.A.; Ferreira, P.M.T.; Coutinho, P.J.G.; Castanheira, E.M.S. Magnetoliposomes Incorporated in Peptide-Based Hydrogels: Towards Development of Magnetolipogels. *Nanomaterials* **2020**, *10*, 1702. [CrossRef] [PubMed]
6. Luo, T.; Gao, J.; Lin, N.; Wang, J. Effects of Two Kinds of Iron Nanoparticles as Reactive Oxygen Species Inducer and Scavenger on the Transcriptomic Profiles of Two Human Leukemia Cells with Different Stemness. *Nanomaterials* **2020**, *10*, 1951. [CrossRef] [PubMed]
7. Kumar, H.; Bhardwaj, K.; Nepovimova, E.; Kuča, K.; Dhanjal, D.S.; Bhardwaj, S.; Bhatia, S.K.; Verma, R.; Kumar, D. Antioxidant Functionalized Nanoparticles: A Combat against Oxidative Stress. *Nanomaterials* **2020**, *10*, 1334. [CrossRef] [PubMed]
8. Bai, X.; Su, G.; Zhai, S. Recent Advances in Nanomedicine for the Diagnosis and Therapy of Liver Fibrosis. *Nanomaterials* **2020**, *10*, 1945. [CrossRef] [PubMed]
9. Köse, G.; Darguzyte, M.; Kiessling, F. Molecular Ultrasound Imaging. *Nanomaterials* **2020**, *10*, 1935. [CrossRef] [PubMed]
10. Khalir, W.K.A.W.M.; Shameli, K.; Jazayeri, S.D.; Othman, N.A.; Jusoh, N.W.C.; Hassan, N.M. In-Situ Biofabrication of Silver Nanoparticles in Ceiba pentandra Natural Fiber Using Entada spiralis Extract with Their Antibacterial and Catalytic Dye Reduction Properties. *Nanomaterials* **2020**, *10*, 1104. [CrossRef] [PubMed]
11. Škrátek, M.; Dvurečenskij, A.; Kluknavský, M.; Barta, A.; Bališ, P.; Mičurová, A.; Cigáň, A.; Eckstein-Andicsová, A.; Maňka, J.; Bernátová, I. Sensitive SQUID Bio-Magnetometry for Determination and Differentiation of Biogenic Iron and Iron Oxide Nanoparticles in the Biological Samples. *Nanomaterials* **2020**, *10*, 1993. [CrossRef] [PubMed]
12. Kumar, P.; Saini, M.; Dehiya, B.S.; Sindhu, A.; Kumar, V.; Kumar, R.; Lamberti, L.; Pruncu, C.I.; Thakur, R. Comprehensive Survey on Nanobiomaterials for Bone Tissue Engineering Applications. *Nanomaterials* **2020**, *10*, 2019. [CrossRef] [PubMed]
13. Idrees, H.; Zaidi, S.Z.J.; Sabir, A.; Khan, R.U.; Zhang, X.; Hassan, S. A Review of Biodegradable Natural Polymer-Based Nanoparticles for Drug Delivery Applications. *Nanomaterials* **2020**, *10*, 1970. [CrossRef] [PubMed]
14. Meng, W.; Rey-Rico, A.; Claudel, M.; Schmitt, G.; Speicher-Mentges, S.; Pons, F.; Lebeau, L.; Venkatesan, J.K.; Cucchiarini, M. rAAV-Mediated Overexpression of SOX9 and TGF-β via Carbon Dot-Guided Vector Delivery Enhances the Biological Activities in Human Bone Marrow-Derived Mesenchymal Stromal Cells. *Nanomaterials* **2020**, *10*, 855. [CrossRef] [PubMed]
15. Urich, J.; Cucchiarini, M.; Rey-Rico, A. Therapeutic Delivery of rAAV sox9 via Polymeric Micelles Counteracts the Effects of Osteoarthritis-Associated Inflammatory Cytokines in Human Articular Chondrocytes. *Nanomaterials* **2020**, *10*, 1238. [CrossRef] [PubMed]
16. Pavlova, A.S.; Dovydenko, I.S.; Kupryushkin, M.S.; Grigor'eva, A.E.; Pyshnaya, I.A.; Pyshnyi, D.V. Amphiphilic "Like-A-Brush" Oligonucleotide Conjugates with Three Dodecyl Chains: Self-Assembly Features of Novel Scaffold Compounds for Nucleic Acids Delivery. *Nanomaterials* **2020**, *10*, 1948. [CrossRef] [PubMed]

17. Noske, S.; Karimov, M.; Aigner, A.; Ewe, A. Tyrosine-Modification of Polypropylenimine (PPI) and Polyethylenimine (PEI) Strongly Improves Efficacy of siRNA-Mediated Gene Knockdown. *Nanomaterials* **2020**, *10*, 1809. [CrossRef] [PubMed]
18. Apartsin, E.; Knauer, N.; Arkhipova, V.; Pashkina, E.; Aktanova, A.; Poletaeva, J.; Sánchez-Nieves, J.; de la Mata, F.J.; Gómez, R. pH-Sensitive Dendrimersomes of Hybrid Triazine-Carbosilane Dendritic Amphiphiles-Smart Vehicles for Drug Delivery. *Nanomaterials* **2020**, *10*, 1899. [CrossRef] [PubMed]

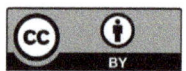

© 2021 by the author. Licensee MDPI, Basel, Switzerland. This article is an open access article distributed under the terms and conditions of the Creative Commons Attribution (CC BY) license (http://creativecommons.org/licenses/by/4.0/).

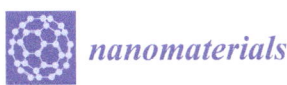

Review

Nanomedicine and Onco-Immunotherapy: From the Bench to Bedside to Biomarkers

Vanessa Acebes-Fernández [1], Alicia Landeira-Viñuela [1], Pablo Juanes-Velasco [1], Angela-Patricia Hernández [1], Andrea Otazo-Perez [1], Raúl Manzano-Román [2], Rafael Gongora [1] and Manuel Fuentes [1,2,*]

[1] Department of Medicine and Cytometry General Service-Nucleus, CIBERONC CB16/12/00400, Cancer Research Centre (IBMCC/CSIC/USAL/IBSAL), 37007 Salamanca, Spain; vanessaacebes@usal.es (V.A.-F.); alavi29@usal.es (A.L.-V.); pablojuanesvelasco@usal.es (P.J.-V.); angytahg@usal.es (A.-P.H.); andreaotazopz@gmail.com (A.O.-P.); rgongora@usal.es (R.G.)
[2] Proteomics Unit, Cancer Research Centre (IBMCC/CSIC/USAL/IBSAL), 37007 Salamanca, Spain; rmanzano@usal.es
* Correspondence: mfuentes@usal.es; Tel.: +34-923-294-811

Received: 3 June 2020; Accepted: 23 June 2020; Published: 29 June 2020

Abstract: The broad relationship between the immune system and cancer is opening a new hallmark to explore for nanomedicine. Here, all the common and synergy points between both areas are reviewed and described, and the recent approaches which show the progress from the bench to the beside to biomarkers developed in nanomedicine and onco-immunotherapy.

Keywords: nanomaterials; nanomedicine; immunotherapy; oncotherapy; immune-checkpoint inhibitors; immunogenic cell death; nano-vaccines; nano-conjugates; immune response

---

1. Introduction

The broad relationship between immune system and cancer has opened novel therapeutic approaches to treat tumours, such as: monoclonal antibodies, adoptive T-cell transfer, vaccination, immune checkpoint inhibitors, and oncolytic virus therapy. These novel immunotherapies are based mainly on the body's self-defense system to fight and defeat cancer. Current research is therefore focused on re-activating the immune system to attack cancer cells with potent cytokines, vaccines, antibodies and immune-stimulatory adjuvants. However, these immunotherapies could have several drawbacks, side effects (due to systemic treatment), low efficacy and resistance, among other things. Hence, nanomedicine is a new field with a strong potential application in immuno-oncology in order to overcome the bottlenecks and to improve the current available immunotherapies. Nanotechnology is a new field that has had a great impact on medicine and biomedical research, as it allows for a high-specific targeted delivery to tumour or immune cells, better clinical outcomes and reduces adverse effects, helping the delivery of vaccines and immunomodulating agents. This is made possible by nanoparticles (NPs), which can be highly variable in structure and function. Bearing all this in mind, it seems highly interesting to explore all these fields (nanotechnology, immune-oncology, immunotherapy, nanomedicines, etc.) in order to find and discover synergies and new opportunities; thus, here, the major features and achievements in these areas are briefly reviewed.

2. Nanomedicine

Nowadays, nanomedicine is an emerging and highly relevant area due to the fact that great advances have been made in the treatment of various diseases, such as cancer, neurodegenerative and cardiovascular diseases, and hormonal problems. To understand the development and possible applications of nanomedicine, it is necessary to define the concept of nanotechnology.

2.1. Nanotechnology: Brief Description

Nanotechnology can be defined as the "development of science and technology at atomic and molecular levels, at the scale of approximately 1–100 nm, to obtain a fundamental understanding of phenomena and materials at that nanoscale and to create and use structures, devices and systems that have new properties and functions because of their size" [1].

Nanotechnology has been emerging in science and technology for the last 20 years. When working at this scale, matter undergoes radical changes in its physical and chemical properties, such as in electrical conductivity, colour, and resistance or elasticity, giving it interesting properties that can be used in many applications in different fields, including electronics, medicine, engineering, environment and energy [1,2]. There are many studies describing a wide number of current nanotechnology applications in multiple fields, such as oil recovery, the formation of conductive films that can be used in electronic devices or even improving anaesthesia in medicine, as just a few examples that illustrate the broad fields of applications [3–6].

2.2. Nanomedicine: Concept

The application of nanotechnology in the health sciences has given rise to nanomedicine, a new discipline that aims to develop tools for diagnosing, preventing and treating diseases at an early stage of their development [1].

Nanomedicine is an interdisciplinary field in which nanoscience, nanoengineering and nanotechnology interact with the life sciences. It is expected that nanomedicine will lead to the development of better devices, drugs and other applications for early diagnosis or treatment of a wide range of diseases with high specificity, efficacy and personalization with the aim of improving the quality of life of patients. Because of its broad scope, it is expected that nanomedicine can be involved in all aspects of medicine, i.e., enter into conventional clinical practice. Nanomedicine differs from other types of conventional medicines in that it involves the development and application of materials and technologies with nanometric length scales [7].

Nanomedicine covers three main areas: nanodiagnosis, controlled drug delivery (nanotherapy), and regenerative medicine. All these areas are briefly described below [1].

Among other nanotechnology strategies, NPs are the key component that allows the development of nanomedicine, and currently there is a great variety of them. The properties of these NPs are affected by their size, shape, and surface bio-functionalization which is relevant for the characterisation of the NPs for each particular medical application. This comprehensive characterisation and precision synthesis allow for these NPs to perform specific functions and these functions can be correlated with specific characteristics of the NPs. In addition to characterization, the development of new methods of separation and purification of NPs is also needed to produce optimal samples for nanomedical applications and to study the behaviour of NPs within biological proximal fluids (serum/plasma, etc.), cells, tissues and the human/animal body. Despite these drawbacks to overcome, NPs are expected to improve the detection and early diagnosis of diseases, and also to help to provide personalised medicines [7].

NPs have a wide range of applications in nanomedicine (Figure 1). NPs can be designed to provide contrast at the targeted zone and report information about the local environment after administration into the body, which also offers the possibility to label tissues with selected markers and enables the local read-out of concentration of targeted molecules, which helps to analyse diseases directly inside the human body. Another application of NPs consists of the in vitro analysis of human proximal body fluids (such as ones of the major sources for biomarkers), participating in massive diagnostic strategies with the aim of detecting molecular alterations. Through NPs, multiple biomarkers can be analysed simultaneously, improving diagnostic accuracy and reproducibility [7].

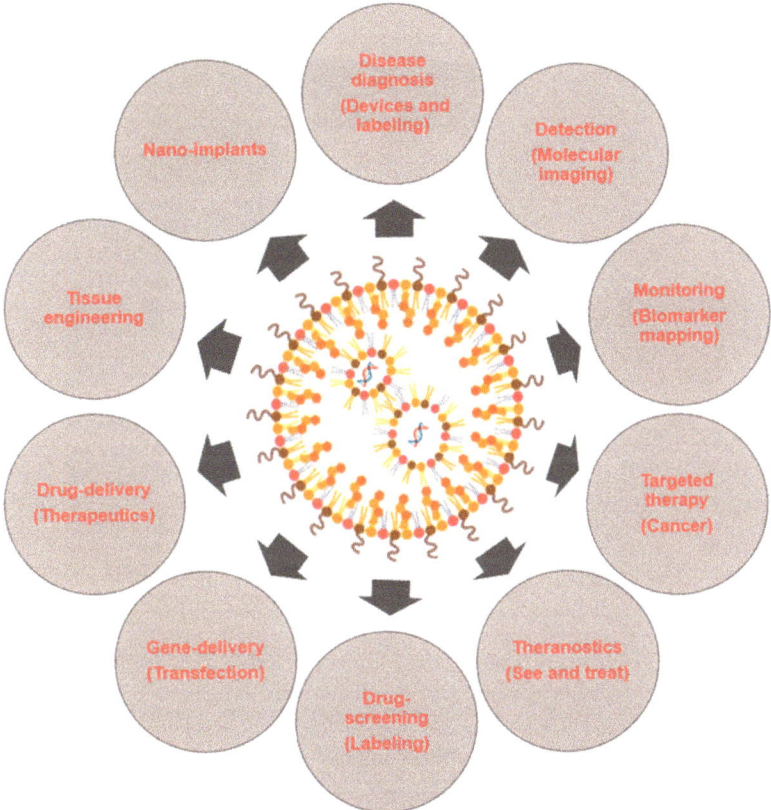

Figure 1. Diagram displaying multiple applications of nanotechnology in Medicine.

NPs are also used for the treatment of diseases, either as drug delivery vehicles, as bioactive materials or as components in implants [8,9]. In addition, nanomedicine is being implemented in the development of new matrices, support or surfaces for the design of implantable and electronic sensors or systems to aid in tissue regeneration; i.e., NPs are beginning to be used in regenerative medicine [7].

Here, several highlights of the major interested areas (nanodiagnostic, targeted drug release, regenerative therapy) about this topic covered by nanomedicine are briefly described.

2.2.1. Nanodiagnostics

In general, nanodiagnosis is considered as the design and development of analytical and imaging systems that allow for the detection of disease or abnormal cell function in early stages, both in vivo and in vitro [1].

Nanomaterials can be used for in vivo diagnosis, being used as contrast agents to visualize tissue structures inside the human body and to delimit healthy vs. pathological tissues. To this end, NPs are designed with different contrast properties for different modalities, such as computed tomography (CT), magnetic resonance imaging (MRI), positron emission tomography (PET), single photon emission computed tomography (SPECT) or fluorescence imaging. NPs will be designed to target specific tissues and generate the contrast. Then, to illustrate the applications, some of these examples are described below (Figure 2) [7].

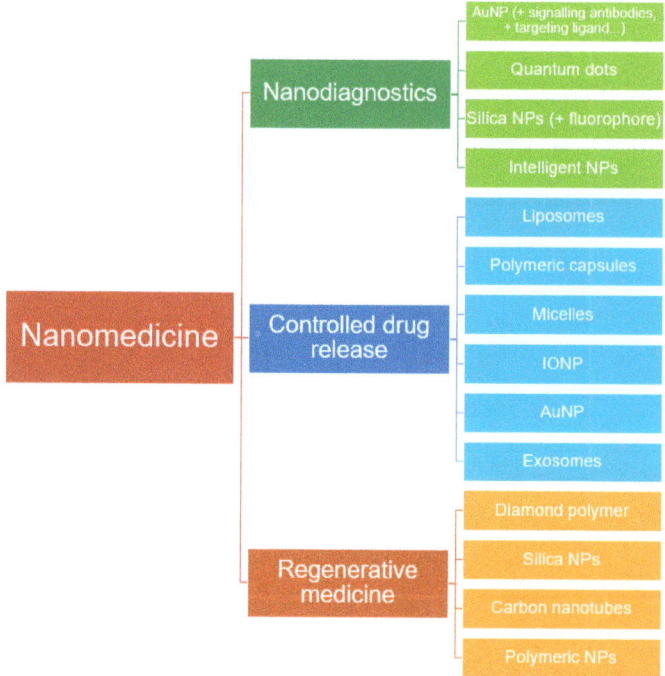

Figure 2. Current nanoparticle (NP) involvement in the multiple applications of nanomedicine.

In the case of CT, X-ray imaging takes advantage of tissue-specific attenuation to generate contrast on X-rays screenings, i.e., bone generates more contrast than soft tissue due to a higher relative electron density in the bone. To increase the contrast of these soft tissues, elements such as iodine or barium, which have a high electron density, were used, but to increase the low sensitivity, NPs were developed as contrast agents [7]. Among these NPs, AuNPs, which have a high electron density, stand out [10]. AuNPs have directional ligands like folic acid to bind to different tissue structures through their corresponding receptor composed of other types of materials that have a high atomic number are also suitable for CT. NP-based CT imaging technologies may change the way clinical diagnosis based on CT is performed [11]. In the case of iodine or barium, the doses required are very high, the contrast agents are usually non-specific and do not bind to cellular biomarkers or accumulate in tissues of interest, so the aim is to design NPs with high atomic number materials conjugated with targeting molecules that allow for different cell types to be specifically marked in vivo [7].

In the MRI example, contrast agents based on biocompatible NPs have advantages over the conventional contrast, such as the ability to adapt their size, shape, composition, circulation time, target cells, and optical and physical properties to optimize the images [7].

There are "smart" NPs that are activated by certain stimuli, such as pH, temperature, redox reactions, ions, proteases or light. These NPs respond to a change in the tumour microenvironment (TME) and allow for the selection of the diagnostic and therapeutic mechanism, which is highly relevant in oncology, because the TME regulates the progression of the tumour and its metastasis. In the case of MRI, probes of these "smart" NPs have been designed that are sensitive to pH, since it is a very important physiological parameter and its deregulation might be a biomarker of cancer. Additionally, hypoxia in the TME results in the production of lactic acid and therefore in acidic conditions, which also constitute a Damage-Associated Molecular Pattern (DAMP). Other probes of these types of NPs used in MRI are the temperature sensitive ones, since in tumours, differences in temperature between tissues are very common [7].

NPs could also be used for in vitro diagnosis, i.e., the detection of molecules, cells and tissues outside the human body. In this case, the function of NPs is to identify unique biological molecules in biological fluids that are associated with the health of patients and are useful for diagnosis. In this case, NPs are coated with ligands and biomolecules to allow for bio-recognition of biological molecules in such fluids [7]. Following the example of AuNPs, in this case they are modified with ligands that bind to a specific complementary protein, causing the agglutination of these NPs, which can be observed colorimetrically [12]. This knowledge has also been used in the detection of colorimetric DNA. The AuNPs diagnostic technique is used in the clinic to analyse patient samples [13]. Hence, AuNPs also serve as biosensors, conjugated with antibodies against signalling proteins, such as anti-CA15-3-HRP, to test CA15-3, which is an important tumour biomarker for breast cancer follow-up. The use of magnetic NPs as proximity sensors in MRI is known as diagnostic magnetic resonance imaging (DMR) [2,14,15].

Another example is the use of QD as fluorescence markers in proteins or nucleic acid assays, such as the detection of antigen surface epitopes [16]. Organic and inorganic polymer NPs have been used in intracellular detection applications. An example is silica NPs carrying fluorophores for intracellular detection of oxygen, pH or metal ion levels [17].

2.2.2. Controlled Drug Release

Bearing in mind the complexity, the conventional drug delivery system cannot deliver the chemotherapeutic agents in the most effective concentration to cause tumour cell death, and debilitating side effects occur. This has led to the development of NPs as a drug delivery system (Figure 2), with the aim of achieving tumour specificity and improving the therapeutic index and pharmacokinetic profile of chemotherapeutic agents [18]. Thus, nanotherapy may allow for target active nanosystems containing recognition elements to act or transport and release drugs specifically on affected areas or cells, with the goal of achieving more effective treatment with fewer side effects [1].

Although NPs have been designed to treat various diseases, their most important application has been in cancer. Many of the NPs formulations for cancer treatment have already been approved by regulatory agencies and used in the clinic, but although they produce fewer adverse effects than naked drugs, their therapeutic effectiveness sometimes does not improve substantially. Therefore, the objective is to develop systems with greater therapeutic efficacy [7].

For nanomedicine to have a high therapeutic efficacy in the administration of drugs against cancer, it must comply in the most efficient way with the five steps of the CAPIR cascade: blood Circulation, Accumulation and Penetration in the tumour, cell Internalization and intracellular Release of the drug (CAPIR) [19]. The current approach to nanomedicine development is to adapt the basic physicochemical properties of NPs (size, surface properties and stability, among others) to achieve the CAPIR cascade. As a consequence of the enhanced permeability-retention effect (EPR), it has been proven that passive diffusion allows for tumour localization of nano-chemotherapeutics, but within the TME the localization of nano-chemotherapeutics can be obstructed by different parameters, such as high interstitial fluid pressure, altered extracellular matrix structure, increased cell division or altered lymphatic drainage. Therefore, there is a need to understand the barriers of TME and modulate it to improve the delivery of these drugs [18].

Different types of available NPs are suitable as drug delivery vehicles, which can be passively or actively targeted at tumour tissues to improve the selectivity of these drugs and reduce their side effects. One of the FDA-approved delivery vehicles is liposomes, which are already used in several cancer therapies (i.e., Doxil) [20]. Polymer nanocapsules, which are made of completely hydrophilic polymers, are used to encapsulate hydrophilic drugs. Polymeric micelles are also used for drug delivery, which involves the self-assembly of amphiphilic molecules. The encapsulation of the anti-tumoral drug in these micelles reduces toxicity and improves circulation [7]. An example is the loading of cisplatin into micelles formed by polyethylene glycol (PEG), which increases the time of drug circulation by reducing acute renal accumulation of polymeric micelles [21].

Platinum-derived anti-cancer drugs are of great use, applied in the treatment of cancer, and now a few of them are back in the spotlight because of the recent developments of onco-immunotherapy. In the study conducted by Díez P. et al., a bile-cysplatin acid derivative conjugated to IONPs (iron oxide NPs) was obtained that improves selective cytotoxic activity and promotes the usefulness of IONPs as drug carriers in tumoral cell lines, where platinum derivatives have shown low efficacy. The use of these IONPs may be of great interest in cancer therapies, as they can be designed to bind tumour cells and release the drug in a specific way [22].

Gold-NP, polymer NP or liposomes are also used as carriers of tumour-peptide vaccines that play an important role in tumour immunotherapy [2,23,24]. Chemotherapy based on platinum (II), ruthenium and gold (III) compounds also kills tumour cells [25,26]. One of the most studied gold (III) compounds is the anti-rheumatic drug Auranofin as a cancer treatment [2,27].

Another type of structure involved in nanomedicine are the exosomes, which are naturally occurring nanosized vesicles secreted endogenously by the cells themselves [28]. They are involved in intercellular and tissue-level communication through the transfer of biological material between cells. Exosomes have great potential for use as nano-carriers for various therapies in both inflammatory diseases and cancer, as well as for diagnosis [7].

In general, for controlled drug release, NPs must be designed to escape immune clearance, but they must also be able to adhere to the target tissues and be absorbed or interact with the desired cells in vivo. They can accumulate in the tissues actively or passively, either through transport by intra-organic pressure or through adhesion to specific biological structures in the target tissue by recognition of surface-bound ligands by molecules [29]. In addition to adapting the surface properties of NPs, the optimization of NPs size is also necessary for their accumulation and penetration into tumours and to ensure treatment efficacy [7]. In addition to passive targeting, the active targeting of NPs is also being developed. One example is the design of integrin-targeted nanomedicines using RGD-modified liposomes, which have been shown to result in elevated intracellular levels of doxorubicin [30]. In this sense, novel ligands are being developed against tumour targets, using different targeting biomolecular motifs. There is still discussion about the benefits of active versus passive targeting [31]. Many different controlled release systems are also being developed, which selectively control the rate of drug release by acting on the diseased cells [8].

Another alternative delivery strategy is the combination of multiple antitumour drugs in a single carrier [32]. Co-administration of chemotherapeutic drugs and nucleic acids has led to promising results in overcoming resistance to multiple drugs. Combining therapies against more than one tumour target improves the therapeutic outcome [33]. One of the advantages of nanomedicines is that they can be administered locally, unlike most chemotherapeutics, which are administered systemically.

2.2.3. Regenerative Medicine

Regenerative medicine aims to repair or replace damaged tissues and organs using nanotechnology tools [1]. Nanomaterials designed to deliver drugs or perform some action on diseased tissue are programmed to degrade later, but nanomaterials that are not removed and remain performing their function continuously are also being synthesized. These nanomaterials will allow for surface modelling and provide new functions in tissue engineering, such as new properties of implants (Figure 2). One example is carbon nanostructures, which are biocompatible and support the growth and proliferation of different cell types [7].

Diamond polymer composites are used in implant nano-engineering, which have the potential to restore damaged tissue [7]. They have very good mechanical properties, which together with the administration of drugs and biological molecules and their biocompatibility, allow for the re-enforcement of implantable polymers, creating the support of multifunctional tissues [9]. Furthermore, they are non-toxic and their production is scalable.

For the application of these types of implants, the interface between the implanted devices and the surrounding cells and tissues is also important. This is where the geometry of the selected device comes into play [7]. Another application is found in neuronal systems, where carbon nanotubes (CNT) are used, which influence the electrical activity of the neurons by improving neural signalling, inducing the formation of a greater number of synaptic contacts and promoting the growth of nerve fibers [34–36].

Biological implants, such as cell-based therapies, are also of great importance in regenerative medicine. One example is the administration of stem cells to regenerate defective tissue [37]. Here, nanotechnology helps to create culture substrates that enable the adhesive properties of the cells to be activated and de-activated. Nanotechnology is also being used in the engineering of artificial organs for regenerative medicine [7].

Nanoconstructions can also be used to control or lead directly cell behaviour, such as nanoscale silicate materials that induce targeted differentiation of mesenchymal stem cells (MSCs) in osteogenic targets [38]. Polymer NPs can be used to release growth factors and cytokines in a controlled manner, such as the release of angiogenic factors (CEGF and PDGF) that induce blood vessel formation [7].

With a better understanding of how nanoscale devices interact with cells, together with the ability to design more controllable nanomaterials, a new era of nanomedicine can be reached for applications in regenerative medicine.

2.3. Nanomaterials in Medicine

At the nanoscale level, properties exist in all materials, both natural and synthetic, but only synthetic materials are generally considered to be part of "nanoscience and engineering" [7]. A wide variety of NPs are currently available, and many of the nanomaterials used can mimic the functions of globular biological macromolecules. These materials include lipid micelles, polymer nanostructures, protein constructions, ribonucleic acid NP, carbon dots, nanodiamonds, carbon nanotubes, graphene, and some inorganic materials such as mesoporous silica NP, superparamagnetic iron oxide NPs, and quantum dots. (Figure 3) [39–44]. These types of materials have unique optical, electronic and magnetic properties depending on size and shape [45].

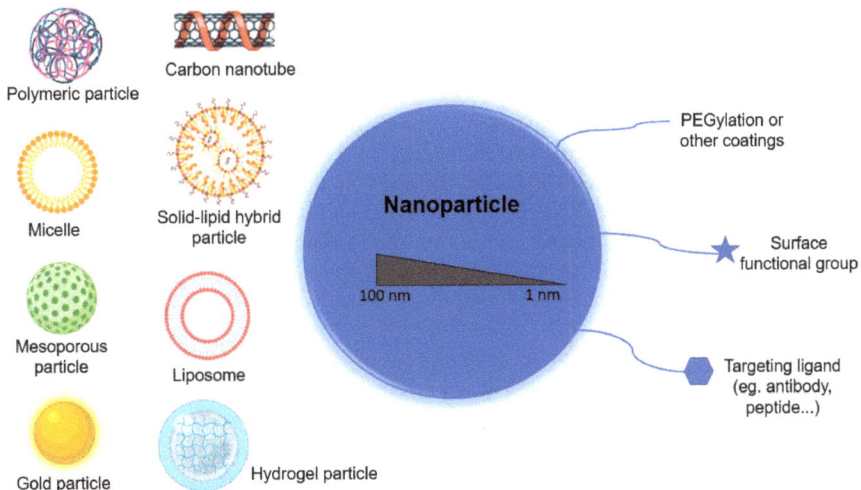

Figure 3. Nanomaterials currently used in the design of NPs, and the available surface modifications.

In recent years, the understanding of MSD-mediated immunotherapy in cancer treatment has improved and a variety of nanomaterials have been developed to regulate MSD. The following is a description of multiple types of NPs composed of a variety of nanomaterials that are used to enhance some of the immunotherapies that are discussed in more detail in this review.

In the case of nanovaccines, for example, the size of these NPs is associated with the mechanism of cellular absorption and the subsequent endocytic pathway, which in turn determines the effect and outcome of the NPs on the cells. The smaller PNPs (25–40 nm) drain into the nodes through the tissue barrier faster than the larger NPs (100 nm), which have to be transported by dendritic cells (DCs). The shape of the NPs is also important in cellular uptake and bio-distribution [46]. Non-spherical NPs have been shown to prevent non-specific cellular phagocytosis by prolonging their systemic circulation, but spherical NPs are more easily transported by DCs [47]. Another important parameter is the charge of NPs, since it influences their internalization and further induction of immune response. Cationic NPs are absorbed more rapidly by macrophages or DCs and have a higher lysosomal escape potential, but they adsorb more serum proteins, reacting with negatively charged components, reducing the permeability of tumour tissues. The NPs that have the better circulation and best penetration into tumours are neutrally net charged NPs [48].

One of the most promising NPs are biodegradable NPs, which generally use poly (lactic-co-glycolic acid) (PLGA), which also has the advantage of a protective effect on antigens [49]. The size of these NPs is the same as that of pathogens, so they are better absorbed by antigen-presenting cells (APCs).

Inorganic and metallic NPs are also used as nano-vaccines. In this case, functional ligands are conjugated with mesoporous silica, calcium phosphate and gold NPs. Peptide micelles, dendrimers, oncolytic viruses and artificial exosomes are also being developed as DC-based nanovaccines [46].

Another type of NPs that allow for the improved recognition of TSAs by the immune system are polymeric NPs that contain large amounts of adjuvant and are membrane-coated by tumour cells with various types of TSAs [50]. Then, depending of properties of polymeric NPs and the type of immunotherapies, several applications have been developed which here are briefly described: i. In the case of aAPCs, dextran-conjugated superparamagnetic iron oxide NPs with major histocompatibility complex (MHC)-Ig dimer and anti-CD28 antibody are used. Magnetic field-induced aAPCs stimulate the activation and proliferation of antigen-specific T-lymphocytes [46]. ii. For cellular immunotherapy, polyNPs (β-amino ester) with a CAR-coding plasmid DNA load are used to enhance chimeric antigen receptor-modified T cells (CAR-T) cells [51]. iii. As for checkpoint inhibitors, zinc pyrophosphate (ZnP) NPs loaded with photosensitizing pyrolipid (ZnP @ pyro) for photodynamic therapy (PDT) have been shown to improve tumour sensitivity to PD-L1 (programmed death-ligand 1) blocking immunotherapy and induce immunogenic cell death [52]. iv. For cytokines, NPs with a self-assembly derived from PEGylated polylactic acid and cationic phospholipid have been designed for targeted administration of IL-12 plasmid DNA [53]. v. Another example is directed AuNPs loaded with endostatin, which blocks neovascularization and normalizes tumour vasculature [54].

Polymeric nano-carriers are used to deliver adjuvant, which accumulates at the site of the tumour through permeability and retention. An example is the use of polyethylene glycol (PEG)-PLGA NPs to encapsulate R837 and a near-infrared dye via an oil-in-water emulsion [55]. PLGA NPs are also used to improve the supply of monoclonal antibodies (mAb) and enhance the activation of T cells [56]. An example is the chemical conjugation of mAb against OX40 (tumour necrosis factor receptor) with PLGA NPs [57].

Another polymer under study is acetylated dextran, which enhances the properties of traditional polymers by allowing for the loading of hydrophilic drugs in a very efficient way, and it is biodegradable and pH-responsive, dissolving under acidic conditions but remaining stable under physiological conditions [56].

Liposomes are also nano-carriers, which allow for a more specific delivery of cytokines and mAb to the site of the tumour. The payloads can be conjugated on the liposomal membrane or charged in the center of the particle. An example is IL-2 and anti-CD137 sticky liposomes [58].

Water-in-oil emulsions are also used, which are large in size and provide a reservoir for the local release of therapeutic agents [56]. An example is the use of these water-in-oil emulsions to deliver anti-CTLA-4 antagonistic antibodies and anti-CD40 agonist antibodies [59].

Another type of material used is hydrogels, which are particularly suitable for delivering biomolecules [56]. They can be generated by the self-assembly of amphiphilic polysaccharides, and cholesterol-bearing pullulan (CHP)-based platforms are also being studied in immunotherapy [60]. Hydroxypropyl cellulose (HPC) nanogels have been shown to drain nearby lymph nodes after skin administration and release their antigen payload into the APCs, enhancing antitumour immunity [61]. Another example is the bioreducible cationic alginate-polyethylenimine nanogel, used to encapsulate ovalbumin as a vaccine that is absorbed by dendritic cells, facilitating antigenic presentation and activating immune responses [62]. Nanogels can also be used in the administration of cytokines, such as murine IL-12 that is incorporated into a CHP nanogel, allowing its sustained release into the bloodstream [63].

AuNPs show great promise due to their safety and adjustable nature, and increase the potency and decrease the toxicity of immunotherapeutics through improved patency and retention [56]. AuNPs conjugated to a tumour peptide that binds to CD13 in the tumour endothelium have been shown to transport and release TNF-α more effectively in vivo [64]. AuNPs can also be used as contrast agents in CT. As an example, the administration of anti-PD-L1-conjugated AuNPs in mice generated a CT signal that correlated with tumour growth, so these NPs can be used to predict responses to immunotherapy treatments [65].

Because of their porous structures, mesoporous silica NPs (MSNs) have a high intrinsic payload encapsulation capacity [56]. An example is the use of liposome-coated MSNs loaded with doxorubicin and oxoplatin (apoptosis inducers) and indoximod (an adjuvant that interferes with immunosuppressive pathways in MSDs), increasing their half-life in circulation and tumour targeting [66]. MSNs have also been designed with large pores that induce a potent immune response when it is combined with photothermal agents and model antigens [56,67].

Other nanoplatforms that are starting to be used are biomimetic nano-carriers, which further improve delivery efficiency and subsequent immune responses. Natural debris can be used to design these NPs, modifying their surface and improving their absorption by the target cells [56]. An example is mannose modification, which has an affinity for receptors present in APC [68]. Galactose modification is another example of biomimetic targeting [69]. These natural carriers also include virus-like particles (VLPs), e.g., cowpea mosaic virus (CPMV)-based VLPs, which combined with an antigenic peptide of human epidermal growth factor receptor 2 (HER2) protein can be used as a vaccine in the treatment of cancer of HER2+ tumours [70].

Heat shock proteins (HSP) also interact with APC receptors and improve antigenic presentation. An example is the use of HSP96-bound antigenic peptides, which are used as a vaccine in colorectal liver metastases [71].

Lipoprotein-based nanoporters are also used, such as the synthetic high-density lipoprotein-mimicking nanodisc that has been used in the targeted vaccination of neo-antigens [72].

Briefly, delivery platforms and their biomimetic modifications provide different advantages in cancer immunotherapy. In addition, many of these nanoplatforms are located at the interface of the natural and the synthetic nanomaterials. Despite the advantages, there are several challenges for these nano-carriers, which include the cost-effective supply of biological nanomaterials, their large-scale production at the pharmaceutical level and the optimisation of long-term storage conditions [56].

The great development of these nanomaterials and the importance they have acquired in the field of immuno-oncology makes it necessary to study both disciplines simultaneously. Furthermore, these disciplines currently have enormous potential for development, and therefore the feedback of knowledge between them must be constant in order to achieve common objectives. The following is a more detailed description of fundamental aspects of immuno-oncology, which helps us to understand its relationship with nanomedicine and also might aid in finding novel applications and new actors in the field.

3. Immuno-Oncology

The generation of T cell-mediated anti-tumour immunity requires a series of steps that constitute a process which is called the cancer immune cycle. The understanding of the cellular and molecular mechanisms involved in these processes allows for the development of several types of immunotherapies that assist in immune activation by modulating regulatory or activating mechanisms, directing these steps to achieve an improved immune response. In contrast, cancer also employs mechanisms that delay or stop this anti-tumour immunity, called immune avoidance mechanisms. Each of these mechanisms is a part of the "cancer hallmarks" that together allow cells to acquire malignancy and then tumour development. Therefore, new approaches to improve the immune response against cancer consist of blocking these immune evasion mechanisms.

Since the cancer immune cycle was described, several strategies have been used to improve the immune processes are grouped into two types: the first one is the use of effector cells/molecules of the immune system to directly attack the tumour cells, as it is named passive immunotherapy, which includes targeted monoclonal antibodies, adoptive cell therapy, and chimeric antigen receptor-modified T cells (CAR-T). The second strategy is to improve the activation of the immune system by modulating immune regulatory mechanisms or endogenous activators, which is called active immunotherapy. In this case, different steps of the immune response can be improved, such as the absorption, processing and presentation of antigens by APCs, the activation and expansion of naive T cells or increasing the efficacious phase of the immune response. Cytokines and different types of vaccines are involved in this type of immunotherapy. Another type of active immunotherapy that is proving very successful is checkpoint inhibitors, which aim to unblock a blocked immune response to increase anti-tumour responses [73].

All of these strategies are discussed in the following sections, but first, a more thorough understanding of the "cancer hallmarks" and "cancer immune cycle" is briefly commented on, as described below.

3.1. Cancer Hallmarks

Tumorigenesis in humans is a multi-step process, reflecting genetic alterations that progressively lead to a continuous transformation of normal cells into highly malignant cells. Tumour genomes are altered at multiple sites, either by point mutations or by more obvious alterations, such as changes in chromosomal complement. Observations in human cancers and animal models indicate that tumour development is driven by a succession of genetic changes, which confer one or another type of growth advantage, resulting in a progressive conversion of normal cells to cancer cells. Cancer cells have defects in the signalling pathways that regulate normal cell proliferation and homeostasis. However, the cancer cells of different tumours have very broad genotype diversity. Based on this complexity, Hanahan and Weinberg proposed that these genotypes were the result of six main essential alterations: self-sufficiency in growth signals, insensitivity to growth-inhibiting signals, avoidance of programmed cell death (apoptosis), unlimited replicative potential, sustained angiogenesis, and tissue invasion and metastasis. Each of these physiological changes are capabilities acquired during tumour development that escape a cancer defence mechanism connected to cells and tissues. These six abilities are shared by most types of human tumours. These capabilities are called the "hallmarks of cancer" [74].

Later, in 2011, they determined that tumours are not just island masses of proliferating cancer cells, but are complex tissues composed of different cellular types that interact with each other. Normal cells recruited to the site of the tumour form the tumour-associated stroma and are actively involved in tumorigenesis. The biology of tumours cannot be understood by just listing the features of the cancer cells; the involvement of the tumour microenvironment must be taken into account. Four other features shared by tumours have been described: genomic instability and mutation, cellular energy dysregulation, escape from immune destruction, and tumour-promoted inflammation (Figure 4) [75]; which are also very relevant to understand the pathology to decipher therapeutically targets and also as a source for diagnostic and prognostic biomarkers.

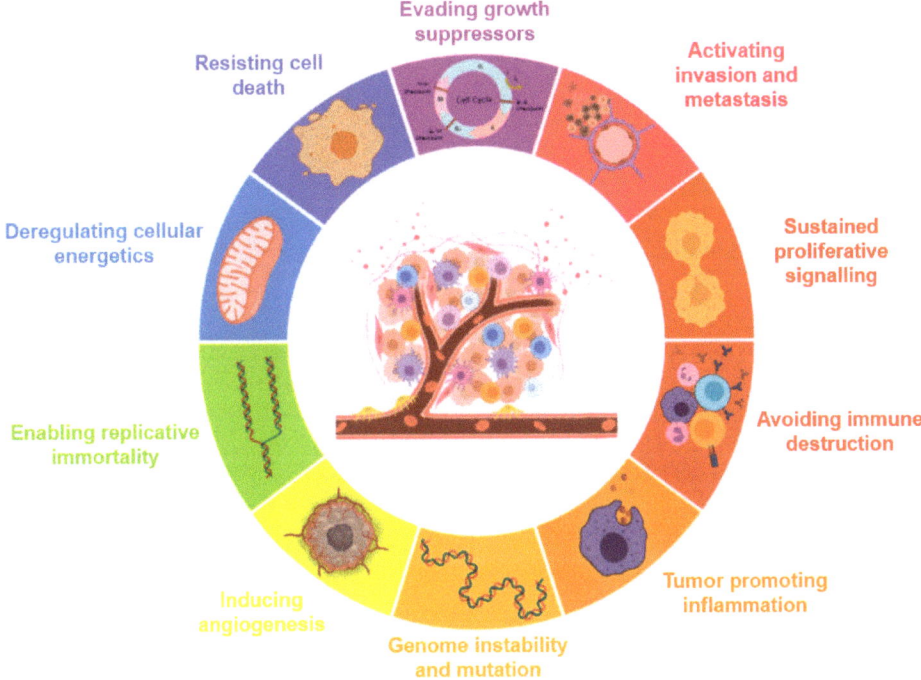

Figure 4. Scheme about the described hallmarks of cancer.

The development of targeted therapies to treat cancer is currently very important and is based on research into the mechanisms of cancer pathogenesis. Different targeted therapies can be classified according to their effects on one or more cancer hallmarks and the efficacy of these drugs is a validation of each hallmark described.

3.2. Immune Cycle in Cancer

For the immune response against cancer to be effective in destroying/eliminating cancer cells, certain events must occur in a staggered and continuous manner. These events are also steps in the "cancer immune cycle" (Figure 5).

The release of neo-antigens (formed from the oncogenesis) is subsequently captured by the dendritic cells (DC) to be processed (Step 1). For this to produce an anticancer T-cell response, it must be accompanied by signals that specify immunity, thus avoiding the induction of peripheral tolerance to tumour antigens. These signals can be pro-inflammatory cytokines and factors released by damaged tumour cells. DCs then present the neoantigens on MHC-I and MHC-II molecules to T cells (step 2). Antigenic presentation on MHC molecules activates effector T cells against specific cancer antigens (step 3). It is in this step that the nature of the immune response is determined, establishing a balance between effector T cells and regulatory T cells. The effector T cells then migrate to the tumour site (step 4), infiltrating the tumour bed (step 5). Once here, the T cells specifically recognize the cancer cells and bind to them through the interaction between the T Cell Receptor (TCR) and its related antigen bound to MHC-I (step 6). Finally, the T cells kill the target cancer cell (step 7). Killing the cancer cell will release tumour-associated antigens (TAAs), causing the cycle to restart. This increases the breadth and depth of subsequent responses [76].

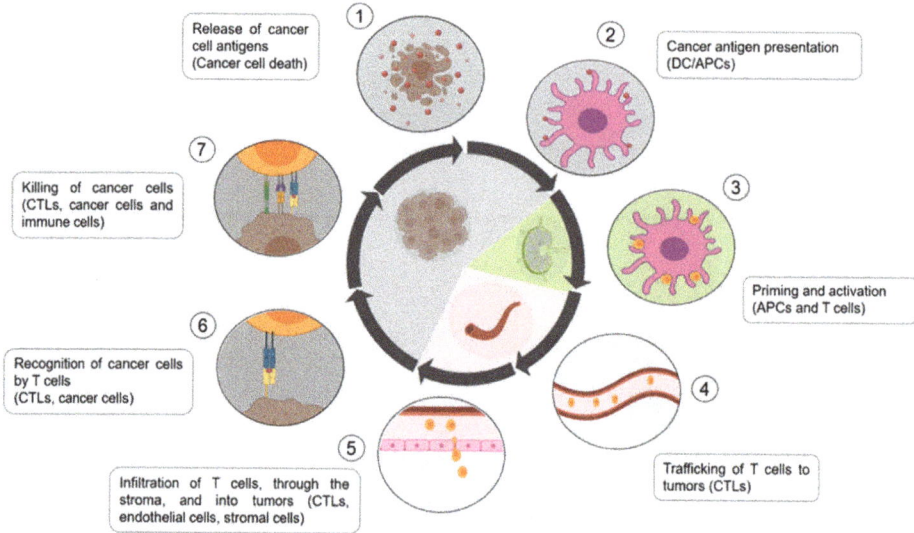

Figure 5. Schematic description of cancer immune cycle.

In cancer patients, this cycle does not work properly, with errors in the different steps described above: tumour antigens are not detected, DCs and T cells do not treat the antigens as foreign, the response is greater in regulatory T cells than in effector cells, T cells do not infiltrate tumours adequately, or even multiple factors in the tumour microenvironment may inhibit effector T cells. Bearing this in mind, the goal of cancer immunotherapy is to initiate a self-reliant cycle of cancer immunity that can amplify and spread without generating an unchecked auto-immune inflammatory response. To achieve this, immunotherapy must escape negative feedback mechanisms (checkpoints and inhibitors). Although amplifying the entire cell cycle provides anti-cancer activity, it generates damage to normal cells and tissues in return which might be drawback or source for resistance to the treatment. Recently, several clinical studies suggest that a common rate-limiting step is "immunostat function", which is the immunosuppression that occurs in the tumour microenvironment [76].

As discussed above, different immunotherapies can act on the several phases of the cancer immune cycle to ensure that an effective immune response is generated against the tumour cells.

3.3. Cancer Immunotherapy

Once the immune cycle and cancer hallmarks are described, the different immunotherapies should act and also new ones could be designed according to them. Hence, most of these immunotherapies is described briefly (from the conventional to the novel ones) (Figure 6).

3.3.1. Cytokines

Cytokines are polypeptides or glycoproteins that cause growth, differentiation and inflammatory or anti-inflammatory signals to different types of cells, which are released at a particular time in response to a specific stimulus and have a limited half-life time in the circulation [77]. Target cells of cytokines express high affinity membrane receptors, which activate intracellular signalling when they bind to cytokines, producing modifications in gene transcription that will determine the cellular response. The receptors receive information about the concentration and time of exposure to different cytokines, which implies a high degree of complexity. Due to all these features, cytokines play important roles as modulating agents that are involved in immune homeostasis by regulating inflammatory response, specific immune response, tolerance mechanisms, and promoting effective pathogen control. Hence, the administration of cytokines allows for the manipulation of the immune system in auto-immune disorders, infectious diseases, increasing the efficiency of the vaccines (due to inherent adjuvants disorders) and in the therapy of cancer [78].

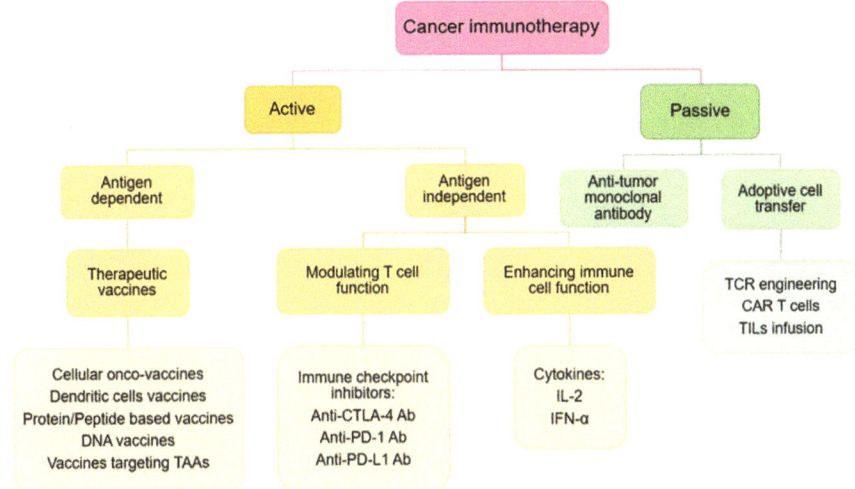

Figure 6. Schematic classification of immunotherapies designed for cancer.

The ability of cytokines to enhance the immune response against cancer and the development of recombinant DNA technology has allowed for preclinical and clinical investigation of the anti-tumoral activity of several recombinant human cytokines since the 1980s [77]. Several cytokines, among others including IL-2, IL-12, IL-15, IL-21, GM-CSF and INF-α, have demonstrated efficacy in preclinical models of murine cancer [79]; however, cytokines have shown limitations, such as their short half-life and narrow therapeutic framework, with low anti-tumour efficacy in their use as monotherapy agent. So far, only a few cytokines showed clinical benefit, which were IL-2 and IFN-α, being approved by the Food and Drug Administration (FDA) as anti-tumoral therapies. In the case of IL-2, it was approved for the treatment of advanced renal cell carcinoma and metastatic melanoma; regarding IFN-α, it was approved for the treatment of hairy cell leukemia, follicular non-Hodgkin's lymphoma, melanoma, and AIDS-related Kaposi's sarcoma [77].

In the case of IL-2, which has been approved by FDA for the treatment of advanced renal cell carcinoma and metastatic melanoma. The identification of IL-2 as a therapeutic agent began in the 1960s, when a factor capable of stimulating lymphocyte division in antigen-activated leukocyte culture supernatants was discovered. In 1969, it was demonstrated that human lymphocyte media contained this factor and could be used to maintain T-cell cultures for more than nine months without the need for repetitive antigenic stimulation. This technique was used to cultivate tumour-reactive cytotoxic T cells. This allowed a more in-depth study of this lymphocyte growth factor, thus giving it the name IL-2 [80], which was approved for the treatment of metastatic renal cell cancer in 1992 and advanced melanoma in 1998. IL-2 has opposite functions, acting as a T-cell growth factor during the initiation of the immune response, but is also essential for terminating the T-cell response, maintaining self-tolerance. This cytokine acts as a growth factor for T CD4+ cells and NK cells and promotes the clonal expansion of antigen activated CD8 T cells. In addition, it facilitates the production of antibodies by B cells that have been previously stimulated by factors such as CD40L. With respect to its immune response attenuation function, IL-2 plays an essential role in the maintenance of peripheral Tregs cells, as well as in the Activation-Induced Cell Death (AICD) of Fas-mediated T CD4+ cells. In IACD, receptor-mediated stimulation of T CD4+ cells with high antigen concentrations induces the expression of IL-2 and their receptors, which interacts and activate the T cell cycle. This antigen activation in turn increases transcription and expression of Fas Ligand (FasL), resulting in T cell death [79].

Regarding IFN-α, it was approved for the treatment of hairy cell leukemia, follicular non-Hodgkin's lymphoma, melanoma, and AIDS-related Kaposi's sarcoma. IFN-α belongs to IFN type I, a family of cytokines synthesized by different cells in response to viral infections and immune stimulation [79]. IFNs of this type induce the expression of MHC class I molecules in tumour cells, involved in the maturation of DCs, activate B and T cells and increase the number of cytotoxic cells. Specifically, IFN-α has pro-apoptotic and anti-proliferative activity, but also presents anti-angiogenic activity on the tumour vasculature. The use of IFN-α was approved in 1986 for the treatment of hairy cell leukemia [77], as it produced a sustained improvement in granulocyte, platelet count and hemoglobin levels in 77% of LCH patients treated [81] and has since been used in the treatment of hematologic malignancies and solid tumours [77], such as chronic myeloid leukemia, AIDS-related Kaposi's sarcoma, renal cell cancer, and in the case of stage II and III melanoma has been used as adjuvant therapy [79].

In contrast, administration of IL-2 and IFN-α has a low response rate and high toxicity associated with high doses, making targeted therapy and checkpoint inhibitors a better option currently for these tumours [77].

A drawback of treatments with cytokines is that, for some of them, positive actions are accompanied by the induction of immune checkpoint cytokines, such as the inhibitory factors IL-10 or TGFβ [79]. IL-10 is released by innate and adaptive immune cells to regulate the activity of pro-inflammatory cytokines; but also as an immunosuppressive cytokine, because it decreases the antigen-presenting activity of dendritic cells (DCs) and inhibits cytotoxic function and cytokine release from T and NK cells (depending on the microenvironment). In chronic infections and cancer, CD8+ T cells exhibit autocrine activity mediated by IL-10, inhibiting their antigen-induced apoptosis, thus prolonging the efficacious activity of cytotoxic lymphocytes. TGFβ has a dual role in the tumour process, since at the beginning of tumorigenesis, TGFβ is an inhibitor of tumour development by blocking the cell cycle; nevertheless, in later stages, the cells develop mechanisms of resistance against the TGFβ´s effects. This resistance mechanism begins to promote tumour progression and mediates the epithelium-mesenchyme transition. In addition, TGFβ promotes the release of angiogenic factors (such as vascular endothelial growth factor (VEGF)), and the recruitment of Treg cells, neutrophils, macrophages (with pro-tumour polarization), myeloid-derived suppressor cells (MDSC) and tolerogenic DCs, in turn decreasing the functions of NK cells and CD8 T lymphocytes [77].

In summary, cytokines have demonstrated anti-tumour therapeutic activity in murine models and in the clinical treatment of certain specific human cancers. Moreover, IL-2 and IFN-α have been approved for the treatment of selected malignancies. In contrast, cytokines in monotherapy have not met all the expectations efficiency as has been observed in preclinical experiments. This is because they are often associated with severe dose-limiting toxicities, and are known to induce immunosuppressive humoral factors, suppressive cells and immune checkpoints. Normally, soluble cytokines act over short distances, in a paracrine or autocrine manner; therefore, to achieve effective intra-tumoral concentrations they must be administered parenterally at high doses, which increases the potential for systemic toxicities, such as hypotension, acute renal failure, respiratory failure and neuropsychiatric symptoms in severe situations. They also do not induce a tumour-specific immune response. To avoid these drawbacks, new mutant engineered cytokines (supercins), chimeric antibody-cytokine fusion proteins (immunocins) or even the combination of cytokines with other therapies such as checkpoint inhibitors, among other novel strategies, are being investigated in an attempt to increase their anticancer efficacy [82]. However, due to these limitations, it has been necessary to develop more tumour-specific immunotherapeutic agents with greater effectiveness and less associated toxicity that are currently being used with better results, and the employment of cytokines in immunotherapy has taken a back seat.

3.3.2. Monoclonal Antibodies

The first monoclonal antibodies (mAb) to be clinically tested as a cancer treatment were murine mABs, but their problems of administration in humans limited their clinical usefulness [83]. The success of mAbs therapy came with the development of techniques that allowed the genetic modification of murine mAb to produce murine–human chimeric mAb or humanized mAb, which behaves like human IgG.

These antibodies have some advantages, such as their specific binding to molecular epitopes, interaction with the effector arms of the immune system, their long half-life, the ability to distribute themselves in the intra- and extravascular compartments and that the host tolerates IgGs well as therapeutic agents. In addition, they can be produced in large quantities and at a controlled cost. Due to their effective bio-distribution, systemic mAbs levels last for weeks or months, mediating a prolonged anti-cancer response. mAb can attack tumour cells by binding to tumour-associated antigens (TAAs) and modifying signalling or directing immune effector mechanisms to those tumour cells [84].

There is currently a wide diversity of mAb-based strategies for cancer therapy. The optimal characteristics for a targeted tumour antigen depend on the mAb to be used, the nature of the tumour and the mechanism of action of these mAb.

mAbs that target cell surface antigens can induce apoptosis by direct transmembrane signalling, by complement-mediated cytotoxicity or by inducing antibody-dependent cell cytotoxicity [85,86]. Determining the most appropriate mechanism for each mAb depends on the clinical scenario and is a continuous scientific challenge.

mAb could induce tumour cell death by target cell signalling. However, resistance can arise when cells with alternative or compensatory signalling pathways appear. The use of combination therapy may overcome these resistances. An example is mAbs against the ErbB family of receptors and their ligands, such as Trastuzumab and Pertuzumab [87,88]. The mechanism of these mAbs is complex, as the receptors can have multiple ligands and mAbs can alter the dimerization properties, interfering in different signalling depending on whether it is directed to a homodimer or heterodimer receptor [84].

For mAbs measuring complement-mediated cytotoxicity (CMC), it is known that their ability to bind complement and induce CMC depends on the antigen concentration, membrane orientation and whether the antigen is in monomer or polymer form. CMC also depends on the mAb isotype and the characteristics of the target cell. Some of these mAbs are anti-CD20, in chronic lymphocytic leukemia (CLL), such as rituximab or obinutuzumab. CMC contributes most to the effect of mAb in hematological malignancies, where target cells are exposed to complement system in the circulation [89].

mAbs can also induce antibody-dependent cell cytotoxicity (ADCC), mediated by FcR binding, which is expressed by immune effecting cells such as NK, granulocytes and monocytes/macrophages [90,91]. The mAb binds to the target cell through FcR, which activates intracellular signals through immunoreceptor tyrosine-based activation motifs (ITAM) and induces the activation of the effector cell, thus producing ADCC.

Many of the tumour associated antigens (TAAs) are not expressed on the surface of the tumour cells but are presented by MHC molecules. Therefore, mAbs have been developed that recognize these peptides, which come from intracellular oncoproteins. These antibodies are restricted by MHC and are still under development and further characterisation [84].

Molecule-specific mAbs that have an impact on the host can block tumour angiogenesis, preventing tumour growth, or target immune checkpoints, enhancing the anti-tumour immune response. In the first case, the mAb that blocks angiogenesis is bevacizumab, which blocks vascular endothelial growth factor (VEGF). This has an anti-tumour effect, as it prevents the passage of nutrients and oxygen to the tumour [92]. As these mAbs do not directly target the tumour, they are usually combined with cytotoxic agents [93]. Bevacizumab is effective in colorectal, lung, breast, renal, brain and ovarian cancer. The mAbs targeting immune checkpoints are described in a following section.

Antibody-drug immunoconjugates and radio-immunoconjugates that deliver a toxic load to tumour cells may also be used. Bi-functional antibodies and Chimeric Antigen Receptor T cells (CAR-T cells) can take advantage of the specificity of mAb to guide the cellular immune system to tumour cells [84]. Therefore, improved mAb-based therapeutic agents are being developed with multiple possibilities in cancer immunotherapy.

3.3.3. CAR-T Cells

This modality of immunotherapy is one of the newest adoptive cell therapy (ACT) strategies in cancer treatment. However, before knowing why it has such an impact as a potential cancer immunotherapy treatment, it is necessary to describe how it has been developed from the first ACT attempts.

Based on the idea that tumour-specific T cells could eliminate tumour cells, ACT was developed, which involves the therapeutic use of T cells, passively administrated (Figure 7) [94].

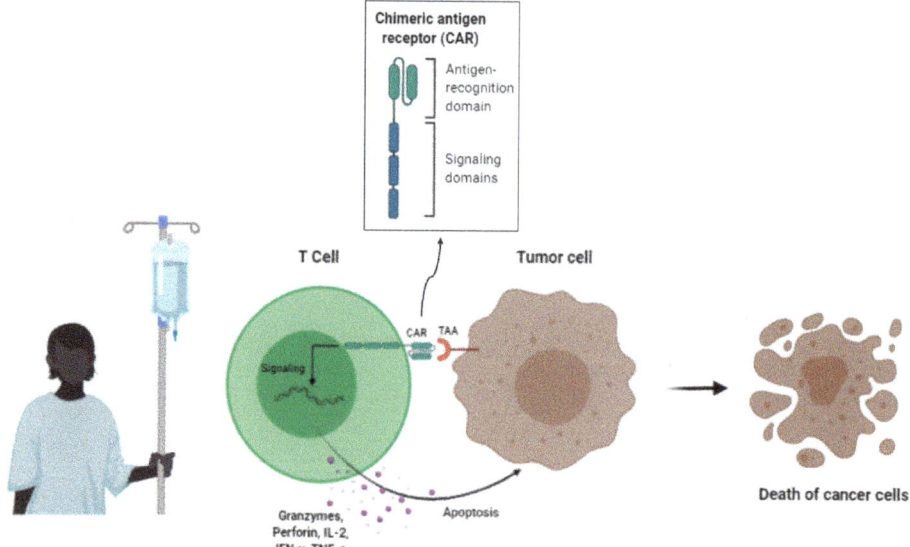

Figure 7. Schematic description of chimeric antigen receptor-modified T cells (CAR-T) cell therapy: structure and mechanism of action.

ACT has some advantages over other approaches to cancer immunotherapy. Large numbers of anti-tumour T cells can be grown in vitro and selected for their high avidity against the desired antigen. In addition, the host can be manipulated prior to administration of these cells to provide a suitable microenvironment in the tumour [95].

Following the use of IL-2 as a T-cell growth factor in the treatment of patients with metastatic melanoma and renal cell cancer (RCC), manipulation of the host immune system has been suggested to elicit an endogenous reaction capable of mediating cancer regression. The most potent cells were tumour infiltrating lymphocytes (TIL) grown from tumour fragments [96]. The first use of TILs was performed by the Surgery Branch, National Cancer Institute (NCI) in 1988 in the treatment of patients with metastatic melanoma [97]. Several TIL studies have shown that cells with anti-tumour activity can be isolated from tumours derived from patients with melanoma, but in most other tumour types these cells are difficult to isolate and spread and do not recognise tumour antigens. Therefore, techniques were developed to introduce anti-tumour T cell receptors (TCR) into autologous lymphocytes for use in therapy. Conventional TCRs $\alpha\beta$ and chimeric antigen receptors (CAR) with anti-tumour specificity can be introduced into normal lymphocytes, providing them with anti-tumour activity. The redirection of T-cell specificity with conventional TCR $\alpha\beta$ receptors is HLA-restricted, limiting treatment to patients expressing a particular HLA haplotype. TCRs, on the other hand, are not restricted to HLA, but are limited by the need for expression of the tumour antigen on the cell surface. In addition, CAR can also recognize carbohydrate and lipid debris, which has greater potential application [95].

Therefore, the use of Chimeric Antigen Receptor modified T cells (CAR-T cells) attempt to combine the high affinity of antibody fragments targeting tumour antigens with the destructive function of T lymphocytes [94].

Essentially, CAR-T cells are synthetic constructions that bind to target cell surface antigens using a single-chain variable fragment recognition (scFv) domain. The first designed generation of CAR-T cells consists of a scFv domain linked to a 3-zeta-strand differentiation cluster (CD3ζ) that induces the activation of T cells after binding to the antigen. This CD3ζ chain can only deliver a single strong intracellular signal (as it does not contain the chains γ, δ and ε that normally make up the TCR-CD3 complex which are required to amplify intracellular signal. In order to improve the CAR molecule, the second and third generation of these CAR-T cells were developed, incorporating other intracellular signalling domains such as CD28, CD137 and ICOS (inducible T cell co-stimulator). Cytokine receptor signalling or inflammatory cytokine expression domains such as IL-12 or IL-18 have been included in fourth and fifth generation CAR-T cells [94].

CAR-T cell therapies have been successful in several hematological malignancies but are less effective in treating most solid tumours. Since 2010, multiple CAR-T cell clinical trials have been conducted targeting CD19 (CD19-CAR-T cells) to promote clinical responses in acute lymphoblastic leukemia (ALL) [98,99], diffuse large B-cell lymphoma (DLBCL) [100], chronic lymphocytic leukemia (CLL) [101], and other non-Hodgkin's B-cell lymphomas [102], with remissions of up to 90% in some cases. This is because CD19 is always expressed in the B cell lineage and attacking CD19 eliminates this cell compartment in patients. Although this advantage may also appear to be a disadvantage, B cell aplasia can be treated with immunoglobulins and is therefore a manageable toxicity [103].

Two constructs of CD19-CAR-T cells have been approved by the FDA for their excellent results in refractory patients to standard therapies. They are Tisagenlecleucel (co-stimulatory domain 4-1BB/CD3ζ), approved in 2017 for B-ALL and in 2018 for DLBCL; and axicabtagene ciloleucel (co-stimulatory domain CD28/ CD3ζ), approved in 2017 for DLBCL. These approvals make CAR-T cells the first FDA-approved personalised gene therapy [104].

In malignant CD19+ refractory B-cell tumours, CD19-CAR-T cells have been shown to be clinically effective. However, these studies have also shown that relapse of the disease is more frequent in antigen-negative tumours, so it is important to determine the loss of antigen for these therapies [94].

On the other hand, monitoring the toxicity of the CAR-T cells is also important. The toxicity associated with this therapy is mainly outside the tumour, which is an obstacle in the clinical development of these therapies, and therefore, it is also very important to select the targets appropriately. The toxicity associated with CAR-T cells must be reversible after the elimination of the target cells or after the exhaustion of the T cells [94].

One of the bottlenecks is that T-lymphocytes are required to be removed from patients' peripheral blood and amplified in vitro, which is complex and time-consuming. To overcome these limitations, the in-situ construction of CAR-T in vivo seems to be the best option. Here, nanomedicine could help to improve the potential of these treatments and overcome mostly of the drawbacks. One of the approaches recently described is based on NPs coated with poly-β-amino-ester with reversible bound plasmid DNA encoding leukemia-specific CAR, which are internalised in the lymphocytes by anti-CD3 antibody-mediated endocytosis. Subsequently, the NPs selectively transfected with CAR genes into the nuclei of the patient's T cells. The T cells programmed by the synthetic NPs were found to in vitro express CAR after 24–48h incubation period. After in vivo administration, the NPs were identified and rapidly bound to the peripheral circulating T cells (abundant in the spleen, lymph nodes and bone marrow of the mice), showing an increase in overall survival rate. Despite the above, it has not yet been verified whether this methodology can effectively produce CAR-T cells and a long-lasting immune response in the human body, as well as whether toxicity problems can occur due to possible off-target effects [46].

Although this success of CAR-T cells has not yet been achieved in patients with solid tumours, the development of CAR-T cells in these solid tumours is still in its early stages. In solid tumours, the first obstacle is to design a CAR-T against an antigen that is expressed in the tumour but not in the normal tissue. Due to this difficulty, CAR-T cells in these tumours have presented serious toxicities until now. Although some tumour specific antigens have been identified, CAR-T cells have had very low efficacy against these target antigens in the clinic [104]. In the case of solid tumours, the effects outside of the tumour could lead to widespread cytokine release, resulting in organ failure. In order to exploit unique neo-antigens in solid tumours, their specific surface accessible expression would be required and combined with the production of immunoglobulins or nano-antibodies (HHV) would have to recognise them in order to generate specific CAR-T cells [105]. In addition, if a perfect antigen is found in solid tumours, CAR-T cell therapies in these types of tumours have to deal with other problems, such as poor traffic to the tumour site or limited persistence and proliferation within the host. The TME of these tumours may also functionally suppress CAR-T cells [104].

Therefore, it could be useful to compromise the microenvironment of solid tumours to delay their growth. The TME of many solid tumours share some characteristics, such as the expression of inhibitory molecules like PD-L1. Hence, a CAR-T cell that recognizes PD-L1 should palliate immune inhibition and allow for the activation of CAR-T cells in the TME, dampening immunosuppressive signals and promoting inflammation [105].

In the solid tumours, the suppressive TME inactivates TILs through the production of immunosuppressive molecules, and inflammatory cytokines are released from the treatment itself (IFN-γ, TNF-α), which is attributed to systemic administration. Targeted therapy based on NPs is required to remodel TME without causing systemic toxicity [46].

Solid tumours depend on the extracellular matrix (ECM) and the neo-vasculature for nutrient supply, which may be another target for T-CAR cells since tumour ECM and new blood vessels have unique antigens that are not present in healthy adults. Based on this, the group led by Yushu Joy Xie has designed a CAR-T cell which can be generated using an HHV that recognizes EIIIB, which is a splice variant of fibronectin that is expressed in a high form in tumoral ECM and neo-vasculature. This may improve the local inflammatory response and drug access to the tumour in otherwise impervious cancers [105].

Both CAR-Ts that recognize PD-L1 and those that recognize EIIIB have been tested in a B16 melanoma model and have shown significant delay in tumour growth and improved survival in both cases [105].

In summary, ACT with CAR-redirected T cells is a potentially curative strategy in patients with tumours resistant to standard treatments. CAR-T cells have demonstrated their potency in hematologic cancers, as reflected by their FDA approval for B-ALL and DLBCL. On the other hand, for solid tumours, this therapy is still in an early stage of development and may require a new approach to improve its effectiveness.

3.3.4. Therapeutic Onco-Vaccines

Another therapeutic strategy is onco-vaccines. Onco-vaccines represent one of the viable options for active immunotherapy against cancer by using the patient's own immune system. Different to prophylactic vaccines, which are administered to healthy individuals, therapeutic vaccines are administered to cancer patients with the aim of eradicating the cancer cells [106].

In general, onco-vaccines are classified depending on their format/content: cellular vaccines, protein/peptide vaccines and genetic vaccines (DNA, RNA and viruses) (Figure 8) [106,107].

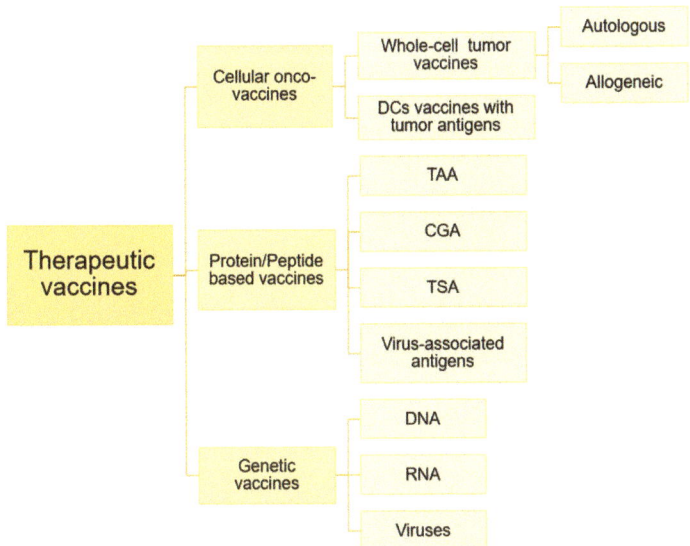

Figure 8. Schematic classification of currently available onco-vaccines.

The main characteristics of each group are:

1. *i. Cellular onco-vaccines*: Within cell-based vaccines there are two types: (i) autologous or allogeneic whole-cell tumour vaccines and (ii) autologous dendritic cells, pulsed or transfected with tumour antigens (contained in tumour lysates, purified proteins, peptides, DNA or RNA) [108]. Autologous cell-based vaccines are based on patient-derived tumour cells, which are irradiated and combined with an immunostimulatory adjuvant and administered to the same individual from whom the cells were extracted and isolated [109]. These vaccines have been tested in a variety of solid cancers, including lung cancer, colorectal cancer, melanoma, renal cell cancer, and prostate cancer [106], showing potent antitumour immunity in preclinical animal models and, in early human clinical trials, have shown relative safety, as well as the induction of tumour-specific immune responses and evidence of antitumour activity, obtaining clinical benefit, although objective response rates remain low [110–113]. One of the advantages of this type of vaccine is that it has a high potential to deliver the full spectrum of Tumour-Associated Antigens (TAAs) and, in addition, autologous tumour cells can be modified to acquire more potent immunostimulatory characteristics [106]. However, there are some disadvantages, such as requiring an enough tumour sample and potentially inducing autoimmunity, as tumours also express patient-specific proteins [114]. Allogeneic tumour cell vaccines typically contain two or three human tumour cell lines, and have the advantage that they contain unlimited sources of tumour antigens and can produce standardized, large-scale vaccines [106]. An example is Canvaxin, which contains three melanoma lines combined with Bacillus Calmatte-Guerin (BCG) as an adjuvant [115]. In 2010, the first cell-based vaccine was approved by the FDA, based on dendritic cell vaccine called provenge (sipuleucel-T), which targets Prostatic Acid Phosphatase (PAP) antigen in castration-resistant metastatic prostate cancer. PAP is an TAA, which gives the vaccine some specificity and therefore improves the anti-cancer effect [116]. Other vaccines that use whole tumour cells as antigens are OncoVAX for colon cancer and GVAX for prostate cancer [117,118]. These cells can also be genetically modified to produce immune molecules, as in the case of Lucanix for NSCLC [119]. The disadvantage of cell-based vaccines is that they are expensive and, in the case of autologous vaccines, it is difficult to produce them on a large scale [107].

2. ii. *Dendritic Cell (DC) Vaccines*: These vaccines are based on the main characteristic of DCs, which are professional antigen-presenting cells. DCs act in the peripheral tissues, where they absorb, process and present antigenic peptides of the pathogen or host to the virgin T lymphocytes in the lymphoid organs through the MHC. Therefore, DCs are important for connecting innate and adaptive immunity. Functional characterisation in DCs determine that three signals are necessary for complete activation of DCs: 1. adequate loading of MHC–peptide complexes in DC for priming of T cells; 2. positive regulation of co-stimulatory molecules such as CD40, CD80 and CD86, 3. production of cytokines that polarize the Th1/Tc1 immune response [106]. Ex vivo generated DCs are used as cancer vaccines. For this purpose, human DCs can be generated in culture from CD34+ hematopoietic progenitors or peripheral blood monocytes [120]. DC vaccines are achieved by loading TAAs antigens on autologous DCs from patients, which are then treated with adjuvants (Figure 9) [106]. For example, GM-CSF is essential for ex vivo generation of monocyte-derived DC [121]. These cells required a maturation process, which is associated with morphological and functional changes in the DC, allowing improved expression of MHC-I and -II, co-stimulatory molecules and increased cytokine production [122]. These ex vivo DCs are then administered to patients to induce anti-tumour immunity. Thus, T cell activation is regulated by co-stimulatory molecules expressed in DC, so the potency of the DC vaccine can be improved by modifying the expression levels of these inhibitory or activating molecules. DCs need stimulation of CD40 by active CD4+ T cells, so human DCs expressing high CD40L lead to increased activation of reactive T cells with low immunogenic tumour antigens. The activating molecules expressed in DC are related to the response of pro-inflammatory T cells, while suppressor molecules contribute to the tolerance or suppression of T cells [106]. The first work that laid the foundation for DC vaccine development was carried out by Inaba et al. in 1992. They cultivated mouse DC ex vivo from bone marrow precursors [123]. One of the first trials testing the immunogenicity of DC was performed on metastatic prostate cancer. Patients received autologous pulsed DCs with peptides restricted to HLA-A0201 derived from the prostate-specific membrane antigen (PSMA). Antigen-specific cellular responses and reduced PSA levels were observed in some patients [124]. These vaccines have also been tested in clinical trials for the treatment of prostate cancer, melanoma, renal cell carcinoma, and glioma [125–131]. The results of these studies are mixed but ultimately indicate that, although studies in mice demonstrate a potent ability of DCs to induce antitumour immunity and autologous DCs generated from peripheral blood in humans are a safe and promising approach, further studies are still needed to demonstrate their clinical efficacy and impact on the survival of patients with these types of cancers. As mentioned above, the DC vaccine Sipuleucel-T (Provenge TM) is the first therapeutic cancer vaccine approved by the FDA and has succeeded in increasing survival with a favourable toxicity profile, opening up new paradigms in cancer treatment [106]. *iii. Protein or peptide-based vaccines*: These vaccines are based on tumour-associated antigens (TAA), cancer germline antigens (CGA), virus-associated antigens or tumour-specific antigens (TSA), along with some adjuvants. Those composed of synthetic peptides generally contain between 20 and 30 amino acids directed at specific epitopes of tumour antigens. Antigens can be modified to bind cytokines, antibodies or immunogenic peptides in these vaccines [107]. In this group of vaccines, a few representative examples are Oncophage, which is used in kidney cancer, melanoma, and brain cancer; and MUC1, which is used in breast cancer and NSCLC [132,133]. These types of vaccines are not very expensive and are also very stable but have the limitation that known peptide epitopes are required to be candidates for use in vaccines. Other disadvantages are immune suppression and the weak immunogenicity of these antigens [134]. Recombinant vaccines based on TAA peptides are classified into different categories: 1. antigens encoded by genes that are normally silenced in adult tissues, but which are transcriptionally reactivated in tumour cells (testicular cancer antigens, such as melanoma associated antigen (MAGE) and SSX-2), 2. Tissue-differentiating antigens, which have a normal tissue origin and appear in both normal and tumour tissue

(melanoma, breast carcinomas and prostate cancer, such as gp100, mammaglobin-A and PSA, respectively), 3. Tissue differentiation antigens similar to the above, but which, compared to their normal homologous tissues, are very high in tumour tissues (MUC-1, HER2, p53, hTERT, etc.), 4. tumour-specific antigens, which are normally mutated oncogenes (e.g., Ras, B-Raf) and 5. molecules associated with tumour stem cells or with the epithelium-mesenchyme transition process [106]. This type of vaccine is more cost-effective than individualized vaccines, but also has the disadvantage of targeting only one or a few epitopes of the TAAs. To improve the immunogenicity of an auto-antigen, the peptide sequence of TAAs can be altered by introducing agonist-enhancing epitopes that increase peptide binding to MHC or TCR, enhancing the T cell response against the target [106]. Immuno-stimulatory adjuvants are also used when the TAA display of a weak immunogenic nature. Aluminium salts have been used as adjuvants to promote humoral immunity but are not effective in diseases requiring cellular immunity. To induce the adaptive immune response, activation of innate immunity is necessary, which has led to questions about theories of how adjuvants promote adaptive immunity [106]. Charles Janeway demonstrated that adaptive immune responses are dependent on innate immune receptors activated by microbial components [135]. Pattern-Associated Molecular Pattern Recognition (PAMPs) through pattern recognition receptors (PRRs) involves the coordination of innate and adaptive immunity to microbial pathogens or infected cells. TLR-mediated activation of DC is very important in this process, which is why many vaccines include PAMPs as part of therapeutic immunizations against cancer. That is, these molecules are used as adjuvants, facilitating the development of vaccines. Some examples are the use of BCG to treat bladder carcinoma, by activating TLR2 and TLR4, or LPS, which is a natural ligand of TLR4 [106].

3. *iv. DNA Vaccines:* These are vaccines in the form of genes use either DNA, such as plasmids, or RNA, such as mRNA [107]. Viral DNA vectors can transfuse infiltrated somatic cells or DCs as part of the inflammatory response to vaccination [106]. APCs absorb genetic material and translate peptide and proteins as cancer-specific antigens, stimulating the immune response [107]. Currently, there are some DNA vaccines include mammaglobin-A for breast cancer, PAP for prostate cancer, and gp100 and gp75 DNA for melanoma [136–139]. Disadvantages may be the method of DNA/RNA delivery and the efficiency of absorption, which may limit transcription and antigenic presentation by APCs [107]. These vaccines have been administered using viral vectors and electroporation, which are effective but difficult to apply in the clinical routine [140,141]. It should also be noted that the administration of live virus may cause side effects and decrease the effectiveness of antiviral antibodies in patients [140].

4. *v. Vaccines targeting TAAs*: To achieve tumour-specific death, cancer vaccines must target restricted epitopes of MHC-I that activate CD8+ T cells, as these are the most potent cells and when activated recognize TSAs and distinguish normal cells from cancer cells [142]. This involves the following processes: degradation of ubiquitous proteins by the proteasome, interaction of peptides with Hsp90 in the cytosol, which acts as a chaperone, active transport into the endoplasmic reticulum by the TAP transporter, modification of peptides by ERAP to an appropriate length, which are subsequently loaded into the peptide-binding cleft of MHC class I molecules with the help of chaperones such as tapain and transport to the cell surface, and can thus be recognised by the CD8+ T-cell receptor [143]. There are different types of tumour antigens that can be targeted in immunotherapy: (i) tumour-associated antigens (TAA), which are over-expressed on tumour cells and are expressed to a lesser extent on normal cells, (ii) cancer germ-line antigens (CGA), which on normal adult cells are found only in reproductive tissues, but are expressed selectively on several types of tumours, (iii) virus-associated antigens, which arise in tumour cells from oncogenic viral proteins; and (iv) tumour-specific antigens (TSAs), which are the neo-antigens and are only found in tumour cells, as they arise from non-anonymous somatic mutations [107]. Commonly, cancer vaccines should target the broadest possible antigen repertoire, which can be achieved by using autologous tumour lysates, whole-tumour-derived mRNA, irradiated

autologous tumour cells, or allogeneic tumour cell lines [144,145]. In addition, effective responses in response to an antigen can result in the immunogenic release of additional endogenous antigens by tumour cell destruction, leading to a broader immune response. This is known as "epitope spread" [146]. Vaccines targeting TAAs have not been very successful so far and are still under development, mainly because many TAAs are also expressed on normal cells, which show central and peripheral tolerance, and the affinity of TCR for these antigens might be very low [147]. In addition, autoimmune toxicities may take place during treatment. Despite this, some AATs are used as targets Despite the weak points on this approach; Currently, several approaches has been quite promising and help to open more studies exploring the full potential, for example: CD19-directed CAR-T therapy in acute lymphoblastic leukemia (ALL), which results in complete remission in a large number of patients [148]. CGAs, such as melanoma associated antigen 3 (MAGE-A3) and NY-ESO-1 antigen, are expressed selectively in some cancers, but when used as a target they result in high toxicities. In particular, severe neurological toxicities and death occur when MAGE-A3 is targeted [149]. On the other hand, virus-coded antigens are only present on tumour cells, not on normal cells, as some cancers are associated with virus infection. Viral oncogenes encode oncoproteins that cause cell transformation. An example is the human papilloma virus (HPV), which is associated with cervical cancer [150]. This method has been effective in treating cancer, but there are also virus-associated antigens with the ability to escape from the immune system [151]. In the approach of these vaccines, the critical and important key aspect is the selection of tumour-specific antigens (TSA), which are the neo-antigens. These are peptides that arise from non-anonymous mutations, alterations in genomic codons, editing, processing and antigen presentation in tumour cells [107]. Among all non-synonymous mutations, a part of them is distributed clonally by the tumour and generates peptides containing mutations (neo-epitopes) that can be recognised by cytotoxic T cells. Deletions and insertions are also highly predictive of response [121]. The use of these mutant derived epitopes is based initially on the responses to checkpoint inhibitors, which are proportional to the mutational load of each tumour [152]. Neoantigens are presented by MHC on the cell surface in order to be recognised by the T lymphocytes of the immune system. TSAs are the best therapeutic targets for cancer vaccines and T-cell-based immunotherapy because they are different from the germline and are not considered proprietary by the immune system. In addition, they are not subject to central or peripheral tolerance, as normal cells do not express them, so they will not cause auto-immunity problems either [107]. To identify immunogenic neo-epitopes in each patient, a combination of genomic sequencing of the tumour, RNA sequencing and bioinformatic tools with algorithms that allow for the prediction of the mutations are required, which will be presented to the T cells based on the processing by the proteasome and the affinity of the molecules for human leukocyte antigen (HLA). The resulting sequences can be synthesized as mRNA or as peptides for use as a vaccine. This methodology has been validated in preclinical trials, demonstrating that mutanome-derived neoantigens can induce an immune response against autologous tumours [153]. There are also phase 1 trials showing the immunogenicity and viability of the vaccine against the neo-antigen in metastatic melanoma [154]. The disadvantage of this customized approach is that it is a lengthy process and is therefore only suitable for certain patients. Neo-antigens have already been identified in different types of cancer such as melanoma, lung cancer, liver and renal cancer [155]. Adoptive cell transfer (ACT) studies of autologous tumour infiltrating lymphocytes (TIL) have shown that an effective antitumour immune response occurs in the presence of tumour specific T cells [156]. Isolated T cell clones or TCR-designed T lymphocytes have demonstrated the epitope patterns of neoantigens that are recognised by T cells [157]. Increasingly, cancer vaccines are being designed based on neo-antigens, targeting immunogenic mutations unique to each patient. Customized RNA mutanome vaccines and peptide-based vaccines have been tested and found to be safe and capable of eliciting T cell responses to neo-epitopes in melanoma patients [154,158]. When neo-epitopes are presented by antigen-presenting cells (APCs), such as dendritic cells and tumour cells themselves, cross presentation—whereby antigen-presenting cells phagocytize exogenous antigens and process them for presentation by MHC-I—plays an important role [159]. For a sufficient response of T cells to a neo-epitope, it is important to consider the affinity of the TCR for its related antigen [142]. Because neo-antigens are small pieces of peptides that contain tumour mutations, immunization with these antigens requires the assistance of other immune-stimulatory agents to produce an efficient immune response. On their own, peptides as vaccines may not be able to stimulate the immune system in a potent way, so they are used in combination with adjuvants [160]. Generally, to activate cytotoxic T cells and obtain a potent immune response, the stimulation of T helper cells is also required [142]. Even peptides with epitopes capable of activating cytotoxic T cells and helper T cells need an adjuvant to obtain an effective vaccine, so containing a potent immune-stimulator is very important to obtain an effective response. Then, CD8+ T cells are induced [161]. The appropriate adjuvant must be able to induce the production of cytokines and co-stimulator molecules from APC and also be able to deliver the optimal amount of antigen, to maintain a balance between antigen persistence, antigen concentration and antigen distribution [162]. In addition, the adjuvant must enhance cell-mediated immunity polarized to type 1 [121]. Adjuvants can function in several ways: gradually releasing the antigen, stimulating pattern recognition receptors in APCs, protecting antigens from rapid degradation, and extending antigen presentation time [142]. Different types of cells with neo-epitopes have also been pressed for immunization, such as B cells, macrophages, splenocytes or dendritic cells, which serve as delivery and adjuvant systems [142]. Since dendritic cells are capable of efficiently capturing, processing and presenting the antigen, initiating the immune response, they are also considered natural adjuvants, but the number of dendritic cells presented in peripheral blood in cancer patients is very low, in addition, this DCs may not be functional due to the effect of TME, so one of the goals is to provide enough functional DCs for each patient. It is also important to determine the DC subtype that works best as an adjuvant, the number of DCs injected, their stage of maturation or the location of the injection [163].

5. The identification of neo-epitopes is the most specific approach to cancer treatment, since it allows for a targeted immune response against specific tumour epitopes, but with this approach, no clinically determinant results have been achieved, since these strategies are conditioned by the TME, T-cell depletion, regulation of the immune checkpoint, tumour heterogeneity, etc. For this reason, it is necessary to find an ideal combination of neo-epitope vaccines, chemotherapy, radiotherapy, checkpoint blocking therapies, etc., specific to each patient [142].

3.3.5. Checkpoints Inhibitors

T cells play a critical role in the recognition together with the effector cells of the acquired immune response, and their activation requires the presence of two signals: the antigen-specific signal, mediated by TCR and MHC, and the co-stimulatory signal, mediated by membrane protein molecules expressed on the surface of the T cells and their ligands. The co-stimulatory molecules of the T cell activation signals enhance the immune responses mediated by TCR signalling. These molecules initiate, stimulate, amplify and enhance the immune response at different stages, also controlling its extension and duration. In tumour tissues, negative regulatory checkpoints predominate, inhibiting T cell activation, thus allowing tumour cells to evade the immune response and generating an immune tolerance of the tumour. Therefore, immune checkpoints (ICs) are key to maintaining self-tolerance, protecting the body against autoimmunity and inflammation by interfering with the cytotoxic T cell (CTL) immune response. Pathways that inhibit the immune checkpoint are always activated in inflammatory MSDs, allowing tumour cells to evade immune surveillance, also eradicating the immune response of TILs. Different types of Immune Checkpoint Inhibitors (ICIs) have been developed to reactivate these dysfunctional T cells [46].

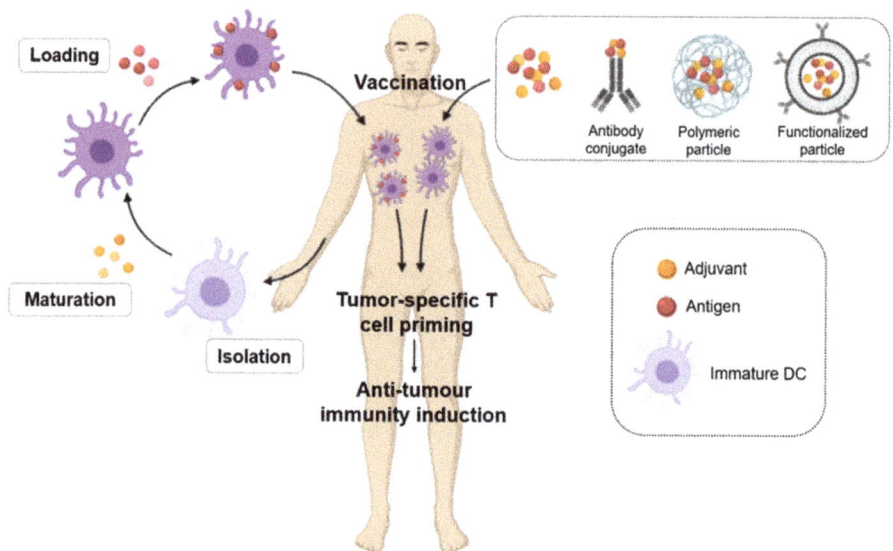

Figure 9. Inducing anti-tumour immune responses by dendritic cell (DC) vaccination through infusing patients with ex vivo antigen loaded DCs (left) or targeting antigens and adjuvants directly to DCs in vivo (right).

Checkpoint inhibitors are monoclonal antibodies that block CTLA-4 (Cytotoxic T-Lymphocyte-associated Antigen 4), PD-1 (Programmed cell Death receptor) or its ligand PD-L1 (Figure 10) [77].

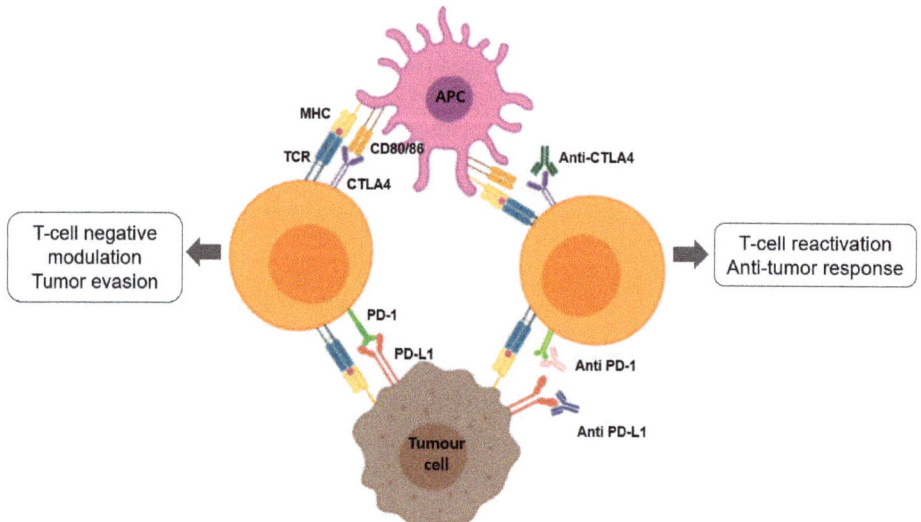

Figure 10. Schematic representation of the mechanisms of immune-checkpoint inhibitors (ICIs).

- CTLA-4:

CTLA-4 is a leukocyte differentiation antigen and a transmembrane receptor on T cells, which shares the B7 ligand with its co-stimulator molecule receptor (CD28). When CTLA-4 binds to B7 it stimulates

T-cell anergy, i.e., it participates in the negative regulation of the immune response by inducing a lack of T-cell response and preventing T-cell activation. The antibody to CTLA-4 has the following anti-tumour mechanisms: (1) modulation of tumour-specific immune effector cells, such as CD8+ T cells, to promote their clonal proliferation, (2) removal of Tregs to reduce inhibition of tumour-associated immune response [46].

- PD1/PD-L1:

The PD-1 and PD-L1 checkpoints limit the excessive immune response to antigens and prevent autoimmunity. PD-1 is expressed in different immune cells such as NK cells, B-lymphocytes, T-lymphocytes, DC and activated monocytes. PD-L1 is overexpressed on tumour cells and promotes cancer avoidance of immune surveillance by inhibiting CTLs. The PD-1/PD-L1 pathway modulates immunosuppression by the following mechanisms: (1) the binding of PD-L1 on the surface of tumour cells and myeloid-derived suppressor cells (MDSCs) to PD-1 on the surface of tumour-specific T cells induces apoptosis and depletion of TIL in MSD; (2) activated PD-1 prevents T cells from proliferating, by selectively inhibiting RAS/MEK/ERK and PI3K/AKT signalling pathways, blocking cell cycle-related gene transcription and protein expression; (3) the expression of PD-L1 on the surface of APCs promotes the transformation of CD4+ T cells into induced Tregs (iTregs) and maintains immunosuppressive function by down-regulating the levels of mTOR, AKT, S6 and ERK2 phosphorylation and up-regulating the expression of PTEN in CD4+ T cells. This is the reason why blocking the PD-1/PD-L1 signalling pathway is expected to restore the function of the effector CD8+ T cells, while suppressing the function of the Tregs and MDSCs, improving the anti-tumour effect of the immune system [46].

This type of immunotherapy has been approved by the FDA for the treatment of melanoma, non-small cell lung cancer, colon and rectal cancer, Hodgkin's lymphoma, Merkel cell carcinoma, head and neck cancer, and bladder cancer [77].

- Combination of immune checkpoint inhibitors (ICIs):

The synergistic combination of monoclonal anti-CTLA-4 and anti-PD-1 antibodies is also used for the treatment of advanced melanoma, metastatic colorectal cancer that is deficient in highly unstable microsatellite repair, and colon and rectal cancer, as it has been shown to improve the overall patient response rate. For this reason, cytokines are being included in combined clinical trials with monoclonal anti-PD-1 and anti-PD-L1 antibodies [77].

On the other hand, the use of immune checkpoint inhibitors presents some problems, such as the appearance of primary and adaptive resistances to ICI monotherapy in some patients. It is therefore important to combine ICIs with other types of anti-tumoral treatment such as chemotherapy or radiotherapy, thus increasing their effectiveness. Another limitation is that some cancers do not respond to PD-1/PD-L1 immunotherapy and systemic administration of these inhibitors has immune-related adverse effects (irAE) [46].

Since the approval of ipilimumab, a CTLA-4-blocking antibody, by the FDA in 2011 for the treatment of metastatic melanoma [164], six other checkpoint inhibitory antibodies, in this case targeting the PD-1/PD-L1 axis, have been approved: nivolumab, pembrolizumab, cemiplimab, atezolizumab, durvalumab, and avelumab. These ICIs act on a wide range of cancers: melanoma, NSCLC, hepatocellular carcinoma, squamous cell head and neck carcinoma, Hodgkin's lymphoma, urothelial carcinoma, etc. [165–168]. In 2015, the FDA approved the combination of ipilimumab with nivolumab (anti-PD-1 antibody), as it showed an improved response rate compared to any monotherapy in the treatment of melanoma [169]. In addition, there are several active clinical trials of ICI combination therapies [170,171]. The identification and validation of more reliable biomarkers would allow for more appropriate selection of patients with cancer that would improve the response rate [172].

3.4. Limitations of Immunotherapy

The previously described immunotherapy strategies (Figure 11) have some limitations and face different challenges.

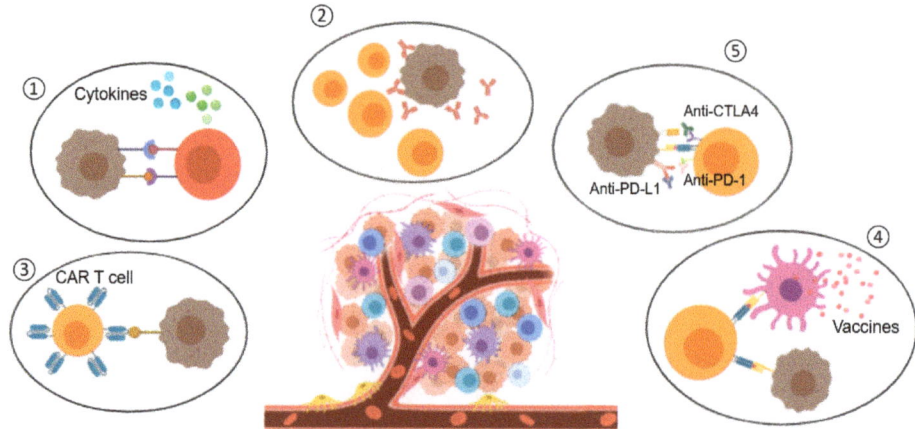

Figure 11. Summary of the different immunotherapies described above. (1) Cytokines, (2) monoclonal antibodies (mAb), (3) CAR-T cells, (4) onco-vaccines and (5) ICIs [173].

Although cytokines were the first approach for immunotherapy introduced in the clinic, they also have some drawbacks. Cytokine treatments consist of high-dose injections, as their half-life is short, resulting in vascular leakage and cytokine release syndrome. In addition, cytokines can promote the survival of regulatory T cells and induce death in stimulated T cells, resulting in autoimmunity against healthy tissues [174].

As for agonist antibodies, they have dose-limiting toxicities, as do cytokines, since they can induce activity on unwanted immune cell subtypes, and immune activity towards healthy cells. In addition, some of these antibodies induce regulatory activity on T cells [175]. Therefore, it is necessary to evaluate dose-associated toxicities and develop delivery platforms. One example is anti-4-1BB antibodies, which—when anchored to liposomal NPs—have a higher intra-tumoral accumulation and lower toxicity than antibodies released freely in mouse models [176].

In the case of CAR-T cells, unlike other treatments, they are unique therapies and the cells can maintain their activity for several years after injection. Despite this, the long-term effects of therapy with CAR-T cells are still being investigated [177]. Other disadvantages of this therapy are that the production of CAR-T cells is expensive, technically complex and time-consuming. In certain tumours, especially solid tumours, depending on their microenvironment, the infused cells do not persist and need combination therapies and new drug delivery systems to improve T-cell survival [175].

CAR-T cells and TCR cells can cause cytokine release syndrome and neurotoxicity [177]. Another problem is making these modified cells effective in solid tumours. One of the solid tumours that has been successfully treated with CAR-T cells is glioblastoma [58], but it expresses the target antigen (EGFRvIII) at much higher levels in the tumour cells than normal cells, which is unusual. As for T cells with high affinity TCR, their toxicity is difficult to predict [178].

In the case of vaccines, those based on DCs have demonstrated high safety profiles, while in clinical trials they have shown a lack of efficacy [179]. The efficacy could be improved by identifying subsets of dendritic cells expressing high levels of specific antigens and by improving the supply to the lymph nodes [180]. As for DNA- or RNA-based vaccines, the former have been tested in clinical trials but are often not successful due to nuclear supply barriers and immunogenicity [181]. mRNA vaccines also have some drawbacks, such as the fact that mRNA can be degraded by nucleases and not internalized into cells. The use of delivery pathways to mediate intracellular internalization may be a good option [182]. Neoantigen vaccines cover an unlimited number of neoantigens, but delivery platforms can improve their efficacy by increasing the stability of the encapsulated molecules and by housing several neoantigens within one platform to treat heterogeneous cancers [175].

For ICIs administered by the systemic route, they can have serious side effects in several organs [183,184]. In addition, many patients do not respond to this treatment, which may be due to a low number of tumour-infiltrating T cells, dysregulation of the checkpoint axes or adapted resistance to checkpoint inhibition [185]. Different tumour microenvironments also have different mechanisms of immunosuppression that require new approaches for effective treatment.

The TME, in the case of solid tumours, is a challenge in the implementation of the above-mentioned immunotherapies. The TME of these tumours can be classified as immunologically "hot" (high immunogenicity) or "cold" (low immunogenicity), with high or low levels of cytotoxic lymphocyte infiltration, respectively. "Hot" tumours have better responses to ICIs than "cold" tumours; then, delivery technologies might be exploited to modulate immunogenicity for "cold" tumours [186].

Another drawback of immunotherapies is related to the systemic toxicity, which can be reduced by delivery platforms by limiting drug exposure in specific tissues, thus allowing for the delivery of otherwise highly toxic combination therapies [187]. The study by Wantong Song et al. shows that NPs allow for the administration of combination immunotherapy treatments, making "cold" tumours susceptible to immunotherapy [188]. Nanomedicines can be designed to respond to the tumour microenvironment and increase site penetration in both "hot" and "cold" solid tumours, overcoming the limitations of immunotherapy [189].

Immunotherapies that require intracellular administration, such as genetic vaccines, must overcome extra- and intracellular barriers with minimal systemic toxicity [190]. Administration and delivery technologies, such as NPs, would allow for the therapeutic burden of such immunotherapies to be encapsulated and protected until they can be released into the cytosol of the target cells [191,192].

4. Nanomedicine and Immunotherapy: Synergy Combination

In order to improve the effectiveness and minimize the toxicity associated with cancer immunotherapy, new strategies have been attempted, including the use of nanomaterials to increase host immunity. Nanomedicine can play a role in improving both active and passive immunotherapy, depending on the functions for which the different NPs have been designed and the processes in which they participate (Figure 12). These NPs can be designed as delivery platforms for immunotherapy, i.e., as delivery vehicles which allow for more efficient and specific transport of immunostimulatory agents, which we will call passive nanomedicine; or they can be designed with nanomaterials which have intrinsic immunomodulatory properties that help to increase anti-tumour immune responses by selectively regulating signalling pathways in different immune cell populations, called active nanomedicine.

4.1. Passive Immune Nanomedicine

Passive immune nanomedicine involves NPs conjugated with growth factors, cytokines and nucleic acids, which intervene by stimulating the maturation, activation or inhibition of some cells of the innate immune response, as well as enhancing the antigenic presentation, with the final objective of activating the adaptive immune response.

Synthetic and natural NPs have physical and chemical ideal properties that make them optimal drug carrier platforms for targeted delivery, such as allowing their pharmacokinetic and pharmacodynamic properties to be modified without altering their anti-tumour effect. The surface of these NPs is directly modified with chemical motifs for selective and/or oriented coupling/immobilization of different biomolecular targets. Commonly, among chemical moieties, a plethora of biomolecules could be bound to the surfaces such as: antibodies, peptides or recombinant proteins, DNA probes, in order to facilitate the selective accumulation of drugs within the tumour tissues when they are released from the internal nucleus of the NP, where they are encapsulated [193].

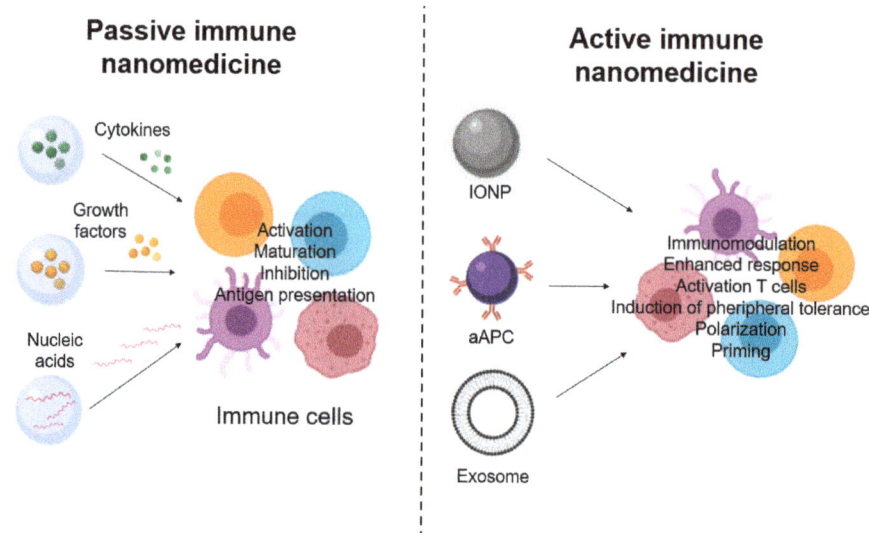

Figure 12. Classification of nanomedicines according to the function caused/promoted on the immune cells [193].

Here, a few of the most representative NPs involved in the multiple functions mentioned above will be further discussed in order to reflect the advantages in oncotherapy.

Lipid-based and polymer-based NPs allow effective delivery of antigens or viral peptides to APC to stimulate memory T-cell responses to tumours. Self-assembled NPs increase the production of inflammatory cytokines such as IL-2 and IFN-γ in activated leukocytes, generating powerful immune responses to low immunogenic tumours.

In this area, another described application of NPs is to produce direct delivery of cytokines, cell growth factors or stimulant cocktails to activate specific or particular functions of immune cells. NPs capable of delivering nucleic acids such as siRNAs or Cas9 mRNAs have also begun to be used to intervene in transcriptional modifications or repair genes associated with disease [193].

One example is the reprogramming of circulating T cells to the anti-tumour phenotype by inserting chimeric antigen receptor (CAR) genes for leukemia into the nucleus using containing synthetic DNA coupled to NPs [194], which offers some advantages over current CAR-T cell therapy, such as replacing the ex vivo expansion of T cells isolated from the patient. In the case of RNA, sequences encoding viral neo-antigens or mutants are used [193], and it is encapsulated in lipid NPs that protect it from degradation by extracellular ribonuclease, ensuring its internalization into APCs so that they express in vivo engineered antigenic peptides [195]. The use of the latter type of NPs has been shown to induce anti-tumour effects and memory T cells, through the activation of INF-α, and induced strong anti-tumour anti-specific responses in three melanoma patients [51].

NPs present another potential advantage, namely targeted immunization, since they are mostly captured (by different mechanisms such as phagocytosis, pinocytosis, and endocytosis) by innate immune cells such as macrophages, monocytes and dendritic cells. The surface of these NPs is a binding substrate for serum proteins such as albumin, apolipoproteins and complement system, forming a biological corona that interacts with different receptors that are expressed in membrane of professional phagocytic cells (i.e., macrophages, DCs, etc.). Although this non-specific absorption by phagocytic cells may be a disadvantage in the case of conventional nanomedicine because it reduces the accessibility and availability of encapsulated drugs in tumour tissues; however in the case of immune nanomedicine it may be an advantage, since these NPs can thus reach lymphoid organs such as the spleen and produce their immunomodulatory effect there.

These properties make NPs outstanding candidates for the administration of tumour vaccines and/or vaccine adjuvants, as they improve their potential while reducing side effects by preventing the systemic distribution of these adjuvants and prolonging their role in lymph node drainage [193].

The intervention of NPs in the different processes of innate immunity can improve the efficacy of passive immunotherapy, and it is therefore necessary to develop new strategies to exploit the full potential of nanomaterials combined with different immunotherapeutics. Passive nanomedicine is an approach that offers many possibilities for improving cancer treatment, which should be further investigated with the aim of transferring its benefits to the clinic.

4.2. Active Immune Nanomedicine

In active immune nanomedicine, different synthetic nanoconstructions or natural nanostructures are used which, due to their intrinsic immunomodulating properties, increase the responses of immune cells, in this case interacting with adaptive immunity cells in a more specific way. In this case, there are many different designs and modifications of NPs that can be used. Some are described below as conjugated NPs, exosomes, artificial antigen-presenting cells or iron oxide NPs (IONPs), among the most promising strategies.

4.2.1. NP Conjugates

One of the novel applications of NPs is their possible role as immunomodulating agents for the treatment of patients with cancer or auto-immune disorders. Liposomal or polymer NPs are designed to mimic biological interactions between APCs and T cells, which can also act as specific subcellular granules to promote anti-tumour immunity [193]. One example is polydimethylsiloxane (PDMS) particles, modified with antibodies to CD3 and CD28, which activate and enhance the in vitro expansion of TCD4+ and CD8+ cells [196].

For instance, NPs could also be designed for direct dependency on immune cells to target and attack different tumour cells [193]. For example, different NPs loaded with chemotherapeutic agents that reduce local recurrences may be delivered via neutrophils, as these cells will be recruited to the tumour resection bed by the inflammatory cytokines released after surgery in the case of brain tumours [197]. Other types of innate immune response cells, such as platelets conjugated with anti-PD-L1 antibodies on their membrane, which also accumulate in the tumour bed after surgery, can also be used to reduce local recurrence [198].

It should be noted that various studies have revealed the importance of the size, shape, density, rigidity and spatial organization of the MHC, among other characteristics [193], since it has been shown that, in the case of NPs used as a substrate for artificial APCs, their size is fundamental for the activation of T cells [2,199].

Another employed NPs are super-paramagnetic, such as those based on fucoidan-dextran, which can be modified with antibodies that inhibit PD-L1 and activate T cells to generate a multifunctional complex. Hence, magnetic field orientation in vivo towards the tumour is achieved by the properties of the nucleus and its effect outside the nucleus is minimised, while the tumour immune response is enhanced by the above-mentioned antibodies [200].

Beyond the modification of nanomaterial compositions, the NPs can also be engineered to enhance tumour cell phagocytosis and subsequent antigenic presentation by macrophages. For example, in HER2-positive breast cancer, bio-specific nanoparticle systems that recruit macrophages to tumour cells with the HER2 receptor can be used [201].

Taking into account the multiple possibilities of conjugation of the nanomaterials and biomolecules described above to design NPs, some of the most important ones, such as aAPCs or iron oxide NPs, are described below. In addition, exosomes, which are nanovesicles that come from cells and transmit information between tissue microenvironments, will be reviewed [202]. In other words, exosomes are vesicles of completely natural origin that can also be used in nanomedicine.

4.2.2. Exosomes

As it was described previously, exosomes are also considered NPs that are originate from cells and transmit information between tissue microenvironments and can influence the function and differentiation of target cells. They are secreted by all cell types, including immune cells (such as B and T cells, DC cells), cancer cells, stem cells and endothelial cells; in addition, exosomes and are present in the human proximal fluids such as blood, urine and breast milk. In general, exosomes are constitutively released by tumour cells or in a regulated manner by immune cells (i.e., B cells). Exosomes biogenesis is produced by internal germination of late endosomes and produce multivessel bodies that fuse with the plasma membrane and are released into the microenvironment [203]. Structurally exosomes are composed of a lipid bilayer expressing ligands and surface receptors, which contains a hydrophilic nucleus. In the nucleus, there is a high rich content from RNA, proteins and other components that come from the source cells. Thus, exosomes carry information in the form of mRNA and miRNA that will correspond to the normal or pathogenic processes of the cells from which they come [202], such as the elimination of unwanted proteins, the presentation of antigens, genetic exchange, immune responses, angiogenesis, inflammation, tumour metastasis and the spread of pathogens or oncogenes [204,205].

Regarding the content on membrane proteins, exosomes contain very interested ligands such as integrines, tetraspanines, and receptors in native conformations, including the co-receptors needed for in vivo signalling [206], among others. The adhesion molecules (i.e., integrines, selectins, etc.) contained in exosomes are known to be expressed on the cells from which they originate; for example, DC-derived exosomes express CD80 and CD86 [207], B-cell derivatives express CD19 [208]. From the proteome point of view, exosome proteomes have been analysed in several studies because, although they constitute only a small part of the total plasma proteome, they are enriched in altered proteins under different pathological conditions and might therefore be considered diagnostic markers [203,209]. Therefore, in lung cancer, colorectal cancer and diabetes, specific expression patterns of serum miRNA have been identified as biomarkers for the detection of these diseases in human physiological proximal fluids [210].

Bearing in mind all these inherent properties of exosomes, they seem ideal biological nano-carriers. Moreover, due to origin, exosomes present biocompatible, such as immune tolerance, which allows them to avoid elimination through adaptive response [206]. They also escape phagocytosis, because they could fuse with cell membranes and avoid lysosome envelopes, and are more stable in the blood [211]. These exosomes can be modified either endogenously at the cellular level or exogenously in cell cultures. Endogenous modification is based on modifying exosome components, such as proteins, at the level of production of the cell from which they originate [206]. Exogenous modifications are important in understanding the extent to which the contents and function of exosomes of different biological origins could be manipulated. These exogenous modifications provide information on how exosomes target and interact with tissue-specific microenvironments in vivo, which would allow for new applications in diagnosis and therapy. The structure of exosomes allows for three types of exogenous modifications: 1.-modifying exosome surface molecules to allow specific targeting and monitoring of exosomes, 2.-loading hydrophobic therapies onto the membrane, and 3.-loading hydrophilic drugs or therapeutic cargo into the nucleus. These modifications facilitate the use of exosomes as nanomedicine approaches in immune-onco-therapy [202].

One of the described applications, it is based on the pre-existing surface receptors themselves, which could be also adapted for use in therapeutic applications. In one recent study, it was shown that mesenchymal stem cell (MSC) exosomes can transmit membrane and ligand receptors to attenuate the function of self-reactive CD4 T cells isolated from mice with experimental autoimmune encephalitis. The ligand PD-L1, TGF-β and galectin-1 were transferred to the T cells and decreased secretion of IL-17 and IFN-γ by 50% by the T cells after treatment with the exosomes [212].

MSCs produce a greater number of exosomes than other cell types and this production is not compromised in terms of quantity or quality thanks to the immortalization of these cells to generate permanent cell lines that guarantee the reproducible and sustainable production of exosomes from

MSCs [213]. These exosomes, in addition to surface markers CD9 and CD81, express adhesion molecules that are also expressed on the MSC membrane, such as CD29, CD44 and CD73. MSCs recruit and regulate T cells, either by cell to cell contact or paracrine. Cytokine secretion and ligand–receptor inhibitory interactions are believed to be an important function of MSCs [203]. Exosomes derived from these cells act as mediators that induce peripheral tolerance of self-reactive cells by carrying MSC-specific tolerance molecules such as PD-L1, Gal-1 and TGF-β. These exosomes have been shown to inhibit the proliferation of self-reactive lymphocytes and promote the secretion of anti-inflammatory cytokines such as IL-10 and TGF-β, among others [214]. Therefore, MSC-derived exosomes are mediators that induce peripheral tolerance and modulate immune responses, and could therefore be used in the treatment of auto-immune diseases [81]. These exosomes have also been used in graft-versus-host disease (GVDH), which has been shown to delay its appearance in mouse models and to increase Tregs cells [215].

Another relevant study, described by Bo Yu et al., was based on the idea that MSCs have different effects on tumour growth, as they may favor tumour initiation or inhibit the progression of established tumours. Thus, exosomes released by MSCs also have varied effects [203]. One effect is the increased incidence and growth of tumours induced by certain cell lines, which indicates that MSC-derived exosomes promote tumour progression as do MSCs in vivo [216]. Another study showed that MSC-derived exosomes suppress tumour progression and angiogenesis by negatively regulating VEGF expression in in vitro and in vivo tumours. The miRNA-16 is believed to be responsible for the anti-angiogenic effect, as MSC-derived exosomes are enriched in this miRNA which targets VEGF [217].

Another exosome modification strategy is using in RNA administration mediated by in exosome. Exosomes have the inherent ability to transmit mRNA and miRNA between cells [218]. Among other methods, electroporation facilitates the loading of exogenous siRNA into exosomes. The efficiency of electroporation depends on the concentration of exosomes and the applied voltage. Using this method, Wahlgren et al. found that plasma-derived exosomes loaded with MAPK-1 siRNAs suppressed the levels of MAPK-1 mRNAs in monocytes and lymphocytes [219].

Momen-Heravi et al. charged B-cell exosomes with the miRNA-155 inhibitor by electroporation. When cells were stimulated with LPS, miRNA-155 increased their production of TNF-α. Exosomes loaded with the miRNA-155 inhibitor were able to reduce the production of TNF-α by LPS-treated macrophages. This strategy allows reducing the negative inflammatory component in different disease processes. The importance of choosing the correct exosome subpopulations for the therapeutic application of interest is highlighted. In this case, the isolation of exosomes was performed using anti-CD36 immunomagnetic microspheres [220]. This type of isolation and enrichment is very useful to separate exosome subpopulations for biomarker studies [221].

Exosomes may also be used as immunotolerant nano-carriers for hydrophilic chemotherapeutic load, such as doxorubicin [202]. Tian et al. designed immunotolerant immature dendritic cell (iDC) exosomes that expressed a chimeric Lamp2b fusion protein and the integrin-specific iRGD peptide α-V. Electroporation was used to load doxorubicin into the exosomes and the encapsulation efficiency was 20%. The iDC exosomes were able to target and accumulate in breast tumours expressing α-V integrin in mice and inhibit their growth. In contrast, free doxorubicin or untargeted doxorubicin exosomes had no effect on tumour growth. In addition, tumour growth inhibition with iDC exosomes did not result in observable toxicity and therefore the use of iDC exosomes as biocompatible nanoporters was validated [222].

Another recent study, it has also been conducted with modified exosomes to treat NSCLC. Here, exosomes loaded with paclitaxel were modified with PEG and AA (ligand) to increase blood circulation time and attack lung metastases. In this way, the drug selectively targets the target cancer cells and increases the survival rate of patients with lung cancer [223].

B-lymphocyte-derived exosomes have also been shown to have immunomodulatory function, triggering specific CD4+ T-cell responses and thus performing a role as transporters of MHC class II peptide complexes between immune cells [224]. In the case of DC-derived exosomes, they have been shown to express MHC class I, class II and co-stimulatory T-cell molecules and to suppress the growth of T-cell-dependent murine tumours [225]. For this reason, these exosomes may begin to be considered as cell-free "vaccines" in cancer immunotherapy [226].

Attempts are still being made to determine the endogenous function of the various exosome subtypes and subpopulations. This is even more important in the design of nano-carriers with tumour exosome subtypes that may have a pathogenic burden, which must be neutralized so that it does not impede the therapeutic efficacy of these exosomes [206]. In contrast, tumour antigen retention may also be beneficial for the development of tumour exosome-based immunotherapies [227]. The various therapeutic applications will require the selection of the optimal exosome subtype for conversion to nano-carriers and this requires an understanding of the normal function of exosomes and the ability to predict the function of modified exosomes.

4.2.3. Artificial Antigen Presentation Cells (aAPC)

Artificial antigen-presenting cells (aAPC) deliver stimulation signals to cytotoxic T cells and are a powerful tool for active and adoptive immunotherapy [228].

In fact, the induction of specific cytotoxic T cell (CTL) responses is a potent therapy against pathogens and tumours. Specific CTLs produce robust responses and generate long-term memory [229]. As an active immunotherapy, CTLs can be activated in vivo.

Two signals are required from APCs for T cell activation, the first being a related antigenic peptide presented on MHC molecules that binds to the TCR, and the second a series of co-stimulatory receptors that modulate T cell response [230]. In immunotherapy, modified NPs that function as artificial antigen-presenting cells (aAPCs) are being used to rapidly expand tumour-specific T cells from naïve precursors and responses to predicted neo-epitopes [231].

Naïve tumour-specific precursors are rare and APC-based methods for the expansion of naïve tumour-specific cells will require continued stimulation during multiple tabletop sessions, followed by T-cell selection and subcloning to generate the number of tumour-specific cells required for adoptive immunotherapy. Therefore, the development of the ideal T-cell expansion platform is required, which generates robust expansion, minimizing culture time and costs [231].

As an example, the study described by Karlo Perica et al., iron-dextran NPs were used and a chimeric immunoglobulin-MHC dimer (MHC-Ig) loaded with a specific peptide is used to generate signal 1 and B7.1 (natural T-cell receptor ligand CD28) or an activating antibody against CD28 is used for signal 2. These molecules are chemically bonded to the surface of the microspheres to generate these aAPCs. It was found that the aAPCs induced antigen-specific T cell expansion in vitro and that both signals were essential for optimal expansion, and also induced anti-tumour activity in vivo. In addition, the amount and density of antigen presented by APCs are known to influence T cell behaviour, proliferation and cell death, and therefore are important parameters to consider in aAPC stimulation [228].

The potential sites where aAPCs may be most effective are the lymph nodes, where the naive and memory T cells are found, and the site of the tumour [228]. In addition, aAPCs may overcome one of the major obstacles in cancer immunotherapy: the tumour's immunosuppressive microenvironment. This is because they deliver the immunostimulatory signal in situ [232]. aAPCs are known to activate T cells by specific receptor-ligand bonds at the cell-sphere interface, but such interactions are not defined at the nanoscale level [233].

Although nanoscale aAPCs have been shown to induce anti-tumour naïve T-cell populations in vivo, the ability of these nanostructures to mediate the rejection of established tumours in highly immunosuppressive microenvironments has not been determined. It is not yet well-known whether a local stimulating signal could overcome several stages of tumour immunosuppression, or even whether aAPC-based stimulation could be enhanced by other immunomodulatory therapies such as checkpoint blocking strategies [228].

Although autologous APCs (DC, monocytes and activated B cells) have originally been used to generate tumour-specific T cells in vitro, this requires regular access to patients' blood and, in addition, the quantity and quality of each patient's autologous APCs is variable. APCAs overcome these problems, are easy to produce and allow reliable expansion of antigen-specific T-cell populations, as we have already seen, making them a promising technology for cancer immunotherapy [234,235].

4.2.4. Iron Oxide NPs (IOPNs)

Currently, there is a growing requirement for image-guided cancer therapy to design personalised therapies in cancer patients, for which advances in the translational development of IONPs may have a significant impact on the clinical and prognostic outcome of these cancer patients [236]. Several approaches based on IONPs have super-paramagnetic properties that are very useful in MRI and are used as contrast agents for diagnostic applications [237].

In recent years, several studies have been conducted to improve the properties of magnetic IONPs with the aim of making them suitable for human biomedical applications, in particular for immunotherapies. One example is surface modifications to reduce non-specific absorption of IONPs by macrophages in the reticuloendothelial system, such as polyethylene glycol (PEG) coating. To increase the efficiency of delivery, magnetic IONPs have been conjugated with different targeting ligands (antibodies, peptides, natural ligands, small molecules, etc.) directed to highly expressed cell receptors on tumour vasculatures, stromal cells and tumour cells [236]. Many preclinical studies have been performed with ligand conjugated IONPs targeting tumours with therapeutic agents for disease detection and treatment applications [238], and the effects on tumour imaging of these types of IONPs have been demonstrated in mouse models [239]. Appropriate targeting ligands and surface modifications have been shown to result in improved accumulation of IONPs in tumour tissues in animal models, while reducing nonspecific accumulation in the liver and spleen [240]. In contrast, IONPs that have been approved by the FDA are untargeted IONPs, and they have been used in humans as contrast agents in MRIs [236].

The properties of IONPs provide an enhanced effect of MRI contrast so that through this methodology drug delivery can be controlled, treatment responses evaluated, and drug delivery controlled by the external magnetic field [241]. Therefore, IONPs are a good candidate for the development of new tumour imaging, targeted drug delivery, and image-guided therapy, which have great potential in new clinical applications.

4.3. NP Biosafety: A Critical Aspect in Nanomedicine and Immunotherapy

To guarantee the effective and safe use of nanomaterials used in Nanomedicine, it is necessary to characterise the interaction between a material and the biological system involved. These are biocompatibility studies that have to be performed with a focus on the environment in which the biomaterial will be administered [242]. To ensure the drug delivery, it is necessary to evaluate this biocompatibility, ensuring the safe release of the medicine and minimizing its toxicity. For example, NPs that have not been modified on their surface are absorbed by phagocytic cells, which can lead to undesirable interactions with the immune system, decreasing the bioavailability of the drug [243].

Biocompatibility is defined as "the ability of a material to function with an appropriate host response in a specific situation" [244]. The employed material has to fulfil its intended functions, the reaction induced has to be appropriate to the intended application, and the nature of the reaction to a material and its suitability may be different in different contexts. The high degree of compatibility is achieved when a material interacts with the body without causing toxic, immunogenic or carcinogenic responses [243]. Importantly, biocompatibility is anatomically dependent, so a biomaterial can cause adverse effects in one type of tissue and will not cause the same response in another [245,246]. The half-life of exposure is also determinant and, therefore, the clearance of each NPs as well. Biocompatibility is subjective, as it is based on the risk-benefit ratio.

Currently, a few studies on biological processes in response to foreign materials or on the nature of the methods available for biocompatibility, so there is a strong need to evaluate the biocompatibility of each material individually and specifically for each tissue and application [243]. An example of this type of studies is the analysis realized by Mikhail V. Zyuzin et al., who proved the immunocompatibility of polyelectrolyte capsules synthesized by layer-by-layer deposition through the incubation of different cell lines with this capsules [247].

NPs are delivered into the bloodstream and are therefore exposed to many biomolecules that will give rise to a protein crown around them [248]. This causes NPs to undergo changes in their physicochemical properties, and therefore it is necessary to study NP–protein interactions in nanomedicine. Proteins in the biological environment are adsorbed to NPs by affinity and protein–protein interactions [2]. The first proteins to bind are those found in high concentrations, although they have low affinity, and are subsequently replaced by proteins with higher affinity that are found in lower concentrations. This phenomenon is called the Vroman effect [249]. The protein crown is classified into hard or soft crown depending on the duration of protein replacement. The hard crown is formed by high affinity proteins with a long exchange time and is the innermost layer. The soft crown is made up of proteins with low affinity and a rapid exchange of proteins [250].

Both the characteristics of NPs and protein concentration, and the biological environment will determine the formation of the protein crown. Therefore, it is important to understand the relationship between the properties of nanomaterials and the biological environment to understand the behaviour and viability of the NPs used.

4.4. Immunogenic Cell Death: A Merge Point of Nanomedicine and Immunotherapy

The maintenance of homeostasis in the human body involves the continuous replacement of different cell compartments, which does not activate the immune system under normal conditions. Instead, the death of some pathogen-infected cells may generate a strong immune response, further establishing a long-term immune memory. Conventionally, only the "self/non-self" model was used to differentiate homeostatic from pathogen-associated cell death, respectively. However, in the 1990s it was demonstrated that some endogenous entities were capable of initiating an immune response in certain circumstances. This means that there would be another factor other than antigenicity that would determine the immunogenic capacity of the different forms of cell death [251].

The Microbe-Associated Molecular Patterns, called MAMPs, are detected by multiple cells of the innate immune system, such as monocytes, macrophages and DC, before the pathogens activate the adaptive response [252]. MAMPs function as adjuvants, interacting with PRRs, which allow the establishment of the first line of defense while generating favourable conditions to initiate the specific immune response [253]. Signalling through PRRs is of great importance, since these receptors are activated by Damage-Associated Molecular Patterns (DAMPs) (Table 1). DAMPs are produced by cells that are in the process of dying and act as adjuvants, informing the body of the danger situation [254]. Under normal conditions, these DAMPs do not activate the adaptive immune response, but when the dying cells are highly antigenic, this occurs, as new antigenic epitopes ("called neo-epitopes) are detected that have not previously produced tolerance. These neo-epitopes can be expressed from microbial genes or from mutated host genes, as in the case of oncogenesis [255]. Therefore, the other factor determining cell death immunogenicity is adjuvancy, which involves MAMPs and DAMPs [251]. Thus, tumours with a high mutational load respond better to some types of immunotherapy, such as immune checkpoint inhibitors (ICIs), than tumours with a low number of somatic mutations [156].

Table 1. Molecules that act as Damage-Associated Molecular Pattern (DAMPs), associated pattern recognition receptors (PRRs) and described biological functions.

Danger Signal	PRR	Function
CALR HSP70 HSP90	LRP1	Promotes the uptake of dead cell-asociated antigens.
Extracellular ATP	P2RX7/P2RY2	Favours the recruitment of APCs and their activation.
HMGB1 dsRNA Cellular RNA LPS Flagellin ssRNA CpG DNA Viral RNA dsDNA	TLR2/TLR4 TLR3 TLR3 TLR4 TLR5 TLR7 TLR9 RLRs CDSs	Activate the synthesis of pro-inflammatory factors (type I IFNs).
Type I IFNs	IFNAR	Promotes CXCL10 secretion by cancer cells and has immune-stimulatory effects.
ANXA1	FPR1	Guides the final approach of APCs to dying cells.
CXCL10	CXCR3	Favours T cell recruitment.

Caption: ANXA1, annexin A1; APC, antigen-presenting cell; CALR, calreticulin; CDS, cytosolic DNA sensor; CXCL10, CXC-chemokine ligand 10; CXCR3, CXC-chemokine receptor 3; ds, double-stranded; FPR1, formyl peptide receptor 1; HMGB1, high-mobility group box 1; HSP70, heat shock protein 70 kDa; HSP90, heat shock protein 90 kDa; IFN, interferon; IFNAR, interferon α/β-receptor; LRP1, LDL receptor related protein 1; P2RX7, purinergic receptor P2X7; P2RY2, purinergic receptor P2Y2; RLR, RIG-I-like receptor; ss, single-stranded; TLR, Toll-like recept.

In the past, cell death was classified only in apoptosis as a physiological process and in necrosis as a pathological and immunogenic process. Nowadays, it is now known that these differences between the two processes are not as clear, as regulated forms of necrosis are involved in tissue development and homeostasis, and apoptotic cells can trigger antigen-specific immune responses [251]. ICD is therefore a type of immune-stimulatory apoptosis that is characterised by the ability of dying cells to elicit powerful adaptive immune responses to altered auto-antigens/neo-epitope derived from tumour cells in the case of cancer [256]. Based on a specific panel of multiple DAMPs four types of ICDs have been described (Figure 13):

1. Pathogen-induced ICD: It is defined as a defence mechanism against pathogens, such as obligatory intracellular bacteria and viruses. After infection, the cells detect MAMPs through specific PRRs, which will send danger signals to neighbouring cells. Intracellular hazard signalling is generated, which will activate autophagy, and microenvironmental hazard signalling, which will induce the secretion of pro-inflammatory cytokines, including TNF and type I interferons. The adaptive immune response is activated when infected cells die and their bodies are internalized in APC, which will present the various non-self-antigenic epitopes in MHC molecules, thus activating CD8+ and CD4+ T cells [251].

2. ICD caused by chemotherapy and/or targeted onco-therapy: Exposure to certain chemotherapeutic agents used in the clinic has been shown to produce ICD in mouse tumour cells [257]. This ICD is based on eIF2A phosphorylation-dependent exposure of endoplasmic reticulum chaperones in the membrane of these tumour cells. Processes such as autophagy-mediated ATP secretion, IFN type I activation, secretion of chemokine ligands such as CXCL10, etc. are also involved. These processes also occur in human tumour cells after chemotherapy. Chemotherapeutic agents that are unable to promote the release of DAMPs do not produce ICD. The degree of antigenicity among tumour cells is very heterogeneous, which may condition the activation of adaptive immunity after ICD. However, the lower level of mutational load associated with oncogenesis has been found to be sufficient to activate this immunogenicity, which is due to the fact that

tumour cells express neoantigens that are different from their own and are therefore not subject to tolerance [251,258].

3. ICD activated by physical signals: There are three physical interventions that trigger ICDs: irradiation, hypericin-based photodynamic therapy (PDT), and high hydrostatic pressure [251,258]. DCs loaded with irradiated tumour cells have been shown to produce strong immune responses in mice and cancer patients [259]. ICD due to hypericin-based PDT or high hydrostatic pressure shows exposure of ER chaperones on the plasma membrane, ATP secretion, and high-mobility group box 1 (HMGB1) [260,261]. DCs exposed to cells suffering from these two types of ICDs induce positive regulation of DC-activation markers and pro-inflammatory cytokine secretion, resulting in priming of tumour-specific CD8+ T cells [251].

4. Necroptotic ICD: This is a form of programmed cell death, initiated by phosphorylation catalyzed by the serine/threonine kinase 3 (RIPK3) protein, which activates the pseudokinase mixed lineage kinase domain-like (MLKL) receptor, which forms oligomers that produce irreversible plasma membrane permeation [262]. Necroptosis is highly pro-inflammatory and is also capable of activating the adaptive immune system, generating a specific antigen response [251]. This has been demonstrated in studies with the mouse cell lines TC-1 and EL4 of lung carcinoma and CT26 of colorectal carcinoma, which were exposed to necroptosis inducers [263,264].

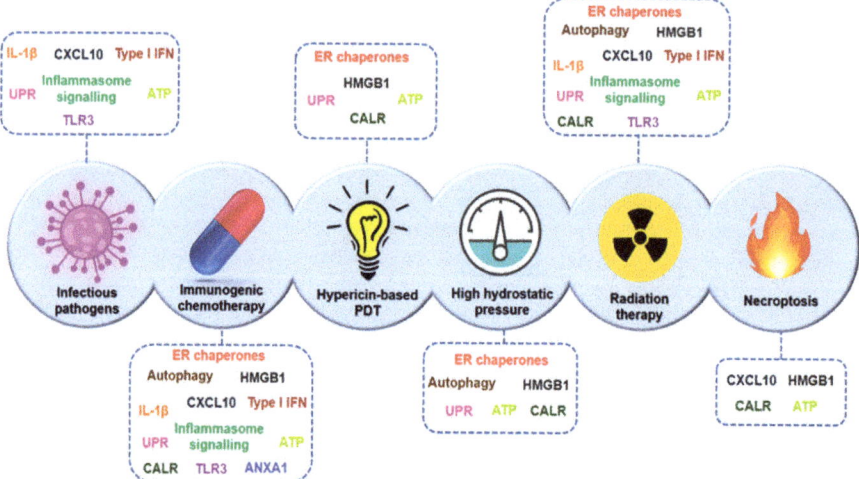

Figure 13. Schematic representation of Immunogenic Cell Death (ICD) classification and their associated DAMPs.

The characteristics of the ICD, such as the exposure of CRT and other ER proteins on the cell surface, the release of HMGB1 or the secretion of ATP, allow for the prediction of the capacity of anti-cancer drugs to stimulate therapeutic immune responses by ICD [265].

For example, calreticulin (CRT) is an ER-associated chaperone involved in various functions, such as MHC-I assembly or calcium homeostasis. Tumour cells that undergo chemotherapy-induced cell death expose CRT on their surface, causing CRT to internalize tumour material and present tumour antigens, activating tumour-specific cytotoxic T cells [265]. Tumours that do not properly expose CRT have been shown to have reduced efficacy of chemotherapy, so this immunogenic signal is necessary to obtain good immune responses [266]. In the clinic, CRT exposure is related to patient survival. In patients with non-Hodgkin's lymphoma, the therapeutic benefit of a pulsed DC vaccine with primary lymphoma cells that undergo ICD is correlated with CRT exposure [267]. For patients with acute myeloid leukemia, CRT exposure by tumour cells is known to predict anti-tumour T-cell responses and improve patient survival [268]. Colorectal cancers that do not express CRT have a worse prognosis [269]. Therefore, the expression of CRT affects the immune responses to the cancer in an important way.

Another important factor is that the tumours are competent in autophagy, since these tumours, in response to chemotherapy, recruit macrophages, DC and T lymphocytes more effectively. This is because autophagy is essential for the immunogenic release of ATP by dying cells, which is a potent chemotherapeutic agent [265]. When autophagy is inhibited in cancer, the recruitment of immune effectors to the tumour bed fails, so it may be an escape mechanism from immune surveillance. Inhibiting enzymes that degrade ATP may improve antineoplastic therapies when autophagy is deactivated [270].

In the case of HMGB1, it is a potent pro-inflammatory stimulus whose release can be induced by most antineoplastic agents [271]. HMGB1 activates the release of pro-inflammatory cytokines by monocytes and macrophages. It has been observed that its neutralization with antibodies prevents cross-presentation of tumour antigens by DC in co-culture experiments, therefore its release is a critical determinant of ICD [272].

The induction of ICD in vivo also generates a TME dominated by Th1 and Th17 cytokines [273], which is expected to increase the efficacy of anti-tumour vaccines and therapies designed to reagent TILs, such as ICI.

But once again, these approaches also encounter some obstacles in the tumour cells. Pathogenic viruses and bacteria have developed different mechanisms to prevent the release or detection of DAMPs to escape the immune response. To this end, they express functional orthopaedics of some molecules and inhibitors of different processes that would be necessary for manifest pathogenicity, mainly limiting adjuvancy. The same occurs with tumour cells, which although they present a high antigenicity, control immunogenicity by acting on the adjuvancy, inhibiting the different processes related to the emission of DAMPs, which impairs the efficacy of treatments such as chemotherapy or immunotherapy [251].

Nanomedicine can also act at the level of ICDs and DAMPs (damage associated molecular patterns), with the aim of restraining the immunogenicity of tumour cells. The NPs can be used to enhance the "danger signals" that are released by these tumour cells. Adjuvant-charged NPs are used and placed in the cells suffering from ICD, thus promoting the transmission of these signals [274]. Another application is the targeted delivery of ICD inducers by other NPs, in the form of discs, which allow them to accumulate in the tumour and positively regulate the danger signals, thus enhancing the response of T cells to neo-antigens, tumour-associated antigens and whole tumour cells [275]. Some NPs also have intrinsic properties to induce ICD, such as gold NPs, which release endogenous immune-stimulatory molecules and facilitate DCs activation [276]. NPs combined with chemotherapy and PDT can also be used to induce ICD or to capture TAAs that are released after radiotherapy, with the goal of enhancing T-cell response when treated with ICIs such as anti-PD-L1 [277,278].

Therefore, the immunotherapeutic strategies described above could benefit from the concept of ICD, avoiding some of the drawbacks that occur in the clinic and enhancing an effective immune response, since the different molecules that determine ICD are involved in multiple processes of the immune cycle against cancer. Pre-clinical and clinical studies have already been conducted that could lay the foundations for the design of combined therapies that restore cellular immunogenicity [279,280].

The concept of ICD can also be used to identify biomarkers to predict therapeutic responses in cancer patients. The distinctive features of ICD in tissues need to be identified and correlated with immunological and clinical observations. It is also important to determine what changes in the immune infiltrate of tumours are caused by the ICD and how they affect therapeutic responses.

5. Biomarkers in Onco-Immunotherapy

As we have already described, immunotherapies are one of the most promising approaches to treat cancer patients, but despite the demonstrated success in a variety of malignant tumours, the responses only occur in a minority of patients. Furthermore, these treatments involve inflammatory toxicity and a high cost. Therefore, determining which patients would derive clinical benefit from immunotherapy is an important goal. This requires the identification and validation of prognostic biomarkers. The integration of multiple tumour and immune response parameters, such as protein expression, genomics and transcriptomics, may be necessary to accurately predict clinical benefit.

5.1. Critical Role of Predictive Biomarkers in Oncology

Progress in the field of immune-oncology has changed traditional treatment models which also the design in clinical trials in order to define objective responses to treatments. With the advent of checkpoint inhibitors, subsets of patients with treatment-resistant metastatic cancers have had long-lasting responses, although many patients still do not respond [281]. Objective responses among patients treated with single-agent regimens are seen in less than half of the patients treated, and combination checkpoint inhibitor therapy increases response rates but also toxicity and cost [282], highlighting the need to identify predictive biomarkers for outcome [281]. The importance of identifying these predictive biomarkers, and not just prognoses, lies in the need to optimise the selection of appropriate tumour types and patients for treatment with immunotherapy, in order to increase efficacy and to avoid unnecessary toxicities, high healthcare costs, etc. This can improve the selection of tumour types and patients that will benefit from immunotherapy, as well as the determination of which patients need a single therapeutic agent, several combined strategies or the development of alternative treatment strategies [282]. Although progress in biomarker research has been rapid, only a few biomarkers have proven to be clinically relevant, including PD-L1. These biomarkers are used to select patients for FDA-approved therapies, but other biomarkers are not yet well-established [281].

Currently, the development of biomarkers in onco-immunotherapy is limited because many of the targets are often inducible and with variability in time and location [282]. This is influenced by the TME and immunoedition. In the TME, there are interactions between various types of infiltrating immune cells (monocytes, granulocytes, DC, T and B cells, mast cells, NK, etc.), heterogeneous tumour cells and tumour-associated stromal cells (macrophages, fibroblasts, endothelial cells). In addition, there is a local variation in oxygenation, perfusion, electrolyte levels and tumour cells that become resistant in conditions of anoxia and lack of nutrients, which generates "microniches" within the tumour microenvironment itself. In addition, clones of tumour cells that are resistant to selective pressure may appear due to incomplete immunoedition and immune escape [283]. The importance of tumour-infiltrating lymphocytes within the tumour microenvironment has been established as containing prognostic value for cancer patients and predictive value for treatment with immunotherapy [282].

Therefore, to target cancer therapy, the variety of biomarkers and trials required is wide. This is due to the great diversity of immunotherapy agents with different mechanisms of action, to tumour heterogeneity, including changes in antigenic profiles over time and the location of each patient, and to the different immunosuppressive mechanisms that are activated in TEM. This complexity requires a profile of the tumour immune interface using multiparametric technologies that encompass the dimensionality and complexity of these interactions, in order to monitor and stratify cancer patients according to individual therapeutic requirements. All this complexity in turn is a rich source of biomarkers [284]. The types of potential biomarkers (Figure 14) and their possible relationship with the tumour immune cycle are described below.

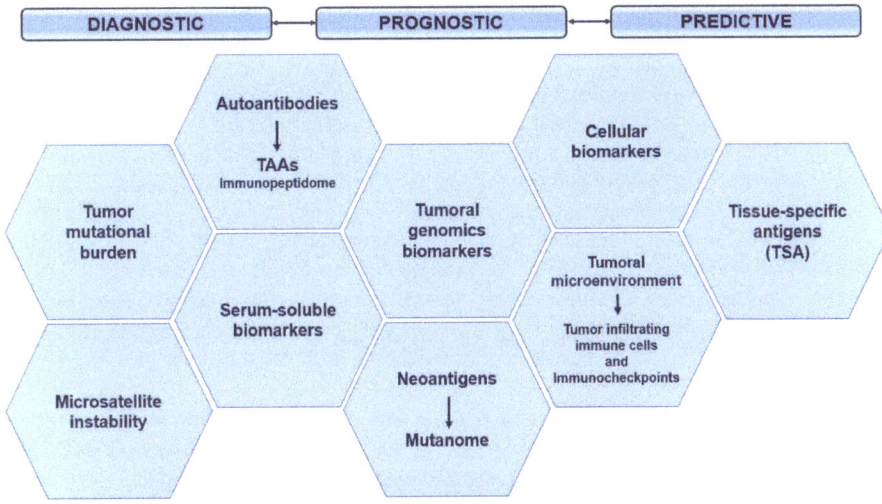

Figure 14. Summary of available biomarkers for Immuno-Oncology.

5.2. Potential Biomarkers in Immuno-Oncology

The FDA defines the concept of biomarker as: "A characteristic that is objectively measurable and evaluable as an indicator of a normal biological process, a pathogenic process, or a pharmacological response to a therapeutic intervention" [285]. Biomarkers are all those molecules that are found in body fluids in small quantities and that are associated with specific health and/or disease processes, and are classified into three types according to their purpose: (1) diagnostic biomarkers: used to detect disease; (2) prognostic biomarkers: used to predict the course of the disease; (3) predictive biomarkers: used to predict the patient's response to treatment. A single biomarker may meet the criteria for different uses [286].

Depending on their nature or location, there are different types of biomarkers, such as soluble factors, tumour-specific factors, host genomic factors, cellular biomarkers, or TME biomarkers [282]. The most important characteristics of the multiple types of potential biomarkers are described below.

5.2.1. Serum-Soluble Biomarkers

Potential biomarkers present in serum, plasma, or peripheral blood are more useful in the clinic; because in general, they should be accurately measurable and reproducible, clinically feasible, cost-effective, and prospectively validated in randomized clinical trials [282].

Soluble serum proteins as possible biomarkers were first suggested in studies of advanced melanoma and colorectal cancer (CRC) patients with high doses of IL-2. High serum levels of IL-6 and C-reactive proteins (CRP) were identified in pre-treatment as possible prognostic markers of treatment failure and shorter overall survival in metastatic CRC after IL-2 therapy [287]. High serum levels of pre-treatment CRP predict resistance to IL-2 therapy in patients with metastatic melanoma [288]. Subsequently, in patients with advanced melanoma, pre-treatment serum VEGF and fibronectin have been shown to be inversely correlated with response to IL-2 treatment [289].

High levels of VEGF and CRP are also inversely correlated with the response of melanoma patients treated with ipilimumab. Elevated serum LDH levels are also a negative predictive value in these patients. If a decrease in LDH and CRP levels occurs during treatment with ipilimumab, at week 12 it is associated with significant disease control [290].

Another potential soluble biomarker is CD25, which has favourable results at low levels, but resistance to treatment with ipilimumab at high levels. However, it is not clear whether this CD25 is a predictive or prognostic biomarker [291].

Circulating predictive biomarkers are expected to include markers of increased type 1 immunity and cytotoxic cell activity [292]. These include cytokines such as IFNγ, IL-12, IL-2 and chemokines such as CXCR3 and CCR5 that are associated with tumour trafficking and stimulate cytotoxic functions [293]. Otherwise, the immunosuppressive pathways of MSD will be disrupted, with molecules such as IDO, MDSCs will increase and immune-regulatory pathways will be stimulated [294].

These types of biomarkers are easily measurable and can be very useful in the clinic, so their identification and validation are essential. So far, most published analyses of these types of biomarkers in immunotherapy have been retrospective [282], although important information has been obtained to determine the mechanisms of clinical benefit. Clinical trials with different approaches still need to be designed to establish the use of these biomarkers in the clinic on a routine basis.

5.2.2. Cellular Biomarkers

Different types of cells in peripheral blood have been studied as prognostic and predictive factors, including T cells, NK cells, DC, macrophages and tumour cells [282]. For example, high numbers of neutrophils and monocytes in peripheral blood are associated with poor survival in metastatic melanoma and serve as prognostic factors for overall survival in IL-2 treated melanoma patients [295].

Lymphocytes are the cells that have been most studied as a predictor of response to immunotherapy [282]. Circulating tumour-reactive lymphocytes can be sampled by multiparametric immunophenotypic analysis with a focus on biomarker development. Thus, immunophenotype by multiparametric flow cytometry allows identification of biomarkers associated with persistence, establishment of antitumour memory, and improvement of clinical outcomes [296,297]. The expression of PD-1 by peripheral lymphocytes correlates with tumour load, which may serve as a biomarker for the response to immunotherapy [298]. Initial lymphopenia and rebound lymphocytosis are known to follow IL-2 treatment. There is a positive association between clinical response and the degree of lymphocytosis following immunotherapy [282].

The presence of induced autoimmunity also serves to predict the response to immunotherapy. In metastatic melanoma, spontaneous antibody formation occurs for several common tumour auto-antigens, including gp100, MAGE-3, or NY-ESO-1 [282]. Patients who are HIV-positive for NY-ESO-1 are most likely to benefit 24 weeks after treatment with ipilimumab [299].

5.2.3. Specific Tumour Antibodies

In the tumour of some malignant neoplasms, B cells are found, organised in germinal centers, which results in the presence of plasma cells. Their function is not yet known, but it is assumed that they are involved in a constant immune reaction at the site of the tumour. In cancer patients, circular antigen-specific auto-antibodies (AAbs) derived from tumour can be detected, which helps to determine immunogenic targets.

Ultimately, cancer sera contain antibodies that react against autologous cell antigens, AATs. Auto-antibodies associated with a particular type of cancer target these abnormal cellular proteins that are involved in tumour transformation, so autoantibodies can be considered as reporters that identify aberrant cellular mechanisms in tumorigenesis [300]. By examining the sera of cancer patients, new TAAs can be identified, such as p62 and p90 [301,302], which have already been identified with this approach. The sensitivity and specificity of different antigen-antibody systems as markers in cancer can also be evaluated to develop TAAs array systems for diagnosis, prediction, and follow-up in cancer patients [300].

The detection of tumour-associated target-specific IgG could act as a substitute for the presence of T cells [294]. It is difficult for these auto-antibodies to have a direct antitumour role, as most of the antigens they target are intracellular [303]. In the example of checkpoint inhibitors, the presence of NY-ESO-1 specific autoantibodies are known to be associated with increased clinical benefit in patients with advanced melanoma who are treated with ipilimumab [299]. This suggests that tumour-specific antibodies may be an indicator of the presence of tumour-specific T cells in the tumour microenvironment and patients with pre-existing ability to react to tumours would be favourably disposed to immunomodulatory therapy [294].

The presence of tertiary lymphoid structures, consisting of germ-center-organised B cells, plasma cells, and T cells, is highly predictive of progression-free survival and overall survival in solid tumours such as melanoma and NSCLC [304,305]. These structures are close to the tumour tissue, so they are believed to play an important role in local immunogenicity and infiltrating B and T cells are known to have tumour specificity. When B cells isolated from NSCLC tumours differentiate in vitro to plasma cells, they produce antibodies to tumour-associated antigens such as NY-ESO-1, TP53, or XAGE-1 [305]. Therefore, these tumour antigen-specific B cells participate in immune mechanisms and are potential targets for the application of immunotherapy. Associating the presence of local antibodies with systemic humoral immunity will be key to establishing serology as a prognostic or predictive marker [294].

For patients with breast cancer who present difficult to interpret mammography, Provista Diagnostics has developed a kit called Videssa ® Breast that, through a blood extraction, allows a more accurate and improved diagnosis, avoiding unnecessary biopsies. It is based on proteomic technology to analyse multiple biomarkers of serum tumour proteins and tumour-associated auto-antibodies (TAAbs) associated with cancer. This kit incorporates nine serum proteins as biomarkers and 20 TAAbs. It allows detecting the presence or absence of breast cancer in women between 25 and 75 years old, with a sensitivity of 93.3% and a specificity of 63.8%. If this test is combined with image diagnosis, 100% of breast cancers can be detected. In all trials performed so far, all breast cancers were identified at an early stage [306]. This demonstrates the importance of detecting specific AAbs for TAAs to improve the diagnosis of patients with cancer.

5.2.4. Tumoral Microenvironment as Biomarker

An important biomarker within the TME is tumour infiltrating immune cells. Tumours with effector T cell infiltration have an active immune microenvironment and respond better to immunotherapy [282]. Phenotypically, two classes of TME can be distinguished: those with a high prevalence of T cells and those without T cells [307].

Inflamed T-cell tumours have large numbers of T cells in the tumour periphery, plus increased expression of T-cell activation markers, type 1 interferons, and high levels of Th1 cytokines that recruit T cells. Because the cells that promote antitumour immunity are CD8+ T cells, CD4+ Th1 cells, NK cells, and mature DCs, tumours that have this predominant infiltration pattern respond better to antitumour immunotherapy [282]. Although tumour infiltrating lymphocytes are sometimes dysfunctional, their presence indicates that there is no inhibition of recruitment [294].

Tumours with a non-inflammatory T-cell microenvironment have few or no effector T cells, but contain chronic inflammation with tumour-associated macrophages, MDSCs, CD4 + FoxP3 + regulatory T cells, and Th2 cytokines, which form an immunosuppressed microenvironment that allows tumour progression, which is associated with a poorer prognosis.

Factors that may mediate the type of phenotype presented by the TME include some soluble and tumour-derived cell-membrane factors, but the mechanisms are not yet known [282].

The prognostic importance of T cells has been seen in some solid tumours, including colorectal, hepatocellular, pancreatic, esophageal, ovarian, non-small cell lung, brain metastases, melanoma, and head and neck cancer [282,294].

Antigen-specific T-cell recognition by MHC class I tetramer staining in situ or analysis of TCR's Vβ repertoire are used to characterise MSD T cells for their specificity [308,309]. Advances in multiplex IHC technologies in tumour tissue also provide information on the nature of immune infiltration into the tumour, depending on the type, number and qualitative characteristics of the immune cells present, and their interaction with tumour and stromal cells, which is related to disease progression and prognosis [294]. In biopsies from patients who respond favourably to checkpoint inhibition, they have a higher number of proliferating CD8+ T cells associated with high levels of expression of PD-L1 as assessed by IHC and higher expression of IFNγ as determined by the gene expression profile [310,311].

5.2.5. Immunocheckpoints (ICs) as Biomarkers

Other important biomarkers being worked with are PD-1 and PD-L1. PD-1 is expressed on most tumour infiltrating T cells, including antigen-specific CD8+ T cells. PD-1 is expressed after T-cell activation and results in the elimination of T cells after they have exerted their function. PD-1 is therefore a checkpoint and serves as a marker for T-cell depletion. Its ligand, PD-L1, is expressed in melanoma tumour cells, non-small cell lung cancer, CRC, bladder cancer, gastric cancer, ovarian cancer, B-cell lymphoma, Merkel cell carcinoma and Hodgkin's lymphoma. If the interaction between PD-1 and its ligand is inhibited by antibodies, the T cells will remain active, mediating antitumour activity [282,312].

Tumour infiltrating immune cells that express PD-1 or PD-L1 are predictive biomarkers for tumours that may respond to T-cell checkpoint blocking. Tumours that have low levels of expression of these molecules have a low response rate to this treatment [282].

Expression of PD-L1 before treatment in tumour cells and immune cells correlates with improved response rates, progression-free survival, and overall survival in pembrilizumab-treated melanoma patients [281].

But the use of PD-1 and PD-L1 still has some drawbacks, such as the expression of PD-L1 is heterogeneous and dynamic within each individual, and even its expression may be induced by activated tumour specific T cells. Its expression may also vary between the primary lesion and its metastasis. In addition, other cell types present in the tumour may express PD-L1, including lymphocytes and macrophages [282,313].

5.2.6. Tumoral Genomics Biomarkers

Effective immune responses to T-cell checkpoint inhibitors in some cancers correlate with the mutational load on the tumour cell [152,314]. Many of these mutations are likely to be transient and will be influencing the process of immunoedition by exerting selective pressure on the immune system. Mutational load or the emergence of neoantigens could be predictive biomarkers for the tumour response to immunotherapy agents if this hypothesis is ultimately established [282].

In one study, the entire exome was sequenced to analyse the effect of cancer genomes on the response to ipilimumab in melanoma patients. A high mutational load and the number of non-anonymous mutations per exome were found to correlate with improved overall survival. In addition, they identified 101 motifs of tetrapeptides in nonameric peptides located in the peptide-binding cleft of MHC class I molecules. These tetrapeptides were shared exclusively by patients who had long-term clinical benefit [315]. In another study, the exome of non-small cell lung cancer treated with pembrolizumab was sequenced and a high burden of non-synonymous mutations in the tumours was seen. Clinical response correlates with the molecular signatures of tobacco-related carcinogenic mutations, increased neoantigen load, and mutations in the DNA repair pathway. Pembrolizumab improved the reactivity of neo-antigen-specific CD8+ T cells and is associated with tumour regression [152].

With expression microarray technologies, genes that play an important role in immune cell biology and are highly expressed in the tumour expression profiles of some patients have been identified. These genes reflect the relative abundance of different populations of tumour-infiltrating leukocytes. From this, robust and reproducible associations between immune gene signatures in solid tumours and clinical outcomes have been identified, providing prognostic information [294]. For example, high gene expression reflecting T, B, and NK cell involvement in metastatic melanoma is associated with prolonged overall survival and survival without metastasis [316].

Immune genes have predictive potential in the context of immunotherapy. These genes include T cell surface markers (CD3, CD277, CD27, CD38), cytotoxic factors (GZMB), and tissue-rejection-related cytokines (CXCL9, CXCL10, CCL4, CCL5) [294,317].

5.3. Tumour Mutational Burden as Biomarkers

In different clinical studies, a high tumour mutation burden (TMB) has been associated with better response rates and improved survival of patients treated with immunotherapies such as ICI. Therefore, TMB is beginning to be used as a biomarker of response to these immunotherapy agents [318].

TMB is the total number of somatic mutations in a defined region of a tumour genome and varies by tumour type and among patients [319–321].

The mutational load of a tumour contributes to its immunogenicity. Tumours that have high TMB, such as melanoma and lung cancers, are thought to be more likely to express neoantigens and induce a stronger immune response after treatment with ICI [322]. Highly mutated tumours ("hot" tumours) have a histological immune signature of depleted immunosuppressive cells and high expression of immune inhibitory molecules. Less mutated tumours ("cold" tumours) have amplified immunosuppressive cells, negative regulation of MHC molecules, and low expression of immune inhibitory molecules. The adaptive immune response is very accurate in predicting patient outcome [294], so it is important to identify whether the presence of effector T cells in MSD is related to antigen-specific T cells [152,323]. For some tumours, this parameter may be a suitable clinical biomarker for making immunotherapy treatment decisions [324,325]. STM is a quantifiable measure of the number of mutations in a tumour, which is an advantage over neoantigens, since not all mutations result in immunogenic neoantigens and it is difficult to determine which mutations may induce these neoantigens, thus new techniques and strategies are required to discover new TAAs as biomarkers [156,320].

Neo-antigens are currently more easily identified by complete exome sequencing. The sequencing of new generation tumours allows the identification of mutations and, using computer algorithms, the identification of mutated peptides that bind to MHC molecules, which helps in the choice of targets to improve the response of T cells [294].

Antigenic peptides are the result of abnormal transcription, translation of alternative open reading frames or post-translational modifications. This diversity of peptides also involves the mechanism of peptide splicing by the proteasome [326]. A variety of human leukocyte antigens are involved in the processing of antigenic peptides [156]. O-glycosylation of cancer-associated aberrant proteins can modify antigenic processing and the immune response [327], and phosphopeptides associated with MHC class I are targets of memory immunity. Phosphopeptide-specific immunity has an important role in tumour recognition and control [294,328].

TMB was first determined using complete exome sequencing, but this method is expensive and has a long response time, so panel-specific sequencing is now used. The implementation of TMB implies a solid clinical and analytical validation. In addition, bioinformatic analysis is also important for its successful implementation in the clinic, since the measurement of BTM is based on new generation sequencing (NGS) techniques [329].

For ICI therapy, expression of PD-L1 correlates with an increased response to therapy and may be a predictor [330]. In contrast, not all patients who express PD-L1 respond well to ICI treatment [331]. Therefore, other MSD factors, such as LIL, also play an important role [332].

In the study by Yu-Pei Chen et al., it was proposed to classify the different types of tumour microenvironments according to the expression of PD-L1 and the presence or absence of LILs, in order to design appropriate combination immunotherapies for cancer [322,333,334]. This study attempted to establish a classification model based on analysis of mRNA expression of PD-L1 and CD8A, and evaluated the applicability of this classification to predict response to ICI treatment, i.e., its correlation with mutation load and number of neoantigens, using RNA-seq [322].

PD-L1 positive MSDs with LILs were generally associated with high BMT or number of neoantigens in multiple tumours, so these cancers would benefit from anti-PD-1/PD-L1 therapies, as these tumours have evidence of pre-existing intra-tumoral T cells being inactivated by compromised PD-L1 [322,334]. In contrast, MSDs that have low expression of PD-L1 and little infiltration of LILs will have a worse prognosis, as no immune reaction is detected. Combination therapy to attract LILs to MSDs, along with ICI, may be a good option in these cases [335]. For MSDs with high expression of PD-L1 but low infiltration of LILs, radiotherapy- mediated immunogenic cell death to release antigens and induce T-cell responses, together with ani-PD-1/PD-L1 inhibitors, may also be a beneficial approach [322,336].

In recent years, studies evaluating TMB as a predictive marker have increased significantly for the response to ICI, demonstrating the importance of this approach in selecting patients to benefit from immunotherapy.

5.4. TCR diversity and MHC Molecules

Thanks to the diversity of the TCR, T cells can recognise a multitude of different epitopes through TCR–MHC interaction, which is associated with effective control of viral infections, other pathogens and tumour cells. This diversity is generated by a complex mechanism based on genetic recombination of DNA, leading to different antigenic specificities [294].

Following immunotherapy based on checkpoint inhibitors, there has been increased interest in analysing TCR diversity, as it allows for a better understanding of the patient's immune system. TCR diversity is estimated to be 10^8–10^{15} and can be evaluated by NS, spectrometry, qPCR multiplex or immune phenotyping. The impact and clinical outcome of immunotherapy has been shown to be related to the diversity of TCR in peripheral blood [294]. Blocking CTLA-4 with tremelimumab has been shown to diversify the peripheral T cell pool, highlighting the effect of this class of immunomodulatory antibodies [337].

The effective response generated by antigen-specific T cells after recognition of tumour antigens expressed on MHC class I molecules can be affected by germline and somatic MHC class I genotype variations [281]. Patients with advanced melanoma and NSCLC treated with checkpoint inhibitors who were heterozygous at the MHC class I locus had better overall survival than those who were homozygous [338]. This is associated with increased clonality of TCR and clonal expansion of T cells following the use of this immunotherapy. The somatic loss of MHC class I heterozygosity in these patients results in poor outcome, which is associated with impaired recognition of neo-antigens by CD8+ T cells due to structural changes at the class I locus [281].

It is necessary to analyse the diversity of TCR and MHC molecules and their interactions in order to achieve a personalised and beneficial immunotherapeutic treatment for each type of cancer, as it has been shown that the basal diversity of TCR in peripheral blood is associated with clinical outcomes [294,339].

5.5. Neoantigens as Biomarkers

There is clear evidence that human tumour cells express antigenic determinants (epitopes) that are recognised by patients' autologous T cells. The short peptides that enable this recognition and the specific removal of the tumour cells occur on MHC molecules and are called immunopeptidomes. T-lymphocytes target epitopes that are formed by epigenetic, translational and post-translational alterations of tumour cells. These TAAs have been exploited for therapeutic purposes, as we have seen, with good but controversial results [340].

It was later shown that tumour cells have mutated endogenous proteins that distinguish them from other cells and can be processed into peptides, presented on the cell surface and recognised by the immune system in vivo, which recognizes them as foreign. These proteins are what are called neoantigens. Neoantigens are very specific, so targeting them would allow for immune cells to distinguish tumour cells from normal ones, thus preventing autoimmunity [340].

Results in mice and humans show that CD8+ and CD4+ T cells are reactive against neoantigens [341–344]. Central T cells are not tolerant of these neoantigens because they are tumour-specific; in fact, these neoantigen-specific T cells have a high functional avidity. In contrast, the reactivity of T cells to autoantigens is reduced and is only achieved when tolerance to these antigens is not fully developed. It has been shown that in cancer patients, TAAs are recognised by T cells with reduced functional avidity [342]. In the case of neoantigens, T cell responses will not produce autoimmune toxicity against healthy tissues, so therapeutic vaccination with neoantigens may be very promising. The problem is that neoantigens are patient-specific and it is unlikely that a vaccine targeting neoantigens shared by large groups of patients can be developed with current knowledge [345].

Neoantigen-reactive T cells have been identified in human cancers such as melanoma, leukemia, ovarian cancer, and cholangiocarcinoma [342,343,346]. For melanoma and NSCLC, TMB was correlated with clinical outcome after anti-CTLA-4 and anti-PD-1 immunotherapy, respectively [152,323]. In addition, the frequency of neoantigen-specific T cells increased in patients who responded to therapy, which correlated with a favourable clinical outcome [342,343,346]. This indicates that the recognition of neoantigens is an important factor in the response to clinical immunotherapies.

Mass sequencing can identify the spectrum of individual tumour mutations (mutanome) with great accuracy and speed. These sequencing data hold great promise for identifying unique targets and designing customized immunotherapy strategies to enhance adaptive mutation-specific immunity [340].

In the post-genome era, bioinformatic technologies and tools have been developed to identify the mutanome. Neo-epitopes can be identified by different means. Neural network algorithms, such as NetMHC, are commonly used to predict in silico the affinity of neo-epitopes derived from mutated sequences that patients bind to MHC class I molecules [341]. The predicted peptides can be synthesized and are used for dilution of patient immunity. This is called reverse identification and can generate large numbers of candidate neo-epitopes that can be further selected by bioinformatic tools based on other parameters. Currently only peptides presented in MHC-I can be predicted, as prediction of CD4 T cell epitopes by algorithms is still limited [347]. Another limitation of reverse identification is that it is not known whether neoepitopes are presented by tumour cells.

Thus, direct identification by MHC ligandome analysis of tumour cells is possible. This requires elution of the peptides presented in MHC molecules derived from the patient's tumour tissue, reverse-phase HPLC fractionation and mass spectrometry. This approach allows the identification of CD8+ and CD4+ T cell neo-epitopes, although validation with exome and transcriptome sequencing data is still required. Although the sensitivity of neoantigen identification by this method has not yet been improved, it is likely to be a very important tool in antigen discovery in the near future [340].

To demonstrate the potential of candidate peptides for neoantigens, experimental validation of their immunogenicity using autologous T cells from the patient is necessary. Functional assays of T cells can be performed with short peptides predicted in silica for CD8+ T cells, or long peptides and mRNA for CD8+ or CD4+ T cells. Several studies have detected neoantigen-specific CD4+ T cells whose induction can control the tumour and, in murine models, the spread of antigen [344].

One strategy for identifying neo-antigens from immunogenic T cells is based on transfecting autologous APCs with RNA or DNA encoding a 12-amino acid mutated gene sequence. The APCs are incubated with autologous T cells (TILs) and the responding T cells can propagate. It is important to define the minimum length of T-cell epitopes and their MHC restriction. For this purpose, APCs expressing only one MHC molecule must be used and pulsed with predicted synthetic peptides. The problem is that large quantities of autologous T cells are required and a massive expansion of these cells.

There are currently several active clinical trials of cancer vaccines targeting neoantigens following different strategies, including poly-epitopic RNA and peptide vaccines based on high-throughput sequencing (HTS) and in silico prediction for metastatic melanoma, peptide vaccines based on HTS data with MS data in glioblastoma and poly-epitope plasmid DNA and RNA vaccines in triple-negative breast cancer.

Mutated T cells are an important component of TILs that spread in vivo and can be used for ACT in patients with melanoma. In addition, neoantigens can be used in passive immunotherapy strategies. Neoantigen-specific T cells can be isolated and expanded to re-infuse into patients. Genetically modified T cells with neoantigen-specific CRT or CAR may also be used [340].

Despite these advances, this type of personalised immunotherapy, which targets unique mutations, has limitations. Most of these mutations are unique to each specific tumour and must be identified and validated in each patient, which requires the development of massive methodologies. Later on, in silico analysis will overcome the need for massive peptide screening. Another important factor is to identify driver mutations, which are the ideal targets for cancer immunotherapy, since they are critical for tumour development, but in most tumours these mutations have not yet been identified. Therefore, the identification of neo-antigens is one of the great challenges of current immunotherapy to develop effective personalised treatments.

5.6. Microsatellite-Unstable Tumours

As described above, it is believed that the set of neoantigens in a tumour is highly individual. This characteristic is what differentiates them from tissue-specific antigens, tumour-associated antigens (TAAs) or other tumour-selective antigens that are considered to be shared. The exception to this is some cancers that possess a high mutational load, including microsatellite-unstable tumours, which have shared neo-antigens due to preferential mutations of several genetic regions called microsatellites.

Cancers with hereditary defects in genes involved in DNA repair have high frequencies of non-synonymous mutations, resulting in a wide variety of tumour neoantigens. In some cases, insertions and deletions also accumulate in DNA hot spots that are prone to mutations with repeating base-pair sequences, called microsatellite instability (MSI). This has made it possible to identify genes with a high mutation frequency in patients with MSI. These recurrent neoantigens can be prime targets for immunotherapy, particularly frame-shifting mutations containing multiple new epitopes that are recognised by several MHC haplotypes [348]. Patients with these types of defects are highly mutational and therefore form immune escape variants. Defects in antigenic presentation by MHC molecules and in molecules associated with MHC expression have been found in patients with MSI tumours [349]. Unstable microsatellite tumours are recognised as a subset of tumours with different prognostic and predictive characteristics.

5.7. Immunopeptidome as Biomarkers

The presentation of peptides in MHC molecules is a mechanism that allows the adaptive immune system to differentiate healthy cells from cancerous or infected cells.

Both MHC class I and MHC class II molecules present peptide antigens to T cells, but structurally and functionally they are different. MHC-I is constitutively expressed on all nucleated cells, including tumour cells. Despite this, some tumour cells may lose the expression of MHC-I as an immune escape mechanism. Loss of MHC-I expression is usually a trigger for NK-mediated cell death, but many tumours can still evade immune-vigilance without MHC-I expression [350]. Loss of MHC-I expression has also been reported as a mechanism of resistance to anti-PD-1 therapy [351]. Some of the tumours that lose expression of MHC-I, maintain expression of MHC-II, but their functional significance in these cases is unclear [352]. In addition, some melanoma cell lines that do not express MHC-II have high levels of MHC-I expression [353]. This suggests that MHC-I and MHC-II are independently regulated in cancer and their expression may have different implications for cancer immunotherapy [350]. In this review we will only consider the peptide load presented by MHC molecules, regardless of possible changes in expression of these molecules.

The antigenic processing machinery is complex and flexible, so predictions using binding motifs or binding affinities for the deduction of MHC-restricted peptides are complicated. MHC peptidomics data based on mass spectrometry and training of prediction algorithms have led to improvements in MHC binding prediction. The precise identification and selection of new MHC peptides as targets for cancer immunotherapy must be an integrated, comprehensive and deep mapping analysis of MHC binding in both healthy and pathological tissues of all types (Figure 15). The depth of the analysis is important since antigen-specific immunotherapies are restricted to certain MHC haplotypes, reducing the fraction of detected ligands that will bind to the same MHC. Once the possible ligands have been defined, their tumour specificity must be confirmed in vivo. Neoantigens already fulfil this characteristic in themselves [354].

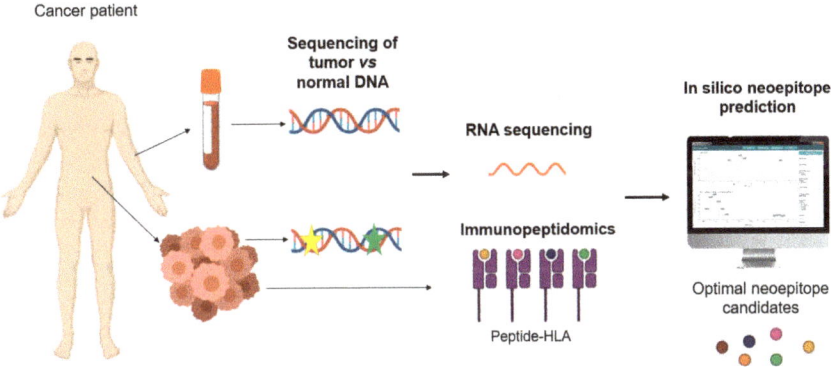

Figure 15. Schematic representation of tumour neoantigen screening: non-synonymous mutations determined by whole-exome or genome sequencing of tumour. These mutations can then be filtered by expression (RNA sequencing) or presentation (immunopeptidomics). In silico algorithms are used to predict and filter optimal neoepitope candidates.

When these targets are selected and validated, predictive biomarkers need to be defined that allow for the identification of positive target patients with the aim of personalizing therapy and treating only those patients who can obtain clinical benefit [355]. This is performed by quantifying mRNA expression using qPCR, since it is assumed that MHC peptide presentation and mRNA expression are correlated. It has been shown that very abundant transcripts generally result in a greater number of MHC class I peptides bound [356], but this is not necessarily true for each peptide-mRNA pair [357]. Mass spectrometry is used to establish the association between peptide presentation and mRNA expression for individual peptides. In addition, this association can be translated from LC-MS/MS to RNA-seq for qPCR data, with the aim of defining predictive biomarkers that allow for precision medicine through the personalised analysis of immunopeptidome-guided mRNA expression, as shown in the study by Jens Fritsche et al. [354].

Briefly, mass spectrometry allows in-depth analysis of human immunopeptidome, expanding the number of targets available for immunotherapy. In addition, it allows the identification of predictive biomarkers based on mRNA, which can be used as complementary diagnostics to qPCR to define positive populations for the target peptide, being able to establish a personalised peptidomic. These biomarkers will improve the efficacy of precision treatment in cancer immunotherapies.

As mentioned above, MHC peptidomes have been studied to identify cancer-specific peptides, for the development of tumour immunotherapies and as a source of information on protein synthesis and degradation patterns within tumour cells. However, it is also known that the levels of soluble MHC class I molecules (sMHC-I) are increased in serum of people affected by pathologies such as cancer, autoimmunity, allergy or viral infections. In the study by Michal Bassani-Sternberg et al. [358] it was postulated that if a significant proportion of sMHC molecules in plasma are released from diseased cells (multiple myeloma, acute myeloid leukaemia and acute lymphoblastic leukaemia) and also carry their original peptide load, analysis of sMHC peptidomes may be an ideal source of biomarkers in various diseases, considering that sMHC peptidomes are similar to membrane MHC peptidomes.

It has been concluded that sMHCs carry defined sets of peptides derived primarily from tumour cells. sMHCs are released from healthy and pathological cells, so it is expected that as the patient's tumour load increases, larger fractions of sMHC peptidomas will originate in plasma from tumour cells. Tumour cells release more sMHC into the circulation than healthy cells, possibly to evade the T-cell immune response. Diseased cells are expected to contribute differently to sMHC peptidomas, depending on the size of the tumour, its type, and its tendency to release sMHC into the circulation. An escape mechanism from immune surveillance related to elevated sMHC levels has also been described, and this characterisation would help to identify peptides involved in this mechanism [359]. Finally, analysis of sMHC peptidomas resulted in the identification of thousands of peptides, including potential biomarkers of disease that would need to be validated clinically [358].

Following this line, the Human Proteome Organization initiated the Human Immuno-Peptidome Project (HUPO-HIPP) in 2015 as a new initiative of the Biology/Disease-Human Proteome Project (B/D-HPP) with the final goal of mapping the entire repertoire of peptides presented at MHC, using mass spectrometry. In addition, this analysis is intended to be accessible to any researcher. The basis of this project is the development of methods and technologies, standardization, effective data exchange and education [360].

Currently there are already multiple databases that collect data on the immunopeptidome presented at MHC analysed by mass spectrometry. One of these is the SysteMHC Atlas (https://systemhcatlas.org), which contains raw immunopeptidomics MS data. They are processed through bioinformatic tools to identify, annotate and validate the peptides in MHC. This generates libraries with the lists of MHC peptide ligands and allele and sample specific peptide spectra. Each project is labelled as HIPP, being a sub-project of B/D-HPP [361].

The aim of this type of database is to allow basic scientists and clinicians to access a large catalogue of MHC-associated peptides to obtain new ideas about the composition of the immunopeptidome; to allow computational scientists to use this data to develop new algorithms for immunopeptidomic analysis; and to allow access to these libraries to facilitate analysis by next-generation MS [361].

Peptide binding affinity prediction tools allow for the detection of peptides in silica for the purpose of identifying T cell epitopes that match MHC-II molecules from a particular host. One of these tools are NetMHCII and NetMHCIIpan [362,363], which are based on ensembles of artificial neural networks that are trained on quantitative peptide binding affinity data from Immune Epitope Database (IEDB) [364]. These types of tools can improve MHC-II binding predictions and reduce experimental costs in epitope-based vaccine design. Understanding peptide–MHC interactions is key to the cellular immune response.

5.8. TAAs as Biomarkers

Autoantibodies are useful biomarkers in clinical diagnosis and are biological agents used to isolate and study the function of intracellular molecules that are self-antigens targets [365]. In other words, they make it possible to characterise their related antigens and clarify the pathogenic mechanisms. These autoantibodies are found in autoimmune diseases but also in cancer [366]. Antibodies to tumour-associated antigens (TAA) in cancer are similar to autoantibodies detected in systemic autoimmune diseases, as these anti-TAAs also have the potential to be diagnostic markers in cancer. The identification of these TAAs in cancer patients allows the study of the mechanisms by which molecular and other alterations of intracellular proteins drive autoimmune responses. Many of the TAAs identified by the autoantibodies of cancer patients have important cellular biosynthetic functions that may be related to carcinogenesis [367]. In addition, there are autoantibody profiles that are unique to each type of cancer and other antibodies are shared. These profiles may serve as diagnostic markers in cancer [365,368].

An example is autoantibodies to p53, which report early carcinogenesis [369]. Anti-p53 has been detected in chronic obstructive pulmonary disease [370], which is prone to the development of lung cancer, as well as in workers exposed to vinyl chloride, who have the same predisposition [371].

Autoantibodies to TAA have also been found in hepatocellular carcinoma [372]. Chronic hepatitis and liver cirrhosis are precursors of hepatocellular carcinoma [367]. After collecting samples from patients with these diseases, the target antigens for antibodies associated with malignancy have been detected. These autoantibodies are usually antinuclear antibodies, and in this case the antigens detected were topoisomer II DNA-α and -β [373]. In addition, in cases where antigens have been identified, these were molecules involved in cell proliferation and gene regulation. Therefore, the patients' immune system appears to be reacting to these factors involved in carcinogenesis [367].

One of the characteristics of TAAs is that they have functions involved in proliferation, transformation and other processes associated with malignancy. Although these molecules are present in most cell types, any alteration of their normal state will only be detectable in malignant cells.

In order to understand how these TAAs acquire immunogenicity, studies have been performed with different TAAs identified, such as p53, p62 or cyclin B1 [367,374]. p62 auto-antibodies to these molecules were detected in patients with hepatocellular carcinoma and their expression was also studied in patients with liver cirrhosis, normal liver biopsies and fetal liver samples. What is observed is that p62 is developmentally regulated and expressed in the fetal liver, but not in the adult, except in malignant liver cells, where it is expressed aberrantly, suggesting that this TAA is an oncofetal antigen [367]. Cyclin B1 has been identified as TAA in patients with hepatocellular carcinoma because it is present in both B-cell and T-cell immune responses and is known to play an important role in the progression of the cell cycle from G2 to M [375].

The importance of TAAs and their autoantibodies in cancer has been seen in both diagnosis and surveillance and in therapy. Many approaches therefore focus on identifying a large number of TAAs, including proteomic approaches such as protein microarrays [367].

To track and understand human autoantigens and to conduct basic and translational research on their functions, databases of human autoantigens have been created. These include AAgAtlas 1.0 (http://biokb.ncpsb.org/aagatlas). This database provides an interface to explore and download human autoantigens and their associated diseases. Human autoantigenic proteins are involved in major diseases, such as the immune system, hypersensitivity reaction or cancer, so these databases are an effective tool to investigate the functions of these proteins and to develop future immunotherapies [376].

Autoantibodies have been integrated as biomarkers with different proteins and are the first protein-based blood test that allows the early detection of cancer after the development of the Videssa® Breast Kit, as discussed above, for breast cancer [306].

Ultimately, cancer immunotherapy is based on the use of peptide antigens derived from amino acid sequences of tumour antigens, focusing on modulating the response of T cells [377]. One of the problems is selecting candidate peptides, since they must be strongly immunogenic to induce the desired response by T cells. To do this, it is important to identify regions of AAD that are recognised by the patient's immune system in order to indicate realistic targets in vivo and to design an immunotherapy that targets these auto-epitopes [367]. These T cell auto-epitopes can be identified from MHC class I molecules [378].

5.9. Techniques for Biomarkers Discovery, Verification and Validation

As we have seen, mass spectrometry is a powerful technology in biological research and allows the characterisation of the plasma proteome in great depth. This has been performed using "triangular strategies", which aim to discover unique biomarker candidates in small cohorts, followed by classical immunoassays in larger validation cohorts. Currently, a "rectangular strategy" is proposed, in which the proteome patterns of large cohorts are correlated with their phenotypes in health and disease. The methodologies developed for biomarker detection are described below [351].

Mass spectrometry (MS) measures the mass spectra and fragmentation of peptides derived from protein digestion very precisely. These sequences are unique, so proteomics is very specific, unlike enzymatic colorimetric tests or immunoassays [379]. In addition, MS allows the analysis of the entire proteome and the quantification of post-translational modifications (PTM). The discovery of PMTs is important as they can form the basis of diagnostic tests.

So far, none of the laboratory tests routinely performed are based on proteins that have been identified by MS and only small molecules (drugs, metabolites) have been used in MS technology [380].

MS has improved its performance in dynamic range and sensitivity, making it optimal for the study of biomarkers. Currently, plasma proteins are the type of molecules most frequently analysed in the clinic, using enzymatic reactions or antibody immunoassays. These methods are the ones selected in the clinic because the time required for the analysis is a few minutes. The main advantage of MS-based proteomics is that it is not necessary to assume the nature or number of potential biomarkers. This strategy allows all possible biomarker studies to be combined for each disease and their relationship to each other [351].

A "triangular strategy" has been proposed to identify biomarkers. This strategy is composed of different steps, in which the number of individuals is increased and the number of proteins is gradually decreased [380]. The first step is to identify peptides following the workflow for hypothesis-free discovery proteomics: enzymatic digestion of proteins by HPLC and peptide analysis by MS/MS, followed by the use of proteomics software platforms to identify and quantify these peptides. The second phase of the strategy triangulates the verification of candidates. In this case, a low number of candidate proteins are tested, selecting a set of peptides, in a larger cohort. Multiple reaction monitoring methods (MRM) are used and only those peptides chosen are fragmented, so that they can be quantified with high sensitivity and specifically. In the third phase, validation with sandwich immunoassays is performed, as they are very specific and have high sensitivity. In this case, only a few candidate biomarkers are validated in a cohort that may consist of thousands of patients [351].

Thanks to the improvements in the LC-MS/MS system and the robustness of bioinformatic analysis, and with the aim of developing a fast and automated workflow that quantifies in depth the plasma proteome in a large number of samples, a "rectangular strategy" has been proposed. In this case, the aim is to measure as many proteins as possible for all possible individuals and conditions. For this purpose, the initial cohort would be much larger and would allow for the identification of significant differences in the proteins. Cohort discovery and validation can be measured by shotgun proteomics, allowing both cohorts to be analysed at the same time. This strategy has the advantage of being able to discover and validate protein patterns characteristic of specific health or disease states and unique biomarker candidates [351].

The goal in proteomics is to achieve sufficient depth in a short time, without exhaustion and with a robust workflow, to allow for the identification of unique biomarkers that can be used in the clinic.

6. Conclusions and Perspectives

The development of anti-cancer drugs has focused on strategies that kill cancer cells directly, such as surgery, radiotherapy, chemotherapy, targeted therapy and immunotherapy. Immunotherapy is based on the recognition of tumour cells as foreign by the immune system. For good results, immunotherapy has to activate and expand tumour-specific T cells. Various approaches have been used for this purpose: direct activation of anti-tumour immunity by means of cancer vaccines (tumour antigens), recombinant cytokines or the infusion of tumour-specific cells. However, these methods did not guarantee that the tumour-specific T cells could nest or perform their function within the tumour. This is due to the existence of tumour-induced immunosuppressive mechanisms in the tumour microenvironment, which prevent the breakdown of immune tolerance to cancer. With the approval of the checkpoint inhibitors, it was demonstrated that an anti-tumour immune response can be initiated by targeting the immune system to break the tolerance to cancer. In contrast, a significant clinical response was only obtained in a few patients with solid tumours such as melanoma, non-small cell lung cancer, kidney or bladder cancer. This is because the response to this treatment depends on the presence of pre-existing tumour-specific CD8 T cells, which correlates with the presence of neoantigens derived from tumour mutations. Because of this relationship, different approaches have been tested that allow for the expansion of anti-tumour T cells along with checkpoint inhibition. These combination therapies have been successful in clinical trials, but the current focus is on targeted therapies to target neoantigens derived from tumour mutations, as the number of mutations in each tumour correlates directly with the efficacy of checkpoint inhibitors. Therefore, it is necessary to establish combined therapies in cancer, among which small molecule inhibitors also stand out. These combination approaches are key to understanding the relationship between the established tumour and the immune system [381]. Combination therapies are useful in inhibiting tumour growth and changing or restoring the TME. Among the most explored are combinations of checkpoint inhibitor (anti-PD1) and targeted (antibody or small molecule) therapies. Rapid lysis of tumour cells with targeted therapies can generate an environment of acute inflammation that enhances tumour immunity, making these therapies additive [73].

On the other hand, programmed physiological cell death, usually in the form of apoptosis, has always been considered a non-immunogenic or even tolerable process. In contrast, the concept of "programmed cell death" (PCD) has assigned immunogenic capabilities to apoptosis. This type of apoptosis is characterised by the ability of dying cells to trigger adaptive immune responses against the altered autoantigens/neo-epitopes derived from cancer, in the case of tumour cells. In addition to antigenicity, adjuvancy, conferred by DAMPs, is necessary.

The pathways that induce ICD can be used to design new therapeutic tools in immunotherapy, to reduce the tumour burden and improve the immunogenic capacity of dying tumour cells, provoking adaptive immune responses in the long term. Various immune-based therapies can benefit from ICD, such as antibody-based therapies, adoptive cell therapy (TIL, NK cell or CAR-T), checkpoint inhibitors, tumour vaccines and combination immunotherapy strategies [256]. One of the most promising strategies is to exploit the ICD concept to obtain highly immunogenic antigen sources for the development of "next generation" DC-based vaccines [382]. ICD inducers can be used to generate immunogenicity in dying tumour cells and to load DC, enhancing their ability to stimulate effector cells and improve T-cell responses to cancer in vivo [99]. This may improve general immunity or create an immune-friendly tumour microenvironment [256]. A number of chemotherapeutic agents are ICD inducers, meaning that many therapeutic strategies have known immunomodulatory or immune-stimulatory effects that should be further investigated to determine if they are associated with the release of DAMPs. The characterisation of new DAMPs may open up new therapeutic targets for targeted chemotherapy [383]. Understanding the molecular pathways involved in these processes would allow for the identification of a new set of potential prognostic biomarkers, but more research is needed to understand the true impact of ICD therapy and exposure to DAMPs [256].

The immune system of the cancer patient detects abnormalities in structure, function, intracellular location, and other cellular alterations during tumorigenesis, which may manifest themselves in humoral or cellular immune responses, which may be the earliest sign of carcinogenesis. The current aim is to use cancer autoantibodies as diagnostic biomarkers, but there is also the possibility that they may be used as monitors of the therapeutic response. If an anti-TAA antibody is detected in the patient, changes in the levels of these antibodies may reflect the status of the tumour, its changes or its tumour load in relation to therapy [367].

Cancer immunotherapy relies heavily on the use of peptide antigens derived from amino acid sequences of tumour antigens and modulates the response of T cells. The problem here is that the peptides selected must be strongly immunogenic and induce a T cell response. Therefore, it would be important to identify the regions of the TAAs that can be recognised by the patient's immune system, which would confirm that they are real targets in vivo and allow for the design of immunotherapies directed to these auto-epitopes. Such auto-epitopes must be able to be identified and isolated from MHC class I molecules [367].

In this sense, T lymphocytes $\alpha\beta$ detect alterations in the host's cellular components, which may be induced by infectious pathogens, chemical or physical damage or oncogenic transformation. The T-lymphocytes generated in the thymus each have a clonally restricted T cell receptor (TCR) [384].

Human tumours contain a high number of somatic mutations, and if peptides containing these mutations occur on MHC class I molecules they may be immunogenic and recognised by the adaptive immune system, which recognizes them as "non-self" neoantigens. Mutant peptides can serve as T cell epitopes [385]. During immune surveillance, each T cell receptor recognizes a different foreign peptide attached to MHC molecules. MS technology allows for the identification of epitopes relevant to different tumours. Molecular CCR cloning methods allow for the molecular quantification of TCR–pMHC interactions [384,386]. This is a major challenge, since MHC-bound peptidoma consists of thousands of different peptides with relevant non-self-antigens often embedded in low numbers, among them the self-peptides, which occur in a greater order of magnitude [384].

In immunogenic tumours, the sequencing of the complete exome and transcriptome of individual tumours, together with mass spectrometry, allows for the identification of mutant peptides to develop vaccines on an individual basis for each patient [385]. In non-immunogenic tumours, the induction of the expression of multiple neoepitopes can direct a polyclonal CTL attack against a cancer. One goal of therapeutic antitumour vaccines is the targeting of CTLs on MHC-bound peptides restricted to cancer cells, increasing the CTLs of high avidity at the site of the tumour [386].

In contrast, few mutant epitopes have been described, as it requires the exploration of the patient's tumour infiltrating lymphocytes based on their ability to recognize antigen libraries created after sequencing of the tumour exome. This requires the use of mass spectrometry combined with transcriptomical or exome sequence analysis to identify neo-epitopes [385].

In short, a large part of the antigens that drive the effectual responses of antitumour CD8 T cells remains unknown. These antigens can be classified into tumour-associated autoantigens and antigens derived from tumour-specific mutant proteins. The presentation of autoantigens in the thymus may result in the elimination of highly avid T cells, thus mutant neo-antigens will be more immunogenic. In contrast, these neoantigens evade identification by mass spectrometry because this method relies on sequence clarification with proteomic databases that do not contain patient-specific mutations. By using transcriptomics and exome sequence analysis to identify mutations, together with the use of MHC class I binding prediction algorithms, too many candidate mutant peptides are detected to be evaluated. Mass spectrometry would allow for the selection of peptides with sufficient expression and presentation by MHC class I, which would be the most immunogenic. By combining both tools, it is possible to identify mutated peptides associated with tumours that present in MHC class I [385].

The immunogenicity of neoepitopes is correlated with the affinity for peptide binding by MHC class I, but other factors such as the interaction of the mutated amino acid with the TCR also play a role, as this is essential for the recognition of the mutated peptide as a stranger [387].

The analysis of MHC peptidoma allows for the identification of peptides derived from the proteolysis of proteins that are generally short-lived in tumour tissues and therefore cannot be identified by conventional proteomic methodologies. One of the current challenges is to find differences between MHC peptidomas from healthy patients and cancer patients, since MHC peptidomas have large amounts of different peptides. Most of these peptides will be from the cellular proteome but also small amounts of cancer-related peptides will be present, which will be different even among different patients presenting the disease. Ultimately, such analysis would allow for the identification of thousands of peptides, including some potential biomarkers of disease. Furthermore, these cancer-related MHC peptides could be used to design patient-specific immunotherapeutics. In other words, the final goal would be to use the MHC peptidoma data to personalize treatments. Mass spectrometry analysis would be a good tool for this purpose, as it is becoming less expensive and faster and can be used in clinical diagnosis on a routine basis [358].

In conclusion, the identification of epitopes that induce the immune response in cancer is necessary to understand and manipulate the immune responses of CD8 T cells for clinical benefit. Tumour-specific mutations are important in shaping the antitumour response, but their identification remains a challenge. The identification of neo-epitopes by combining whole exome sequencing, transcriptome and mass spectrometry analysis strategies, together with a structural prediction algorithm to predict peptide immunogenicity in MHC class I would facilitate the monitoring of tumour-specific T cells, which would be useful in the prognosis of cancer patients, as well as the development of new vaccines [385].

Cancer immunotherapy is undergoing a major transition from traditional approaches that activate systemic immune responses based on understanding the processes of immune activation to more effective and less toxic treatments that target immune normalization in the tumour microenvironment based on tumour-induced immune escape mechanisms [73].

NPs play an important role in these improvements in immunotherapeutic treatments. Nanomaterials applied to nanomedicine would make it possible to increase the effectiveness and reduce the toxicity of practically all the immunotherapeutics described. There are very varied nanoparticle designs that can serve as immunotherapy delivery platforms, allowing for specific and targeted delivery. In addition, NPs can also be designed to enhance the immune response of the host. Due to their great potential, research into these nanomaterials in combination with drugs is necessary to ensure their biosafety and determine their specific functions and applications based on their biocompatibility. Improving these approaches would make it possible to overcome some of the drawbacks of immunotherapy and initiate a new path in cancer treatment.

Author Contributions: V.A.-F. and M.F. designed manuscript outline. V.A.-F. designs and prepares figures and tables. All the authors (V.A.-F., A.L.-V., P.J.-V., A.-P.H., A.O.-P., R.M.-R., R.G., M.F.) participate in writing, discussing and prepare manuscript. All authors have read and agreed to the published version of the manuscript.

Funding: We gratefully acknowledge financial support from the Spanish Health Institute Carlos III (ISCIII) for the grants: FIS PI17/01930 and CB16/12/00400. Fundación Solórzano FS/38-2017. The Proteomics Unit belongs to ProteoRed, PRB3-ISCIII, supported by grant PT17/0019/0023, of the PE I + D + I 2017-2020, funded by ISCIII and FEDER. A. Landeira-Viñuela is supported by VII Centenario-USAL PhD Program, P. Juanes-Velasco is supported by IBSAL PhD Program, V-Acebes-Fernández is supported by "Retención Talentos" Programm sponsored by Ayuntamiento Salamanca (Salamanca, Spain).

Acknowledgments: We thanks GRG. for her help in language edition.

Conflicts of Interest: The authors declare no conflict of interest.

References

1. Lechuga, L. *Nanomedicina: Aplicación de la Nanotecnología en la Salud*; Digital.csic.es.: Madrid, Spain, 2011.
2. Auría-Soro, C.; Nesma, T.; Juanes-Velasco, P.; Landeira-Viñuela, A.; Fidalgo-Gomez, H.; Acebes-Fernandez, V.; Gongora, R.; Parra, M.J.A.; Manzano-Roman, R.; Fuentes, M. Interactions of nanoparticles and biosystems: Microenvironment of nanoparticles and biomolecules in nanomedicine. *Nanomaterials* **2019**, *9*, 1365. [CrossRef]
3. Arab, D.; Pourafshary, P. Nanoparticles-assisted surface charge modification of the porous medium to treat colloidal particles migration induced by low salinity water flooding. *Colloids Surf. A Physicochem. Eng. Asp.* **2013**, *436*, 803–814. [CrossRef]
4. Hashemi, R.; Nassar, N.N.; Pereira Almao, P. Nanoparticle technology for heavy oil in-situ upgrading and recovery enhancement: Opportunities and challenges. *Appl. Energy* **2014**, *133*, 374–387. [CrossRef]
5. Mohammadizadeh, M.; Pourabbas, B.; Mahmoodian, M.; Foroutani, K.; Fallahian, M. Facile and rapid production of conductive flexible films by deposition of polythiophene nanoparticles on transparent poly(ethyleneterephtalate): Electrical and morphological properties. *Mater. Sci. Semicond. Process.* **2014**, *20*, 74–83. [CrossRef]
6. Doyle, D.J. Nanotechnology in Anesthesia and Medicine. *Adv. Anesth.* **2013**, *31*, 181–200. [CrossRef]
7. Pelaz, B.; Alexiou, C.; Alvarez-Puebla, R.A.; Alves, F.; Andrews, A.M.; Ashraf, S.; Balogh, L.P.; Ballerini, L.; Bestetti, A.; Brendel, C.; et al. Diverse Applications of Nanomedicine. *ACS Nano* **2017**, *11*, 2313–2381. [CrossRef]
8. Singh, R.; Lillard, J.W. Nanoparticle-based targeted drug delivery. *Exp. Mol. Pathol.* **2009**, *86*, 215–223. [CrossRef]
9. Zhang, Q.; Mochalin, V.N.; Neitzel, I.; Hazeli, K.; Niu, J.; Kontsos, A.; Zhou, J.G.; Lelkes, P.I.; Gogotsi, Y. Mechanical properties and biomineralization of multifunctional nanodiamond-PLLA composites for bone tissue engineering. *Biomaterials* **2012**, *33*, 5067–5075. [CrossRef]

10. Bao, C.; Conde, J.; Polo, E.; del Pino, P.; Moros, M.; Baptista, P.V.; Grazu, V.; Cui, D.; de la Fuente, J.M. A promising road with challenges: Where are gold nanoparticles in translational research? *Nanomedicine* **2014**, *9*, 2353–2370. [CrossRef]
11. Zhou, S.-A.; Brahme, A. Development of phase-contrast X-ray imaging techniques and potential medical applications. *Phys. Med.* **2008**, *24*, 129–148. [CrossRef]
12. Leuvering, J.H.W.; Thal, P.J.H.M.; Van der Waart, M.; Schuurs, A.H.W.M. A sol particle agglutination assay for human chorionic gonadotrophin. *J. Immunol. Methods* **1981**, *45*, 183–194. [CrossRef]
13. Xu, X.; Daniel, W.L.; Wei, W.; Mirkin, C.A. Colorimetric Cu^{2+} Detection Using DNA-Modified Gold-Nanoparticle Aggregates as Probes and Click Chemistry. *Small* **2010**, *6*, 623–626. [CrossRef]
14. Ambrosi, A.; Airò, F.; Merkoçi, A. Enhanced Gold Nanoparticle Based ELISA for a Breast Cancer Biomarker. *Anal. Chem.* **2010**, *82*, 1151–1156. [CrossRef] [PubMed]
15. Sharifi, M.; Avadi, M.R.; Attar, F.; Dashtestani, F.; Ghorchian, H.; Rezayat, S.M.; Saboury, A.A.; Falahati, M. Cancer diagnosis using nanomaterials based electrochemical nanobiosensors. *Biosens. Bioelectron.* **2019**, *126*, 773–784. [CrossRef]
16. Meng, Z.; Song, R.; Chen, Y.; Zhu, Y.; Tian, Y.; Li, D.; Cui, D. Rapid screening and identification of dominant B cell epitopes of HBV surface antigen by quantum dot-based fluorescence polarization assay. *Nanoscale Res. Lett.* **2013**, *8*, 118. [CrossRef] [PubMed]
17. Koo, Y.-E.L.; Cao, Y.; Kopelman, R.; Koo, S.M.; Brasuel, M.; Philbert, M.A. Real-Time Measurements of Dissolved Oxygen Inside Live Cells by Organically Modified Silicate Fluorescent Nanosensors. *Anal. Chem.* **2004**, *76*, 2498–2505. [CrossRef]
18. Fernandes, C.; Suares, D.; Yergeri, M.C. Tumor Microenvironment Targeted Nanotherapy. *Front. Pharmacol.* **2018**, *9*, 1230. [CrossRef]
19. Tay, C.Y.; Cai, P.; Setyawati, M.I.; Fang, W.; Tan, L.P.; Hong, C.H.L.; Chen, X.; Leong, D.T. Nanoparticles Strengthen Intracellular Tension and Retard Cellular Migration. *Nano Lett.* **2014**, *14*, 83–88. [CrossRef]
20. Stirland, D.L.; Nichols, J.W.; Miura, S.; Bae, Y.H. Mind the gap: A survey of how cancer drug carriers are susceptible to the gap between research and practice. *J. Control. Release* **2013**, *172*, 1045–1064. [CrossRef]
21. MaHam, A.; Tang, Z.; Wu, H.; Wang, J.; Lin, Y. Protein-Based Nanomedicine Platforms for Drug Delivery. *Small* **2009**, *5*, 1706–1721. [CrossRef] [PubMed]
22. Díez, P.; González-Muñoz, M.; González-González, M.; Dégano, R.M.; Jara-Acevedo, R.; Sánchez-Paradinas, S.; Piñol, R.; Murillo, J.L.; Lou, G.; Palacio, F.; et al. Functional insights into the cellular response triggered by a bile-acid platinum compound conjugated to biocompatible ferric nanoparticles using quantitative proteomic approaches. *Nanoscale* **2017**, *9*, 9960–9972. [CrossRef] [PubMed]
23. Maleki Dizaj, S.; Barzegar-Jalali, M.; Zarrintan, M.H.; Adibkia, K.; Lotfipour, F. Calcium carbonate nanoparticles as cancer drug delivery system. *Expert Opin. Drug Deliv.* **2015**, *12*, 1649–1660. [CrossRef] [PubMed]
24. Johnstone, T.C.; Suntharalingam, K.; Lippard, S.J. The Next Generation of Platinum Drugs: Targeted Pt(II) Agents, Nanoparticle Delivery, and Pt(IV) Prodrugs. *Chem. Rev.* **2016**, *116*, 3436–3486. [CrossRef]
25. Magherini, F.; Fiaschi, T.; Valocchia, E.; Becatti, M.; Pratesi, A.; Marzo, T.; Massai, L.; Gabbiani, C.; Landini, I.; Nobili, S.; et al. Antiproliferative effects of two gold(I)-N-heterocyclic carbene complexes in A2780 human ovarian cancer cells: A comparative proteomic study. *Oncotarget* **2018**, *9*, 28042–28068. [CrossRef]
26. Centi, S.; Tatini, F.; Ratto, F.; Gnerucci, A.; Mercatelli, R.; Romano, G.; Landini, I.; Nobili, S.; Ravalli, A.; Marrazza, G.; et al. In vitro assessment of antibody-conjugated gold nanorods for systemic injections. *J. Nanobiotechnol.* **2014**, *12*, 1–10. [CrossRef]
27. Marzo, T.; Massai, L.; Pratesi, A.; Stefanini, M.; Cirri, D.; Magherini, F.; Becatti, M.; Landini, I.; Nobili, S.; Mini, E.; et al. Replacement of the Thiosugar of Auranofin with Iodide Enhances the Anticancer Potency in a Mouse Model of Ovarian Cancer. *ACS Med. Chem. Lett.* **2019**, *10*, 656–660. [CrossRef]
28. Sun, J.; Zhang, L.; Wang, J.; Feng, Q.; Liu, D.; Yin, Q.; Xu, D.; Wei, Y.; Ding, B.; Shi, X.; et al. Tunable Rigidity of (Polymeric Core)-(Lipid Shell) Nanoparticles for Regulated Cellular Uptake. *Adv. Mater.* **2015**, *27*, 1402–1407. [CrossRef]
29. Sugahara, K.N.; Teesalu, T.; Karmali, P.P.; Kotamraju, V.R.; Agemy, L.; Greenwald, D.R.; Ruoslahti, E. Coadministration of a Tumor-Penetrating Peptide Enhances the Efficacy of Cancer Drugs. *Science 80* **2010**, *328*, 1031–1035. [CrossRef]

30. Liu, X.; Chen, Y.; Li, H.; Huang, N.; Jin, Q.; Ren, K.; Ji, J. Enhanced Retention and Cellular Uptake of Nanoparticles in Tumors by Controlling Their Aggregation Behavior. *ACS Nano* **2013**, *7*, 6244–6257. [CrossRef]
31. Dai, W.; Yang, T.; Wang, Y.; Wang, X.; Wang, J.; Zhang, X.; Zhang, Q. Peptide PHSCNK as an integrin α5β1 antagonist targets stealth liposomes to integrin-overexpressing melanoma. *Nanomed. Nanotechnol. Biol. Med.* **2012**, *8*, 1152–1161. [CrossRef] [PubMed]
32. Skirtach, A.G.; Muñoz Javier, A.; Kreft, O.; Köhler, K.; Piera Alberola, A.; Möhwald, H.; Parak, W.J.; Sukhorukov, G.B. Laser-Induced Release of Encapsulated Materials inside Living Cells. *Angew. Chem. Int. Ed.* **2006**, *45*, 4612–4617. [CrossRef] [PubMed]
33. Ochs, M.; Carregal-Romero, S.; Rejman, J.; Braeckmans, K.; De Smedt, S.C.; Parak, W.J. Light-Addressable Capsules as Caged Compound Matrix for Controlled Triggering of Cytosolic Reactions. *Angew. Chem. Int. Ed.* **2013**, *52*, 695–699. [CrossRef]
34. Kim, Y.; Zhu, J.; Yeom, B.; Di Prima, M.; Su, X.; Kim, J.-G.; Yoo, S.J.; Uher, C.; Kotov, N.A. Stretchable nanoparticle conductors with self-organized conductive pathways. *Nature* **2013**, *500*, 59–63. [CrossRef] [PubMed]
35. Lovat, V.; Pantarotto, D.; Lagostena, L.; Cacciari, B.; Grandolfo, M.; Righi, M.; Spalluto, G.; Prato, M.; Ballerini, L. Carbon Nanotube Substrates Boost Neuronal Electrical Signaling. *Nano Lett.* **2005**, *5*, 1107–1110. [CrossRef]
36. Mattson, M.P.; Haddon, R.C.; Rao, A.M. Molecular Functionalization of Carbon Nanotubes and Use as Substrates for Neuronal Growth. *J. Mol. Neurosci.* **2000**, *14*, 175–182. [CrossRef]
37. Shin, S.R.; Jung, S.M.; Zalabany, M.; Kim, K.; Zorlutuna, P.; Kim, S.; Nikkhah, M.; Khabiry, M.; Azize, M.; Kong, J.; et al. Carbon-Nanotube-Embedded Hydrogel Sheets for Engineering Cardiac Constructs and Bioactuators. *ACS Nano* **2013**, *7*, 2369–2380. [CrossRef]
38. Lee, J.; Kotov, N.A. Notch Ligand Presenting Acellular 3D Microenvironments for ex vivo Human Hematopoietic Stem-Cell Culture made by Layer-By-Layer Assembly. *Small* **2009**, *5*, 1008–1013. [CrossRef]
39. Torchilin, V.P. Micellar Nanocarriers: Pharmaceutical Perspectives. *Pharm. Res.* **2006**, *24*, 1–16. [CrossRef]
40. Lee, Y.; Fukushima, S.; Bae, Y.; Hiki, S.; Ishii, T.; Kataoka, K. A Protein Nanocarrier from Charge-Conversion Polymer in Response to Endosomal pH. *J. Am. Chem. Soc.* **2007**, *129*, 5362–5363. [CrossRef]
41. Colombo, M.; Carregal-Romero, S.; Casula, M.F.; Gutiérrez, L.; Morales, M.P.; Böhm, I.B.; Heverhagen, J.T.; Prosperi, D.; Parak, W.J. Biological applications of magnetic nanoparticles. *Chem. Soc. Rev.* **2012**, *41*, 4306. [CrossRef] [PubMed]
42. Baughman, R.H. Carbon Nanotubes–the Route Toward Applications. *Science 80* **2002**, *297*, 787–792. [CrossRef]
43. Yu, S.-J.; Kang, M.-W.; Chang, H.-C.; Chen, K.-M.; Yu, Y.-C. Bright Fluorescent Nanodiamonds: No Photobleaching and Low Cytotoxicity. *J. Am. Chem. Soc.* **2005**, *127*, 17604–17605. [CrossRef] [PubMed]
44. Guo, P. The emerging field of RNA nanotechnology. *Nat. Nanotechnol.* **2010**, *5*, 833–842. [CrossRef] [PubMed]
45. Sapsford, K.E.; Tyner, K.M.; Dair, B.J.; Deschamps, J.R.; Medintz, I.L. Analyzing Nanomaterial Bioconjugates: A Review of Current and Emerging Purification and Characterization Techniques. *Anal. Chem.* **2011**, *83*, 4453–4488. [CrossRef] [PubMed]
46. Gao, S.; Yang, D.; Fang, Y.; Lin, X.; Jin, X.; Wang, Q.; Wang, X.; Ke, L.; Shi, K. Engineering nanoparticles for targeted remodeling of the tumor microenvironment to improve cancer immunotherapy. *Theranostics* **2019**, *9*, 126–151. [CrossRef]
47. Decuzzi, P.; Godin, B.; Tanaka, T.; Lee, S.Y.; Chiappini, C.; Liu, X.; Ferrari, M. Size and shape effects in the biodistribution of intravascularly injected particles. *J. Control. Release* **2010**, *141*, 320–327. [CrossRef]
48. He, C.; Hu, Y.; Yin, L.; Tang, C.; Yin, C. Effects of particle size and surface charge on cellular uptake and biodistribution of polymeric nanoparticles. *Biomaterials* **2010**, *31*, 3657–3666. [CrossRef] [PubMed]
49. Heo, M.B.; Lim, Y.T. Programmed nanoparticles for combined immunomodulation, antigen presentation and tracking of immunotherapeutic cells. *Biomaterials* **2014**, *35*, 590–600. [CrossRef] [PubMed]
50. Yang, R.; Xu, J.; Xu, L.; Sun, X.; Chen, Q.; Zhao, Y.; Peng, R.; Liu, Z. Cancer Cell Membrane-Coated Adjuvant Nanoparticles with Mannose Modification for Effective Anticancer Vaccination. *ACS Nano* **2018**, *12*, 5121–5129. [CrossRef]
51. Smith, T.T.; Stephan, S.B.; Moffett, H.F.; McKnight, L.E.; Ji, W.; Reiman, D.; Bonagofski, E.; Wohlfahrt, M.E.; Pillai, S.P.S.; Stephan, M.T. In situ programming of leukaemia-specific t cells using synthetic DNA nanocarriers. *Nat. Nanotechnol.* **2017**, *12*, 813–822. [CrossRef] [PubMed]

52. Duan, X.; Chan, C.; Guo, N.; Han, W.; Weichselbaum, R.R.; Lin, W. Photodynamic Therapy Mediated by Nontoxic Core-Shell Nanoparticles Synergizes with Immune Checkpoint Blockade To Elicit Antitumor Immunity and Antimetastatic Effect on Breast Cancer. *J. Am. Chem. Soc.* **2016**, *138*, 16686–16695. [CrossRef]
53. Liu, X.; Gao, X.; Zheng, S.; Wang, B.; Li, Y.; Zhao, C.; Muftuoglu, Y.; Chen, S.; Li, Y.; Yao, H.; et al. Modified nanoparticle mediated IL-12 immunogene therapy for colon cancer. *Nanomed. Nanotechnol. Biol. Med.* **2017**, *13*, 1993–2004. [CrossRef] [PubMed]
54. Li, W.; Zhao, X.; Du, B.; Li, X.; Liu, S.; Yang, X.Y.; Ding, H.; Yang, W.; Pan, F.; Wu, X.; et al. Gold Nanoparticle-Mediated Targeted Delivery of Recombinant Human Endostatin Normalizes Tumour Vasculature and Improves Cancer Therapy. *Sci. Rep.* **2016**, *6*, 30619. [CrossRef] [PubMed]
55. Chen, Q.; Xu, L.; Liang, C.; Wang, C.; Peng, R.; Liu, Z. Photothermal therapy with immune-adjuvant nanoparticles together with checkpoint blockade for effective cancer immunotherapy. *Nat. Commun.* **2016**, *7*, 1–13. [CrossRef] [PubMed]
56. Zhuang, J.; Holay, M.; Park, J.H.; Fang, R.H.; Zhang, J.; Zhang, L. Nanoparticle delivery of immunostimulatory agents for cancer immunotherapy. *Theranostics* **2019**, *9*, 7826–7848. [CrossRef]
57. Chen, W.L.; Liu, S.J.; Leng, C.H.; Chen, H.W.; Chong, P.; Huang, M.H. Disintegration and cancer immunotherapy efficacy of a squalane-in-water delivery system emulsified by bioresorbable poly(ethylene glycol)-block-polylactide. *Biomaterials* **2014**, *35*, 1686–1695. [CrossRef]
58. Zhang, Y.; Li, N.; Suh, H.; Irvine, D.J. Nanoparticle anchoring targets immune agonists to tumors enabling anti-cancer immunity without systemic toxicity. *Nat. Commun.* **2018**, *9*, 1–15. [CrossRef]
59. Rahimian, S.; Fransen, M.F.; Kleinovink, J.W.; Amidi, M.; Ossendorp, F.; Hennink, W.E. Polymeric microparticles for sustained and local delivery of antiCD40 and antiCTLA-4 in immunotherapy of cancer. *Biomaterials* **2015**, *61*, 33–40. [CrossRef]
60. Akiyoshi, K.; Deguchi, S.; Moriguchi, N.; Yamaguchi, S.; Sunamoto, J. Self-Aggregates of Hydrophobized Polysaccharides in Water. Formation and Characteristics of Nanoparticles. *Macromolecules* **1993**, *26*, 3062–3068. [CrossRef]
61. Muraoka, D.; Harada, N.; Hayashi, T.; Tahara, Y.; Momose, F.; Sawada, S.I.; Mukai, S.A.; Akiyoshi, K.; Shiku, H. Nanogel-based immunologically stealth vaccine targets macrophages in the medulla of lymph node and induces potent antitumor immunity. *ACS Nano* **2014**, *8*, 9209–9218. [CrossRef] [PubMed]
62. Li, P.; Luo, Z.; Liu, P.; Gao, N.; Zhang, Y.; Pan, H.; Liu, L.; Wang, C.; Cai, L.; Ma, Y. Bioreducible alginate-poly(ethylenimine) nanogels as an antigen-delivery system robustly enhance vaccine-elicited humoral and cellular immune responses. *J. Control. Release* **2013**, *168*, 271–279. [CrossRef] [PubMed]
63. Shimizu, T.; Kishida, T.; Hasegawa, U.; Ueda, Y.; Imanishi, J.; Yamagishi, H.; Akiyoshi, K.; Otsuji, E.; Mazda, O. Nanogel DDS enables sustained release of IL-12 for tumor immunotherapy. *Biochem. Biophys. Res. Commun.* **2008**, *367*, 330–335. [CrossRef] [PubMed]
64. Curnis, F.; Fiocchi, M.; Sacchi, A.; Gori, A.; Gasparri, A.; Corti, A. NGR-tagged nano-gold: A new CD13-selective carrier for cytokine delivery to tumors. *Nano Res.* **2016**, *9*, 1393–1408. [CrossRef] [PubMed]
65. Meir, R.; Shamalov, K.; Sadan, T.; Motiei, M.; Yaari, G.; Cohen, C.J.; Popovtzer, R. Fast Image-Guided Stratification Using Anti-Programmed Death Ligand 1 Gold Nanoparticles for Cancer Immunotherapy. *ACS Nano* **2017**, *11*, 11127–11134. [CrossRef]
66. Lu, J.; Liu, X.; Liao, Y.P.; Salazar, F.; Sun, B.; Jiang, W.; Chang, C.H.; Jiang, J.; Wang, X.; Wu, A.M.; et al. Nano-enabled pancreas cancer immunotherapy using immunogenic cell death and reversing immunosuppression. *Nat. Commun.* **2017**, *8*, 1–14. [CrossRef]
67. Ding, B.; Shao, S.; Yu, C.; Teng, B.; Wang, M.; Cheng, Z.; Wong, K.L.; Ma, P.; Lin, J. Large-Pore Mesoporous-Silica-Coated Upconversion Nanoparticles as Multifunctional Immunoadjuvants with Ultrahigh Photosensitizer and Antigen Loading Efficiency for Improved Cancer Photodynamic Immunotherapy. *Adv. Mater.* **2018**, *30*, 1802479. [CrossRef]
68. Irache, J.M.; Salman, H.H.; Gamazo, C.; Espuelas, S. Mannose-targeted systems for the delivery of therapeutics. *Expert Opin. Drug Deliv.* **2008**, *5*, 703–724. [CrossRef]
69. Wang, C.; Li, P.; Liu, L.; Pan, H.; Li, H.; Cai, L.; Ma, Y. Self-adjuvanted nanovaccine for cancer immunotherapy: Role of lysosomal rupture-induced ROS in MHC class I antigen presentation. *Biomaterials* **2016**, *79*, 88–100. [CrossRef]

70. Shukla, S.; Jandzinski, M.; Wang, C.; Gong, X.; Bonk, K.W.; Keri, R.A.; Steinmetz, N.F. A Viral Nanoparticle Cancer Vaccine Delays Tumor Progression and Prolongs Survival in a HER2 + Tumor Mouse Model. *Adv. Ther.* **2019**, *2*, 1800139. [CrossRef]
71. Crane, C.A.; Han, S.J.; Ahn, B.; Oehlke, J.; Kivett, V.; Fedoroff, A.; Butowski, N.; Chang, S.M.; Clarke, J.; Berger, M.S.; et al. Individual patient-specific immunity against high-grade glioma after vaccination with autologous tumor derived peptides bound to the 96 KD chaperone protein. *Clin. Cancer Res.* **2013**, *19*, 205–214. [CrossRef]
72. Kuai, R.; Ochyl, L.J.; Bahjat, K.S.; Schwendeman, A.; Moon, J.J. Designer vaccine nanodiscs for personalized cancer immunotherapy. *Nat. Mater.* **2017**, *16*, 489–498. [CrossRef]
73. Sanmamed, M.F.; Chen, L. A Paradigm Shift in Cancer Immunotherapy: From Enhancement to Normalization. *Cell* **2018**, *175*, 313–326. [CrossRef] [PubMed]
74. Hanahan, D.; Weinberg, R.A. The hallmarks of cancer. *Cell* **2000**, *100*, 57–70. [CrossRef]
75. Hanahan, D.; Weinberg, R.A. Hallmarks of cancer: The next generation. *Cell* **2011**, *144*, 646–674. [CrossRef]
76. Chen, D.S.; Mellman, I. Oncology meets immunology: The cancer-immunity cycle. *Immunity* **2013**, *39*, 1–10. [CrossRef] [PubMed]
77. Berraondo, P.; Sanmamed, M.F.; Ochoa, M.C.; Etxeberria, I.; Aznar, M.A.; Pérez-Gracia, J.L.; Rodríguez-Ruiz, M.E.; Ponz-Sarvise, M.; Castañón, E.; Melero, I. Cytokines in clinical cancer immunotherapy. *Br. J. Cancer* **2019**, *120*, 6–15. [CrossRef] [PubMed]
78. Christian, D.A.; Hunter, C.A. Particle-mediated delivery of cytokines for immunotherapy. *Immunotherapy* **2012**, *4*, 425–441. [CrossRef] [PubMed]
79. Waldmann, T.A. Cytokines in cancer immunotherapy. *Cold Spring Harb. Perspect. Biol.* **2018**, *10*, a028472. [CrossRef] [PubMed]
80. Wrangle, J.M.; Patterson, A.; Johnson, C.B.; Neitzke, D.J.; Mehrotra, S.; Denlinger, C.E.; Paulos, C.M.; Li, Z.; Cole, D.J.; Rubinstein, M.P. IL-2 and beyond in Cancer Immunotherapy. *J. Interf. Cytokine Res.* **2018**, *38*, 45–68. [CrossRef]
81. Ratain, M.J.; Golomb, H.M.; Vardiman, J.W.; Vokes, E.E.; Jacobs, R.H.; Daly, K. Treatment of Hairy Cell Leukemia With Recombinant Alpha2 Interferon. *Blood* **1985**, *65*, 644–648. [CrossRef]
82. Conlon, K.C.; Miljkovic, M.D.; Waldmann, T.A. Cytokines in the Treatment of Cancer. *J. Interf. Cytokine Res.* **2019**, *39*, 6–21. [CrossRef] [PubMed]
83. Meeker, T.C.; Lowder, J.; Maloney, D.G.; Miller, R.A.; Thielemans, K.; Warnke, R.; Levy, R. A clinical trial of anti-idiotype therapy for B cell malignancy. *Blood* **1985**, *65*, 1349–1363. [CrossRef] [PubMed]
84. Weiner, G.J. Building better monoclonal antibody-based therapeutics. *Nat. Rev. Cancer* **2015**, *15*, 361–370. [CrossRef] [PubMed]
85. Tutt, A.L.; French, R.R.; Illidge, T.M.; Honeychurch, J.; McBride, H.M.; Penfold, C.A.; Fearon, D.T.; Parkhouse, R.M.E.; Klaus, G.G.B.; Glennie, M.J. Monoclonal antibody therapy of B cell lymphoma: Signaling activity on tumor cells appears more important than recruitment of effectors. *J. Immunol.* **1998**, *161*, 3176–3185.
86. Clynes, R.; Takechi, Y.; Moroi, Y.; Houghton, A.; Ravetch, J.V. Fc receptors are required in passive and active immunity to melanoma. *Proc. Natl. Acad. Sci. USA* **1998**, *95*, 652–656. [CrossRef]
87. Yarden, Y.; Pines, G. The ERBB network: At last, cancer therapy meets systems biology. *Nat. Rev. Cancer* **2012**, *12*, 553–563. [CrossRef]
88. Franklin, M.C.; Carey, K.D.; Vajdos, F.F.; Leahy, D.J.; De Vos, A.M.; Sliwkowski, M.X. Insights into ErbB signaling from the structure of the ErbB2-pertuzumab complex. *Cancer Cell* **2004**, *5*, 317–328. [CrossRef]
89. Pawluczkowycz, A.W.; Beurskens, F.J.; Beum, P.V.; Lindorfer, M.A.; van de Winkel, J.G.J.; Parren, P.W.H.I.; Taylor, R.P. Binding of Submaximal C1q Promotes Complement-Dependent Cytotoxicity (CDC) of B Cells Opsonized with Anti-CD20 mAbs Ofatumumab (OFA) or Rituximab (RTX): Considerably Higher Levels of CDC Are Induced by OFA than by RTX. *J. Immunol.* **2009**, *183*, 749–758. [CrossRef] [PubMed]
90. Lefebvre, M.L.; Krause, S.W.; Salcedo, M.; Nardin, A. Ex vivo-activated human macrophages kill chronic lymphocytic leukemia cells in the presence of rituximab: Mechanism of antibody-dependent cellular cytotoxicity and impact of human serum. *J. Immunother.* **2006**, *29*, 388–397. [CrossRef]
91. Dall'ozzo, S.; Tartas, S.; Paintaud, G.; Cartron, G.; Colombat, P.; Bardos, P.; Watier, H.; Thibault, G. Rituximab-Dependent Cytotoxicity by Natural Killer Cells: Influence of FCGR3A Polymorphism on the Concentration-Effect Relationship. *Cancer Res.* **2004**, *64*, 4664–4669.

92. Ferrara, N.; Hillan, K.J.; Gerber, H.P.; Novotny, W. Discovery and development of bevacizumab, an anti-VEGF antibody for treating cancer. *Nat. Rev. Drug Discov.* **2004**, *3*, 391–400. [CrossRef] [PubMed]
93. Sennino, B.; McDonald, D.M. Controlling escape from angiogenesis inhibitors. *Nat. Rev. Cancer* **2012**, *12*, 699–709. [CrossRef] [PubMed]
94. Benmebarek, M.R.; Karches, C.H.; Cadilha, B.L.; Lesch, S.; Endres, S.; Kobold, S. Killing mechanisms of chimeric antigen receptor (CAR) T cells. *Int. J. Mol. Sci.* **2019**, *20*, 1283. [CrossRef] [PubMed]
95. Feldman, S.A.; Assadipour, Y.; Kriley, I.; Goff, S.L.; Rosenberg, S.A. Adoptive Cell Therapy—Tumor-Infiltrating Lymphocytes, T-Cell Receptors, and Chimeric Antigen Receptors. *Semin. Oncol.* **2015**, *42*, 626–639. [CrossRef]
96. Rosenberg, S.A.; Spiess, P.; Lafreniere, R. A new approach to the adoptive immunotherapy of cancer with tumor-infiltrating lymphocytes. *Science 80* **1986**, *233*, 1318–1321. [CrossRef]
97. Rosenberg, S.A.; Packard, B.S.; Aebersold, P.M.; Solomon, D.; Topalian, S.L.; Toy, S.T.; Simon, P.; Lotze, M.T.; Yang, J.C.; Seipp, C.A.; et al. Use of Tumor-Infiltrating Lymphocytes and Interleukin-2 in the Immunotherapy of Patients with Metastatic Melanoma. *N. Engl. J. Med.* **1988**, *319*, 1676–1680. [CrossRef]
98. Grupp, S.A.; Kalos, M.; Barrett, D.; Aplenc, R.; Porter, D.L.; Rheingold, S.R.; Teachey, D.T.; Chew, A.; Hauck, B.; Wright, J.F.; et al. Chimeric antigen receptor-modified T cells for acute lymphoid leukemia. *N. Engl. J. Med.* **2013**, *368*, 1509–1518. [CrossRef]
99. Brentjens, R.J.; Davila, M.L.; Riviere, I.; Park, J.; Wang, X.; Cowell, L.G.; Bartido, S.; Stefanski, J.; Taylor, C.; Olszewska, M.; et al. CD19-targeted T cells rapidly induce molecular remissions in adults with chemotherapy-refractory acute lymphoblastic leukemia. *Sci. Transl. Med.* **2013**, *5*, 177ra38. [CrossRef]
100. Kochenderfer, J.N.; Dudley, M.E.; Kassim, S.H.; Somerville, R.P.T.; Carpenter, R.O.; Maryalice, S.S.; Yang, J.C.; Phan, G.Q.; Hughes, M.S.; Sherry, R.M.; et al. Chemotherapy-refractory diffuse large B-cell lymphoma and indolent B-cell malignancies can be effectively treated with autologous T cells expressing an anti-CD19 chimeric antigen receptor. *J. Clin. Oncol.* **2015**, *33*, 540–549. [CrossRef]
101. Porter, D.L.; Levine, B.L.; Kalos, M.; Bagg, A.; June, C.H. Chimeric antigen receptor-modified T cells in chronic lymphoid leukemia. *N. Engl. J. Med.* **2011**, *365*, 725–733. [CrossRef] [PubMed]
102. Kochenderfer, J.N.; Dudley, M.E.; Feldman, S.A.; Wilson, W.H.; Spaner, D.E.; Maric, I.; Stetler-Stevenson, M.; Phan, G.Q.; Hughes, M.S.; Sherry, R.M.; et al. B-cell depletion and remissions of malignancy along with cytokine-associated toxicity in a clinical trial of anti-CD19 chimeric-antigen-receptor–transduced T cells. *Blood* **2012**, *119*, 2709–2720. [CrossRef]
103. Doan, A.; Pulsipher, M.A. Hypogammaglobulinemia due to CAR T-cell therapy. *Pediatr. Blood Cancer* **2018**, *65*, e26914. [CrossRef]
104. Knochelmann, H.M.; Smith, A.S.; Dwyer, C.J.; Wyatt, M.M.; Mehrotra, S.; Paulos, C.M. CAR T Cells in Solid Tumors: Blueprints for Building Effective Therapies. *Front. Immunol.* **2018**, *9*, 1740. [CrossRef] [PubMed]
105. Xie, Y.J.; Dougan, M.; Jailkhani, N.; Ingram, J.; Fang, T.; Kummer, L.; Momin, N.; Pishesha, N.; Rickelt, S.; Hynes, R.O.; et al. Nanobody-based CAR T cells that target the tumor microenvironment inhibit the growth of solid tumors in immunocompetent mice. *Proc. Natl. Acad. Sci. USA* **2019**, *116*, 7624–7631. [CrossRef] [PubMed]
106. Guo, C.; Manjili, M.H.; Subjeck, J.R.; Sarkar, D.; Fisher, P.B.; Wang, X.Y. Therapeutic cancer vaccines. Past, present, and future. In *Advances in Cancer Research*; Academic Press Inc.: Cambridge, MA, USA, 2013; Volume 119, pp. 421–475.
107. Pan, R.-Y.; Chung, W.-H.; Chu, M.-T.; Chen, S.-J.; Chen, H.-C.; Zheng, L.; Hung, S.-I. Recent Development and Clinical Application of Cancer Vaccine: Targeting Neoantigens. *J. Immunol. Res.* **2018**, *2018*. [CrossRef]
108. Galluzzi, L.; Vacchelli, E.; Bravo-San Pedro, J.M.; Buqué, A.; Senovilla, L.; Baracco, E.E.; Bloy, N.; Castoldi, F.; Abastado, J.P.; Agostinis, P.; et al. Classification of current anticancer immunotherapies. *Oncotarget* **2014**, *5*, 12472–12508. [CrossRef]
109. Berger, M.; Kreutz, F.T.; Horst, J.L.; Baldi, A.C.; Koff, W.J. Phase I Study with an Autologous Tumor Cell Vaccine for Locally Advanced or Metastatic Prostate Cancer. *J. Pharm. Pharm. Sci.* **2007**, *10*, 144–152.
110. Hanna, M.G.; Hoover, H.C.; Vermorken, J.B.; Harris, J.E.; Pinedo, H.M. Adjuvant active specific immunotherapy of stage II and stage III colon cancer with an autologous tumor cell vaccine: First randomized phase III trials show promise. In *Proceedings of the Vaccine*; Elsevier: Amsterdam, The Netherlands, 2001; Volume 19, pp. 2576–2582.

111. Rüttinger, D.; van den Engel, N.K.; Winter, H.; Schlemmer, M.; Pohla, H.; Grützner, S.; Wagner, B.; Schendel, D.J.; Fox, B.A.; Jauch, K.W.; et al. Adjuvant therapeutic vaccination in patients with non-small cell lung cancer made lymphopenic and reconstituted with autologous PBMC: First clinical experience and evidence of an immune response. *J. Transl. Med.* **2007**, *5*, 43. [CrossRef]
112. Berd, D.; Maguire, H.C.; McCue, P.; Mastrangelo, M.J. Treatment of metastatic melanoma with an autologous tumor-cell vaccine: Clinical and immunologic results in 64 patients. *J. Clin. Oncol.* **1990**, *8*, 1858–1867. [CrossRef]
113. Antonia, S.J.; Seigne, J.; Diaz, J.; Muro-Cacho, C.; Extermann, M.; Farmelo, M.J.; Friberg, M.; Alsarraj, M.; Mahany, J.J.; Pow-Sang, J.; et al. Phase I trial of a B7-1 (CD80) gene modified autologous tumor cell vaccine in combination with systemic interleukin-2 in patients with metastatic renal cell carcinoma. *J. Urol.* **2002**, *167*, 1995–2000. [CrossRef]
114. Butterfield, L.H. Cancer vaccines. *BMJ* **2015**, *350*, h988. [CrossRef] [PubMed]
115. Morton, D.L.; Foshag, L.J.; Hoon, D.S.B.; Nizze, J.A.; Wanek, L.A.; Chang, C.; Davtyan, D.G.; Gupta, R.K.; Elashoff, R.; Irie, R.F.; et al. Prolongation of survival in metastatic melanoma after active specific immunotherapy with a new polyvalent melanoma vaccine. In Proceedings of the Annals of Surgery; Lippincott, Williams, and Wilkins: Philadelphia, PA, USA, 1992; Volume 216, pp. 463–482.
116. Cheever, M.A.; Higano, C.S. PROVENGE (sipuleucel-T) in prostate cancer: The first FDA-approved therapeutic cancer vaccine. *Clin. Cancer Res.* **2011**, *17*, 3520–3526. [CrossRef] [PubMed]
117. Hanna, M.G. Immunotherapy with autologous tumor cell vaccines for treatment of occult disease in early stage colon cancer. *Hum. Vaccines Immunother.* **2012**, *8*, 1156–1160. [CrossRef] [PubMed]
118. Geary, S.M.; Salem, A.K. Prostate cancer vaccines update on clinical development. *Oncoimmunology* **2013**, *2*, e24523. [CrossRef] [PubMed]
119. Zappa, C.; Mousa, S.A. Non-small cell lung cancer: Current treatment and future advances. *Transl. Lung Cancer Res.* **2016**, *5*, 288–300. [CrossRef] [PubMed]
120. Banchereau, J.; Palucka, A.K. Dendritic cells as therapeutic vaccines against cancer. *Nat. Rev. Immunol.* **2005**, *5*, 296–306. [CrossRef]
121. Vermaelen, K. Vaccine strategies to improve anticancer cellular immune responses. *Front. Immunol.* **2019**, *10*, 8. [CrossRef]
122. Van Willigen, W.W.; Bloemendal, M.; Gerritsen, W.R.; Schreibelt, G.; De Vries, I.J.M.; Bol, K.F. Dendritic cell cancer therapy: Vaccinating the right patient at the right time. *Front. Immunol.* **2018**, *9*, 2265. [CrossRef]
123. Inba, K.; Inaba, M.; Romani, N.; Aya, H.; Deguchi, M.; Ikehara, S.; Muramatsu, S.; Steinman, R.M. Generation of large numbers of dendritic cells from mouse bone marrow cultures supplemented with granulocyte/macrophage colony-stimulating factor. *J. Exp. Med.* **1992**, *176*, 1693–1702. [CrossRef]
124. Murphy, G.P.; Tjoa, B.; Ragde, H.; Kenny, G.; Boynton, A. Phase I clinical trial: T-cell therapy for prostate cancer using autologous dendritic cells pulsed with HLA-A0201-specific peptides from prostate-specific membrane antigen. *Prostate* **1996**, *29*, 371–380. [CrossRef]
125. Small, E.J.; Schellhammer, P.F.; Higano, C.S.; Redfern, C.H.; Nemunaitis, J.J.; Valone, F.H.; Verjee, S.S.; Jones, L.A.; Hershberg, R.M. Placebo-controlled phase III trial of immunologic therapy with Sipuleucel-T (APC8015) in patients with metastatic, asymptomatic hormone refractory prostate cancer. *J. Clin. Oncol.* **2006**, *24*, 3089–3094. [CrossRef] [PubMed]
126. Kantoff, P.W.; Higano, C.S.; Shore, N.D.; Berger, E.R.; Small, E.J.; Penson, D.F.; Redfern, C.H.; Ferrari, A.C.; Dreicer, R.; Sims, R.B.; et al. Sipuleucel-T immunotherapy for castration-resistant prostate cancer. *N. Engl. J. Med.* **2010**, *363*, 411–422. [CrossRef] [PubMed]
127. Nestle, F.O.; Alijagic, S.; Gilliet, M.; Sun, Y.; Grabbe, S.; Dummer, R.; Burg, G.; Schadendorf, D. Vaccination of melanoma patients with peptide- or tumor lysate-pulsed dendritic cells. *Nat. Med.* **1998**, *4*, 328–332. [CrossRef]
128. Romano, E.; Rossi, M.; Ratzinger, G.; De Cos, M.A.; Chung, D.J.; Panageas, K.S.; Wolchock, J.D.; Houghton, A.N.; Chapman, P.B.; Heller, G.; et al. Peptide-loaded langerhans cells, despite increased IL15 secretion and T-cell activation in vitro, elicit antitumor T-cell responses comparable to peptide-loaded monocyte-derived dendritic cells in vivo. *Clin. Cancer Res.* **2011**, *17*, 1984–1997. [CrossRef]
129. Thurner, B.; Haendle, I.; Röder, C.; Dieckmann, D.; Keikavoussi, P.; Jonuleit, H.; Bender, A.; Maczek, C.; Schreiner, D.; Von Den Driesch, P.; et al. Vaccination with Mage-3A1 peptide-pulsed nature, monocyte-derived

dendritic cells expands specific cytotoxic T cells and induces regression of some metastases in advanced stage IV melanoma. *J. Exp. Med.* **1999**, *190*, 1669–1678. [CrossRef]
130. Yu, J.S.; Liu, G.; Ying, H.; Yong, W.H.; Black, K.L.; Wheeler, C.J. Vaccination with tumor lysate-pulsed dendritic cells elicits antigen-specific, cytotoxic T-cells in patients with malignant glioma. *Cancer Res.* **2004**, *64*, 4973–4979. [CrossRef]
131. Höltl, L.; Rieser, C.; Papesh, C.; Ramoner, R.; Herold, M.; Klocker, H.; Radmayr, C.; Stenzl, A.; Bartsch, G.; Thurnher, M. Cellular and humoral immune responses in patients with metastatic renal cell carcinoma after vaccination with antigen pulsed dendritic cells. *J. Urol.* **1999**, *161*, 777–782. [CrossRef]
132. di Pietro, A.; Tosti, G.; Ferrucci, P.F.; Testori, A. Oncophage: Step to the future for vaccine therapy in melanoma. *Expert Opin. Biol. Ther.* **2008**, *8*, 1973–1984. [CrossRef]
133. Xia, W.; Wang, J.; Xu, Y.; Jiang, F.; Xu, L. L-BLP25 as a peptide vaccine therapy in non-small cell lung cancer: A review. *J. Thorac. Dis.* **2014**, *6*, 1513–1520.
134. Mocellin, S.; Pilati, P.; Nitti, D. Peptide-Based Anticancer Vaccines: Recent Advances and Future Perspectives. *Curr. Med. Chem.* **2009**, *16*, 4779–4796. [CrossRef] [PubMed]
135. Janeway, C.A. The immune system evolved to discriminate infectious nonself from noninfectious self. *Immunol. Today* **1992**, *13*, 11–16. [CrossRef]
136. FLEMING, T.P.; WATSON, M.A. Mammaglobin, a Breast-Specific Gene, and Its Utility as a Marker for Breast Cancer. *Ann. N. Y. Acad. Sci.* **2006**, *923*, 78–79. [CrossRef] [PubMed]
137. Johnson, L.E.; Brockstedt, D.; Leong, M.; Lauer, P.; Theisen, E.; Sauer, J.D.; McNeel, D.G. Heterologous vaccination targeting prostatic acid phosphatase (PAP) using DNA and Listeria vaccines elicits superior anti-tumor immunity dependent on CD4+ T cells elicited by DNA priming. *Oncoimmunology* **2018**, *7*, e1456603. [CrossRef]
138. Schwartzentruber, D.J.; Lawson, D.H.; Richards, J.M.; Conry, R.M.; Miller, D.M.; Treisman, J.; Gailani, F.; Riley, L.; Conlon, K.; Pockaj, B.; et al. gp100 peptide vaccine and interleukin-2 in patients with advanced melanoma. *N. Engl. J. Med.* **2011**, *364*, 2119–2127. [CrossRef]
139. Ghanem, G.; Fabrice, J. Tyrosinase related protein 1 (TYRP1/gp75) in human cutaneous melanoma. *Mol. Oncol.* **2011**, *5*, 150–155. [CrossRef]
140. Osada, T.; Morse, M.A.; Hobeika, A.; Lyerly Kim, H. Novel recombinant alphaviral and adenoviral vectors for cancer immunotherapy. *Semin. Oncol.* **2012**, *39*, 305–310. [CrossRef]
141. Lee, S.H.; Danishmalik, S.N.; Sin, J.I. DNA vaccines, electroporation and their applications in cancer treatment. *Hum. Vaccines Immunother.* **2015**, *11*, 1889–1900. [CrossRef]
142. Brennick, C.A.; George, M.M.; Corwin, W.L.; Srivastava, P.K.; Ebrahimi-Nik, H. Neoepitopes as cancer immunotherapy targets: Key challenges and opportunities. *Immunotherapy* **2017**, *9*, 361–371. [CrossRef]
143. Srivastava, P.K. Peptide-binding heat shock proteins in the endoplasmic reticulum: Role in immune response to cancer and in antigen presentation. *Adv. Cancer Res.* **1993**, *62*, 153–177. [CrossRef]
144. Keenan, B.P.; Jaffee, E.M. Whole cell vaccines—Past progress and future strategies. *Semin. Oncol.* **2012**, *39*, 276–286. [CrossRef]
145. Chiang, C.L.L.; Coukos, G.; Kandalaft, L.E. Whole tumor antigen vaccines: Where are we? *Vaccines* **2015**, *3*, 344–372. [CrossRef] [PubMed]
146. Gulley, J.; Madan, R.; Pachynski, R.; Mulders, P.; Sheikh, N.; Trager, J.; CG, D. Role of antigen spread and distinctive characteristics of immunotherapy in cancer treatment. *JNCI J. Natl. Cancer Inst.* **2017**, *109*, djw261. [CrossRef] [PubMed]
147. Stone, J.D.; Harris, D.T.; Kranz, D.M. TCR affinity for p/MHC formed by tumor antigens that are self-proteins: Impact on efficacy and toxicity. *Curr. Opin. Immunol.* **2015**, *33*, 16–22. [CrossRef]
148. Mullard, A. FDA approves first CAR T therapy. *Nat. Rev. Drug Discov.* **2017**, *16*, 669. [CrossRef] [PubMed]
149. Morgan, R.A.; Chinnasamy, N.; Abate-Daga, D.; Gros, A.; Robbins, P.F.; Zheng, Z.; Dudley, M.E.; Feldman, S.A.; Yang, J.C.; Sherry, R.M.; et al. Cancer regression and neurological toxicity following anti-MAGE-A3 TCR gene therapy. *J. Immunother.* **2013**, *36*, 133–151. [CrossRef]
150. Gillison, M.L.; Koch, W.M.; Capone, R.B.; Spafford, M.; Westra, W.H.; Wu, L.; Zahurak, M.L.; Daniel, R.W.; Viglione, M.; Symer, D.E.; et al. Evidence for a Causal Association Between Human Papillomavirus and a Subset of Head and Neck Cancers. *J. Natl. Cancer Inst.* **2000**, *92*, 709–720. [CrossRef] [PubMed]

151. Wang, X.G.; Revskaya, E.; Bryan, R.A.; Strickler, H.D.; Burk, R.D.; Casadevall, A.; Dadachova, E. Treating Cancer as an Infectious Disease—Viral Antigens as Novel Targets for Treatment and Potential Prevention of Tumors of Viral Etiology. *PLoS ONE* **2007**, *2*, e1114. [CrossRef] [PubMed]
152. Rizvi, N.A.; Hellmann, M.D.; Snyder, A.; Kvistborg, P.; Makarov, V.; Havel, J.J.; Lee, W.; Yuan, J.; Wong, P.; Ho, T.S.; et al. Mutational landscape determines sensitivity to PD-1 blockade in non-small cell lung cancer. *Science 80* **2015**, *348*, 124–128. [CrossRef]
153. Kreiter, S.; Castle, J.C.; Türeci, Ö.; Sahin, U. Targeting the tumor mutanome for personalized vaccination therapy. *Oncoimmunology* **2012**, *1*, 768–769. [CrossRef]
154. Sahin, U.; Derhovanessian, E.; Miller, M.; Kloke, B.P.; Simon, P.; Löwer, M.; Bukur, V.; Tadmor, A.D.; Luxemburger, U.; Schrörs, B.; et al. Personalized RNA mutanome vaccines mobilize poly-specific therapeutic immunity against cancer. *Nature* **2017**, *547*, 222–226. [CrossRef] [PubMed]
155. Li, L.; Goedegebuure, S.P.; Gillanders, W.E. Preclinical and clinical development of neoantigen vaccines. *Ann. Oncol.* **2017**, *28*, xii11–xii17. [CrossRef] [PubMed]
156. Schumacher, T.N.; Schreiber, R.D. Neoantigens in cancer immunotherapy. *Science 80* **2015**, *348*, 69–74. [CrossRef] [PubMed]
157. Strønen, E.; Toebes, M.; Kelderman, S.; Van Buuren, M.M.; Yang, W.; Van Rooij, N.; Donia, M.; Böschen, M.L.; Lund-Johansen, F.; Olweus, J.; et al. Targeting of cancer neoantigens with donor-derived T cell receptor repertoires. *Science 80* **2016**, *352*, 1337–1341. [CrossRef]
158. Ott, P.A.; Hu, Z.; Keskin, D.B.; Shukla, S.A.; Sun, J.; Bozym, D.J.; Zhang, W.; Luoma, A.; Giobbie-Hurder, A.; Peter, L.; et al. An immunogenic personal neoantigen vaccine for patients with melanoma. *Nature* **2017**, *547*, 217–221. [CrossRef]
159. Kovacsovics-Bankowski, M.; Rock, K.L. A phagosome-to-cytosol pathway for exogenous antigens presented on MHC class I molecules. *Science 80* **1995**, *267*, 243–246. [CrossRef]
160. Janeway, C.A. Approaching the asymptote? Evolution and revolution in immunology. In *Proceedings of the Cold Spring Harbor Symposia on Quantitative Biology*; Cold Spring Harbor Laboratory Press: New York, NY, USA, 1989; Volume 54, pp. 1–13.
161. Apetoh, L.; Smyth, M.J.; Drake, C.G.; Abastado, J.P.; Apte, R.N.; Ayyoub, M.; Blay, J.Y.; Bonneville, M.; Butterfield, L.H.; Caignard, A.; et al. Consensus nomenclature for CD8+ T cell phenotypes in cancer. *Oncoimmunology* **2015**, *4*, e998538. [CrossRef]
162. Khong, H.; Overwijk, W.W. Adjuvants for peptide-based cancer vaccines. *J. Immunother. Cancer* **2016**, *4*, 56. [CrossRef]
163. Sabado, R.L.; Bhardwaj, N. Cancer immunotherapy: Dendritic-cell vaccines on the move. *Nature* **2015**, *519*, 300–301. [CrossRef]
164. Hodi, F.S.; O'Day, S.J.; McDermott, D.F.; Weber, R.W.; Sosman, J.A.; Haanen, J.B.; Gonzalez, R.; Robert, C.; Schadendorf, D.; Hassel, J.C.; et al. Improved survival with ipilimumab in patients with metastatic melanoma. *N. Engl. J. Med.* **2010**, *363*, 711–723. [CrossRef]
165. Wei, S.C.; Duffy, C.R.; Allison, J.P. Fundamental mechanisms of immune checkpoint blockade therapy. *Cancer Discov.* **2018**, *8*, 1069–1086. [CrossRef] [PubMed]
166. Markham, A.; Duggan, S. Cemiplimab: First Global Approval. *Drugs* **2018**, *78*, 1841–1846. [CrossRef] [PubMed]
167. Lee, H.T.; Lee, S.H.; Heo, Y.S. Molecular interactions of antibody drugs targeting PD-1, PD-L1, and CTLA-4 in immuno-oncology. *Molecules* **2019**, *24*, 1190. [CrossRef] [PubMed]
168. Sunshine, J.; Taube, J.M. PD-1/PD-L1 inhibitors. *Curr. Opin. Pharmacol.* **2015**, *23*, 32–38. [CrossRef]
169. Carlino, M.S.; Long, G.V. Ipilimumab combined with nivolumab: A standard of care for the treatment of advanced melanoma? *Clin. Cancer Res.* **2016**, *22*, 3992–3998. [CrossRef]
170. Song, M.; Chen, X.; Wang, L.; Zhang, Y. Future of anti-PD-1/PD-L1 applications: Combinations with other therapeutic regimens. *Chin. J. Cancer Res.* **2018**, *30*, 157–172. [CrossRef] [PubMed]
171. Liu, Y.L.; Zamarin, D. Combination Immune Checkpoint Blockade Strategies to Maximize Immune Response in Gynecological Cancers. *Curr. Oncol. Rep.* **2018**, *20*, 94. [CrossRef]
172. Nishino, M.; Ramaiya, N.H.; Hatabu, H.; Hodi, F.S. Monitoring immune-checkpoint blockade: Response evaluation and biomarker development. *Nat. Rev. Clin. Oncol.* **2017**, *14*, 655–668. [CrossRef]

173. Emens, L.A.; Ascierto, P.A.; Darcy, P.K.; Demaria, S.; Eggermont, A.M.M.; Redmond, W.L.; Seliger, B.; Marincola, F.M. Cancer immunotherapy: Opportunities and challenges in the rapidly evolving clinical landscape. *Eur. J. Cancer* **2017**, *81*, 116–129. [CrossRef]
174. Lee, S.; Margolin, K. Cytokines in Cancer Immunotherapy. *Cancers* **2011**, *3*, 3856–3893. [CrossRef]
175. Riley, R.S.; June, C.H.; Langer, R.; Mitchell, M.J. Delivery technologies for cancer immunotherapy. *Nat. Rev. Drug Discov.* **2019**, *18*, 175–196. [CrossRef] [PubMed]
176. Porter, D.L.; Hwang, W.T.; Frey, N.V.; Lacey, S.F.; Shaw, P.A.; Loren, A.W.; Bagg, A.; Marcucci, K.T.; Shen, A.; Gonzalez, V.; et al. Chimeric antigen receptor T cells persist and induce sustained remissions in relapsed refractory chronic lymphocytic leukemia. *Sci. Transl. Med.* **2015**, *7*, 303ra139. [CrossRef]
177. O'Rourke, D.M.; Nasrallah, M.P.; Desai, A.; Melenhorst, J.J.; Mansfield, K.; Morrissette, J.J.D.; Martinez-Lage, M.; Brem, S.; Maloney, E.; Shen, A.; et al. A single dose of peripherally infused EGFRvIII-directed CAR T cells mediates antigen loss and induces adaptive resistance in patients with recurrent glioblastoma. *Sci. Transl. Med.* **2017**, *9*, 399. [CrossRef] [PubMed]
178. Linette, G.P.; Stadtmauer, E.A.; Maus, M.V.; Rapoport, A.P.; Levine, B.L.; Emery, L.; Litzky, L.; Bagg, A.; Carreno, B.M.; Cimino, P.J.; et al. Cardiovascular toxicity and titin cross-reactivity of affinity-enhanced T cells in myeloma and melanoma. *Blood* **2013**, *122*, 863–871. [CrossRef] [PubMed]
179. Rosenberg, S.A.; Yang, J.C.; Restifo, N.P. Cancer immunotherapy: Moving beyond current vaccines. *Nat. Med.* **2004**, *10*, 909–915. [CrossRef] [PubMed]
180. Garg, A.D.; Coulie, P.G.; Van den Eynde, B.J.; Agostinis, P. Integrating Next-Generation Dendritic Cell Vaccines into the Current Cancer Immunotherapy Landscape. *Trends Immunol.* **2017**, *38*, 577–593. [CrossRef] [PubMed]
181. Yang, B.; Jeang, J.; Yang, A.; Wu, T.C.; Hung, C.F. DNA vaccine for cancer immunotherapy. *Hum. Vaccines Immunother.* **2014**, *10*, 3153–3164. [CrossRef]
182. Kauffman, K.J.; Webber, M.J.; Anderson, D.G. Materials for non-viral intracellular delivery of messenger RNA therapeutics. *J. Control. Release* **2016**, *240*, 227–234. [CrossRef]
183. June, C.H.; Warshauer, J.T.; Bluestone, J.A. Is autoimmunity the Achilles' heel of cancer immunotherapy? *Nat. Med.* **2017**, *23*, 540–547. [CrossRef]
184. Byun, D.J.; Wolchok, J.D.; Rosenberg, L.M.; Girotra, M. Cancer immunotherapy-immune checkpoint blockade and associated endocrinopathies. *Nat. Rev. Endocrinol.* **2017**, *13*, 195–207. [CrossRef]
185. Restifo, N.P.; Smyth, M.J.; Snyder, A. Acquired resistance to immunotherapy and future challenges. *Nat. Rev. Cancer* **2016**, *16*, 121–126. [CrossRef]
186. Binnewies, M.; Roberts, E.W.; Kersten, K.; Chan, V.; Fearon, D.F.; Merad, M.; Coussens, L.M.; Gabrilovich, D.I.; Ostrand-Rosenberg, S.; Hedrick, C.C.; et al. Understanding the tumor immune microenvironment (TIME) for effective therapy. *Nat. Med.* **2018**, *24*, 541–550. [CrossRef]
187. Milling, L.; Zhang, Y.; Irvine, D.J. Delivering safer immunotherapies for cancer. *Adv. Drug Deliv. Rev.* **2017**, *114*, 79–101. [CrossRef] [PubMed]
188. Song, W.; Shen, L.; Wang, Y.; Liu, Q.; Goodwin, T.J.; Li, J.; Dorosheva, O.; Liu, T.; Liu, R.; Huang, L. Synergistic and low adverse effect cancer immunotherapy by immunogenic chemotherapy and locally expressed PD-L1 trap. *Nat. Commun.* **2018**, *9*. [CrossRef] [PubMed]
189. Wong, C.; Stylianopoulos, T.; Cui, J.; Martin, J.; Chauhan, V.P.; Jiang, W.; Popovíc, Z.; Jain, R.K.; Bawendi, M.G.; Fukumura, D. Multistage nanoparticle delivery system for deep penetration into tumor tissue. *Proc. Natl. Acad. Sci. USA* **2011**, *108*, 2426–2431. [CrossRef] [PubMed]
190. McNamara, M.A.; Nair, S.K.; Holl, E.K. RNA-Based Vaccines in Cancer Immunotherapy. *J. Immunol. Res.* **2015**, *2015*. [CrossRef] [PubMed]
191. Zhu, G.; Zhang, F.; Ni, Q.; Niu, G.; Chen, X. Efficient Nanovaccine Delivery in Cancer Immunotherapy. *ACS Nano* **2017**, *11*, 2387–2392. [CrossRef] [PubMed]
192. Lopez-Bertoni, H.; Kozielski, K.L.; Rui, Y.; Lal, B.; Vaughan, H.; Wilson, D.R.; Mihelson, N.; Eberhart, C.G.; Laterra, J.; Green, J.J. Bioreducible Polymeric Nanoparticles Containing Multiplexed Cancer Stem Cell Regulating miRNAs Inhibit Glioblastoma Growth and Prolong Survival. *Nano Lett.* **2018**, *18*, 4086–4094. [CrossRef]
193. Liu, Z.; Jiang, W.; Nam, J.; Moon, J.J.; Kim, B.Y.S. Immunomodulating Nanomedicine for Cancer Therapy. *Nano Lett.* **2018**, *18*, 6655–6659. [CrossRef]

194. Oberli, M.A.; Reichmuth, A.M.; Dorkin, J.R.; Mitchell, M.J.; Fenton, O.S.; Jaklenec, A.; Anderson, D.G.; Langer, R.; Blankschtein, D. Lipid Nanoparticle Assisted mRNA Delivery for Potent Cancer Immunotherapy. *Nano Lett.* **2017**, *17*, 1326–1335. [CrossRef]
195. Kranz, L.M.; Diken, M.; Haas, H.; Kreiter, S.; Loquai, C.; Reuter, K.C.; Meng, M.; Fritz, D.; Vascotto, F.; Hefesha, H.; et al. Systemic RNA delivery to dendritic cells exploits antiviral defence for cancer immunotherapy. *Nature* **2016**, *534*, 396–401. [CrossRef] [PubMed]
196. Lambert, L.H.; Goebrecht, G.K.E.; De Leo, S.E.; O'Connor, R.S.; Nunez-Cruz, S.; De Li, T.; Yuan, J.; Milone, M.C.; Kam, L.C. Improving T Cell Expansion with a Soft Touch. *Nano Lett.* **2017**, *17*, 821–826. [CrossRef]
197. Xue, J.; Zhao, Z.; Zhang, L.; Xue, L.; Shen, S.; Wen, Y.; Wei, Z.; Wang, L.; Kong, L.; Sun, H.; et al. Neutrophil-mediated anticancer drug delivery for suppression of postoperative malignant glioma recurrence. *Nat. Nanotechnol.* **2017**, *12*, 692–700. [CrossRef]
198. Wang, C.; Sun, W.; Ye, Y.; Hu, Q.; Bomba, H.N.; Gu, Z. In situ activation of platelets with checkpoint inhibitors for post-surgical cancer immunotherapy. *Nat. Biomed. Eng.* **2017**, *1*, 1–10. [CrossRef]
199. Hickey, J.W.; Vicente, F.P.; Howard, G.P.; Mao, H.Q.; Schneck, J.P. Biologically Inspired Design of Nanoparticle Artificial Antigen-Presenting Cells for Immunomodulation. *Nano Lett.* **2017**, *17*, 7045–7054. [CrossRef] [PubMed]
200. Chiang, C.S.; Lin, Y.J.; Lee, R.; Lai, Y.H.; Cheng, H.W.; Hsieh, C.H.; Shyu, W.C.; Chen, S.Y. Combination of fucoidan-based magnetic nanoparticles and immunomodulators enhances tumour-localized immunotherapy. *Nat. Nanotechnol.* **2018**, *13*, 746–754. [CrossRef] [PubMed]
201. Yuan, H.; Jiang, W.; Von Roemeling, C.A.; Qie, Y.; Liu, X.; Chen, Y.; Wang, Y.; Wharen, R.E.; Yun, K.; Bu, G.; et al. Multivalent bi-specific nanobioconjugate engager for targeted cancer immunotherapy. *Nat. Nanotechnol.* **2017**, *12*, 763–769. [CrossRef] [PubMed]
202. Hood, J.L. Post isolation modification of exosomes for nanomedicine applications. *Nanomedicine* **2016**, *11*, 1745–1756. [CrossRef]
203. Yu, B.; Zhang, X.; Li, X. Exosomes derived from mesenchymal stem cells. *Int. J. Mol. Sci.* **2014**, *15*, 4142–4157. [CrossRef]
204. Zöller, M. Tetraspanins: Push and pull in suppressing and promoting metastasis. *Nat. Rev. Cancer* **2009**, *9*, 40–55. [CrossRef]
205. Théry, C.; Ostrowski, M.; Segura, E. Membrane vesicles as conveyors of immune responses. *Nat. Rev. Immunol.* **2009**, *9*, 581–593. [CrossRef] [PubMed]
206. Hood, J.L.; Wickline, S.A. A systematic approach to exosome-based translational nanomedicine. *Wiley Interdiscip. Rev. Nanomed. Nanobiotechnol.* **2012**, *4*, 458–467. [CrossRef] [PubMed]
207. Munich, S.; Sobo-Vujanovic, A.; Buchser, W.J.; Beer-Stolz, D.; Vujanovic, N.L. Dendritic cell exosomes directly kill tumor cells and activate natural killer cells via TNF superfamily ligands. *Oncoimmunology* **2012**, *1*, 1074–1083. [CrossRef] [PubMed]
208. Saunderson, S.C.; Schuberth, P.C.; Dunn, A.C.; Miller, L.; Hock, B.D.; MacKay, P.A.; Koch, N.; Jack, R.W.; McLellan, A.D. Induction of Exosome Release in Primary B Cells Stimulated via CD40 and the IL-4 Receptor. *J. Immunol.* **2008**, *180*, 8146–8152. [CrossRef]
209. Raimondo, F.; Morosi, L.; Chinello, C.; Magni, F.; Pitto, M. Advances in membranous vesicle and exosome proteomics improving biological understanding and biomarker discovery. *Proteomics* **2011**, *11*, 709–720. [CrossRef]
210. Chen, X.; Ba, Y.; Ma, L.; Cai, X.; Yin, Y.; Wang, K.; Guo, J.; Zhang, Y.; Chen, J.; Guo, X.; et al. Characterization of microRNAs in serum: A novel class of biomarkers for diagnosis of cancer and other diseases. *Cell Res.* **2008**, *18*, 997–1006. [CrossRef]
211. Bunggulawa, E.J.; Wang, W.; Yin, T.; Wang, N.; Durkan, C.; Wang, Y.; Wang, G. Recent advancements in the use of exosomes as drug delivery systems. *J. Nanobiotechnol.* **2018**, *16*, 1–13. [CrossRef]
212. Mokarizadeh, A.; Delirezh, N.; Morshedi, A.; Mosayebi, G.; Farshid, A.-A.; Dalir-Naghadeh, B. Phenotypic modulation of auto-reactive cells by insertion of tolerogenic molecules via MSC-derived exosomes. *Vet. Res. Forum Int. Q. J.* **2012**, *3*, 257–25761.
213. Yeo, R.W.Y.; Lai, R.C.; Zhang, B.; Tan, S.S.; Yin, Y.; Teh, B.J.; Lim, S.K. Mesenchymal stem cell: An efficient mass producer of exosomes for drug delivery. *Adv. Drug Deliv. Rev.* **2013**, *65*, 336–341. [CrossRef]

214. Mokarizadeh, A.; Delirezh, N.; Morshedi, A.; Mosayebi, G.; Farshid, A.A.; Mardani, K. Microvesicles derived from mesenchymal stem cells: Potent organelles for induction of tolerogenic signaling. *Immunol. Lett.* **2012**, *147*, 47–54. [CrossRef]
215. Zhang, B.; Yin, Y.; Lai, R.C.; Tan, S.S.; Choo, A.B.H.; Lim, S.K. Mesenchymal stem cells secrete immunologically active exosomes. *Stem Cells Dev.* **2014**, *23*, 1233–1244. [CrossRef] [PubMed]
216. Zhu, W.; Huang, L.; Li, Y.; Zhang, X.; Gu, J.; Yan, Y.; Xu, X.; Wang, M.; Qian, H.; Xu, W. Exosomes derived from human bone marrow mesenchymal stem cells promote tumor growth in vivo. *Cancer Lett.* **2012**, *315*, 28–37. [CrossRef]
217. Lee, J.K.; Park, S.R.; Jung, B.K.; Jeon, Y.K.; Lee, Y.S.; Kim, M.K.; Kim, Y.G.; Jang, J.Y.; Kim, C.W. Exosomes derived from mesenchymal stem cells suppress angiogenesis by down-regulating VEGF expression in breast cancer cells. *PLoS ONE* **2013**, *8*, e84256. [CrossRef]
218. Valadi, H.; Ekström, K.; Bossios, A.; Sjöstrand, M.; Lee, J.J.; Lötvall, J.O. Exosome-mediated transfer of mRNAs and microRNAs is a novel mechanism of genetic exchange between cells. *Nat. Cell Biol.* **2007**, *9*, 654–659. [CrossRef]
219. Wahlgren, J.; Karlson, T.D.L.; Brisslert, M.; Vaziri Sani, F.; Telemo, E.; Sunnerhagen, P.; Valadi, H. Plasma exosomes can deliver exogenous short interfering RNA to monocytes and lymphocytes. *Nucleic Acids Res.* **2012**, *40*, e130. [CrossRef] [PubMed]
220. Momen-Heravi, F.; Bala, S.; Bukong, T.; Szabo, G. Exosome-mediated delivery of functionally active miRNA-155 inhibitor to macrophages. *Nanomed. Nanotechnol. Biol. Med.* **2014**, *10*, 1517–1527. [CrossRef] [PubMed]
221. Witwer, K.W.; Buzás, E.I.; Bemis, L.T.; Bora, A.; Lässer, C.; Lötvall, J.; Nolte-'t Hoen, E.N.; Piper, M.G.; Sivaraman, S.; Skog, J.; et al. Standardization of sample collection, isolation and analysis methods in extracellular vesicle research. *J. Extracell. Vesicles* **2013**, *2*, 20360. [CrossRef] [PubMed]
222. Tian, Y.; Li, S.; Song, J.; Ji, T.; Zhu, M.; Anderson, G.J.; Wei, J.; Nie, G. A doxorubicin delivery platform using engineered natural membrane vesicle exosomes for targeted tumor therapy. *Biomaterials* **2014**, *35*, 2383–2390. [CrossRef] [PubMed]
223. Kim, M.S.; Haney, M.J.; Zhao, Y.; Yuan, D.; Deygen, I.; Klyachko, N.L.; Kabanov, A.V.; Batrakova, E.V. Engineering macrophage-derived exosomes for targeted paclitaxel delivery to pulmonary metastases: In vitro and in vivo evaluations. *Nanomed. Nanotechnol. Biol. Med.* **2018**, *14*, 195–204. [CrossRef] [PubMed]
224. Raposo, G.; Nijman, H.W.; Stoorvogel, W.; Leijendekker, R.; Harding, C.V.; Melief, C.J.M.; Geuze, H.J. B lymphocytes secrete antigen-presenting vesicles. *J. Exp. Med.* **1996**, *183*, 1161–1172. [CrossRef]
225. Zitvogel, L.; Regnault, A.; Lozier, A.; Wolfers, J.; Flament, C.; Tenza, D.; Ricciardi-Castagnoli, P.; Raposo, G.; Amigorena, S. Eradication of established murine tumors using a novel cell-free vaccine: Dendritic cell-derived exosomes. *Nat. Med.* **1998**, *4*, 594–600. [CrossRef] [PubMed]
226. Conlan, R.S.; Pisano, S.; Oliveira, M.I.; Ferrari, M.; Mendes Pinto, I. Exosomes as Reconfigurable Therapeutic Systems. *Trends Mol. Med.* **2017**, *23*, 636–650. [CrossRef] [PubMed]
227. Wolfers, J.; Lozier, A.; Raposo, G.; Regnault, A.; Théry, C.; Masurier, C.; Flament, C.; Pouzieux, S.; Faure, F.; Tursz, T.; et al. Tumor-derived exosomes are a source of shared tumor rejection antigens for CTL cross-priming. *Nat. Med.* **2001**, *7*, 297–303. [CrossRef] [PubMed]
228. Perica, K.; De León Medero, A.; Durai, M.; Chiu, Y.L.; Bieler, J.G.; Sibener, L.; Niemöller, M.; Assenmacher, M.; Richter, A.; Edidin, M.; et al. Nanoscale artificial antigen presenting cells for T cell immunotherapy. *Nanomed. Nanotechnol. Biol. Med.* **2014**, *10*, 119–129. [CrossRef]
229. Zhang, N.; Bevan, M.J. CD8+ T Cells: Foot Soldiers of the Immune System. *Immunity* **2011**, *35*, 161–168. [CrossRef]
230. Smith-Garvin, J.E.; Koretzky, G.A.; Jordan, M.S. T Cell Activation. *Annu. Rev. Immunol.* **2009**, *27*, 591–619. [CrossRef]
231. Perica, K.; Bieler, J.G.; Schütz, C.; Varela, J.C.; Douglass, J.; Skora, A.; Chiu, Y.L.; Oelke, M.; Kinzler, K.; Zhou, S.; et al. Enrichment and Expansion with Nanoscale Artificial Antigen Presenting Cells for Adoptive Immunotherapy. *ACS Nano* **2015**, *9*, 6861–6871. [CrossRef]
232. Rabinovich, G.A.; Gabrilovich, D.; Sotomayor, E.M. Immunosuppressive Strategies that are Mediated by Tumor Cells. *Annu. Rev. Immunol.* **2007**, *25*, 267–296. [CrossRef]

233. Nel, A.E.; Mädler, L.; Velegol, D.; Xia, T.; Hoek, E.M.V.; Somasundaran, P.; Klaessig, F.; Castranova, V.; Thompson, M. Understanding biophysicochemical interactions at the nano-bio interface. *Nat. Mater.* **2009**, *8*, 543–557. [CrossRef]
234. Butler, M.O.; Hirano, N. Human cell-based artificial antigen-presenting cells for cancer immunotherapy. *Immunol. Rev.* **2014**, *257*, 191–209. [CrossRef]
235. Rhodes, K.R.; Green, J.J. Nanoscale artificial antigen presenting cells for cancer immunotherapy. *Mol. Immunol.* **2018**, *98*, 13–18. [CrossRef] [PubMed]
236. Zhu, L.; Zhou, Z.; Mao, H.; Yang, L. Magnetic nanoparticles for precision oncology: Theranostic magnetic iron oxide nanoparticles for image-guided and targeted cancer therapy. *Nanomedicine* **2017**, *12*, 73–87. [CrossRef] [PubMed]
237. Mahmoudi, M.; Sant, S.; Wang, B.; Laurent, S.; Sen, T. Superparamagnetic iron oxide nanoparticles (SPIONs): Development, surface modification and applications in chemotherapy. *Adv. Drug Deliv. Rev.* **2011**, *63*, 24–46. [CrossRef] [PubMed]
238. Petros, R.A.; Desimone, J.M. Strategies in the design of nanoparticles for therapeutic applications. *Nat. Rev. Drug Discov.* **2010**, *9*, 615–627. [CrossRef]
239. Bonnemain, B. Superparamagnetic agents in magnetic resonance imaging: Physicochemical characteristics and clinical applications. A review. *J. Drug Target.* **1998**, *6*, 167–174. [CrossRef] [PubMed]
240. Yu, M.K.; Park, J.; Jon, S. Targeting strategies for multifunctional nanoparticles in cancer imaging and therapy. *Theranostics* **2012**, *2*, 3–44. [CrossRef] [PubMed]
241. Wang, C.; Sun, X.; Cheng, L.; Yin, S.; Yang, G.; Li, Y.; Liu, Z. Multifunctional theranostic red blood cells for magnetic-field-enhanced in vivo combination therapy of cancer. *Adv. Mater.* **2014**, *26*, 4794–4802. [CrossRef]
242. Williams, D.F. On the mechanisms of biocompatibility. *Biomaterials* **2008**, *29*, 2941–2953. [CrossRef]
243. Naahidi, S.; Jafari, M.; Edalat, F.; Raymond, K.; Khademhosseini, A.; Chen, P. Biocompatibility of engineered nanoparticles for drug delivery. *J. Control. Release* **2013**, *166*, 182–194. [CrossRef]
244. Guerrero, S.; Herance, J.R.; Rojas, S.; Mena, J.F.; Gispert, J.D.; Acosta, G.A.; Albericio, F.; Kogan, M.J. Synthesis and in vivo evaluation of the biodistribution of a 18F-labeled conjugate gold-nanoparticle-peptide with potential biomedical application. *Bioconjug. Chem.* **2012**, *23*, 399–408. [CrossRef]
245. Jiang, W.; Gupta, R.K.; Deshpande, M.C.; Schwendeman, S.P. Biodegradable poly(lactic-co-glycolic acid) microparticles for injectable delivery of vaccine antigens. *Adv. Drug Deliv. Rev.* **2005**, *57*, 391–410. [CrossRef] [PubMed]
246. Anderson, J.M.; Rodriguez, A.; Chang, D.T. Foreign body reaction to biomaterials. *Semin. Immunol.* **2008**, *20*, 86–100. [CrossRef] [PubMed]
247. Zyuzin, M.V.; Díez, P.; Goldsmith, M.; Carregal-Romero, S.; Teodosio, C.; Rejman, J.; Feliu, N.; Escudero, A.; Almendral, M.J.; Linne, U.; et al. Comprehensive and Systematic Analysis of the Immunocompatibility of Polyelectrolyte Capsules. *Bioconjug. Chem.* **2017**, *28*, 556–564. [CrossRef] [PubMed]
248. Peng, Q.; Zhang, S.; Yang, Q.; Zhang, T.; Wei, X.Q.; Jiang, L.; Zhang, C.L.; Chen, Q.M.; Zhang, Z.R.; Lin, Y.F. Preformed albumin corona, a protective coating for nanoparticles based drug delivery system. *Biomaterials* **2013**, *34*, 8521–8530. [CrossRef] [PubMed]
249. Hirsh, S.L.; McKenzie, D.R.; Nosworthy, N.J.; Denman, J.A.; Sezerman, O.U.; Bilek, M.M.M. The Vroman effect: Competitive protein exchange with dynamic multilayer protein aggregates. *Colloids Surf. B Biointerfaces* **2013**, *103*, 395–404. [CrossRef]
250. Liu, W.; Rose, J.; Auffan, M.; Bottero, J.-Y. Protein corona formation for nanomaterials and proteins of a similar size: Hard or soft corona? View project. *Nanoscale* **2014**, *5*, 1658–1665. [CrossRef]
251. Galluzzi, L.; Buqué, A.; Kepp, O.; Zitvogel, L.; Kroemer, G. Immunogenic cell death in cancer and infectious disease. *Nat. Rev. Immunol.* **2017**, *17*, 97–111. [CrossRef]
252. Broz, P.; Monack, D.M. Newly described pattern recognition receptors team up against intracellular pathogens. *Nat. Rev. Immunol.* **2013**, *13*, 551–565. [CrossRef]
253. Cao, X. Self-regulation and cross-regulation of pattern-recognition receptor signalling in health and disease. *Nat. Rev. Immunol.* **2016**, *16*, 35–50. [CrossRef]
254. Fuchs, Y.; Steller, H. Live to die another way: Modes of programmed cell death and the signals emanating from dying cells. *Nat. Rev. Mol. Cell Biol.* **2015**, *16*, 329–344. [CrossRef] [PubMed]
255. Van Kempen, T.S.; Wenink, M.H.; Leijten, E.F.A.; Radstake, T.R.D.J.; Boes, M. Perception of self: Distinguishing autoimmunity from autoinflammation. *Nat. Rev. Rheumatol.* **2015**, *11*, 483–492. [CrossRef]

256. Serrano-del Valle, A.; Anel, A.; Naval, J.; Marzo, I. Immunogenic cell death and immunotherapy of multiple myeloma. *Front. Cell Dev. Biol.* **2019**, *7*, 50. [CrossRef] [PubMed]
257. Dudek, A.M.; Garg, A.D.; Krysko, D.V.; De Ruysscher, D.; Agostinis, P. Inducers of immunogenic cancer cell death. *Cytokine Growth Factor Rev.* **2013**, *24*, 319–333. [CrossRef] [PubMed]
258. Li, X. The inducers of immunogenic cell death for tumor immunotherapy. *Tumori J.* **2018**, *104*, 1–8. [CrossRef] [PubMed]
259. Kurokawa, T.; Oelke, M.; Mackensen, A. Induction and clonal expansion of tumor-specific cytotoxic T lymphocytes from renal cell carcinoma patients after stimulation with autologous dendritic cells loaded with tumor cells. *Int. J. Cancer* **2001**, *91*, 749–756. [CrossRef]
260. Fucikova, J.; Moserova, I.; Truxova, I.; Hermanova, I.; Vancurova, I.; Partlova, S.; Fialova, A.; Sojka, L.; Cartron, P.F.; Houska, M.; et al. High hydrostatic pressure induces immunogenic cell death in human tumor cells. *Int. J. Cancer* **2014**, *135*, 1165–1177. [CrossRef]
261. Garg, A.D.; Krysko, D.V.; Vandenabeele, P.; Agostinis, P. Hypericin-based photodynamic therapy induces surface exposure of damage-associated molecular patterns like HSP70 and calreticulin. *Cancer Immunol. Immunother.* **2012**, *61*, 215–221. [CrossRef]
262. Wang, H.; Sun, L.; Su, L.; Rizo, J.; Liu, L.; Wang, L.F.; Wang, F.S.; Wang, X. Mixed Lineage Kinase Domain-like Protein MLKL Causes Necrotic Membrane Disruption upon Phosphorylation by RIP3. *Mol. Cell* **2014**, *54*, 133–146. [CrossRef]
263. Yang, H.; Ma, Y.; Chen, G.; Zhou, H.; Yamazaki, T.; Klein, C.; Pietrocola, F.; Vacchelli, E.; Souquere, S.; Sauvat, A.; et al. Contribution of RIP3 and MLKL to immunogenic cell death signaling in cancer chemotherapy. *Oncoimmunology* **2016**, *5*, e1149673. [CrossRef]
264. Aaes, T.L.; Kaczmarek, A.; Delvaeye, T.; De Craene, B.; De Koker, S.; Heyndrickx, L.; Delrue, I.; Taminau, J.; Wiernicki, B.; De Groote, P.; et al. Vaccination with Necroptotic Cancer Cells Induces Efficient Anti-tumor Immunity. *Cell Rep.* **2016**, *15*, 274–287. [CrossRef]
265. Kroemer, G.; Galluzzi, L.; Kepp, O.; Zitvogel, L. Immunogenic Cell Death in Cancer Therapy. *Annu. Rev. Immunol.* **2013**, *31*, 51–72. [CrossRef] [PubMed]
266. Obeid, M.; Tesniere, A.; Ghiringhelli, F.; Fimia, G.M.; Apetoh, L.; Perfettini, J.L.; Castedo, M.; Mignot, G.; Panaretakis, T.; Casares, N.; et al. Calreticulin exposure dictates the immunogenicity of cancer cell death. *Nat. Med.* **2007**, *13*, 54–61. [CrossRef]
267. Zappasodi, R.; Pupa, S.M.; Ghedini, G.C.; Bongarzone, I.; Magni, M.; Cabras, A.D.; Colombo, M.P.; Carlo-Stella, C.; Gianni, A.M.; Di Nicola, M. Improved clinical outcome in indolent B-cell lymphoma patients vaccinated with autologous tumor cells experiencing immunogenic death. *Cancer Res.* **2010**, *70*, 9062–9072. [CrossRef] [PubMed]
268. Wemeau, M.; Kepp, O.; Tesnière, A.; Panaretakis, T.; Flament, C.; De Botton, S.; Zitvogel, L.; Kroemer, G.; Chaput, N. Calreticulin exposure on malignant blasts predicts a cellular anticancer immune response in patients with acute myeloid leukemia. *Cell Death Dis.* **2010**, *1*, e104. [CrossRef]
269. Peng, R.Q.; Chen, Y.B.; Ding, Y.; Zhang, R.; Zhang, X.; Yu, X.J.; Zhou, Z.W.; Zeng, Y.X.; Zhang, X.S. Expression of calreticulin is associated with infiltration of T-cells in stage III B colon cancer. *World J. Gastroenterol.* **2010**, *16*, 2428–2434. [CrossRef] [PubMed]
270. Michaud, M.; Martins, I.; Sukkurwala, A.Q.; Adjemian, S.; Ma, Y.; Pellegatti, P.; Shen, S.; Kepp, O.; Scoazec, M.; Mignot, G.; et al. Autophagy-dependent anticancer immune responses induced by chemotherapeutic agents in mice. *Science 80* **2011**, *334*, 1573–1577. [CrossRef]
271. Andersson, U.; Tracey, K.J. HMGB1 Is a Therapeutic Target for Sterile Inflammation and Infection. *Annu. Rev. Immunol.* **2011**, *29*, 139–162. [CrossRef]
272. Apetoh, L.; Ghiringhelli, F.; Tesniere, A.; Obeid, M.; Ortiz, C.; Criollo, A.; Mignot, G.; Maiuri, M.C.; Ullrich, E.; Saulnier, P.; et al. Toll-like receptor 4–dependent contribution of the immune system to anticancer chemotherapy and radiotherapy. *Nat. Med.* **2007**, *13*, 1050–1059. [CrossRef]
273. Ma, Y.; Aymeric, L.; Locher, C.; Mattarollo, S.R.; Delahaye, N.F.; Pereira, P.; Boucontet, L.; Apetoh, L.; Ghiringhelli, F.; Casares, N.; et al. Contribution of IL-17-producing $\gamma\delta$ T cells to the efficacy of anticancer chemotherapy. *J. Exp. Med.* **2011**, *208*, 869. [CrossRef]
274. Fan, Y.; Kuai, R.; Xu, Y.; Ochyl, L.J.; Irvine, D.J.; Moon, J.J. Immunogenic Cell Death Amplified by Co-localized Adjuvant Delivery for Cancer Immunotherapy. *Nano Lett.* **2017**, *17*, 7387–7393. [CrossRef]

275. Kuai, R.; Yuan, W.; Son, S.; Nam, J.; Xu, Y.; Fan, Y.; Schwendeman, A.; Moon, J.J. Elimination of established tumors with nanodisc-based combination chemoimmunotherapy. *Sci. Adv.* **2018**, *4*, eaao1736. [CrossRef] [PubMed]
276. Bear, A.S.; Kennedy, L.C.; Young, J.K.; Perna, S.K.; Mattos Almeida, J.P.; Lin, A.Y.; Eckels, P.C.; Drezek, R.A.; Foster, A.E. Elimination of Metastatic Melanoma Using Gold Nanoshell-Enabled Photothermal Therapy and Adoptive T Cell Transfer. *PLoS ONE* **2013**, *8*, e69073. [CrossRef] [PubMed]
277. He, C.; Duan, X.; Guo, N.; Chan, C.; Poon, C.; Weichselbaum, R.R.; Lin, W. Core-shell nanoscale coordination polymers combine chemotherapy and photodynamic therapy to potentiate checkpoint blockade cancer immunotherapy. *Nat. Commun.* **2016**, *7*, 1–12. [CrossRef] [PubMed]
278. Min, Y.; Roche, K.C.; Tian, S.; Eblan, M.J.; McKinnon, K.P.; Caster, J.M.; Chai, S.; Herring, L.E.; Zhang, L.; Zhang, T.; et al. Antigen-capturing nanoparticles improve the abscopal effect and cancer immunotherapy. *Nat. Nanotechnol.* **2017**, *12*, 877–882. [CrossRef] [PubMed]
279. Menger, L.; Vacchelli, E.; Adjemian, S.; Martins, I.; Ma, Y.; Shen, S.; Yamazaki, T.; Sukkurwala, A.Q.; Michaud, M.; Mignot, G.; et al. Cardiac glycosides exert anticancer effects by inducing immunogenic cell death. *Sci. Transl. Med.* **2012**, *4*, 143ra99. [CrossRef]
280. Martins, I.; Kepp, O.; Schlemmer, F.; Adjemian, S.; Tailler, M.; Shen, S.; Michaud, M.; Menger, L.; Gdoura, A.; Tajeddine, N.; et al. Restoration of the immunogenicity of cisplatin-induced cancer cell death by endoplasmic reticulum stress. *Oncogene* **2011**, *30*, 1147–1158. [CrossRef]
281. Tray, N.; Weber, J.S.; Adams, S. Predictive biomarkers for checkpoint immunotherapy: Current status and challenges for clinical application. *Cancer Immunol. Res.* **2018**, *6*, 1122–1128. [CrossRef]
282. Spencer, K.R.; Wang, J.; Silk, A.W.; Ganesan, S.; Kaufman, H.L.; Mehnert, J.M. Biomarkers for Immunotherapy: Current Developments and Challenges. *Am. Soc. Clin. Oncol. Educ. B.* **2016**, e493–e503. [CrossRef]
283. Nelson, D.; Fisher, S.; Robinson, B. The "Trojan Horse" Approach to Tumor Immunotherapy: Targeting the Tumor Microenvironment. *J. Immunol. Res.* **2014**, *2014*, 789069. [CrossRef]
284. Masucci, G.V.; Cesano, A.; Hawtin, R.; Janetzki, S.; Zhang, J.; Kirsch, I.; Dobbin, K.K.; Alvarez, J.; Robbins, P.B.; Selvan, S.R.; et al. Validation of biomarkers to predict response to immunotherapy in cancer: Volume I-pre-analytical and analytical validation. *J. Immunother. Cancer* **2016**, *4*, 76. [CrossRef]
285. FDA-NIH Biomarker Working Group. *BEST (Biomarkers, EndpointS, and Other Tools)*; Food and Drug Administration (US): New York, NY, USA, 2017; Volume 55. [CrossRef]
286. Califf, R.M. Biomarker definitions and their applications. *Exp. Biol. Med.* **2018**, *243*, 213–221. [CrossRef] [PubMed]
287. May, J.Y.; Negrier, S.; Combaret, V.; Attali, S.; Goillot, E.; Mercatello, A.; Ravault, A.; Tourani, J.M.; Moskovtchenko, J.F.; Philip, T.; et al. Serum Level of Interleukin 6 as a Prognosis Factor in Metastatic Renal Cell Carcinoma. *Cancer Res.* **1992**, *52*, 3317–3322.
288. Tartour, E.; Blay, J.Y.; Dorval, T.; Escudier, B.; Mosseri, V.; Douillard, J.Y.; Deneux, L.; Gorin, I.; Negrier, S.; Mathiot, C.; et al. Predictors of clinical response to interleukin-2-based immunotherapy in melanoma patients: A French multiinstitutional study. *J. Clin. Oncol.* **1996**, *14*, 1697–1703. [CrossRef] [PubMed]
289. Sabatino, M.; Kim-Schulze, S.; Panelli, M.C.; Stroncek, D.; Wang, E.; Taback, B.; Kim, D.W.; DeRaffele, G.; Pos, Z.; Marincola, F.M.; et al. Serum vascular endothelial growth factor and fibronectin predict clinical response to high-dose interleukin-2 therapy. *J. Clin. Oncol.* **2009**, *27*, 2645–2652. [CrossRef] [PubMed]
290. Simeone, E.; Gentilcore, G.; Giannarelli, D.; Grimaldi, A.M.; Caracò, C.; Curvietto, M.; Esposito, A.; Paone, M.; Palla, M.; Cavalcanti, E.; et al. Immunological and biological changes during ipilimumab treatment and their potential correlation with clinical response and survival in patients with advanced melanoma. *Cancer Immunol. Immunother.* **2014**, *63*, 675–683. [CrossRef] [PubMed]
291. Hannani, D.; Vétizou, M.; Enot, D.; Rusakiewicz, S.; Chaput, N.; Klatzmann, D.; Desbois, M.; Jacquelot, N.; Vimond, N.; Chouaib, S.; et al. Anticancer immunotherapy by CTLA-4 blockade: Obligatory contribution of IL-2 receptors and negative prognostic impact of soluble CD25. *Cell Res.* **2015**, *25*, 208–224. [CrossRef]
292. Fridman, W.H.; Pagès, F.; Sautès-Fridman, C.; Galon, J. The immune contexture in human tumours: Impact on clinical outcome. *Nat. Rev. Cancer* **2012**, *12*, 298–306. [CrossRef]
293. Galon, J.; Angell, H.K.; Bedognetti, D.; Marincola, F.M. The Continuum of Cancer Immunosurveillance: Prognostic, Predictive, and Mechanistic Signatures. *Immunity* **2013**, *39*, 11–26. [CrossRef]

294. Gnjatic, S.; Bronte, V.; Brunet, L.R.; Butler, M.O.; Disis, M.L.; Galon, J.; Hakansson, L.G.; Hanks, B.A.; Karanikas, V.; Khleif, S.N.; et al. Identifying baseline immune-related biomarkers to predict clinical outcome of immunotherapy. *J. Immunother. Cancer* **2017**, *5*, 1–18. [CrossRef]
295. Schmidt, H.; Bastholt, L.; Geertsen, P.; Christensen, I.J.; Larsen, S.; Gehl, J.; Von Der Maase, H. Elevated neutrophil and monocyte counts in peripheral blood are associated with poor survival in patients with metastatic melanoma: A prognostic model. *Br. J. Cancer* **2005**, *93*, 273–278. [CrossRef]
296. Powell, D.J.; Dudley, M.E.; Robbins, P.F.; Rosenberg, S.A. Transition of late-stage effector T cells to CD27+ CD28+ tumor-reactive effector memory T cells in humans after adoptive cell transfer therapy. *Blood* **2005**, *105*, 241–250. [CrossRef] [PubMed]
297. Ochsenbein, A.F.; Riddell, S.R.; Brown, M.; Corey, L.; Baerlocher, G.M.; Lansdorp, P.M.; Greenberg, P.D. CD27 Expression Promotes Long-Term Survival of Functional Effector–Memory CD8+Cytotoxic T Lymphocytes in HIV-infected Patients. *J. Exp. Med.* **2004**, *200*, 1407–1417. [CrossRef] [PubMed]
298. MacFarlane, A.W.; Jillab, M.; Plimack, E.R.; Hudes, G.R.; Uzzo, R.G.; Litwin, S.; Dulaimi, E.; Al-Saleem, T.; Campbell, K.S. PD-1 Expression on Peripheral Blood Cells Increases with Stage in Renal Cell Carcinoma Patients and Is Rapidly Reduced after Surgical Tumor Resection. *Cancer Immunol. Res.* **2014**, *2*, 320–331. [CrossRef] [PubMed]
299. Yuan, J.; Adamow, M.; Ginsberg, B.A.; Rasalan, T.S.; Ritter, E.; Gallardo, H.F.; Xu, Y.; Pogoriler, E.; Terzulli, S.L.; Kuk, D.; et al. Integrated NY-ESO-1 antibody and CD8 + T-cell responses correlate with clinical benefit in advanced melanoma patients treated with ipilimumab. *Proc. Natl. Acad. Sci. USA* **2011**, *108*, 16723–16728. [CrossRef]
300. Zhang, J.Y.; Looi, K.S.; Tan, E.M. Identification of tumor-associated antigens as diagnostic and predictive biomarkers in cancer. *Methods Mol. Biol.* **2009**, *520*, 1–10. [CrossRef]
301. Lu, M.; Nakamura, R.M.; Dent, E.D.B.; Zhang, J.Y.; Nielsen, F.C.; Christiansen, J.; Chan, E.K.L.; Tan, E.M. Aberrant expression of fetal RNA-binding protein p62 in liver cancer and liver cirrhosis. *Am. J. Pathol.* **2001**, *159*, 945–953. [CrossRef]
302. Hoo, L.S.; Zhang, J.Y.; Chan, E.K.L. Cloning and characterization of a novel 90 kDa "companion" auto-antigen of p62 overexpressed in cancer. *Oncogene* **2002**, *21*, 5006–5015. [CrossRef]
303. Noguchi, T.; Kato, T.; Wang, L.; Maeda, Y.; Ikeda, H.; Sato, E.; Knuth, A.; Gnjatic, S.; Ritter, G.; Sakaguchi, S.; et al. Intracellular Tumor-Associated Antigens Represent Effective Targets for Passive Immunotherapy. *AACR* **2012**, *72*, 1672–1682. [CrossRef]
304. Germain, C.; Gnjatic, S.; Dieu-Nosjean, M.-C. Tertiary Lymphoid Structure-Associated B Cells are Key Players in Anti-Tumor Immunity. *Front. Immunol.* **2015**, *6*, 67. [CrossRef]
305. Germain, C.; Gnjatic, S.; Tamzalit, F.; Knockaert, S.; Remark, R.; Erémyer´erémy Goc, J.; Lepelley, A.; Becht, E.; Katsahian, S.; Bizouard, G.; et al. Presence of B Cells in Tertiary Lymphoid Structures Is Associated with a Protective Immunity in Patients with Lung Cancer. *Am. J. Respir. Crit. Care Med.* **2014**, *189*, 832–844. [CrossRef]
306. Videssa Breast | Detección de Cáncer de Mama a Base de Sangre. Available online: https://www.provistadx.com/videssa-breast (accessed on 16 May 2020).
307. Gajewski, T.F.; Schreiber, H.; Fu, Y.X. Innate and adaptive immune cells in the tumor microenvironment. *Nat. Immunol.* **2013**, *14*, 1014–1022. [CrossRef]
308. De Vries, I.J.M.; Bernsen, M.R.; van Geloof, W.L.; Scharenborg, N.M.; Lesterhuis, W.J.; Rombout, P.D.M.; Van Muijen, G.N.P.; Figdor, C.G.; Punt, C.J.A.; Ruiter, D.J.; et al. In situ detection of antigen-specific T cells in cryo-sections using MHC class I tetramers after dendritic cell vaccination of melanoma patients. *Cancer Immunol. Immunother.* **2007**, *56*, 1667–1676. [CrossRef] [PubMed]
309. Robins, H.S.; Campregher, P.V.; Srivastava, S.K.; Wacher, A.; Turtle, C.J.; Kahsai, O.; Riddell, S.R.; Warren, E.H.; Carlson, C.S. Comprehensive assessment of T-cell receptor β-chain diversity in αβ T cells. *Blood* **2009**, *114*, 4099–4107. [CrossRef]
310. Ji, R.-R.; Chasalow, S.D.; Wang, L.; Hamid, O.; Schmidt, H.; Cogswell, J.; Alaparthy, S.; Berman, D.; Jure-Kunkel, M.; Siemers, N.O.; et al. An immune-active tumor microenvironment favors clinical response to ipilimumab. *Cancer Immunol. Immunother.* **2012**, *61*, 1019–1031. [CrossRef] [PubMed]
311. Herbst, R.S.; Soria, J.-C.; Kowanetz, M.; Fine, G.D.; Hamid, O.; Gordon, M.S.; Sosman, J.A.; McDermott, D.F.; Powderly, J.D.; Gettinger, S.N.; et al. Predictive correlates of response to the anti-PD-L1 antibody MPDL3280A in cancer patients. *Nature* **2014**, *515*, 563–567. [CrossRef] [PubMed]

312. Ahmadzadeh, M.; Johnson, L.A.; Heemskerk, B.; Wunderlich, J.R.; Dudley, M.E.; White, D.E.; Rosenberg, S.A. Tumor antigen-specific CD8 T cells infiltrating the tumor express high levels of PD-1 and are functionally impaired. *Blood* **2009**, *114*, 1537–1544. [CrossRef]
313. Meng, X.; Huang, Z.; Teng, F.; Xing, L.; Yu, J. Predictive biomarkers in PD-1/PD-L1 checkpoint blockade immunotherapy. *Cancer Treat. Rev.* **2015**, *41*, 868–876. [CrossRef]
314. Van Allen, E.M.; Miao, D.; Schilling, B.; Shukla, S.A.; Blank, C.; Zimmer, L.; Sucker, A.; Hillen, U.; Foppen, M.H.G.; Goldinger, S.M.; et al. Genomic correlates of response to CTLA-4 blockade in metastatic melanoma. *Science 80* **2015**, *350*, 207–211. [CrossRef]
315. Chan, T.A.; Wolchok, J.D.; Snyder, A. Correction: Genetic basis for clinical response to CTLA-4 blockade in melanoma: To the editor. *N. Engl. J. Med.* **2015**, *373*, 1984. [CrossRef]
316. Cirenajwis, H.; Ekedahl, H.; Lauss, M.; Harbst, K.; Carneiro, A.; Enoksson, J.; Rosengren, F.; Werner-Hartman, L.; Törngren, T.; Kvist, A.; et al. Molecular stratification of metastatic melanoma using gene expression profiling: Prediction of survival outcome and benefit from molecular targeted therapy. *Oncotarget* **2015**, *6*, 12297–12309. [CrossRef]
317. Stoll, G.; Enot, D.; Mlecnik, B.; Galon, J.; Zitvogel, L.; Kroemer, G. Immune-related gene signatures predict the outcome of neoadjuvant chemotherapy. *Oncoimmunology* **2014**, *3*, e27884. [CrossRef] [PubMed]
318. Stenzinger, A.; Allen, J.D.; Maas, J.; Stewart, M.D.; Merino, D.M.; Wempe, M.M.; Dietel, M. Tumor mutational burden standardization initiatives: Recommendations for consistent tumor mutational burden assessment in clinical samples to guide immunotherapy treatment decisions. *Genes Chromosom. Cancer* **2019**, *58*, 578–588. [CrossRef] [PubMed]
319. Lawrence, M.S.; Stojanov, P.; Polak, P.; Kryukov, G.V.; Cibulskis, K.; Sivachenko, A.; Carter, S.L.; Stewart, C.; Mermel, C.H.; Roberts, S.A.; et al. Mutational heterogeneity in cancer and search for new cancer genes. *Nature* **2013**, *499*, 214–218. [CrossRef] [PubMed]
320. Chalmers, Z.R.; Connelly, C.F.; Fabrizio, D.; Gay, L.; Ali, S.M.; Ennis, R.; Schrock, A.; Campbell, B.; Shlien, A.; Chmielecki, J.; et al. Analysis of 100,000 human cancer genomes reveals the landscape of tumor mutational burden. *Genome Med.* **2017**, *9*, 34. [CrossRef]
321. Health, N.; Bank, B.B.; Nahmani, A.; Cancer, P.; Trust, R.T.H.; Foundation, P.; Ministry, S. Signatures of mutational processes in human cancer. *Nature* **2013**, *500*, 1–108. [CrossRef]
322. Chen, Y.P.; Zhang, Y.; Lv, J.W.; Li, Y.Q.; Wang, Y.Q.; He, Q.M.; Yang, X.J.; Sun, Y.; Mao, Y.P.; Yun, J.P.; et al. Genomic Analysis of Tumor Microenvironment Immune Types across 14 Solid Cancer Types: Immunotherapeutic Implications. *Theranostics* **2017**, *7*, 3585. [CrossRef]
323. Snyder, A.; Makarov, V.; Merghoub, T.; Yuan, J.; Zaretsky, J.M.; Desrichard, A.; Walsh, L.A.; Postow, M.A.; Wong, P.; Ho, T.S.; et al. Genetic Basis for Clinical Response to CTLA-4 Blockade in Melanoma. *N. Engl. J. Med.* **2014**, *371*, 2189–2199. [CrossRef]
324. Yarchoan, M.; Hopkins, A.; Jaffee, E.M. Tumor mutational burden and response rate to PD-1 inhibition. *N. Engl. J. Med.* **2017**, *377*, 2500–2501. [CrossRef]
325. Sharma, P.; Allison, J.P. The future of immune checkpoint therapy. *Science 80* **2015**, *348*, 56–61. [CrossRef]
326. Vigneron, N.; Stroobant, V.; Chapiro, J.; Ooms, A.; Degiovanni, G.; Morel, S.; Van Der Bruggen, P.; Boon, T.; Van Den Eynde, B.J. An Antigenic Peptide Produced by Peptide Splicing in the Proteasome. *Science 80* **2004**, *304*, 587–590. [CrossRef]
327. Madsen, C.B.; Petersen, C.; Lavrsen, K.; Harndahl, M.; Buus, S.; Clausen, H.; Pedersen, A.E.; Wandall, H.H. Cancer Associated Aberrant Protein O-Glycosylation Can Modify Antigen Processing and Immune Response. *PLoS ONE* **2012**, *7*, e50139. [CrossRef] [PubMed]
328. Cobbold, M.; De La Pena, H.; Norris, A.; Polefrone, J.M.; Qian, J.; English, A.M.; Cummings, K.L.; Penny, S.; Turner, J.E.; Cottine, J.; et al. MHC Class I-Associated Phosphopeptides Are the Targets of Memory-like Immunity in Leukemia. *Sci. Transl. Med.* **2013**, *5*, 203ra125. [CrossRef] [PubMed]
329. Meléndez, B.; Van Campenhout, C.; Rorive, S.; Remmelink, M.; Salmon, I.; D'Haene, N. Methods of measurement for tumor mutational burden in tumor tissue. *Transl. Lung Cancer Res.* **2018**, *7*, 661–667. [CrossRef] [PubMed]
330. Zou, W.; Wolchok, J.D.; Chen, L. PD-L1 (B7-H1) and PD-1 pathway blockade for cancer therapy: Mechanisms, response biomarkers, and combinations. *Sci. Transl. Med.* **2016**, *8*, 328rv4. [CrossRef]

331. Garon, E.B.; Rizvi, N.A.; Hui, R.; Leighl, N.; Balmanoukian, A.S.; Eder, J.P.; Patnaik, A.; Aggarwal, C.; Gubens, M.; Horn, L.; et al. Pembrolizumab for the treatment of non-small-cell lung cancer. *N. Engl. J. Med.* **2015**, *372*, 2018–2028. [CrossRef]
332. Taube, J.M.; Klein, A.; Brahmer, J.R.; Xu, H.; Pan, X.; Kim, J.H.; Chen, L.; Pardoll, D.M.; Topalian, S.L.; Anders, R.A. Association of PD-1, PD-1 ligands, and other features of the tumor immune microenvironment with response to anti-PD-1 therapy. *Clin. Cancer Res.* **2014**, *20*, 5064–5074. [CrossRef]
333. Ock, C.Y.; Keam, B.; Kim, S.; Lee, J.S.; Kim, M.; Kim, T.M.; Jeon, Y.K.; Kim, D.W.; Chung, D.H.; Heo, D.S. Pan-Cancer Immunogenomic Perspective on the Tumor Microenvironment Based on PD-L1 and CD8 T-Cell Infiltration. *Clin. Cancer Res.* **2016**, *22*, 2261–2270. [CrossRef]
334. Teng, M.W.L.; Ngiow, S.F.; Ribas, A.; Smyth, M.J. Classifying Cancers Based on T-cell Infiltration and PD-L1. *Cancer Res* **2015**, *75*, 2139–2145. [CrossRef]
335. Bald, T.; Landsberg, J.; Lopez-Ramos, D.; Renn, M.; Glodde, N.; Jansen, P.; Gaffal, E.; Steitz, J.; Tolba, R.; Kalinke, U.; et al. Immune cell-poor melanomas benefit from PD-1 blockade after targeted type I IFN activation. *Cancer Discov.* **2014**, *4*, 674–687. [CrossRef]
336. Kalbasi, A.; June, C.H.; Haas, N.; Vapiwala, N. Radiation and immunotherapy: A synergistic combination. *J. Clin. Investig.* **2013**, *123*, 2756–2763. [CrossRef]
337. Robert, L.; Tsoi, J.; Wang, X.; Emerson, R.; Homet, B.; Chodon, T.; Mok, S.; Huang, R.R.; Cochran, A.J.; Comin-Anduix, B.; et al. CTLA4 blockade broadens the peripheral T-cell receptor repertoire. *Clin. Cancer Res.* **2014**, *20*, 2424–2432. [CrossRef] [PubMed]
338. Chowell, D.; Morris, L.G.T.; Grigg, C.M.; Weber, J.K.; Samstein, R.M.; Makarov, V.; Kuo, F.; Kendall, S.M.; Requena, D.; Riaz, N.; et al. Patient HLA class I genotype influences cancer response to checkpoint blockade immunotherapy. *Science 80* **2018**, *359*, 582–587. [CrossRef]
339. Robert, L.; Harview, C.; Emerson, R.; Wang, X.; Mok, S.; Homet, B.; Comin-Anduix, B.; Koya, R.C.; Robins, H.; Tumeh, P.C.; et al. Distinct immunological mechanisms of CTLA-4 and PD-1 blockade revealed by analyzing TCR usage in blood lymphocytes. *Oncoimmunology* **2014**, *3*, e29244. [CrossRef] [PubMed]
340. Bobisse, S.; Foukas, P.G.; Coukos, G.; Harari, A. Neoantigen-based cancer immunotherapy. *Ann. Transl. Med.* **2016**, *4*, 14. [CrossRef] [PubMed]
341. Castle, J.C.; Kreiter, S.; Diekmann, J.; L€Ower, M.; Van De Roemer, N.; De Graaf, J.; Selmi, A.; Diken, M.; Boegel, S.; Paret, C.; et al. Exploiting the Mutanome for Tumor Vaccination. *AACR* **2012**, *72*, 1081–1091. [CrossRef]
342. van Rooij, N.; van Buuren, M.M.; Philips, D.; Velds, A.; Toebes, M.; Heemskerk, B.; van Dijk, L.J.A.; Behjati, S.; Hilkmann, H.; el Atmioui, D.; et al. Tumor Exome Analysis Reveals Neoantigen-Specific T-Cell Reactivity in an Ipilimumab-Responsive Melanoma. *J. Clin. Oncol.* **2013**, *31*, e439–e442. [CrossRef]
343. Wick, D.A.; Webb, J.R.; Nielsen, J.S.; Martin, S.D.; Kroeger, D.R.; Milne, K.; Castellarin, M.; Twumasi-Boateng, K.; Watson, P.H.; Holt, R.A.; et al. Surveillance of the Tumor Mutanome by T Cells during Progression from Primary to Recurrent Ovarian Cancer. *Hum. Cancer Biol.* **2014**, *20*, 1125–1134. [CrossRef]
344. Kreiter, S.; Vormehr, M.; van de Roemer, N.; Diken, M.; Löwer, M.; Diekmann, J.; Boegel, S.; Schrörs, B.; Vascotto, F.; Castle, J.C.; et al. Mutant MHC class II epitopes drive therapeutic immune responses to cancer. *Nature* **2015**, *520*, 692–696. [CrossRef]
345. Vogelstein, B.; Papadopoulos, N.; Velculescu, V.E.; Zhou, S.; Diaz, L.A.; Kinzler, K.W. Cancer Genome Landscapes. *Science 80* **2013**, *339*, 1546–1558. [CrossRef]
346. Rajasagi, M.; Shukla, S.A.; Fritsch, E.F.; Keskin, D.B.; DeLuca, D.; Carmona, E.; Zhang, W.; Sougnez, C.; Cibulskis, K.; Sidney, J.; et al. Systematic identification of personal tumor-specific neoantigens in chronic lymphocytic leukemia. *Blood* **2014**, *124*, 453–462. [CrossRef]
347. Lundegaard, C.; Lund, O.; Nielsen, M. Prediction of epitopes using neural network based methods. *J. Immunol. Methods* **2011**, *374*, 26–34. [CrossRef]
348. Wirth, T.C.; Kühnel, F. Neoantigen targeting—Dawn of a new era in cancer immunotherapy? *Front. Immunol.* **2017**, *8*, 1848. [CrossRef]
349. Kloor, M.; Michel, S.; Von Knebel Doeberitz, M. Immune evasion of microsatellite unstable colorectal cancers. *Int. J. Cancer* **2010**, *127*, 1001–1010. [CrossRef]
350. Axelrod, M.L.; Cook, R.S.; Johnson, D.B.; Balko, J.M. Biological consequences of MHC-II expression by tumor cells in cancer. *Clin. Cancer Res.* **2019**, *25*, 2392–2402. [CrossRef] [PubMed]

351. Geyer, P.E.; Holdt, L.M.; Teupser, D.; Mann, M. Revisiting biomarker discovery by plasma proteomics. *Mol. Syst. Biol.* **2017**, *13*, 942. [CrossRef] [PubMed]
352. Rodig, S.J.; Gusenleitner, D.; Jackson, D.G.; Gjini, E.; Giobbie-Hurder, A.; Jin, C.; Chang, H.; Lovitch, S.B.; Horak, C.; Weber, J.S.; et al. MHC proteins confer differential sensitivity to CTLA-4 and PD-1 blockade in untreated metastatic melanoma. *Sci. Transl. Med.* **2018**, *10*, eaar3342. [CrossRef]
353. Johnson, D.B.; Estrada, M.V.; Salgado, R.; Sanchez, V.; Doxie, D.B.; Opalenik, S.R.; Vilgelm, A.E.; Feld, E.; Johnson, A.S.; Greenplate, A.R.; et al. Melanoma-specific MHC-II expression represents a tumour-autonomous phenotype and predicts response to anti-PD-1/PD-L1 therapy. *Nat. Commun.* **2016**, *7*, 10582. [CrossRef] [PubMed]
354. Fritsche, J.; Rakitsch, B.; Hoffgaard, F.; Römer, M.; Schuster, H.; Kowalewski, D.J.; Priemer, M.; Stos-Zweifel, V.; Hörzer, H.; Satelli, A.; et al. Translating Immunopeptidomics to Immunotherapy-Decision-Making for Patient and Personalized Target Selection. *Proteomics* **2018**, *18*, 1700284. [CrossRef] [PubMed]
355. Britten, C.M.; Singh-Jasuja, H.; Flamion, B.; Hoos, A.; Huber, C.; Kallen, K.J.; Khleif, S.N.; Kreiter, S.; Nielsen, M.; Rammensee, H.G.; et al. The regulatory landscape for actively personalized cancer immunotherapies. *Nat. Biotechnol.* **2013**, *31*, 880–882. [CrossRef] [PubMed]
356. Fortier, M.H.; Caron, É.; Hardy, M.P.; Voisin, G.; Lemieux, S.; Perreault, C.; Thibault, P. The MHC class I peptide repertoire is molded by the transcriptome. *J. Exp. Med.* **2008**, *205*, 595–610. [CrossRef] [PubMed]
357. Weinzierl, A.O.; Lemmel, C.; Schoor, O.; Müller, M.; Krüger, T.; Wernet, D.; Hennenlotter, J.; Stenzl, A.; Klingel, K.; Rammensee, H.G.; et al. Distorted relation between mRNA copy number and corresponding major histocompatibility complex ligand density on the cell surface. *Mol. Cell. Proteom.* **2007**, *6*, 102–113. [CrossRef] [PubMed]
358. Bassani-Sternberg, M.; Barnea, E.; Beer, I.; Avivi, I.; Katz, T.; Admon, A. Soluble plasma HLA peptidome as a potential source for cancer biomarkers. *Proc. Natl. Acad. Sci. USA* **2010**, *107*, 18769–18776. [CrossRef]
359. Zavazava, N.; Kronke, M. Soluble HLA class I molecules induce apoptosis in alloreactive cytotoxic T lymphocytes. *Nat. Med.* **1996**, *2*, 1267. [CrossRef] [PubMed]
360. HUPO-Proyecto de Inmunopéptido Humano. Available online: https://hupo.org/human-immuno-peptidome-project/ (accessed on 18 May 2020).
361. Shao, W.; Pedrioli, P.G.A.; Wolski, W.; Scurtescu, C.; Schmid, E.; Vizcaíno, J.A.; Courcelles, M.; Schuster, H.; Kowalewski, D.; Marino, F.; et al. The SysteMHC Atlas project. *Nucleic Acids Res.* **2018**, *46*, D1237–D1247. [CrossRef] [PubMed]
362. Andreatta, M.; Karosiene, E.; Rasmussen, M.; Stryhn, A.; Buus, S.; Nielsen, M. Accurate pan-specific prediction of peptide-MHC class II binding affinity with improved binding core identification. *Immunogenetics* **2015**, *67*, 641–650. [CrossRef] [PubMed]
363. Nielsen, M.; Lund, O. NN-align. An artificial neural network-based alignment algorithm for MHC class II peptide binding prediction. *BMC Bioinform.* **2009**, *10*, 296. [CrossRef]
364. Vita, R.; Overton, J.A.; Greenbaum, J.A.; Ponomarenko, J.; Clark, J.D.; Cantrell, J.R.; Wheeler, D.K.; Gabbard, J.L.; Hix, D.; Sette, A.; et al. The immune epitope database (IEDB) 3.0. *Nucleic Acids Res.* **2015**, *43*, D405–D412. [CrossRef]
365. Tan, E.M. Antinuclear Antibodies: Diagnostic Markers for Autoimmune Diseases and Probes for Cell Biology. *Adv. Immunol.* **1989**, *44*, 93–151. [CrossRef]
366. Crawford, L.V.; Pim, D.C.; Bulbrook, R.D. Detection of antibodies against the cellular protein p53 in sera from patients with breast cancer. *Int. J. Cancer* **1982**, *30*, 403–408. [CrossRef]
367. Tan, E.M.; Zhang, J. Autoantibodies to tumor-associated antigens: Reporters from the immune system. *Immunol. Rev.* **2008**, *222*, 328–340. [CrossRef]
368. Tan, E.M.; Shi, F.D. Relative paradigms between autoantibodies in lupus and autoantibodies in cancer. *Clin. Exp. Immunol.* **2003**, *134*, 169–177. [CrossRef] [PubMed]
369. Lubin, R.; Zalcman, G.; Bouchet, L.; Tr É Daniel, J.; Legros, Y.; Cazals, D.; Hirsch, A.; Soussi, T. Serum p53 antibodies as early markers of lung cancer. *Nat. Med.* **1995**, *1*, 701–702. [CrossRef]
370. Trivers, G.E.; De Benedetti, V.M.G.; Cawley, H.L.; Caron, G.; Harrington, A.M.; Bennett, W.P.; Jett, J.R.; Colby, T.V.; Tazelaar, H.; Pairolero, P.; et al. Anti-p53 Antibodies in Sera from Patients with Chronic Obstructive Pulmonary Disease Can Predate a Diagnosis of Cancer. *Clin. Cancer Res.* **1996**, *2*, 1767–1775.

371. Trivers, G.E.; Cawley, H.L.; Debenedetti, V.M.G.; Hollstein, M.; Marion, M.J.; Bennett, W.P.; Hoover, M.L.; Prives, C.C.; Tamburro, C.C.; Harris, C.C. Anti-p53 antibodies in sera of workers occupationally exposed to vinyl chloride. *J. Natl. Cancer Inst.* **1995**, *87*, 1400–1407. [CrossRef] [PubMed]
372. Imai, H.; Nakano, Y.; Kiyosawa, K.; Tan, E.M. Increasing titers and changing specificities of antinuclear antibodies in patients with chronic liver disease who develop hepatocellular carcinoma. *Cancer* **1993**, *71*, 26–35. [CrossRef]
373. Woessner, R.D.; Mattern, M.R.; Mirabelli, C.K.; Johnson, R.K.; Drake, F.H. Proliferation- and cell cycle-dependent differences in expression of the 170 kilodalton and 180 kilodalton forms of topoisomerase II in NIH-3T3 cells. *Cell Growth Differ.* **1991**, *2*, 209–214. [PubMed]
374. Winter, S.F.; Minna, J.D.; Johnson, B.E.; Takahashi, T.; Gazdar, A.F.; Carbone, D.P. Development of antibodies against p53 in lung cancer patients appears to be dependent on the type of p53 mutation. *Cancer Res.* **1992**, *52*, 4168–4174. [PubMed]
375. Suzuki, H.; Graziano, D.F.; McKolanis, J.; Finn, O.J. T cell-dependent antibody responses against aberrantly expressed cyclin B1 protein in patients with cancer and premalignant disease. *Clin. Cancer Res.* **2005**, *11*, 1521–1526. [CrossRef]
376. Wang, D.; Yang, L.; Zhang, P.; LaBaer, J.; Hermjakob, H.; Li, D.; Yu, X. AAgAtlas 1.0: A human autoantigen database. *Nucleic Acids Res.* **2017**, *45*, D769–D776. [CrossRef]
377. Soares, M.M.; Mehta, V.; Finn, O.J. Three Different Vaccines Based on the 140-Amino Acid MUC1 Peptide with Seven Tandemly Repeated Tumor-Specific Epitopes Elicit Distinct Immune Effector Mechanisms in Wild-Type Versus MUC1-Transgenic Mice with Different Potential for Tumor Rejection. *J. Immunol.* **2001**, *166*, 6555–6563. [CrossRef]
378. Kao, H.; Marto, J.A.; Hoffmann, T.K.; Shabanowitz, J.; Finkelstein, S.D.; Whiteside, T.L.; Hunt, D.F.; Finn, O.J. Identification of cyclin B1 as a shared human epithelial tumor-associated antigen recognized by T cells. *J. Exp. Med.* **2001**, *194*, 1313–1323. [CrossRef]
379. Wild, D. *The Immunoassay Handbook: Theory and Applications of Ligand Binding, ELISA and Related Techniques*; Newnes: Oxford, UK, 2013; ISBN 9780080970370.
380. Vogeser, M.; Seger, C. Mass spectrometry methods in clinical diagnostics—State of the art and perspectives. *TrAC-Trends Anal. Chem.* **2016**, *84*, 1–4. [CrossRef]
381. Pedersen, A.W.; Kopp, K.L.; Andersen, M.H.; Zocca, M.-B. Immunoregulatory antigens—Novel targets for cancer immunotherapy. *Chin. Clin. Oncol.* **2018**, *7*, 8. [CrossRef]
382. Montico, B.; Lapenta, C.; Ravo, M.; Martorelli, D.; Muraro, E.; Zeng, B.; Comaro, E.; Spada, M.; Donati, S.; Santini, S.M.; et al. Exploiting a new strategy to induce immunogenic cell death to improve dendritic cell-based vaccines for lymphoma immunotherapy. *Oncoimmunology* **2017**, *6*, e1356964. [CrossRef] [PubMed]
383. Garg, A.D.; Nowis, D.; Golab, J.; Vandenabeele, P.; Krysko, D.V.; Agostinis, P. Immunogenic cell death, DAMPs and anticancer therapeutics: An emerging amalgamation. *Biochim. Biophys. Acta-Rev. Cancer* **2010**, *1805*, 53–71. [CrossRef]
384. Das, D.K.; Feng, Y.; Mallis, R.J.; Li, X.; Keskin, D.B.; Hussey, R.E.; Brady, S.K.; Wang, J.H.; Wagner, G.; Reinherz, E.L.; et al. Force-dependent transition in the T-cell receptor β-subunit allosterically regulates peptide discrimination and pMHC bond lifetime. *Proc. Natl. Acad. Sci. USA* **2015**, *112*, 1517–1522. [CrossRef]
385. Yadav, M.; Jhunjhunwala, S.; Phung, Q.T.; Lupardus, P.; Tanguay, J.; Bumbaca, S.; Franci, C.; Cheung, T.K.; Fritsche, J.; Weinschenk, T.; et al. Predicting immunogenic tumour mutations by combining mass spectrometry and exome sequencing. *Nature* **2014**, *515*, 572–576. [CrossRef] [PubMed]
386. Reinherz, E.L. αβ TCR-mediated recognition: Relevance to tumor-antigen discovery and cancer immunotherapy. *Cancer Immunol. Res.* **2015**, *3*, 305–312. [CrossRef]
387. Sette, A.; Vitiello, A.; Reherman, B.; Fowler, P.; Nayersina, R.; Kast, W.M.; Melief, C.J.; Oseroff, C.; Yuan, L.; Ruppert, J.; et al. The relationship between class I binding affinity and immunogenicity of potential cytotoxic T cell epitopes. *J. Immunol.* **1994**, *153*, 5586–5592.

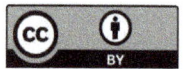

© 2020 by the authors. Licensee MDPI, Basel, Switzerland. This article is an open access article distributed under the terms and conditions of the Creative Commons Attribution (CC BY) license (http://creativecommons.org/licenses/by/4.0/).

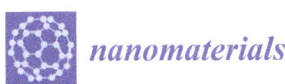

Review

Advances in Gold Nanoparticle-Based Combined Cancer Therapy

Kyle Bromma [1] and Devika B. Chithrani [1,2,3,4,*]

1. Department of Physics and Astronomy, University of Victoria, Victoria, BC V8P 5C2, Canada; kbromma@uvic.ca
2. British Columbia Cancer, Medical Physics, Victoria, BC V8R 6V5, Canada
3. Centre for Advanced Materials and Related Technologies (CAMTEC), University of Victoria, Victoria, BC V8P 5C2, Canada
4. Centre for Biomedical Research, University of Victoria, Victoria, BC V8P 5C2, Canada
* Correspondence: devikac@uvic.ca

Received: 20 July 2020; Accepted: 21 August 2020; Published: 26 August 2020

Abstract: According to the global cancer observatory (GLOBOCAN), there are approximately 18 million new cancer cases per year worldwide. Cancer therapies are largely limited to surgery, radiotherapy, and chemotherapy. In radiotherapy and chemotherapy, the maximum tolerated dose is presently being used to treat cancer patients. The integrated development of innovative nanoparticle (NP) based approaches will be a key to address one of the main issues in both radiotherapy and chemotherapy: normal tissue toxicity. Among other inorganic NP systems, gold nanoparticle (GNP) based systems offer the means to further improve chemotherapy through controlled delivery of chemotherapeutics, while local radiotherapy dose can be enhanced by targeting the GNPs to the tumor. There have been over 20 nanotechnology-based therapeutic products approved for clinical use in the past two decades. Hence, the goal of this review is to understand what we have achieved so far and what else we can do to accelerate clinical use of GNP-based therapeutic platforms to minimize normal tissue toxicity while increasing the efficacy of the treatment. Nanomedicine will revolutionize future cancer treatment options and our ultimate goal should be to develop treatments that have minimum side effects, for improving the quality of life of all cancer patients.

Keywords: gold nanoparticles; radiation; chemotherapy; radiosensitizer; drug delivery system; chemoradiotherapy

1. Introduction

According to American Cancer Society statistics in 2020, there will be an estimated 1.8 million new cancer cases diagnosed and 606,520 cancer deaths in the United States alone. Cancer is an abnormal growth of cells caused by multiple changes in gene expression leading to deregulation of the balance of cell death and proliferation, ultimately leading to an evolving population of cells that can invade tissues and metastasize to other sites [1]. The main types of cancer treatments include surgery, chemotherapy and radiotherapy according to the Canadian Cancer Society [2]. The treatment plan of each cancer patient will vary depending on the type of cancer and the advancement of cancer [2,3]. Radiotherapy is one of the most widely used treatment approaches, being used in approximately 50% of all cancer patients. In radiotherapy, a high dose of ionizing radiation is delivered to the tumor site, which interacts with and excites the atoms inside the cancer cells, causing damage to important structures, ultimately killing the cell [4]. Currently, the clinic mainly employs gamma or X-ray photons, ion-based electrons, or protons as radiation sources in the treatment [5,6]. While radiotherapy is widely used in many different types of cancers, a major issue still present is the normal tissue toxicity [7]. A photon beam will irradiate some of the surrounding healthy tissue no matter how well shaped or conformed the beam is to the dimensions of the tumor, and this dose to normal tissue limits the amount of radiation a patient can receive [8].

Chemotherapy is also used to eradicate micro-metastases and to improve local control of the primary tumor [9]. In chemotherapy, anticancer drugs are administered either orally or intravenously to disrupt the rapid overgrowth of malignant cells [10,11]. Similar to radiotherapy, the side effects caused by anti-cancer drugs remain as one of the important limitations in the advancement of cancer treatment [12,13]. Therefore, we need to improve the bioavailability of the drug in the tumor region, while confining them to this target, to reduce the amount of the drug needed, and thus the number, and severity, of side effects [14]. Some nanoparticle (NP)-based therapeutic systems have already been introduced into the pharmaceutical market. For example, Doxil, a polyethylene glycol (PEG)-liposome containing Doxorubicin, is approved for AIDS-related Kaposi's sarcoma, ovarian cancer, and multiple myeloma [15,16]. Liposomal drugs and polymer drug conjugates account for most of the FDA (Food and Drug Administration, Tulsa, OK, USA)-approved systems so far [17]. However, in radiotherapy, NP-driven radiosensitization strategies that use inorganic high-Z (atomic number) materials have been pursued to improve the local radiation dose and minimize the damage to surrounding healthy tissue [18]. The interaction of high-Z materials with therapeutic X-ray photons results in an increase in the production of cell damaging species, such as free radicals and low energy electrons [19,20]. Inorganic NP systems such as gold nanoparticles (GNPs), silver NPs, gadolinium-based NPs, lanthanide-based NPs, and titanium oxide nanotubes have been reported as radiosensitizers [21–27]. Gadolinium-based NPs offer an innovative approach because of their capacity to act as a radiosensitizer as well as a powerful contrast agent in magnetic resonance imaging [26]. The high Z-nature of silver-based NPs along with their antimicrobial properties made them a good candidate in radiotherapy [27]. However, GNPs are the most widely used NP system in radiotherapy due to their ease of production, high Z-nature, advantageous surface chemistry, and biocompatibility [25,28–30].

There are different gold-based nanotherapeutic systems available, such as spherical GNPs, gold nanorods, gold nanoshells, gold nanoclusters, and GNP-incorporated liposomal nanoparticles, with many new anisotropic geometries being developed regularly. Spherical GNPs are the most commonly used gold-based nanotherapeutic, as their production is relatively simple and alteration of size and surface chemistry, such as conjugation with polyethylene glycol, is easily achieved [31,32]. Further, GNPs are heavily studied for use in the treatment of cancer through X-ray irradiation and as an anticancer drug carrier [33]. The use of gold nano-rods and gold nanoshells for the treatment of cancer involves the induction of hyperthermia, due to their larger cross-section at near-infrared (NIR) frequencies [34,35]. A comprehensive review of the use of gold-based nanomaterials such as gold nanoshells and gold nanorods in photothermal therapy has been described previously by Vines et al. [36]. It has also recently been shown that gold-based nanotherapeutics can absorb radiofrequency (RF) frequencies and generate heat, opening an avenue to treat more deep-set tumors with the use of gold and hyperthermia-based options [37]. Although more research must be completed, the use of RF waves with gold nanomaterials is very promising. Furthermore, due to the surface plasmon resonance effect present in GNPs, visible light irradiation can also allow for hyperthermia via photothermal therapy, recently shown by Mendes et al. with a green laser light in combination with 14 nm GNPs and doxorubicin [38]. However, the penetration depth of green light is even less than NIR and is thus limited in applicability [39]. Due to their theranostic benefits, such as imaging and biosensing, along with therapeutic properties such as drug delivery, gold nanoclusters have emerged as a useful tool [40,41]. The use of gold nanoclusters can allow for molecular imaging, improving diagnostics and imaging in the future [42]. Ultrasmall gold nanoclusters have also emerged as a useful technology due to their near 100% renal clearance, allowing for the improved probing of disease when utilized as a biosensor [43]. Lipid-based nanoparticles are an avenue that is being explored due to their ability to encapsulate GNPs for radiosensitization purposes and simultaneously act as a drug delivery platform [44]. Utilizing liposomal nanoparticles as a 'smart' drug carrier can allow for controlled release of the internalized cargo, such as in response a NIR light source, allowing more control over the treatment process [45].

GNP-based platforms are being researched and have been tested extensively in the field of cancer nanomedicine [46]. For example, a novel nanomedicine that conjugated human tumor necrosis factor alpha (rhTNF) and thiolated PEG onto the surface of colloidal GNPs (named CYT-6091) has been tested in phase 1 clinical trial in cancer patients [47]. The results from the CYT-6091 trial showed that doses up to 600 µg/g of rhTNF were administered without encountering dose-limiting toxicity and was less toxic than a treatment with just rhTNF, as evidenced by a lack of hypertension in patients. Furthermore, the GNPs had gathered in the tumor and mostly avoided healthy tissue. Other phase 1 clinical trials involved the use of PEGylated gold nanoshells around a silica nanoparticle, called AuroLase®, in head and neck, lung, and prostate cancer, with laser irradiation [48–50]. Results have, however, not translated to an effective treatment outcome. Another early phase 1 clinical trial involves the use of NU-0129, a platform consisting of nucleic acids attached to the surface of spherical GNPs [51]. The goal of this study is to use the conjugated nucleic acids to bypass the blood-brain barrier and target the BcL2L12 gene present in recurrent glioblastoma. If successful, this platform could supress this gene, which would lead to reduced proliferation and containing the spread of the tumor. However, translation of GNPs to the clinic is still in progress, and further optimization of protocols will have to be elucidated before the majority of research can move out of the preclinical stage, as described in the extensive review by Schuemann et al. [52].

For patients with locally advanced disease, a combination of treatments, such as surgery with chemotherapy and/or radiotherapy is being used. A combination of chemotherapy and radiotherapy (referred to as chemoradiation) is a logical and reasonable approach that has greatly improved the cure rates of solid tumor [8,53]. This combined treatment modality provides local control of the primary tumor mass through radiation while tumor metastasis is suppressed through anticancer drugs [8]. One of the major limitations of chemoradiation as a treatment option is the normal-tissue toxicity, as either radiotherapy or chemotherapy can cause major normal tissue toxicity, as described previously. In order to overcome the normal tissue toxicity in current cancer treatment modalities mentioned previously, NPs are being used to enhance either the local radiation dose or improve delivery of anticancer drugs, or both, as seen in Figure 1. GNPs are one of the materials extensively tested for both radiotherapy and chemotherapy. Therefore, this review article will be focused on prospects of GNP-mediated cancer therapeutics.

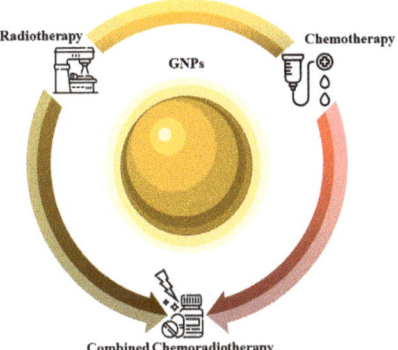

Figure 1. Gold nanoparticle-based cancer therapeutics. Radiotherapy and chemotherapy are the two main modalities, besides surgery, in treating cancer. However, normal tissue toxicity in both methods remains a large issue in limiting the effective dose to the tumor. Thus, gold nanomaterials have been introduced to improve the locally deposited dose into tumors and act as a drug delivery system. The combination of radiotherapy and chemotherapy, called chemoradiotherapy, allows for an optimum platform for eradicating the tumor and improving cancer therapeutics.

Due to the large amount of recent interest in GNPs as a therapeutic agent, there have been many reviews on the topic [33,36,37,52,54–61]. Beik et al. have a recent, extensive review on the use of GNPs in various different modalities, including radiotherapy and chemotherapy, with a larger focus on photothermal therapy and combined treatment options [56]. However, the focus on radiotherapy is limited mainly to kV energy ranges, where GNPs have the largest differential in absorption cross section compared to soft tissue. To be clinically relevant in a larger variety of cancers, the efficacy of GNPs at an MV energy range needs to be explored. As previously mentioned, recent reviews on the use of irradiation in the NIR and RF range with gold nanomaterials for hyperthermia have shown promise [36,37]. Despite continuing research, however, irradiation involving X-rays dominate clinical treatment schemes, occurring in greater than 50% of patients [62]. Of all the gold nano-based therapeutics, spherical GNPs are extensively tested for both radiotherapy and chemotherapy. Therefore, this review article will be focused on prospects of GNP-mediated cancer therapeutics with clinically relevant radiotherapy, chemotherapy, and with a combined modality. This includes information that is necessary in order to improve efficacy, such as an understanding of GNP uptake at a cellular level, and how the size, shape, and functionalization of the GNPs alters effectiveness. In order to better understand the application of GNPs in cancer treatment, an introductory section is presented to understand the behavior of GNPs at a single cell level.

2. Intracellular Fate of Gold Nanoparticles Based on Their Physicochemical Properties

There are different methods of entry into cells for NPs, including clathrin-mediated endocytosis, clathrin-caveolin independent endocytosis, and caveolae-mediated endocytosis [63]. Most NPs, including GNPs, enter the cell mostly via clathrin-mediated, or receptor-mediated, endocytosis (RME) [46,64–68]. The efficiency of the RME process depends on the interaction between molecules on the NP surface (ligands) and the cell membrane receptors. As illustrated in Figure 2A by Jin et al., cell surface receptors bind to molecules on surface of NPs, causing membrane wrapping of the NP with a corresponding increase in elastic energy [64,68]. The receptor-ligand binding immobilizes receptors causing configurational entropy to be reduced. More receptors diffuse to the wrapping site, driven by the local reduction in free energy, allowing the membrane to wrap completely around the particle [69].

RME is therefore an energy dependent process where the path of the NPs within the cell is explained in Figure 2B. NPs first reach the cell membrane and connect with the cell membrane receptors, which are mobile on the surface. Internalization of NPs occurs via invagination of the membrane, which then get trapped in endosomal vesicles. These internalized NPs are sorted inside the vesicle and eventually fuse with lysosomes, which can be seen within the cell as shown in Figure 2C by Ma et al. [70]. NPs are then excreted out of the cell. This intracellular path of NPs was further confirmed by Liu et al. by using a NP complex tagged with a fluorophore [71]. This group suggested that NPs are eventually transported to lysosomes by observing the co-localization of the fluorescently tagged NPs and lysosomes stained with lysotrackers.

The RME is also dependent on the size, shape, and surface properties of NPs. Chithrani et al. investigated the effect of both size and shape on GNP internalization (see Figure 3A,B) [66]. Among the size range of 10–100 nm, bare GNPs of diameter 50 nm had the highest uptake. They also found that the cellular uptake of rod-shaped NPs was lower than their spherical counter parts. This outcome was explained as a result of balance between energy needed for membrane wrapping of NPs and kinetics of receptor diffusion along the cell membrane [67,68]. They used citrate-capped NPs for the study which were not functionalized, where the RME process of the NPs was facilitated via non-specific binding of serum proteins on the NP surface once they were introduced to the tissue culture media [72]. However, it is important to optimize NPs properly for efficient in vivo delivery to the tumor.

There are many factors to consider when optimizing GNPs for use in an in vivo environment. For example, the administration route of the GNPs affects their absorption, toxicity, and tissue distribution [73,74]. Oral and intraperitoneal routes of administration had the largest toxicity, while a tail vein injection had the least, suggesting that an intravenous injection is most promising.

Upon administration, the pharmacokinetics of the GNPs is another factor that must be optimized. GNPs exhibit very complex and varying pharmacokinetics, due the vast number of options in size, shape, and functionalization. Avoidance of opsonization and the reticuloendothelial system (e.g., liver and spleen), while also targeting the tumor, are important goals in nanotechnology [75].

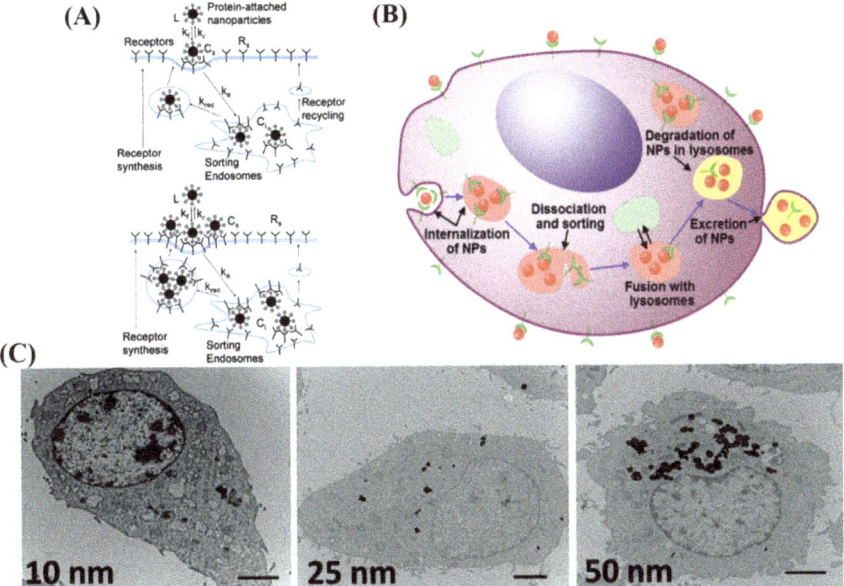

Figure 2. Uptake of GNP by receptor-mediated endocytosis. (A,B) Schematic illustrating pathway of citrate-capped GNP uptake into the cell. (A) Describes the entry and sort mechanism for a single NP and multiple NPs, while (B) describes the entire flow of internalization and excretion. Once GNPs are attached to the receptors on the surface of the cell, membrane invagination occurs followed by budding into the cell, forming a vesicle. The internalized GNPs are sorted inside the vesicle and eventually fuse with lysosomes. GNPs are then excreted out of the cell. (C) Transmission electron microscope images of rat kidney cells treated with three different sizes of GNPs. Scale bar is 2 µm. Reproduced with permission [68,70]. Copyright American Chemical Society, 2009, 2011.

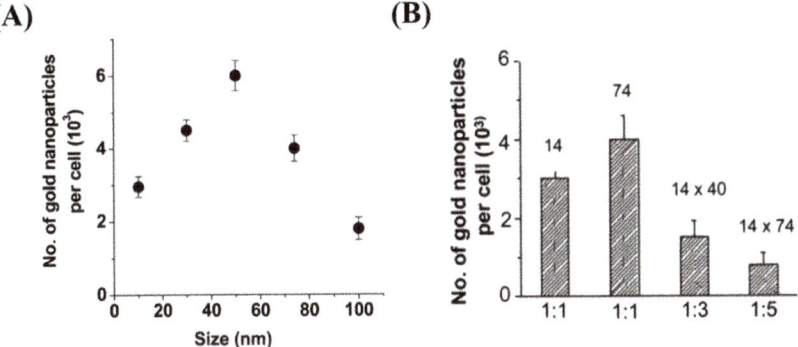

Figure 3. Effect of size and shape on cellular uptake of gold nanoparticles. (A) Dependence of gold nanoparticle cellular uptake as a funtion of their diameter. (B) Comparison of uptake of rod-shaped nanoparticles (aspect ratios 1:3 and 1:5) and spherical nanoparticles (1:1). Reproduced with permission from [66]. Copyright American Chemical Society, 2006.

Prolonged in vivo residency time and preferential localization in tumors are key features of an efficient NP system [76]. If not functionalized properly, the opsonin protein in the blood plasma will attach to the NP surface, leading to the removal of the NP from the circulatory system by macrophages [77,78]. Furthermore, the protein corona that can form from interactions of the GNPs with blood, as a result of size, shape, charge, and functionalization, can alter the behavior of the nanoplatform [79]. Therefore, surface modifications of GNPs are performed to protect the particle from the environment and to target the particle to a specific cell or tissue type. This is critical, because the GNPs need to be present long enough for the process of accumulation within a tumor through its leaky vasculature, known as the enhanced permeability and retention (EPR) effect [80]. Previous studies have shown that the addition of PEG molecules to the surface of NPs increases blood circulation time [80–82]. The process of PEGylation allows for the ethylene glycol to form associations with water molecules, allowing for the formation of a protective hydrating layer, which in turn hinders protein adsorption and clearance by macrophages [83]. The stability of GNPs functionalized with PEG molecules was done by Zhang et al. in Figure 4A, who showed that PEGylated GNPs maintain stability over time, compared to bare GNPs who aggregate quickly [82]. GNPs functionalized with PEG molecules have also shown the capacity to evade the immune system and remain in the blood undetected by macrophages [76]. Further, Zhang et al. showed that GNPs maintained a large blood concentration over time for 20 nm and 40 nm PEGylated GNPs, as seen in Figure 4B [82]. However, the drawback of PEGylating the NP surface is that RME is very much retarded. To overcome this lower uptake of NPs, researchers have added targeting moieties to overcome the reduced NP uptake. One approach was to add a peptide containing arginine-glycine-aspartic acid (RGD) sequence, as performed by Cruje et al. in Figure 4C [77]. The RGD sequence can recognize the integrin $\alpha v \beta 3$ that is highly expressed by several solid tumors and has demonstrably higher uptake than GNPs functionalized with just PEG [76,84]. Depending on the size of the PEG molecule and GNP, the uptake dynamics shown in Figure 4D was changed. For example, it was shown that smaller GNPs had a higher uptake compared to GNPs of diameter 50 nm [76,85]. The peptide and PEG molecules were on the order of 2 kDa and smaller NPs were able to maximize the ligand–receptor interaction of RGD peptide using their higher surface curvature [76,85].

Various factors can affect the pharmacokinetics of the GNPs. Depending on the size, the GNPs will have a different fate in vivo [86]. Smaller PEGylated GNPs of sizes 4 nm and 13 nm had high blood levels for 24 h and were cleared after 7 days, while larger GNPs (100 nm) were completed cleared after 24 h. Furthermore, the accumulation of smaller GNPs in the liver and spleen was peaked after 7 days, and in the mesenteric lymph node after a month, followed by clearance after 6 months. Larger GNPs were taken up into the liver, spleen, and mesenteric lymph node within 30 min. In general, larger GNPs concentrate in the kidney and spleen, and smaller GNPs are found throughout more organs [87]. Ultrasmall GNPs (<10 nm) have been studied due to their improved capabilities to be cleared from the reticuloendothelial system [88]. Further, Bugno et al. showed that that smaller GNPs (2 nm) have a three-fold increased tumor penetration compared to their larger counterparts (4 nm) [89]. As hypoxic regions far from capillaries tend to be the driver for treatment resistance, the ability to reach these regions with GNPs to increase local damage is a very important goal [90]. However, due to the large surface of curvature, despite surface coating with moieties like PEG, ultrasmall GNPs can have gaps that can be filled with blood proteins such as fibrinogen. As a result, smaller GNPs can contribute to an inflammatory response, due to their interactions with these proteins, highlighting the necessity for proper functionalization [91]. Another factor that impacts biodistribution is the surface charge, which can be controlled by various surface conjugations, such as with PEG [92,93]. The addition of PEG to 20 nm glucose-functionalized GNPs has been shown to increase the half-life period from 1.23 h to 6.17 h [94]. Furthermore, Geng et al. found that the functionalization of the GNPs lead to 20 times higher concentration in tumor tissue compared to normal tissue in the same organ, leading to an increase in damage to tumor following radiation [94]. This highlights the importance of proper functionalization to properly target GNPs to the tumor.

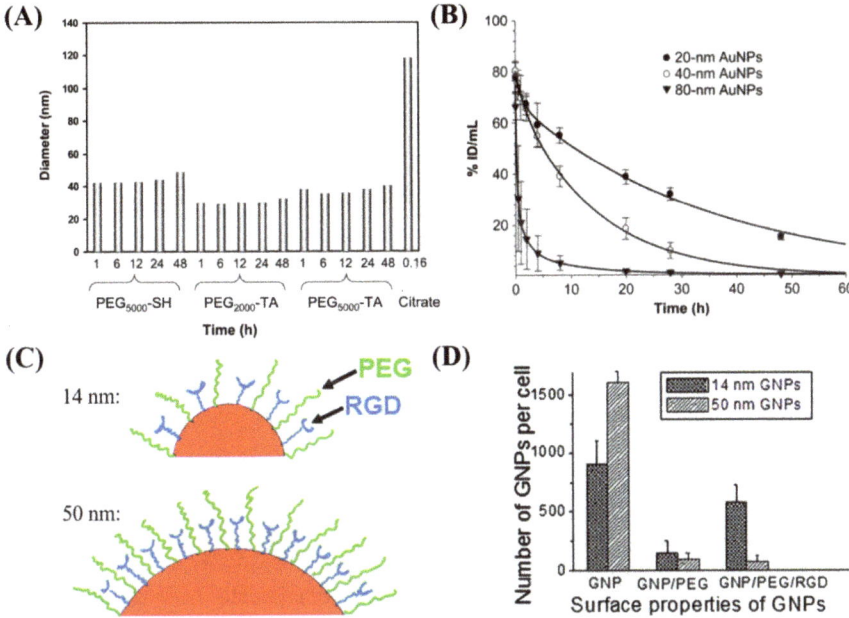

Figure 4. Effect of functionalization on cellular uptake of gold nanoparticles. (A) Diameter as measured using dynamic light scattering of GNPs functionalized with different PEG moieties, compared to bare GNPs. (B) Pharmacokinetics of different sized PEGylated GNPs expressed as a percentage of injected dose per gram of tissue in mice. (C) GNPs can be functionalized with PEG for stability and a peptide containing integrin binding domain RGD for targeting. (D) The use of the RGD functionalized GNPs allowed for improved uptake into tumors cells compared to GNPs functionalized with solely PEG. Reproduced with permission from [76,82]. Copyright Elsevier, 2009; Copyright Royal Society of Chemistry, 2015.

Other functionalization methods have also been tested to effectively target GNPs to tumors. In a variety of different epithelial cancers, epidermal growth factor receptors (EGFRs) can have significantly higher expression on cancer cells compared to normal cells [95]. Cetuximab (C225) is an antibody that allows for EGFR targeting, and has been shown to be effective at improving uptake compared to PEGylated GNPs in-vitro and in-vivo, by Kao et al. [96]. Another method involves the use of aptamer-based targeting. Aptamers are short single-stranded DNA or RNA oligonucleotides that are capable of binding to biological targets [97]. Aptamer-based GNPs can allow for specific targeting as well as aid in diagnostics [98]. Transferrin is a serum glycoprotein that can also be used to target GNPs to tumor cells, as there is an upregulation of receptors on metastatic and drug-resistant malignant cells [99]. The use of transferrin coated GNPs have been shown to improved uptake and allow for specific targeting to improve delivery of therapeutic agents [100]. Folic acid is another targeting molecule that can be employed, as the folate-receptor can be upregulated on human tumors while being minimally expressed on most normal tissue, as evidenced by Zhang et al. [99,101]. While there are many different functionalization modalities that can be employed, it is very important to test the efficiency of functionalized NP systems by varying their size, shape, and surface properties to optimize their internalization within tumor cells to cause the maximum damage. No matter what system that is employed, careful consideration of the functionalized GNPs with the protein corona that can form in vivo can allow for proper targeting and a predictable fate. [102] GNPs have also been associated with anti-inflammatory responses [103]. Thus, the toxicity of GNPs is an important factor that has been explored.

A number of groups studying GNP cytotoxicity concluded that GNP biocompatibility depends on size, surface properties and concentration [104,105]. Many experimental works reported that GNPs are non-toxic. For example, Connor et al. found various sizes (4, 12, 18 nm) and capping agents (citrate, cysteine, glucose, biotin, and cetyltrimethyl ammonium bromide) were nontoxic to K562 human leukemia cell line up to micromolar concentrations based on MTT assays [105]. Steckiewicz et al. found that the shape and concentration of the GNP complexes impact toxicity, with spheroidal GNPs (14 nm) imparting the least toxicity [106]. Sukla et al. observed lysine capped 35 nm GNPs did not show detectable cytotoxicity up to 100 µM concentration in RAW265.7 macrophage cells based on MTT assays [104]. It has been shown that PEGylated 12.1 nm sized GNPs incubated in HeLa cells had an IC_{50} of 0.477 mM [107]. Despite the many reports on non-toxicity of GNPs, contradictory research results are also present [108,109]. The lack of general consensus on NP toxicity is due to different experimental methods employed, incubation conditions (concentrations and exposure time), variability of sizes and functionalities of GNPs, variability of cell lines, and different measures and assays for toxicity [108,110]. However, most current research platforms are working in conditions that have previously been shown to be non-toxic, and future work should focus on maintaining this important constraint.

3. Gold Nanoparticles as Radiosensitizers

The use of high atomic number (Z) material to enhance radiation dose has been studied for more than 50 years. The interest in using high-Z material stems from the production of secondary electrons, such as photoelectrons, Auger electrons, and Compton electrons. These secondary products are effective at damaging DNA as well as ionizing surrounding water molecules, forming free radicals [110]. While the atomic number of tissue is approximately $Z\sim7.5$, materials with a higher atomic number used in the past such as Iodine ($Z = 53$) and gold ($Z = 79$) have a larger cross-section for absorption of radiation. For example, it was demonstrated in vitro that incorporating iodine into cellular DNA using iododeoxyuridine enhanced radiosensitivity at keV ranges by a factor of three [111]. The outcome of the in vitro study was also seen in an in vivo study, where an intratumoral injection of iodine and 200 kVp X-ray radiation suppressed the tumor growth by 80% [112]. In addition to having a great difference in mass attenuation between gold and soft tissue, gold has been shown to be biocompatible, simple, and economical to manufacture in many different shapes and sizes [113].

Radiation dose enhancement due to GNPs was first demonstrated using 1.9 nm GNPs in a mouse model, in one of the pioneering studies in GNP-mediated radiation dose enhancement by Hainfeld et al. [29]. A radiation dose of 30 Gy with 250 kVp X-rays to subcutaneous tumors in mice resulted in a significant decrease in tumor volume. However, the concentration of gold in this study was considerably high, at 2.7 g Au/kg body weight, which is not clinically feasible. Furthermore, the use of kV energies, while allowing for prominent photoelectric absorption in gold, is hindered due to the reduced penetration for deep-set tumors. Thus, as previously discussed, optimization of the internalization of the GNPs into the tumor cells, both in-vitro and in-vivo, is required for ideal efficacy. Whenever gold was internalized in vitro, radiosensitization was achievable at MV energy ranges, at concentrations as low as 1 ng/g [25,114–116]. This was demonstrated by Chithrani et al. in Figure 5A–C, which found a 17% increase in radiosensitization at 6 MV with 50 nm spherical GNPs [25]. When moving to an in vivo environment, radiosensitization was seen at a delivered dose of 10 µg/g of body weight [117]. This was accomplished by Wolfe et al. using targeted GNRs, as seen in Figure 5D–F, where there was a 36% increase in radiosensitization in vitro in PC3 cells, and a significantly enhanced tumor-growth delay when treated in vivo [117]. The treated dose is a $\sim 1 \times 10^6$ improvement over the original treatment seen in Hainfeld's pioneering study. The addition of targeting and improvements in the optimization of uptake has allowed significant progress in facilitating the progress of gold nanomaterials to the clinic.

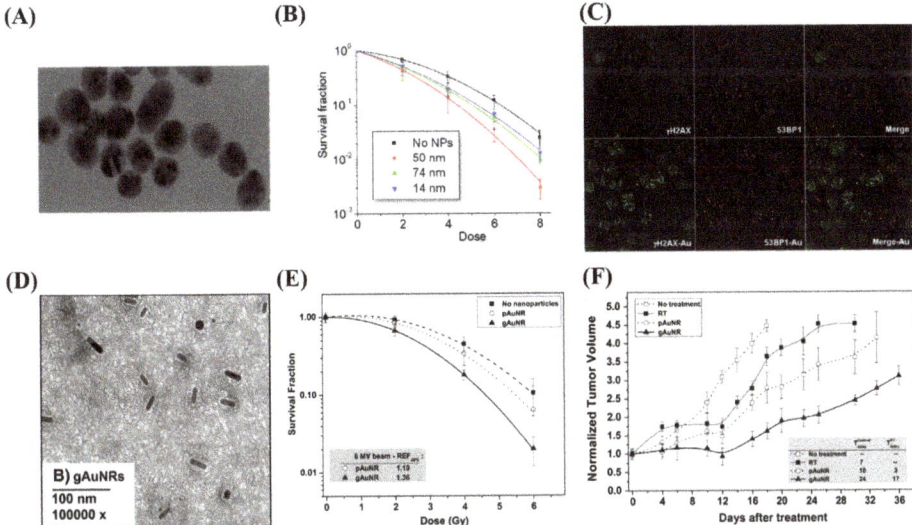

Figure 5. Radiosensitization due to gold nanoparticles. (**A–C**) Spheroidal GNPs improve radiosensitization in vitro, with the largest effect occurring with 50 nm GNPs, as they have the optimum uptake. This can be seen both through clonogenic assays as well as through imaging of double strand break foci with confocal microscopy. (**D–F**) GNRs displayed increased radiosensitization when targeted towards prostate cancer cell lines both in vitro through a clonogenic assay as well as in vivo through tumor volume measurements in a mouse model. Reproduced with permission from [117]. Copyright Elsevier, 2015.

GNPs localized intracellularly increases the probability of ionization events leading to local enhanced deposition of energy causing more damage to tumor cells [25]. The physical mechanism of GNP radiosensitization, seen in Figure 6A, occurs within the first nanoseconds of exposure, and is based on the difference in mass energy absorption coefficients between gold and soft tissue, enabling dose enhancement. The range of electrons released from GNPs is short, only a few micrometers, causing highly localized ionizing events. Thus, to achieve any enhancement from GNPs in radiation therapy, GNPs must be delivered and internalized specifically by tumor cells.

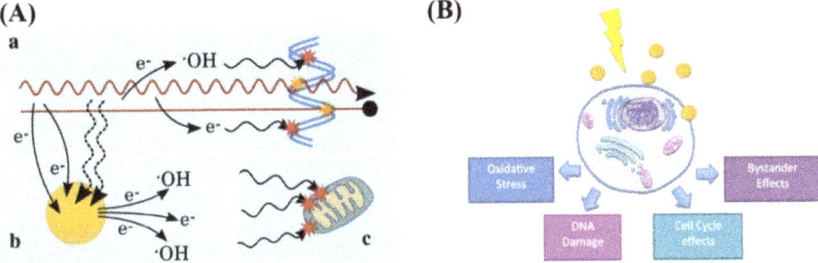

Figure 6. Radiosensitization and radiobiological effects. (**A**) Schematic showing chemical mechanism of GNP radiosensitization. While the radiation causes direct and indirect damage (yellow and red stars, respectively), there can be induction of secondary electrons and reactive oxygen species through gold nanoparticles. This can lead to damage to the DNA as well as secondary parts of the cell, such as the mitochondria. (**B**) GNPs can influence the cell through generation of reactive oxygen species, DNA damage, as well as cell cycle and bystander effects. Reproduced with permission from [110,118]. Copyright Springer Nature, 2016, 2017.

The chemical mechanism of GNP radiosensitization occurs through the radiochemical sensitization of DNA by increasing catalytic surface activity and increasing radical generation from the GNP surface [60]. Despite the prevailing notion that GNPs are chemically inert, there is a growing body of evidence that, due to the electronically active surface of GNPs, they are capable of catalyzing chemical reactions [119]. Catalysis by GNPs occurs mainly through surface interaction with molecular oxygen, generating free radicals [60]. This seems more evident in small GNPs (<5 nm in diameter) where surface to volume ratio is greater [120]. When combined with irradiation, the catalytic effects appear to be enhanced, with smaller GNPs with larger surface areas yielding more ROS [121]. However, it has been shown that at all energy levels, the dose enhancement observed cannot be simply explained by physical or chemical mechanisms [122]. To explain this, a radiobiological effect must be occurring.

The main radiobiological mechanisms involved in the cell's response to irradiated GNPs results are the production of reactive oxygen species (ROS), oxidative stress, DNA damage induction, potential bystander effects, and cell cycle effects, as explained by Rosa et al. in Figure 6B [118]. Oxidative stress can cause cellular damage to the cell, including the oxidation of lipids, proteins, and DNA, which can result in apoptotic and necrotic cell death [123]. The mitochondria do appear to play a role, and the data indicate loss of function due to high intracellular ROS levels. It has been shown that the use of 1.4-nm triphenyl monosulfonate (TPPMS)-coated GNPs resulted in a loss of mitochondrial potential through elevated oxidative stress, resulting in necrotic cell death [122]. There have also been studies suggesting that GNPs may cause cell cycle disruptions and induce apoptosis. Radiosensitivity varies throughout the cell cycle with S phase being where a cell is most radioresistant and G2/M phase being most sensitive [124]. This could also depend on cell type, expression of cyclin kinases, and NP characteristics such as coating and size. For example, the use of 1.9 nm GNPs in DU-145 and MDA-MB-231 resulted in an increase in sub-G1 population in DU-145 population but not in MDA-MB-231 [125].

The biocompatibility of GNPs has already been tested in a phase I clinical trial. Furthermore, both in vitro and in vivo studies have shown the possibility of using GNPs as a radiosensitizer at clinically feasible concentrations, as discussed previously. Radiotherapy can also be combined with chemotherapy (chemoradiation) in cases where the tumor is not localized anymore, but metastasized as well, or to reduce potential micro-metastases spread. We will discuss the recent research conducted towards adding GNPs to this chemoradiation protocol in the next section.

4. Rationale for Gold Nanoparticles in Chemoradiotherapy

Radiotherapy is mainly used to control the tumor locally as discussed previously. Chemotherapy is used to control the tumor metastasis. Therefore, a combination of chemotherapy and radiotherapy (chemoradiation) is being practiced in the clinic to treat patients with locally advanced disease. Considering the variety of drugs available for cancer treatment, the possible choice of sequencing of combined chemotherapy and radiation therapy is countless, and the treatment plan differs between each patient. The standard treatment sequence refers to chemotherapy regimen before a traditional external beam radiation therapy treatment [53]. Chemotherapy used prior to irradiation is expected to cause maximal tumor regression for locally advanced tumors. The major limitation of combining chemotherapy and radiation therapy is normal tissue toxicity, since either modality can cause major normal tissue toxicity [8]. The main problems currently associated with chemotherapy are the biodistribution of pharmaceuticals, the lack of drug-specific affinity towards the tumor, limited plasma half-life, poor solubility and stability in physiological fluids, and nonspecific toxicity [126]. GNPs, due to their high surface area-to-volume ratio, as well as a large number of surface bio conjugation possibilities, are an ideal platform for delivering pharmaceutics for chemotherapy [46,127–129]. The use of GNPs as drug delivery system (DDS) can improve the pharmacokinetics, the pharmacodynamics, and the biodistribution of various drugs, as well as allow for improved targeting to reduce normal tissue toxicity. Beyond being an effective radiosensitizer, GNPs allow for a 100- to 1000-fold increase in ligand density compared to that of liposomal or polymeric DDSs [55]. Thus, the combination of the

GNPs with radiotherapy and chemotherapy is part of the natural progression of the exploration of GNPs as a complete treatment modality.

The conjugation of moieties such as chemotherapeutic agents to the surface of the GNPs can be done using various techniques. The most common method is through the use of thiol group-containing biomolecules [130]. The use of thiolated biomolecules allows for functionalization of the GNPs with various agents, such as DNA, peptides, antibodies, and proteins [131,132]. This is a very robust method, as the majority of anticancer drugs can be thiolated, so as to be compatible with GNPs as a DDS [133,134]. Furthermore, capping agents, such as carboxyl terminated PEG molecules, with a thiol bond can allow for further functionalization techniques [131,135]. A general overview of various drug loading techniques using GNPs was explored by Fratoddi et al. [136]. GNPs, due to their favorable surface chemistry, are a suitable drug carrier for use in chemotherapeutics, and may be available for use in a wide range of drug delivery applications.

GNPs have been conjugated to a large variety of cytotoxic, anticancer drugs, and combined with radiation for improved efficacy. This includes paclitaxel, methotrexate, gemcitabine, doxorubicin, docetaxel, bleomycin, and platinum-based drugs like cisplatin [133,137–141]. Many different drugs can be used for different purposes, a few of which we will expand on. For instance, the antitumor activity of cisplatin was first discovered by Rosenberg and co-workers in 1960s, when they were examining whether electrical currents affect cellular division [142]. The researchers discovered that the inhibition of cellular division observed in the study was not due to electrical current, but platinum hydrolysis products formed from platinum electrodes. They reported that cis-tetrachlorodiammineplatinum (IV), cis-[PtCl$_4$ (NH3)$_2$], was the potent agent responsible for the inhibition. Cisplatin is now used to treat various types of cancers (i.e., cervical cancer, non-small-cell lung cancer, ovarian cancer, germ cell tumors, osteosarcomas, etc.), with a cure rate as high as 90% in testicular cancer [143]. However, long term cisplatin usage results in drug resistance [144]. To counteract this resistance, very high systemic doses of cisplatin should be administered, which results in severe systemic toxicity and poor patient compliance, limiting its clinical use [144–146]. It was shown recently that GNPs can be used to enhance damage caused by platinum-based anticancer drugs [147,148]. Comenge et al. conjugated cisplatin to GNPs and tested the efficacy of this DDS compared to the free drug along, as shown in Figure 7A–C [147]. They found that the use of GNPs led to 300 times more platinum being encapsulated in A549 cells in vitro, and while moving to in vivo, found similar efficacy but largely absent normal tissue toxicity. Yang et al. instead used free cisplatin along with GNPs in a combined chemoradiotherapy modality in vitro, seen in Figure 7D–F [116]. An additive relationship was discovered when treated with GNPs, cisplatin, and radiation in MDA-MB-231 cells. The use of GNPs may be an important avenue to explore when integrating cisplatin into chemoradiation protocols.

Another chemotherapy agent that is limited due to high normal tissue toxicity is docetaxel (DTX). DTX is a cytotoxic member of the taxanes and is an effective antimicrotubular agent that is effective in the treatment of multiple different types of cancers including head and neck, breast, prostate, and non-small-cell lung cancer [149–152]. Docetaxel's mechanism of action is primarily through the ability to enhance microtubule assembly and stabilize free microtubules within the cytoplasm, thus preventing their depolymerization during normal cell division [153]. This has many consequences for the fate of the cell, including inhibition of progression through the cell cycle and inevitably death via mitotic catastrophe, depending on the dose [154]. Francois et al. tested DTX-conjugated GNPs on MCF7 and HCT15 cells and found a 2.5 times more efficient response compared to free DTX [139]. DTX has also been shown to block the cell cycle at the G_2/M phase [155]. This is critical because the G_2/M phase has shown special sensitivity to the ionizing radiation, causing more cell death [156]. Moreover, by arresting tumor cells in the M phase of the cell cycle, it synergizes the lethal effects of radiotherapy, thereby serving as an ideal radiosensitizer. Both in vitro and in vivo studies have demonstrated the synergistic effects of DTX when combined with radiotherapy [157,158]. Furthermore, it has been shown that the uptake of NPs, including GNPs, is increased when the cell population is synchronized in the G_2/M phase [85,159]. This suggests the use of DTX concomitantly with other drugs or radiation, which was tested by Bannister et al. as seen in Figure 8 [160]. DTX used as a synchronizing agent when paired with GNPs lead to higher uptake, a higher localization of the GNPs to the nucleus, and a larger, synergistic response to radiotherapy.

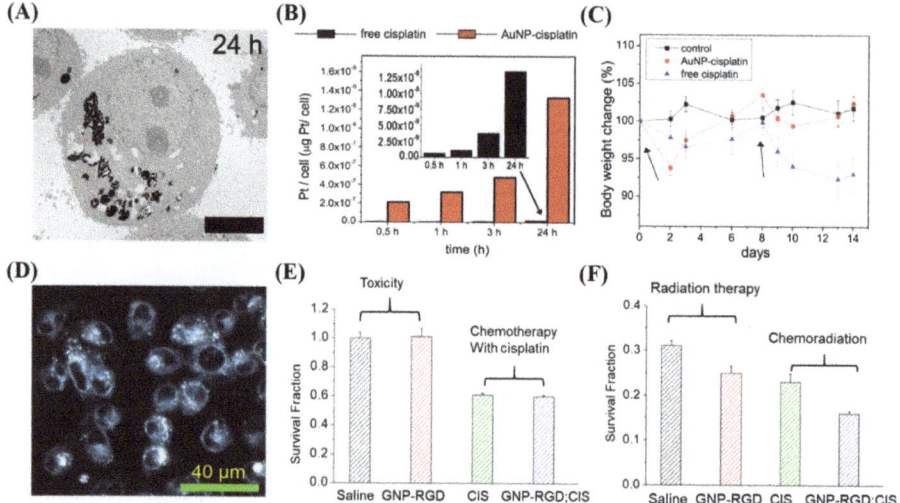

Figure 7. Cisplatin and gold nanoparticles. (**A**–**C**) Cisplatin conjugated GNPs lead to an increased deposition of platinum into A549 cells compared to the free drug in vitro, which led to less side effects in vivo with similar efficacy. Scale bar is 4 µm. (**D**–**F**) The use of free cisplatin to synergize with GNPs in a chemoradiation modality in vitro lead to a synergistic effect. Scale bar is 40 µm. Reproduced with permission from [116,147]. Copyright Public Library of Science, 2012; Copyright Multidisciplinary Digital Publishing Institute, 2018.

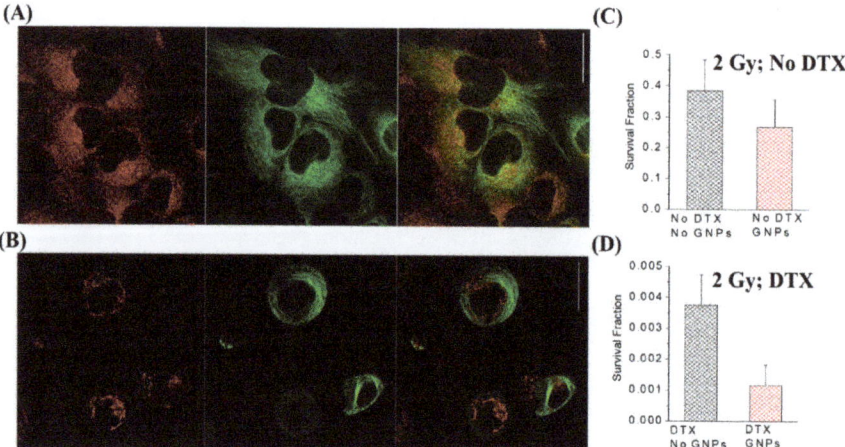

Figure 8. Docetaxel and gold nanoparticles. (**A**) Confocal imaging of GNPs (labelled in red) and the microtubule (MT) structure (labelled in green) in HeLa cells. (**B**) Confocal imaging of GNPs and MTs after treatment with 50 nM of DTX. (**C**) Radiosensitization of GNPs without DTX. (**D**) Radiosensitization of GNPs with 50 nM DTX, showing a synergistic effect. Scale bar is 25 µm. Reproduced with permission from [160]. Copyright British Journal of Radiology, 2020.

Normal tissue toxicity is an issue in escalating current dose regimes in many tumors. However, in pancreatic cancer, despite advancements in chemotherapy and radiotherapy, the current 5 year survival rate is only 9% [161]. Gemcitabine is a pyrimidine analog that is a mainstay treatment of adenocarcinoma of the pancreas, but is also used for treatment of bladder and non-small cell lung cancer [162–164]. Upon cellular encapsulation, gemcitabine is phosphorylated to its active diphosphate and triphosphate metabolites, which inhibit RR and DNA synthesis, respectively [165]. Despite its prominent use in the clinic, only a small portion of the drug is converted to its active forms. Up to 90% of the injected dose is collected from urine one week after treatment, with 75% of that being in the first 24 h [166]. The use of gemcitabine-conjugated GNPs could be an avenue for both improved uptake of the drug as well as improved efficacy in the very deadly pancreatic disease. It has been shown that 20 nm GNPs by themselves can sensitive pancreatic cell to the effects of gemcitabine by Huai et al. [167]. This is explained by showing that GNPs inhibited epithelial to mesenchymal transition and reduced cancer cell stemness—possible causes of anticancer drug resistance [168]. Furthermore, Pal et al. showed in Figure 9 that gemcitabine-conjugated GNPs that specifically target pancreatic cancer cells with a plectin-1 peptide have improved efficacy in situ compared to the free drug alone [169]. The use of gemcitabine with radiotherapy has also been shown to be more effective than the drug alone through clinical trials [170]. Thus, in the future, the addition of gemcitabine-conjugated GNPs to a radiotherapy protocol may prove highly beneficial.

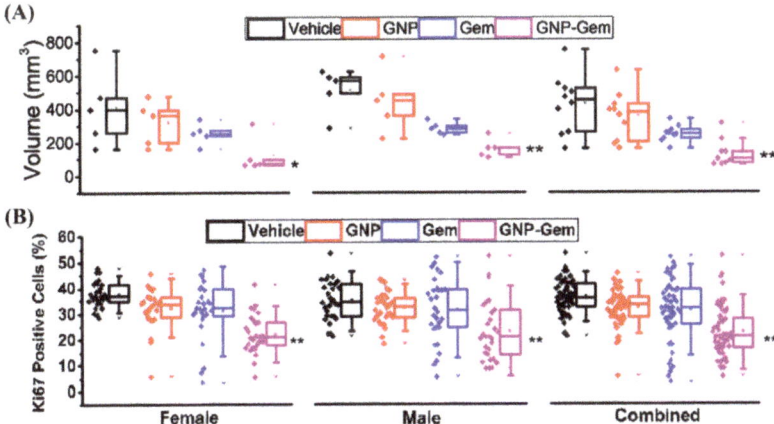

Figure 9. Gold nanoparticle mediated delivery of Gemcitabine. (A) Gemcitabine-conjugated GNPs showed a significant increase in efficacy when treating mice, as measured through volume. (B) KI67, a marker for proliferation, also showed reduced proliferative cells when treated with the GNP complex compared to the free drug alone, signifying improved efficacy. Black = vehicle, Red = GNP, Blue = Gem and Purple = GNP-Gem. * and ** denote $p < 0.05$ and $p < 0.01$ compared to vehicle-treated group respectively. Reproduced with permission from [169]. Copyright Royal Society of Chemistry, 2017.

The use of GNPs as chemotherapeutic DDSs is increasing, and the combination of chemotherapy with radiotherapy remains one of the most effective treatment modalities available in the clinic. A brief summary of recent studies, no older than 2016, involving the use of GNPs with chemotherapy and radiotherapy, can be seen in Table 1. The use of GNPs in combination with anticancer drugs and radiation is still limited in literature; however, the published work thus far shows a trend of improved dose response to the tumor coupled with reduced normal tissue toxicity. Further studies need to be completed, however, before translation to the clinic.

Table 1. Recent applications of anticancer drugs with gold nanoparticles in drug delivery and combined radiation therapy with clinically relevant energies.

Nanoparticle Complex	Treatment Parameters	Modality	Experimental Outcomes	Cell Line/Tumor Model	Ref.
PTX-TNFα-PEG-GNPs	32.6 nm GNPs; 2.5 mg/kg dose	Chemotherapy	Selective delivery of nanoparticles to tumor and improved efficacy	Ovarian Cancer Cell Line (A2780); B16/F10 tumor-bearing C57BL/6 mice	[133]
DOX-PEG-GNPs	41 nm GNPs; 6 mg/kg dose	Chemotherapy	Dramatically reduced normal tissue toxicity	Ovarian Cancer Cell Line (A2780); CD-1 mice	[138]
BLM-DOX-PEG-GNPs	13 nm GNPs; 10–100 nM dose	Chemotherapy	Cancer cell environment-mediated drug release and improve EC50	Cervical Cancer Cell Line (HeLa)	[140]
CIS-GLC-PEG-GNP	20 nm GNPs; 10 mg/kg dose; 25 Gy at 6 MV	Chemo-radiotherapy	Similar effect to free cisplatin; dramatically improve result when combined with radiation	Skin Cancer Cell line (A-431); A-431 tumor-bearing mice	[171]
DOX@GNPs	2 nm GNPs; 5 mg/kg dose	Chemotherapy	Efficient renal clearance with effective targeting. Reduced normal tissue toxicity with improved antitumor efficacy	Breast Cancer Cell lines (MCF-7 and MDA-MB-231); Murine Mammary 4T1; CD-1 Mice	[172]
PDC-PEG-GNPs	25–50 nm GNPs; 0–50 μM dose	Chemotherapy	Improved half-life of drug, similar cytotoxicity towards target cells, and active for longer	Murine Lymphoma cells (A20)	[173]
Alginate co-loaded with GNPs and CIS	44 nm NP; 20 μg/mL dose of GNP with 5 μg/mL CIS; 4 Gy at 6 MV	Chemo-radiotherapy with photothermal therapy	ACA and radiotherapy saw improved efficacy over cisplatin and radiation. The addition of photothermal therapy further improved therapeutic results.	Cervical Cancer Cell line (KB)	[174]
5-FU/GSH-GNPs	9–17 nm GNPs; 0.5–1.5 mg/mL dose	Chemotherapy	Better anticancer effect against the cancer, and reduced drug doses as a result	Colorectal Cancer Cell lines isolated from patients	[175]
CS-GNPs-DOX	21 nm GNPs; 0.05–0.3 mM dose; 0.5, 1, and 3 Gy at 6 MV	Chemo-radiotherapy	Enhanced treatment results including lowered survival fraction, increased apoptosis, and increased DNA damage	Breast Cancer Cell line (MCF-7)	[176]
GNP-PEG-RGD; CIS	10 nm GNPs with 435 nM CIS; 0.3 nM dose; 2 Gy at 6 MV	Chemo-radiotherapy	Improved efficacy of treatment compared to cisplatin and radiation alone	Breast Cancer Cell line (MDA-MB-231)	[116]
GNP-PEG-RGD; DTX	17.2 nm GNPs; 0.2 nM GNPs with 50 nM DTX; 2 Gy at 6 MV	Chemo-radiotherapy	Improved retention of GNPs due to cell synchronicity induced by DTX. Synergistic therapeutic effect found when GNPs and DTX combined	Breast Cancer Cell line (MDA-MB-231) and Cervical Cancer Cell line (HeLa)	[160]

GNP: Gold Nanoparticle; PAC: Paclitaxel; TNF: Tumor Necrosis Factor; PEG: Polyethylene Glycol; DOX: Doxorubicin; BLM: Bleomycin; CIS: Cisplatin; GLC: Glucose; PDC: Peptide-drug-conjugate containing chlorambucil, melphalan, or bendamustine; 5-FU: 5-Fluorouracil; GSH: Glutathione; CS: Chitosan; RGD: arginyl-glycyl-aspartic acid tripeptide; DTX: Docetaxel

5. Future Considerations

A large issue that is plaguing nanotechnology in general is that a very low (~0.7%) portion of the administered dose is being delivered to the tumor [177]. While Wilhelm et al. describe the issue as improving understanding of the processes present in the body that inhibit the uptake of NPs, and then optimizing those processes, a more personalized approach could be introduced. Personalized medicine involves the analysis of a patient's genetic code in order to have a better understanding of the potential response to treatment [178]. This is a very important avenue to explore, as it has been estimated that any class of anticancer drug used is ineffective in 75% of patients [179]. This is a result of no two cancers from different patients being the same. Beyond using genomic information to improve each individual's cancer treatments, the use of an in vitro model that can better mimic the in vivo environment present in a patient may allow for the actual testing of treatment prior to administration. This can be achieved through the use of three-dimensional organoid models [180].

Organoid models have many advantages if implemented into a personalized medicine protocol. The use of a patient's own cells, as described in Figure 10 by Fan et al., allows for the maintenance of the heterogeneity present [181]. Furthermore, normal spheroids can be engineered to have similar genetic alterations present in a patient, as discovered using their genomic information, through the use of gene-editing [182]. There are many other advantages as well, including low-cost generation, and quick (~4 weeks) results can be obtained. The capability of organoids to enable drug screening in an in vitro environment is being widely explored [180]. Furthermore, the use of organoid models has recently been tested on a chemoradiotherapy treatment of advanced rectal cancer and was able to accurately predict the response [183]. In the future, the use of organoids to screen chemoradiotherapy protocols with GNPs may enable an accurate assessment of response and allow for tailored, personalized medical care.

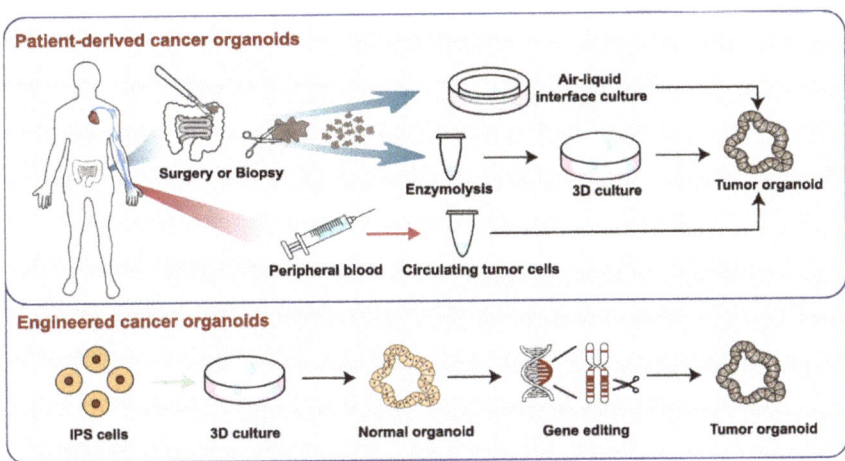

Figure 10. Organoid models toward personalized medicine. Patient-derived cancer organoids can be derived from surgically resected/biopsied tissues and circulating tumor cells. Furthermore, using gene-editing, normal spheroids can be mutated into tumor organoids. Reproduced with permission from [180]. Copyright Springer Nature, 2019.

Spheroids, and patient derived organoids, should be seen as avascular tumors, with limitations. To move towards personalized medical care with GNPs—using organoids as an assessment tool—certain strategies will have to be employed and obstacles overcome [184]. First, many more preclinical studies will have to be undertaken involving the use of GNPs with spheroids and their ability to accurately predict tumor response. This will have to be a large expanse of research, with many different types of treatment options including chemotherapy and radiotherapy as well as combined modalities. Second, scalability is very important: a high throughput method of testing efficacy of drugs and radiation modalities will have to be elucidated, as well as producing the organoids in a large-scale manner. Work is under way to improve production of spheroids as well as protocols for high throughput drug and radiation testing [185–187]. However, translation to the clinic will require more work at the bio–nano interface.

The use of GNPs in this workflow has limited published work, with most research focusing on individual treatment modalities, and not overall high throughput methods for translation to personalized medicine. Towards this, cheap and efficient GNP systems that can be easily functionalized with various moieties such as anticancer drugs or targeting ligands need to be designed for mass-scale production. Furthermore, comparisons of GNP-treated spheroids and organoids with in vivo models must be undertaken for improved confidence for translation to the clinic. Finally, it must be accepted the spheroids are a simplistic model when compared to an in vivo environment and will not be able to predict everything. However, despite this, the use of GNPs with organoid models for personalized medicine may be able to help save lives and improve the quality of lives in the future.

6. Conclusions

In the pursuit of improved cancer therapeutics, the use of GNPs offers the potential of improving on many different facets of the treatment process. Despite progress, the translation of GNPs to clinical practice has been limited due to the lack of coordination between researchers and clinicians. Many advances covered in this review aim to address issues that have arisen in the past, including targeted therapy, and the combination of radiotherapy and chemotherapy paired with GNPs for improved efficacy. However, it is still important to improve upon the current research so that translation to the clinic can be expedited.

Author Contributions: All authors have made substantial contributions in preparation of the manuscript. All authors agreed to be personally accountable for the author's own contributions and to ensure that the questions related to the accuracy or integrity of any part of the work, even ones in which the author was not personally involved, are appropriately investigated, resolved, and the resolution agreement published in the literature. All authors have read and agreed to the published version of the manuscript.

Funding: This research was funded by Natural Sciences and Engineering Research Council of Canada (NSERC), grant number 418453.

Acknowledgments: The authors would like to acknowledge Canada Foundation for Innovation (CFI), the British Columbia government, Natural Sciences and Engineering Research Council of Canada (NSERC), British Columbia Cancer, Vancouver Island (BCC), Centre for Advanced Materials and Related Technologies (CAMTEC), and University of Victoria for their financial support.

Conflicts of Interest: The authors declare no conflict of interest.

References

1. Ruddon, R.W. *Cancer Biology*, 4th ed.; Oxford University Press: Oxford, UK, 2007.
2. Treatment-Canadian Cancer Society. Available online: https://www.cancer.ca/en/cancer-information/diagnosis-and-treatment/treatment/?region=on (accessed on 6 August 2020).
3. Types of Cancer Treatment-National Cancer Institute. Available online: https://www.cancer.gov/about-cancer/treatment/types (accessed on 6 August 2020).
4. Joiner, M.C.; van der Kogel, A.J. *Basic Clinical Radiobiology*, 5th ed.; CRC Press: Boca Raton, FL, USA, 2018; ISBN 9781444179637.
5. Podgorsak, E.B. *Radiation Oncology Physics: A Handbook for Teachers and Students*; International Atomic Energy Agency: Vienna, Austria, 2003.
6. Podgoršak, E.B. *Radiation Physics for Medical Physicists*; Springer International Publishing: Cham, Switzerland, 2016; ISBN 9783319253800.
7. Delaney, G.P.; Barton, M.B. Evidence-based Estimates of the Demand for Radiotherapy. *Clin. Oncol.* **2015**. [CrossRef]

8. Herscher, L.L.; Cook, J.A.; Pacelli, R.; Pass, H.I.; Russo, A.; Mitchell, J.B. Principles of chemoradiation: Theoretical and practical considerations. *Oncology* **1999**, *13*, 11–22.
9. Tannock, I.F.; Hill, R.P.; Bristow, R.G.; Harrington, L. *Basic Science of Oncology*, 5th ed.; McGraw-Hill Education: Beijing, China, 2005; ISBN 0071745203.
10. Hanahan, D.; Weinberg, R.A. Hallmarks of cancer: The next generation. *Cell* **2011**, *144*, 646–674. [CrossRef]
11. Crawford, S. Is it time for a new paradigm for systemic cancer treatment? Lessons from a century of cancer chemotherapy. *Front. Pharmacol.* **2013**, 68. [CrossRef]
12. Jain, R.K. Transport of molecules, particles, and cells in solid tumors. *Annu. Rev. Biomed. Eng.* **1999**, *1*, 241–263. [CrossRef]
13. Georgelin, T.; Bombard, S.; Siaugue, J.-M.; Cabuil, V. Nanoparticle-Mediated Delivery of Bleomycin. *Angew. Chem. Int. Ed.* **2010**, *49*, 8897–8901. [CrossRef]
14. Strebhardt, K.; Ullrich, A. Paul Ehrlich's magic bullet concept: 100 Years of progress. *Nat. Rev. Cancer* **2008**, *8*, 473–480. [CrossRef] [PubMed]
15. Davis, M.E.; Chen, Z.; Shin, D.M. Nanoparticle therapeutics: An emerging treatment modality for cancer. *Nat. Rev. Drug Discov.* **2008**, *7*, 771–782. [CrossRef] [PubMed]
16. Lytton-Jean, A.K.R.; Kauffman, K.J.; Kaczmarek, J.C.; Langer, R. Cancer nanotherapeutics in clinical trials. *Cancer Treat. Res.* **2015**, *166*, 293–322. [CrossRef] [PubMed]
17. Zhang, L.; Gu, F.; Chan, J.; Wang, A.; Langer, R.; Farokhzad, O. Nanoparticles in Medicine: Therapeutic Applications and Developments. *Clin. Pharmacol. Ther.* **2008**, *83*, 761–769. [CrossRef]
18. Retif, P.; Pinel, S.; Toussaint, M.; Frochot, C.; Chouikrat, R.; Bastogne, T.; Barberi-Heyob, M. Nanoparticles for radiation therapy enhancement: The key parameters. *Theranostics* **2015**, *5*, 1030–1044. [CrossRef] [PubMed]
19. Zhang, Z.; Berg, A.; Levanon, H.; Fessenden, R.W.; Meisel, D. On the interactions of free radicals with gold nanoparticles. *J. Am. Chem. Soc.* **2003**, *125*, 7959–7963. [CrossRef] [PubMed]
20. Zheng, Y.; Sanche, L. Low Energy Electrons in Nanoscale Radiation Physics: Relationship to Radiosensitization and Chemoradiation Therapy. *Rev. Nanosci. Nanotechnol.* **2013**, *2*, 1–28. [CrossRef]
21. Townley, H.E.; Kim, J.; Dobson, P.J. In vivo demonstration of enhanced radiotherapy using rare earth doped titania nanoparticles. *Nanoscale* **2012**, *4*, 5043–5050. [CrossRef] [PubMed]
22. Mirjolet, C.; Papa, A.L.; Créhange, G.; Raguin, O.; Seignez, C.; Paul, C.; Truc, G.; Maingon, P.; Millot, N. The radiosensitization effect of titanate nanotubes as a new tool in radiation therapy for glioblastoma: A proof-of-concept. *Radiother. Oncol.* **2013**, *108*, 136–142. [CrossRef] [PubMed]
23. Takahashi, J.; Misawa, M. Analysis of potential radiosensitizing materials for x-ray-induced photodynamic therapy. *Nanobiotechnology* **2007**, *3*, 116–126. [CrossRef]
24. Yang, W.; Read, P.W.; Mi, J.; Baisden, J.M.; Reardon, K.A.; Larner, J.M.; Helmke, B.P.; Sheng, K. Semiconductor Nanoparticles as Energy Mediators for Photosensitizer-Enhanced Radiotherapy. *Int. J. Radiat. Oncol. Biol. Phys.* **2008**, *72*, 633–635. [CrossRef]
25. Chithrani, D.B.; Jelveh, S.; Jalali, F.; Van Prooijen, M.; Allen, C.; Bristow, R.G.; Hill, R.P.; Jaffray, D.A. Gold nanoparticles as radiation sensitizers in cancer therapy. *Radiat. Res.* **2010**. [CrossRef]
26. Le Duc, G.; Miladi, I.; Alric, C.; Mowat, P.; Bräuer-Krisch, E.; Bouchet, A.; Khalil, E.; Billotey, C.; Janier, M.; Lux, F.; et al. Toward an image-guided microbeam radiation therapy using gadolinium-based nanoparticles. *ACS Nano* **2011**, *5*, 9566–9574. [CrossRef]
27. Liu, P.; Huang, Z.; Chen, Z.; Xu, R.; Wu, H.; Zang, F.; Wang, C.; Gu, N. Silver nanoparticles: A novel radiation sensitizer for glioma? *Nanoscale* **2013**, *5*, 11829–11836. [CrossRef]
28. Hainfeld, J.F.; Dilmanian, F.A.; Slatkin, D.N.; Smilowitz, H.M. Radiotherapy enhancement with gold nanoparticles. *J. Pharm. Pharmacol.* **2008**, *60*, 977–985. [CrossRef] [PubMed]
29. Hainfeld, J.F.; Slatkin, D.N.; Smilowitz, H.M. The use of gold nanoparticles to enhance radiotherapy in mice. *Phys. Med. Biol.* **2004**. [CrossRef] [PubMed]
30. Zheng, Y.; Sanche, L. Gold nanoparticles enhance DNA damage induced by anti-cancer drugs and radiation. *Radiat. Res.* **2009**. [CrossRef] [PubMed]
31. Yeh, Y.C.; Creran, B.; Rotello, V.M. Gold nanoparticles: Preparation, properties, and applications in bionanotechnology. *Nanoscale* **2012**, *4*, 1871–1880. [CrossRef]
32. Stiufiuc, R.; Iacovita, C.; Nicoara, R.; Stiufiuc, G.; Florea, A.; Achim, M.; Lucaciu, C.M. One-step synthesis of PEGylated gold nanoparticles with tunable surface charge. *J. Nanomater.* **2013**. [CrossRef]

33. Sztandera, K.; Gorzkiewicz, M.; Klajnert-Maculewicz, B. Gold Nanoparticles in Cancer Treatment. *Mol. Pharm.* **2018**, *16*, 1–23. [CrossRef]
34. Huff, T.B.; Tong, L.; Zhao, Y.; Hansen, M.N.; Cheng, J.X.; Wei, A. Hyperthermic effects of gold nanorods on tumor cells. *Nanomedicine* **2007**. [CrossRef]
35. Rastinehad, A.R.; Anastos, H.; Wajswol, E.; Winoker, J.S.; Sfakianos, J.P.; Doppalapudi, S.K.; Carrick, M.R.; Knauer, C.J.; Taouli, B.; Lewis, S.C.; et al. Gold nanoshell-localized photothermal ablation of prostate tumors in a clinical pilot device study. *Proc. Natl. Acad. Sci. USA* **2019**. [CrossRef]
36. Vines, J.B.; Yoon, J.H.; Ryu, N.E.; Lim, D.J.; Park, H. Gold nanoparticles for photothermal cancer therapy. *Front. Chem.* **2019**, *7*. [CrossRef]
37. Abadeer, N.S.; Murphy, C.J. Recent Progress in Cancer Thermal Therapy Using Gold Nanoparticles. *J. Phys. Chem. C* **2016**, *120*, 4691–4716. [CrossRef]
38. Mendes, R.; Pedrosa, P.; Lima, J.C.; Fernandes, A.R.; Baptista, P.V. Photothermal enhancement of chemotherapy in breast cancer by visible irradiation of Gold Nanoparticles. *Sci. Rep.* **2017**. [CrossRef] [PubMed]
39. Ash, C.; Dubec, M.; Donne, K.; Bashford, T. Effect of wavelength and beam width on penetration in light-tissue interaction using computational methods. *Lasers Med. Sci.* **2017**. [CrossRef] [PubMed]
40. Yang, J.; Wang, F.; Yuan, H.; Zhang, L.; Jiang, Y.; Zhang, X.; Liu, C.; Chai, L.; Li, H.; Stenzel, M. Recent advances in ultra-small fluorescent Au nanoclusters toward oncological research. *Nanoscale* **2019**, *11*, 17967–17980. [CrossRef] [PubMed]
41. Porret, E.; Le Guével, X.; Coll, J.L. Gold nanoclusters for biomedical applications: Toward: In vivo studies. *J. Mater. Chem. B* **2020**, *8*, 2216–2232. [CrossRef]
42. Bouché, M.; Hsu, J.C.; Dong, Y.C.; Kim, J.; Taing, K.; Cormode, D.P. Recent Advances in Molecular Imaging with Gold Nanoparticles. *Bioconjug. Chem.* **2020**, *31*, 303–314. [CrossRef]
43. Loynachan, C.N.; Soleimany, A.P.; Dudani, J.S.; Lin, Y.; Najer, A.; Bekdemir, A.; Chen, Q.; Bhatia, S.N.; Stevens, M.M. Renal clearable catalytic gold nanoclusters for in vivo disease monitoring. *Nat. Nanotechnol.* **2019**. [CrossRef]
44. Bromma, K.; Rieck, K.; Kulkarni, J.; O'Sullivan, C.; Sung, W.; Cullis, P.; Schuemann, J.; Chithrani, D.B. Use of a lipid nanoparticle system as a Trojan horse in delivery of gold nanoparticles to human breast cancer cells for improved outcomes in radiation therapy. *Cancer Nanotechnol.* **2019**. [CrossRef]
45. Mathiyazhakan, M.; Wiraja, C.; Xu, C. A Concise Review of Gold Nanoparticles-Based Photo-Responsive Liposomes for Controlled Drug Delivery. *Nano-Micro Lett.* **2018**. [CrossRef]
46. Chithrani, D.B. Optimization of Bio-Nano Interface Using Gold Nanostructures as a Model Nanoparticle System. *Insci. J.* **2011**. [CrossRef]
47. Libutti, S.K.; Paciotti, G.F.; Byrnes, A.A.; Alexander, H.R.; Gannon, W.E.; Walker, M.; Seidel, G.D.; Yuldasheva, N.; Tamarkin, L. Phase I and pharmacokinetic studies of CYT-6091, a novel PEGylated colloidal gold-rhTNF nanomedicine. *Clin. Cancer Res.* **2010**. [CrossRef]
48. *Clinicaltrials Pilot Study of AuroLase(tm) Therapy in Refractory and/or Recurrent Tumors of the Head and Neck*; U.S. National Library of Medicine: Bethesda, MD, USA; Goodyear: Akron, OH, USA, 2010.
49. Nanospectra Biosciences Inc. *Efficacy Study of AuroLase Therapy in Subjects with Primary and/or Metastatic Lung Tumors*; U.S. National Library of Medicine: Philadelphia, PA, USA, 2016.
50. Nanospectra Biosciences Inc. *MRI/US Fusion Imaging and Biopsy in Combination With Nanoparticle Directed Focal Therapy for Ablation of Prostate Tissue*; U.S. National Library of Medicine: Baltimore, MD, USA, 2016.
51. Northwesten Universty. *NU-0129 in Treating Patients With Recurrent Glioblastoma or Gliosarcoma Undergoing Surgery*; U.S. National Library of Medicine: Chicago, IL, USA, 2019.
52. Schuemann, J.; Bagley, A.; Berbeco, R.; Bromma, K.; Butterworth, K.T.; Byrne, H.; Chithrani, D.B.; Cho, S.H.; Cook, J.R.; Favaudon, V.; et al. Roadmap for metal nanoparticles in radiation therapy: Current status, translational challenges, and future directions. *Phys. Med. Biol.* **2020**. [CrossRef] [PubMed]
53. Rubin, P.; Carter, S.K. Combination Radiation Therapy and Chemotherapy: A Logical Basis for Their Clinical Use. *CA. Cancer J. Clin.* **1976**. [CrossRef] [PubMed]
54. Sharifi, M.; Attar, F.; Saboury, A.A.; Akhtari, K.; Hooshmand, N.; Hasan, A.; El-Sayed, M.A.; Falahati, M. Plasmonic gold nanoparticles: Optical manipulation, imaging, drug delivery and therapy. *J. Control. Release* **2019**, *311*, 170–189. [CrossRef]
55. Dykman, L.A.; Khlebtsov, N.G. Gold nanoparticles in chemo-, immuno-, and combined therapy: Review [Invited]. *Biomed. Opt. Express* **2019**. [CrossRef] [PubMed]

56. Beik, J.; Khateri, M.; Khosravi, Z.; Kamrava, S.K.; Kooranifar, S.; Ghaznavi, H.; Shakeri-Zadeh, A. Gold nanoparticles in combinatorial cancer therapy strategies. *Coord. Chem. Rev.* **2019**, *387*, 299–324. [CrossRef]
57. Elahi, N.; Kamali, M.; Baghersad, M.H. Recent biomedical applications of gold nanoparticles: A review. *Talanta* **2018**, *184*, 537–556. [CrossRef] [PubMed]
58. Riley, R.S.; Day, E.S. Gold nanoparticle-mediated photothermal therapy: Applications and opportunities for multimodal cancer treatment. *Wiley Interdiscip. Rev. Nanomed. Nanobiotechnol.* **2017**, *9*, e1449. [CrossRef]
59. Siddique, S.; Chow, J.C.L. Gold nanoparticles for drug delivery and cancer therapy. *Appl. Sci.* **2020**, *10*, 3824. [CrossRef]
60. Her, S.; Jaffray, D.A.; Allen, C. Gold nanoparticles for applications in cancer radiotherapy: Mechanisms and recent advancements. *Adv. Drug Deliv. Rev.* **2017**, *109*, 84–101. [CrossRef]
61. Kong, F.Y.; Zhang, J.W.; Li, R.F.; Wang, Z.X.; Wang, W.J.; Wang, W. Unique roles of gold nanoparticles in drug delivery, targeting and imaging applications. *Molecules* **2017**, *22*, 1445. [CrossRef]
62. Citrin, D.E. Recent developments in radiotherapy. *N. Engl. J. Med.* **2017**, *377*, 1065–1075. [CrossRef] [PubMed]
63. Foroozandeh, P.; Aziz, A.A. Insight into Cellular Uptake and Intracellular Trafficking of Nanoparticles. *Nanoscale Res. Lett.* **2018**, *13*. [CrossRef] [PubMed]
64. Chithrani, B.D.; Stewart, J.; Allen, C.; Jaffray, D.A. Intracellular uptake, transport, and processing of nanostructures in cancer cells. *Nanomed. Nanotechnol. Biol. Med.* **2009**. [CrossRef] [PubMed]
65. Chithrani, D.B. Intracellular uptake, transport, and processing of gold nanostructures. *Mol. Membr. Biol.* **2010**, *27*, 299–311. [CrossRef]
66. Chithrani, B.D.; Ghazani, A.A.; Chan, W.C.W. Determining the size and shape dependence of gold nanoparticle uptake into mammalian cells. *Nano Lett.* **2006**. [CrossRef] [PubMed]
67. Gao, H.; Shi, W.; Freund, L.B. Mechanics of receptor-mediated endocytosis. *Proc. Natl. Acad. Sci. USA* **2005**. [CrossRef]
68. Jin, H.; Heller, D.A.; Sharma, R.; Strano, M.S. Size-dependent cellular uptake and expulsion of single-walled carbon nanotubes: Single particle tracking and a generic uptake model for nanoparticles. *ACS Nano* **2009**. [CrossRef]
69. Jin, H.; Heller, D.A.; Strano, M.S. Single-particle tracking of endocytosis and exocytosis of single-walled carbon nanotubes in NIH-3T3 cells. *Nano Lett.* **2008**. [CrossRef]
70. Ma, X.; Wu, Y.; Jin, S.; Tian, Y.; Zhang, X.; Zhao, Y.; Yu, L.; Liang, X.J. Gold nanoparticles induce autophagosome accumulation through size-dependent nanoparticle uptake and lysosome impairment. *ACS Nano* **2011**. [CrossRef]
71. Liu, M.; Li, Q.; Liang, L.; Li, J.; Wang, K.; Li, J.; Lv, M.; Chen, N.; Song, H.; Lee, J.; et al. Real-Time visualization of clustering and intracellular transport of gold nanoparticles by correlative imaging. *Nat. Commun.* **2017**. [CrossRef]
72. Chithrani, B.D.; Chan, W.C.W. Elucidating the mechanism of cellular uptake and removal of protein-coated gold nanoparticles of different sizes and shapes. *Nano Lett.* **2007**. [CrossRef] [PubMed]
73. Bednarski, M.; Dudek, M.; Knutelska, J.; Nowiński, L.; Sapa, J.; Zygmunt, M.; Nowak, G.; Luty-Błocho, M.; Wojnicki, M.; Fitzner, K.; et al. The influence of the route of administration of gold nanoparticles on their tissue distribution and basic biochemical parameters: In vivo studies. *Pharmacol. Rep.* **2015**. [CrossRef] [PubMed]
74. Zhang, X.D.; Wu, H.Y.; Wu, D.; Wang, Y.Y.; Chang, J.H.; Zhai, Z.B.; Meng, A.M.; Liu, P.X.; Zhang, L.A.; Fan, F.Y. Toxicologic effects of gold nanoparticles in vivo by different administration routes. *Int. J. Nanomed.* **2010**. [CrossRef] [PubMed]
75. Nie, S. Editorial: Understanding and overcoming major barriers in cancer nanomedicine. *Nanomedicine* **2010**, *5*, 523–528. [CrossRef]
76. Cruje, C.; Yang, C.; Uertz, J.; Van Prooijen, M.; Chithrani, B.D. Optimization of PEG coated nanoscale gold particles for enhanced radiation therapy. *RSC Adv.* **2015**. [CrossRef]
77. Cruje, C.; Chithrani, D.B. Polyethylene Glycol Functionalized Nanoparticles for Improved Cancer Treatment. *Rev. Nanosci. Nanotechnol.* **2014**. [CrossRef]
78. Tenzer, S.; Docter, D.; Kuharev, J.; Musyanovych, A.; Fetz, V.; Hecht, R.; Schlenk, F.; Fischer, D.; Kiouptsi, K.; Reinhardt, C.; et al. Rapid formation of plasma protein corona critically affects nanoparticle pathophysiology. *Nat. Nanotechnol.* **2013**. [CrossRef]

79. Carnovale, C.; Bryant, G.; Shukla, R.; Bansal, V. Gold nanoparticle biodistribution and toxicity: Role of biological corona in relation with nanoparticle characteristics. In *Metal Nanoparticles in Pharma*; Springer International Publishing: Cham, Switzerland, 2017; ISBN 9783319637907.
80. Yang, C.; Bromma, K.; Chithrani, D. Peptide mediated in vivo tumor targeting of nanoparticles through optimization in single and multilayer in vitro cell models. *Cancers (Basel)* **2018**, *10*, 84. [CrossRef]
81. Manson, J.; Kumar, D.; Meenan, B.J.; Dixon, D. Polyethylene glycol functionalized gold nanoparticles: The influence of capping density on stability in various media. *Gold Bull.* **2011**. [CrossRef]
82. Zhang, G.; Yang, Z.; Lu, W.; Zhang, R.; Huang, Q.; Tian, M.; Li, L.; Liang, D.; Li, C. Influence of anchoring ligands and particle size on the colloidal stability and in vivo biodistribution of polyethylene glycol-coated gold nanoparticles in tumor-xenografted mice. *Biomaterials* **2009**. [CrossRef]
83. Milton Harris, J.; Chess, R.B. Effect of pegylation on pharmaceuticals. *Nat. Rev. Drug Discov.* **2003**, *2*, 214–221. [CrossRef] [PubMed]
84. Yin, H.Q.; Bi, F.L.; Gan, F. Rapid synthesis of cyclic RGD conjugated gold nanoclusters for targeting and fluorescence imaging of melanoma A375 cells. *Bioconjug. Chem.* **2015**. [CrossRef] [PubMed]
85. Rieck, K.; Bromma, K.; Sung, W.; Bannister, A.; Schuemann, J.; Chithrani, D.B. Modulation of gold nanoparticle mediated radiation dose enhancement through synchronization of breast tumor cell population. *Br. J. Radiol.* **2019**, *92*. [CrossRef] [PubMed]
86. Cho, W.S.; Cho, M.; Jeong, J.; Choi, M.; Han, B.S.; Shin, H.S.; Hong, J.; Chung, B.H.; Jeong, J.; Cho, M.H. Size-dependent tissue kinetics of PEG-coated gold nanoparticles. *Toxicol. Appl. Pharmacol.* **2010**. [CrossRef] [PubMed]
87. Li, X.; Hu, Z.; Ma, J.; Wang, X.; Zhang, Y.; Wang, W.; Yuan, Z. The systematic evaluation of size-dependent toxicity and multi-time biodistribution of gold nanoparticles. *Colloids Surf. B Biointerfaces* **2018**. [CrossRef] [PubMed]
88. Fan, M.; Han, Y.; Gao, S.; Yan, H.; Cao, L.; Li, Z.; Liang, X.J.; Zhang, J. Ultrasmall gold nanoparticles in cancer diagnosis and therapy. *Theranostics* **2020**, *10*, 494–4957. [CrossRef]
89. Bugno, J.; Poellmann, M.J.; Sokolowski, K.; Hsu, H.J.; Kim, D.H.; Hong, S. Tumor penetration of Sub-10 nm nanoparticles: Effect of dendrimer properties on their penetration in multicellular tumor spheroids. *Nanomed. Nanotechnol. Biol. Med.* **2019**. [CrossRef]
90. Jing, X.; Yang, F.; Shao, C.; Wei, K.; Xie, M.; Shen, H.; Shu, Y. Role of hypoxia in cancer therapy by regulating the tumor microenvironment. *Mol. Cancer* **2019**, *18*, 157. [CrossRef]
91. Kharazian, B.; Lohse, S.E.; Ghasemi, F.; Raoufi, M.; Saei, A.A.; Hashemi, F.; Farvadi, F.; Alimohamadi, R.; Jalali, S.A.; Shokrgozar, M.A.; et al. Bare surface of gold nanoparticle induces inflammation through unfolding of plasma fibrinogen. *Sci. Rep.* **2018**. [CrossRef]
92. Elci, S.G.; Jiang, Y.; Yan, B.; Kim, S.T.; Saha, K.; Moyano, D.F.; Yesilbag Tonga, G.; Jackson, L.C.; Rotello, V.M.; Vachet, R.W. Surface Charge Controls the Suborgan Biodistributions of Gold Nanoparticles. *ACS Nano* **2016**. [CrossRef]
93. Riviere, J.E.; Jaberi-Douraki, M.; Lillich, J.; Azizi, T.; Joo, H.; Choi, K.; Thakkar, R.; Monteiro-Riviere, N.A. Modeling gold nanoparticle biodistribution after arterial infusion into perfused tissue: Effects of surface coating, size and protein corona. *Nanotoxicology* **2018**. [CrossRef]
94. Geng, F.; Xing, J.Z.; Chen, J.; Yang, R.; Hao, Y.; Song, K.; Kong, B. Pegylated glucose gold nanoparticles for improved in-vivo bio-distribution and enhanced radiotherapy on cervical cancer. *J. Biomed. Nanotechnol.* **2014**. [CrossRef] [PubMed]
95. Harding, J.; Burtness, B. Cetuximab: An epidermal growth factor receptor chimeric human-murine monoclonal antibody. *Drugs Today* **2005**, *41*, 107–127. [CrossRef] [PubMed]
96. Kao, H.W.; Lin, Y.Y.; Chen, C.C.; Chi, K.H.; Tien, D.C.; Hsia, C.C.; Lin, W.J.; Chen, F.D.; Lin, M.H.; Wang, H.E. Biological characterization of cetuximab-conjugated gold nanoparticles in a tumor animal model. *Nanotechnology* **2014**. [CrossRef] [PubMed]
97. Ni, X.; Castanares, M.; Mukherjee, A.; Lupold, S.E. Nucleic Acid Aptamers: Clinical Applications and Promising New Horizons. *Curr. Med. Chem.* **2011**. [CrossRef] [PubMed]
98. Jo, H.; Ban, C. Aptamer-nanoparticle complexes as powerful diagnostic and therapeutic tools. *Exp. Mol. Med.* **2016**, *5*. [CrossRef]
99. Byrne, J.D.; Betancourt, T.; Brannon-Peppas, L. Active targeting schemes for nanoparticle systems in cancer therapeutics. *Adv. Drug Deliv. Rev.* **2008**, *15*, 1617–1626. [CrossRef]

100. Choi, C.H.J.; Alabi, C.A.; Webster, P.; Davis, M.E. Mechanism of active targeting in solid tumors with transferrin-containing gold nanoparticles. *Proc. Natl. Acad. Sci. USA* **2010**. [CrossRef]
101. Zhang, Z.; Jia, J.; Lai, Y.; Ma, Y.; Weng, J.; Sun, L. Conjugating folic acid to gold nanoparticles through glutathione for targeting and detecting cancer cells. *Bioorg. Med. Chem.* **2010**, *18*, 5528–5534. [CrossRef]
102. Charbgoo, F.; Nejabat, M.; Abnous, K.; Soltani, F.; Taghdisi, S.M.; Alibolandi, M.; Thomas Shier, W.; Steele, T.W.J.; Ramezani, M. Gold nanoparticle should understand protein corona for being a clinical nanomaterial. *J. Control. Release* **2018**, *272*, 39–53. [CrossRef]
103. de Carvalho, T.G.; Garcia, V.B.; de Araújo, A.A.; da Silva Gasparotto, L.H.; Silva, H.; Guerra, G.C.B.; de Castro Miguel, E.; de Carvalho Leitão, R.F.; da Silva Costa, D.V.; Cruz, L.J.; et al. Spherical neutral gold nanoparticles improve anti-inflammatory response, oxidative stress and fibrosis in alcohol-methamphetamine-induced liver injury in rats. *Int. J. Pharm.* **2018**. [CrossRef] [PubMed]
104. Shukla, R.; Bansal, V.; Chaudhary, M.; Basu, A.; Bhonde, R.R.; Sastry, M. Biocompatibility of gold nanoparticles and their endocytotic fate inside the cellular compartment: A microscopic overview. *Langmuir* **2005**, *23*, 10644–10654. [CrossRef] [PubMed]
105. Connor, E.E.; Mwamuka, J.; Gole, A.; Murphy, C.J.; Wyatt, M.D. Gold nanoparticles are taken up by human cells but do not cause acute cytotoxicity. *Small* **2005**. [CrossRef] [PubMed]
106. Steckiewicz, K.P.; Barcinska, E.; Malankowska, A.; Zauszkiewicz–Pawlak, A.; Nowaczyk, G.; Zaleska-Medynska, A.; Inkielewicz-Stepniak, I. Impact of gold nanoparticles shape on their cytotoxicity against human osteoblast and osteosarcoma in in vitro model. Evaluation of the safety of use and anti-cancer potential. *J. Mater. Sci. Mater. Med.* **2019**. [CrossRef] [PubMed]
107. Zhang, X.D.; Wu, D.; Shen, X.; Chen, J.; Sun, Y.M.; Liu, P.X.; Liang, X.J. Size-dependent radiosensitization of PEG-coated gold nanoparticles for cancer radiation therapy. *Biomaterials* **2012**. [CrossRef]
108. Fratoddi, I.; Venditti, I.; Cametti, C.; Russo, M.V. How toxic are gold nanoparticles? The state-of-the-art. *Nano Res.* **2015**. [CrossRef]
109. Jia, Y.P.; Ma, B.Y.; Wei, X.W.; Qian, Z.Y. The in vitro and in vivo toxicity of gold nanoparticles. *Chin. Chem. Lett.* **2017**. [CrossRef]
110. Haume, K.; Rosa, S.; Grellet, S.; Śmiałek, M.A.; Butterworth, K.T.; Solov'yov, A.V.; Prise, K.M.; Golding, J.; Mason, N.J. Gold nanoparticles for cancer radiotherapy: A review. *Cancer Nanotechnol.* **2016**, *7*. [CrossRef]
111. Nath, R.; Bongiorni, P.; Rockwell, S. Iododeoxyuridine radiosensitization by low- and high-energy photons for brachytherapy dose rates. *Radiat. Res.* **1990**. [CrossRef]
112. Matsudaira, H.; Ueno, A.M.; Furuno, I. Iodine contrast medium sensitizes cultured mammalian cells to X rays but not to γ rays. *Radiat. Res.* **1980**. [CrossRef]
113. Xie, W.Z.; Friedland, W.; Li, W.B.; Li, C.Y.; Oeh, U.; Qiu, R.; Li, J.L.; Hoeschen, C. Simulation on the molecular radiosensitization effect of gold nanoparticles in cells irradiated by x-rays. *Phys. Med. Biol.* **2015**. [CrossRef] [PubMed]
114. Khoo, A.M.; Cho, S.H.; Reynoso, F.J.; Aliru, M.; Aziz, K.; Bodd, M.; Yang, X.; Ahmed, M.F.; Yasar, S.; Manohar, N.; et al. Radiosensitization of Prostate Cancers in Vitro and in Vivo to Erbium-filtered Orthovoltage X-rays Using Actively Targeted Gold Nanoparticles. *Sci. Rep.* **2017**. [CrossRef] [PubMed]
115. Yang, C.; Bromma, K.; Di Ciano-Oliveira, C.; Zafarana, G.; van Prooijen, M.; Chithrani, D.B. Gold nanoparticle mediated combined cancer therapy. *Cancer Nanotechnol.* **2018**. [CrossRef]
116. Yang, C.; Bromma, K.; Sung, W.; Schuemann, J.; Chithrani, D. Determining the radiation enhancement effects of gold nanoparticles in cells in a combined treatment with cisplatin and radiation at therapeutic megavoltage energies. *Cancers (Basel)* **2018**, *10*, 150. [CrossRef] [PubMed]
117. Wolfe, T.; Chatterjee, D.; Lee, J.; Grant, J.D.; Bhattarai, S.; Tailor, R.; Goodrich, G.; Nicolucci, P.; Krishnan, S. Targeted gold nanoparticles enhance sensitization of prostate tumors to megavoltage radiation therapy in vivo. *Nanomed. Nanotechnol. Biol. Med.* **2015**. [CrossRef] [PubMed]
118. Rosa, S.; Connolly, C.; Schettino, G.; Butterworth, K.T.; Prise, K.M. Biological mechanisms of gold nanoparticle radiosensitization. *Cancer Nanotechnol.* **2017**, *8*. [CrossRef]
119. Mikami, Y.; Dhakshinamoorthy, A.; Alvaro, M.; García, H. Catalytic activity of unsupported gold nanoparticles. *Catal. Sci. Technol.* **2013**, *3*, 58–69. [CrossRef]
120. Nel, A.; Xia, T.; Mädler, L.; Li, N. Toxic potential of materials at the nanolevel. *Science* **2006**, *311*, 622–627. [CrossRef]

121. Misawa, M.; Takahashi, J. Generation of reactive oxygen species induced by gold nanoparticles under x-ray and UV Irradiations. *Nanomed. Nanotechnol. Biol. Med.* **2011**. [CrossRef]
122. Butterworth, K.T.; McMahon, S.J.; Currell, F.J.; Prise, K.M. Physical basis and biological mechanisms of gold nanoparticle radiosensitization. *Nanoscale* **2012**. [CrossRef]
123. Pan, Y.; Leifert, A.; Ruau, D.; Neuss, S.; Bornemann, J.; Schmid, G.; Brandau, W.; Simon, U.; Jahnen-Dechent, W. Gold nanoparticles of diameter 1.4 nm trigger necrosis by oxidative stress and mitochondrial damage. *Small* **2009**. [CrossRef] [PubMed]
124. Pawlik, T.M.; Keyomarsi, K. Role of cell cycle in mediating sensitivity to radiotherapy. *Int. J. Radiat. Oncol. Biol. Phys.* **2004**. [CrossRef] [PubMed]
125. Butterworth, K.T.; Coulter, J.A.; Jain, S.; Forker, J.; McMahon, S.J.; Schettino, G.; Prise, K.M.; Currell, F.J.; Hirst, D.G. Evaluation of cytotoxicity and radiation enhancement using 1.9nm gold particles: Potential application for cancer therapy. *Nanotechnology* **2010**. [CrossRef] [PubMed]
126. Elbayoumi, T.A. Nano drug-delivery systems in cancer therapy: Gains, pitfalls and considerations in DMPK and PD. *Ther. Deliv.* **2010**, *1*. [CrossRef]
127. Paciotti, G.F.; Kingston, D.G.I.; Tamarkin, L. Colloidal gold nanoparticles: A novel nanoparticle platform for developing multifunctional tumor-targeted drug delivery vectors. *Drug Dev. Res.* **2006**, *67*, 47–54. [CrossRef]
128. Paciotti, G.F.; Myer, L.; Weinreich, D.; Goia, D.; Pavel, N.; McLaughlin, R.E.; Tamarkin, L. Colloidal gold: A novel nanoparticle vector for tumor directed drug delivery. *Drug Deliv. J. Deliv. Target. Ther. Agents* **2004**. [CrossRef]
129. Ghosh, P.; Han, G.; De, M.; Kim, C.K.; Rotello, V.M. Gold nanoparticles in delivery applications. *Adv. Drug Deliv. Rev.* **2008**, *60*. [CrossRef]
130. Spampinato, V.; Parracino, M.A.; La Spina, R.; Rossi, F.; Ceccone, G. Surface Analysis of Gold Nanoparticles Functionalized with Thiol-Modified Glucose SAMs for Biosensor Applications. *Front. Chem.* **2016**, *4*, 8. [CrossRef]
131. Jazayeri, M.H.; Amani, H.; Pourfatollah, A.A.; Pazoki-Toroudi, H.; Sedighimoghaddam, B. Various methods of gold nanoparticles (GNPs) conjugation to antibodies. *Sens. Bio-Sens. Res.* **2016**, *9*, 17–22. [CrossRef]
132. Awotunde, O.; Okyem, S.; Chikoti, R.; Driskell, J.D. The Role of Free Thiol on Protein Adsorption to Gold Nanoparticles. *Langmuir* **2020**. [CrossRef]
133. Paciotti, G.F.; Zhao, J.; Cao, S.; Brodie, P.J.; Tamarkin, L.; Huhta, M.; Myer, L.D.; Friedman, J.; Kingston, D.G.I. Synthesis and Evaluation of Paclitaxel-Loaded Gold Nanoparticles for Tumor-Targeted Drug Delivery. *Bioconjug. Chem.* **2016**. [CrossRef] [PubMed]
134. Spicer, C.D.; Pashuck, E.T.; Stevens, M.M. Achieving Controlled Biomolecule-Biomaterial Conjugation. *Chem. Rev.* **2018**, *118*, 7702–7743. [CrossRef] [PubMed]
135. Brown, S.D.; Nativo, P.; Smith, J.A.; Stirling, D.; Edwards, P.R.; Venugopal, B.; Flint, D.J.; Plumb, J.A.; Graham, D.; Wheate, N.J. Gold nanoparticles for the improved anticancer drug delivery of the active component of oxaliplatin. *J. Am. Chem. Soc.* **2010**. [CrossRef] [PubMed]
136. Fratoddi, I.; Venditti, I.; Cametti, C.; Russo, M.V. Gold nanoparticles and gold nanoparticle-conjugates for delivery of therapeutic molecules. Progress and challenges. *J. Mater. Chem. B* **2014**, *2*, 4204–4220. [CrossRef] [PubMed]
137. Patra, C.R.; Bhattacharya, R.; Wang, E.; Katarya, A.; Lau, J.S.; Dutta, S.; Muders, M.; Wang, S.; Buhrow, S.A.; Safgren, S.L.; et al. Targeted delivery of gemcitabine to pancreatic adenocarcinoma using cetuximab as a targeting agent. *Cancer Res.* **2008**. [CrossRef]
138. Du, Y.; Xia, L.; Jo, A.; Davis, R.M.; Bissel, P.; Ehrich, M.F.; Kingston, D.G.I. Synthesis and Evaluation of Doxorubicin-Loaded Gold Nanoparticles for Tumor-Targeted Drug Delivery. *Bioconjug. Chem.* **2018**. [CrossRef]
139. François, A.; Laroche, A.; Pinaud, N.; Salmon, L.; Ruiz, J.; Robert, J.; Astruc, D. Encapsulation of docetaxel into PEGylated gold nanoparticles for vectorization to cancer cells. *ChemMedChem* **2011**. [CrossRef]
140. Farooq, M.U.; Novosad, V.; Rozhkova, E.A.; Wali, H.; Ali, A.; Fateh, A.A.; Neogi, P.B.; Neogi, A.; Wang, Z. Gold Nanoparticles-enabled Efficient Dual Delivery of Anticancer Therapeutics to HeLa Cells. *Sci. Rep.* **2018**. [CrossRef]
141. Tan, J.; Cho, T.J.; Tsai, D.H.; Liu, J.; Pettibone, J.M.; You, R.; Hackley, V.A.; Zachariah, M.R. Surface Modification of Cisplatin-Complexed Gold Nanoparticles and Its Influence on Colloidal Stability, Drug Loading, and Drug Release. *Langmuir* **2018**. [CrossRef]

142. Rosenberg, B.; VanCamp, L.; Trosko, J.E.; Mansour, V.H. Platinum compounds: A new class of potent antitumour agents. *Nature* **1969**, *222*, 385–386. [CrossRef]
143. Wang, D.; Lippard, S.J. Cellular processing of platinum anticancer drugs. *Nat. Rev. Drug Discov.* **2005**, *4*, 307–320. [CrossRef] [PubMed]
144. Kelland, L. The resurgence of platinum-based cancer chemotherapy. *Nat. Rev. Cancer* **2007**, *7*, 574–584. [CrossRef] [PubMed]
145. Reedijk, J. New clues for platinum antitumor chemistry: Kinetically controlled metal binding to DNA. *Proc. Natl. Acad. Sci. USA* **2003**, *100*, 3611–3616. [CrossRef] [PubMed]
146. Oliver, T.G.; Mercer, K.L.; Sayles, L.C.; Burke, J.R.; Mendus, D.; Lovejoy, K.S.; Cheng, M.H.; Subramanian, A.; Mu, D.; Powers, S.; et al. Chronic cisplatin treatment promotes enhanced damage repair and tumor progression in a mouse model of lung cancer. *Genes Dev.* **2010**. [CrossRef]
147. Comenge, J.; Sotelo, C.; Romero, F.; Gallego, O.; Barnadas, A.; Parada, T.G.C.; Domínguez, F.; Puntes, V.F. Detoxifying Antitumoral Drugs via Nanoconjugation: The Case of Gold Nanoparticles and Cisplatin. *PLoS ONE* **2012**, *7*, e47562. [CrossRef]
148. Zhao, X.; Pan, J.; Li, W.; Yang, W.; Qin, L.; Pan, Y. Gold nanoparticles enhance cisplatin delivery and potentiate chemotherapy by decompressing colorectal cancer vessels. *Int. J. Nanomed.* **2018**. [CrossRef]
149. Lyseng-Williamson, K.A.; Fenton, C. Docetaxel: A review of its use in metastatic breast cancer. *Drugs* **2005**, *65*, 2513–2531. [CrossRef]
150. Kumar, P. A new paradigm for the treatment of high-risk prostate cancer: Radiosensitization with docetaxel. *Rev. Urol.* **2003**, *5* (Suppl. S3), S71–S77.
151. Scagliotti, G.V.; Turrisi, A.T. Docetaxel-Based Combined-Modality Chemoradiotherapy for Locally Advanced Non-Small Cell Lung Cancer. *Oncologist* **2003**, *8*, 361–374. [CrossRef]
152. Colevas, A.D.; Posner, M.R. Docetaxel in head and neck cancer: A review. *Am. J. Clin. Oncol. Cancer Clin. Trials* **1998**, *21*, 482–486. [CrossRef]
153. Fulton, B.; Spencer, C.M. Docetaxel: A Review of its Pharmacodynamic and Pharmacokinetic Properties and Therapeutic Efficacy in the Management of Metastatic Breast Cancer. *Drugs* **1996**. [CrossRef] [PubMed]
154. Herbst, R.S.; Khuri, F.R. Mode of action of docetaxel - A basis for combination with novel anticancer agents. *Cancer Treat. Rev.* **2003**. [CrossRef]
155. Nehmé, A.; Varadarajan, P.; Sellakumar, G.; Gerhold, M.; Niedner, H.; Zhang, Q.; Lin, X.; Christen, R.D. Modulation of docetaxel-induced apoptosis and cell cycle arrest by all-trans retinoic acid in prostate cancer cells. *Br. J. Cancer* **2001**. [CrossRef] [PubMed]
156. Loibl, S.; Denkert, C.; von Minckwitz, G. Neoadjuvant treatment of breast cancer-Clinical and research perspective. *Breast* **2015**. [CrossRef] [PubMed]
157. Hennequin, C.; Giocanti, N.; Favaudon, V. Interaction of ionizing radiation with paclitaxel (taxol) and docetaxel (taxotere) in HeLa and SQ20B cells. *Cancer Res.* **1996**, *56*, 1842–1850. [PubMed]
158. Mason, K.A.; Hunter, N.R.; Milas, M.; Abbruzzese, J.L.; Milas, L. Docetaxel enhances tumor radioresponse in vivo. *Clin. Cancer Res.* **1997**, *3*, 2431–2438. [PubMed]
159. Kim, J.A.; Aberg, C.; Salvati, A.; Dawson, K.A. Role of cell cycle on the cellular uptake and dilution of nanoparticles in a cell population. *Nat. Nanotechnol.* **2012**. [CrossRef]
160. Bannister, A.H.; Bromma, K.; Sung, W.; Monica, M.; Cicon, L.; Howard, P.; Chow, R.L.; Schuemann, J.; Chithrani, D.B. Modulation of nanoparticle uptake, intracellular distribution, and retention with docetaxel to enhance radiotherapy. *Br. J. Radiol.* **2020**, *93*. [CrossRef]
161. Rawla, P.; Sunkara, T.; Gaduputi, V. Epidemiology of Pancreatic Cancer: Global Trends, Etiology and Risk Factors. *World J. Oncol.* **2019**, *10*, 10–27. [CrossRef]
162. Burris, H.A.; Moore, M.J.; Andersen, J.; Green, M.R.; Rothenberg, M.L.; Modiano, M.R.; Cripps, M.C.; Portenoy, R.K.; Storniolo, A.M.; Tarassoff, P.; et al. Improvements in survival and clinical benefit with gemcitabine as first- line therapy for patients with advanced pancreas cancer: A randomized trial. *J. Clin. Oncol.* **1997**. [CrossRef]
163. Shelley, M.D.; Jones, G.; Cleves, A.; Wilt, T.J.; Mason, M.D.; Kynaston, H.G. Intravesical gemcitabine therapy for non-muscle invasive bladder cancer (NMIBC): A systematic review. *BJU Int.* **2012**, *109*, 496–505. [CrossRef] [PubMed]

164. Kroep, J.R.; Giaccone, G.; Tolis, C.; Voorn, D.A.; Loves, W.J.P.; Van Groeningen, C.J.; Pinedo, H.M.; Peters, G.J. Sequence dependent effect of paclitaxel on gemcitabine metabolism in relation to cell cycle and cytotoxicity in non-small-cell lung cancer cell lines. *Br. J. Cancer* **2000**. [CrossRef] [PubMed]
165. Peters, G.J.; Van Der Wilt, C.L.; Van Moorsel, C.J.A.; Kroep, J.R.; Bergman, A.M.; Ackland, S.P. Basis for effective combination cancer chemotherapy with antimetabolites. *Pharmacol. Ther.* **2000**, *87*, 227–253. [CrossRef]
166. Peters, G.J.; Clavel, M.; Noordhuis, P.; Geyssen, G.J.; Laan, A.C.; Guastalla, J.; Edzes, H.T.; Vermorken, J.B. Clinical phase I and pharmacology study of gemcitabine (2′, 2′-difluorodeoxycytidine) administered in a two-weekly schedule. *J. Chemother.* **2007**. [CrossRef] [PubMed]
167. Huai, Y.; Zhang, Y.; Xiong, X.; Das, S.; Bhattacharya, R.; Mukherjee, P. Gold Nanoparticles sensitize pancreatic cancer cells to gemcitabine. *Cell Stress* **2019**. [CrossRef]
168. Shibue, T.; Weinberg, R.A. EMT, CSCs, and drug resistance: The mechanistic link and clinical implications. *Nat. Rev. Clin. Oncol.* **2017**, *14*, 611–629. [CrossRef]
169. Pal, K.; Al-Suraih, F.; Gonzalez-Rodriguez, R.; Dutta, S.K.; Wang, E.; Kwak, H.S.; Caulfield, T.R.; Coffer, J.L.; Bhattacharya, S. Multifaceted peptide assisted one-pot synthesis of gold nanoparticles for plectin-1 targeted gemcitabine delivery in pancreatic cancer. *Nanoscale* **2017**. [CrossRef]
170. Loehrer, P.J.; Feng, Y.; Cardenes, H.; Wagner, L.; Brell, J.M.; Cella, D.; Flynn, P.; Ramanathan, R.K.; Crane, C.H.; Alberts, S.R.; et al. Gemcitabine alone versus gemcitabine plus radiotherapy in patients with locally advanced pancreatic cancer: An Eastern Cooperative Oncology Group trial. *J. Clin. Oncol.* **2011**. [CrossRef]
171. Davidi, E.S.; Dreifuss, T.; Motiei, M.; Shai, E.; Bragilovski, D.; Lubimov, L.; Kindler, M.J.J.; Popovtzer, A.; Don, J.; Popovtzer, R. Cisplatin-conjugated gold nanoparticles as a theranostic agent for head and neck cancer. *Head Neck* **2018**. [CrossRef]
172. Peng, C.; Xu, J.; Yu, M.; Ning, X.; Huang, Y.; Du, B.; Hernandez, E.; Kapur, P.; Hsieh, J.T.; Zheng, J. Tuning the In Vivo Transport of Anticancer Drugs Using Renal-Clearable Gold Nanoparticles. *Angew. Chem.-Int. Ed.* **2019**. [CrossRef]
173. Kalimuthu, K.; Lubin, B.C.; Bazylevich, A.; Gellerman, G.; Shpilberg, O.; Luboshits, G.; Firer, M.A. Gold nanoparticles stabilize peptide-drug-conjugates for sustained targeted drug delivery to cancer cells. *J. Nanobiotechnol.* **2018**. [CrossRef] [PubMed]
174. Alamzadeh, Z.; Beik, J.; Mirrahimi, M.; Shakeri-Zadeh, A.; Ebrahimi, F.; Komeili, A.; Ghalandari, B.; Ghaznavi, H.; Kamrava, S.K.; Moustakis, C. Gold nanoparticles promote a multimodal synergistic cancer therapy strategy by co-delivery of thermo-chemo-radio therapy. *Eur. J. Pharm. Sci.* **2020**. [CrossRef] [PubMed]
175. Safwat, M.A.; Soliman, G.M.; Sayed, D.; Attia, M.A. Gold nanoparticles enhance 5-fluorouracil anticancer efficacy against colorectal cancer cells. *Int. J. Pharm.* **2016**. [CrossRef]
176. Fathy, M.M.; Mohamed, F.S.; Elbialy, N.S.; Elshemey, W.M. Multifunctional Chitosan-Capped Gold Nanoparticles for enhanced cancer chemo-radiotherapy: An invitro study. *Phys. Med.* **2018**. [CrossRef] [PubMed]
177. Wilhelm, S.; Tavares, A.J.; Dai, Q.; Ohta, S.; Audet, J.; Dvorak, H.F.; Chan, W.C.W. Analysis of nanoparticle delivery to tumours. *Nat. Rev. Mater.* **2016**, *1*. [CrossRef]
178. Verma, M. Personalized medicine and cancer. *J. Pers. Med.* **2012**, *2*, 1–14. [CrossRef] [PubMed]
179. Krzyszczyk, P.; Acevedo, A.; Davidoff, E.J.; Timmins, L.M.; Marrero-Berrios, I.; Patel, M.; White, C.; Lowe, C.; Sherba, J.J.; Hartmanshenn, C.; et al. The growing role of precision and personalized medicine for cancer treatment. *Technology* **2018**. [CrossRef]
180. Fan, H.; Demirci, U.; Chen, P. Emerging organoid models: Leaping forward in cancer research. *J. Hematol. Oncol.* **2019**, *12*. [CrossRef]
181. Fatehullah, A.; Tan, S.H.; Barker, N. Organoids as an in vitro model of human development and disease. *Nat. Cell Biol.* **2016**, *18*, 246–254. [CrossRef]
182. Driehuis, E.; Clevers, H. CRISPR/Cas 9 genome editing and its applications in organoids. *Am. J. Physiol.-Gastrointest. Liver Physiol.* **2017**, *312*, G257–G265. [CrossRef]
183. Yao, Y.; Xu, X.; Yang, L.; Zhu, J.; Wan, J.; Shen, L.; Xia, F.; Fu, G.; Deng, Y.; Pan, M.; et al. Patient-Derived Organoids Predict Chemoradiation Responses of Locally Advanced Rectal Cancer. *Cell Stem Cell* **2020**. [CrossRef] [PubMed]
184. Vives, J.; Batlle-Morera, L. The challenge of developing human 3D organoids into medicines. *Stem Cell Res. Ther.* **2020**, *11*, 1–4. [CrossRef] [PubMed]

185. Dossena, M.; Piras, R.; Cherubini, A.; Barilani, M.; Dugnani, E.; Salanitro, F.; Moreth, T.; Pampaloni, F.; Piemonti, L.; Lazzari, L. Standardized GMP-compliant scalable production of human pancreas organoids. *Stem Cell Res. Ther.* **2020**. [CrossRef] [PubMed]
186. Quereda, V.; Hou, S.; Madoux, F.; Scampavia, L.; Spicer, T.P.; Duckett, D. A Cytotoxic Three-Dimensional-Spheroid, High-Throughput Assay Using Patient-Derived Glioma Stem Cells. *SLAS Discov.* **2018**. [CrossRef]
187. Brüningk, S.C.; Rivens, I.; Box, C.; Oelfke, U.; ter Haar, G. 3D tumour spheroids for the prediction of the effects of radiation and hyperthermia treatments. *Sci. Rep.* **2020**. [CrossRef]

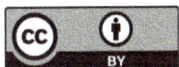

© 2020 by the authors. Licensee MDPI, Basel, Switzerland. This article is an open access article distributed under the terms and conditions of the Creative Commons Attribution (CC BY) license (http://creativecommons.org/licenses/by/4.0/).

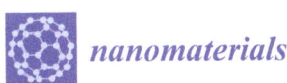

Article

Ultrastructural Features of Gold Nanoparticles Interaction with HepG2 and HEK293 Cells in Monolayer and Spheroids

Boris Chelobanov [†], Julia Poletaeva [†], Anna Epanchintseva, Anastasiya Tupitsyna, Inna Pyshnaya and Elena Ryabchikova *

Institute of Chemical Biology and Fundamental Medicine, Siberian Branch of Russian Academy of Science, Lavrent'ev av., 8, 630090 Novosibirsk, Russia; boris.p.chelobanov@gmail.com (B.C.); fabaceae@yandex.ru (J.P.); annaepanch@gmail.com (A.E.); aysa@ngs.ru (A.T.); pyshnaya@niboch.nsc.ru (I.P.)
* Correspondence: lenryab@yandex.ru; Tel.: +7-383-363-51-63
† These authors contributed equally to this work.

Received: 27 August 2020; Accepted: 13 October 2020; Published: 16 October 2020

Abstract: Use of multicellular spheroids in studies of nanoparticles (NPs) has increased in the last decade, however details of NPs interaction with spheroids are poorly known. We synthesized AuNPs (12.0 ± 0.1 nm in diameter, transmission electron microscopy (TEM) data) and covered them with bovine serum albumin (BSA) and polyethyleneimine (PEI). Values of hydrodynamic diameter were 17.4 ± 0.4; 35.9 ± 0.5 and ±125.9 ± 2.8 nm for AuNPs, AuBSA-NPs and AuPEI-NPs, and Z-potential (net charge) values were −33.6 ± 2.0; −35.7 ± 1.8 and 39.9 ± 1.3 mV, respectively. Spheroids of human hepatocarcinoma (HepG2) and human embryo kidney (HEK293) cells (Corning ®spheroid microplates CLS4515-5EA), and monolayers of these cell lines were incubated with all NPs for 15 min–4 h, and fixed in 4% paraformaldehyde solution. Samples were examined using transmission and scanning electron microscopy. HepG2 and HEK2893 spheroids showed tissue-specific features and contacted with culture medium by basal plasma membrane of the cells. HepG2 cells both in monolayer and spheroids did not uptake of the AuNPs, while AuBSA-NPs and AuPEI-NPs readily penetrated these cells. All studied NPs penetrated HEK293 cells in both monolayer and spheroids. Thus, two different cell cultures maintained a type of the interaction with NPs in monolayer and spheroid forms, which not depended on NPs Z-potential and size.

Keywords: AuNPs; AuPEI-NPs; AuBSA-NPs; electron microscopy; ultrastructure of HepG2 cells and spheroids; ultrastructure of HEK293 cells and spheroids; penetration of NPs into monolayer and spheroids

1. Introduction

Gold nanoparticles have a number of unique physical and chemical properties that, together with a good biocompatibility, makes them a promising tool for nanomedicine. Advantages of using gold nanoparticles (AuNPs) and their various modifications in the treatment and diagnosis of diseases are being actively studied; a number of comprehensive detailed reviews is devoted to this issue [1–6]. Similar to other NPs, AuNPs are studied in cell cultures and in laboratory animals; and in last decade a new experimental model has been developed: multicellular spheroids or micro-tissues (cell cultures in 3D-form); the advantages of spheroids are described in details [7–10]. Spheroids that mimic the structure and functions of various tissues have shown their suitability for studies of different problems in modern biomedicine, including the effects of drugs, drug damage to the liver, toxicity of chemical compounds, and human hepatocarcinoma (HepG2) spheroids are considered in such studies as a practically adequate replacement of primary hepatocytes [11–15]. The advent of commercially available devices for cultivation of spheroids has transformed their obtaining from "high art" into affordable technology, which expanded the scope of their application. Various approaches for obtaining spheroids are reported, which roughly can be divided to scaffold-based and scaffold-free; see reviews [8,12,16–18].

The number of published works on cellular spheroids is already in the thousands, but many details of their structure remain unknown, including the structure of their external surface and the morphological substrate of contact with the environment. Meanwhile, structure of the region adjacent to spheroids surface determine the nature of interaction not only with the culture medium, but also with soluble preparations and NPs containing in that medium. Morphological changes in spheroids treated with NPs or chemical compounds are studied mainly in transmitted light and various fluorescence methods [9,19–21]. The use of electron microscopy is rare and mostly is limited to registration of NPs presence in a cell [22–24] or TEM-illustration of NPs used in a study [9,15,21,25,26]. However, the size of NPs requires studying their interaction with cells at subcellular level, which is realized in a transmission electron microscopy (TEM) of ultrathin sections.

In this work, we examined and compared the morphology of HepG2 and human embryo kidney (HEK293) cell monolayers and spheroids with TEM and scanning electron microscopy (SEM), because we found out an insufficiency of published data. Both cell lines are epithelial in nature; however, HepG2 is well-differentiated line, which possesses structural and morphologic characteristics of hepatocytes, while morphology of HEK 293 cell line does not show tissue-specific features. In this work, we describe structural organization of the spheroids and point out the features specific for each cell type.

It was interesting to find out how HepG2 and HEK293 epithelial cell lines interact with the same NPs in monolayer and spheroids. We incubated the cells in monolayer and spheroids with synthesized AuNPs and their modified variants coated with protein (bovine serum albumin, BSA) or polymer (polyethylenimine, PEI). Here, we present data on features of the penetration of these NPs into HepG2 and HEK293 cells and compare those in spheroids and monolayer.

In common, in this work we present new comparative data on morphology of HepG2 and HEK293 cells in monolayer and spheroids, and their interaction with AuNPs, AuPEI and AuBSA-NPs.

2. Materials and Methods

2.1. Reagents

All used reagents were analytical grade. Ultrapure water of 18.2 MΩ·cm at 25 °C (Simplicity 185 system, Millipore, Burlington, MA, USA) was used in all processes of NPs preparation.

2.2. Preparation of AuNPs, AuBSA-NPs and AuPEI-NPs

AuNPs were synthesized similarly to [27]. In brief, the solution of $Na_3C_6H_5O_7·3H_2O$ (5 mL, 38.8 mM) (Fluka, Charlotte, NC, USA) was added under stirring to the boiled solution of $HAuCl_4·3H_2O$ (45 mL, 1 mM) (Aurat, Moscow, Russia). The mixture was intensively stirred for 20 min and kept at room temperature for 24 h, and then filtered (pore size of 0.45 µm, MDI, Ambala Cantt, India). Extinction coefficient of resultant suspension was $\varepsilon_{260} = 8.78 \times 10^8$ M^{-1} cm^{-1} (Shimadzu, Kyoto, Japan), which corresponds to a concentration of 3.6×10^{-9} M of Au [28]. The suspension was stored at 4 °C.

AuPEI-NPs were prepared by layer-by-layer approach. Initially, the reaction mixture (695 µL) containing AuNPs (3.6 nM) and 0.72 µM oligodeoxyribonucleotide (ON) was incubated for 30 min at 56 °C to prepare non-covalent AuON-NPs serving as an intermediate compound [29]. Oligodeoxyribonucleotide (5′-TTT TTT TTT TTT TTT TTT TTT TTT TT-3′) was synthesized on an ASM-800 (Biosset, Novosibirsk, Russia) by the solid-phase phosphoroamidite protocol using phosphoramidites from ChemGenes (Wilmington, MA USA). The ON was purified by reversed phase high performance liquid chromatography (HPLC) on an Agilent 1200 Series (Santa Clara, CA, USA) using a Zorbax 5 µm Eclipse-XDB-C18 80 Å column (150 × 4.6 mm^2) by Agilent (Santa Clara, CA, USA).

The AuON-NPs were washed with 0.5 mL of 4 mM $Na_3C_6H_5O_7$ solution and precipitated by centrifugation for 30 min at 13,200 rpm. The precipitate was diluted with 0.57 mL of 4 mM $Na_3C_6H_5O_7$ solution, and pH of the suspension was adjusted to 10 with 12.5 µL of 1 M Na_2HPO_4 (AlfaChem Plus, Saint Petersburg, Russia). Solution of 100 µL of 0.8% 11-mercaptoundecanoic acid (MUA) (Sigma-Aldrich, St. Louis, MO, USA) in 10% ethanol (Kemerovo Pharmaceutical factory, Kemerovo, Russia) was added with shaking (1400 rpm) to AuON-NPs, and the mixture was incubated for 30 min at 25 °C to obtain AuON-MUA-NPs. The product was washed with 0.6 mL of 1 mM NaCl (Panreac, Barcelona, Spain), and precipitated by centrifugation for 10 min at 13,200 rpm. The precipitate was diluted with 0.25 mL of 1 mM NaCl. The final step was carried out in several tubes (Eppendorf, Hamburg, Germany). The AuON-MUA-NPs (50 µL) were added with shaking (1400 rpm) to 50 µL of 0.1% branched polyethylenimine (PEI) in each tube. The PEI $(-NHCH_2CH_2-)_x(-N(CH_2CH_2NH_2)CH_2CH_2-)_y$, 10 kDa of molecular weight, was 99% of purity (Alfa Aesar, Ward Hill, MA, USA). The mixture was incubated for 30 min at 25 °C. Resulting product was washed with 0.5 mL of 1 mM NaCl, and then precipitated by centrifugation for 10 min at 13,200 rpm. The precipitate was diluted in 50 µL of 1 mM NaCl. The concentration of AuON-MUA-PEI-NPs (further designated as AuPEI-NPs) in the resulting suspension was 10 nM of AuNPs.

AuNPs coated with BSA were obtained by incubation of 250 µL 3 nM AuNPs with 50 µL of 10% BSA (Sigma, St. Louis, MO, USA) for 24 h on a Multi-rotator Multi Bio RS-24 at 10 rpm (Biosan, Riga, Latvia) [30]. The resulting AuBSA-NPs were washed with 1 mL of PBS (Sigma-Aldrich, St. Louis, MO, USA) and separated from the excess BSA by centrifugation for 30 min at 13,000 rpm on a Heraeus Biofuge pico (Thermo Fisher Scientific, Waltham, MA, USA). The AuBSA-NPs precipitate was suspended in PBS and the volume was brought to a concentration of AuNPs 10 nM. The stability of the AuBSA-NPs was confirmed by the absence of color changes when adding an equal volume of 3 M NaCl. The preparation was stored at 4 °C.

2.3. Physicochemical Characterization of Nanoparticles

All prepared NPs were examined in transmission electron microscope (TEM) (see Section 2.6). Optical extinction spectra were recorded on a Clariostar plate fluorimeter (BMG, Labtech Ortenberg, Germany) in the range of 400–800 nm according to manufacturer's instructions.

Hydrodynamic characteristics of the NPs were evaluated by method of photon correlation spectroscopy on a Malvern Zetasizer Nano-ZS instrument (Malvern Instruments, Malvern, UK). The measurements were performed at least 5 times for each sample.

All prepared NPs were subjected to agarose gel electrophoresis. Samples containing 5 µL (0.5 pmol) of each kind of NPs and 1 µL glycerol/water (1:1, v/v) were loaded into the wells of 0.8% agarose (Lonza Rockland, ME, USA) in Tris-Glycine buffer (250 mM glycine, 25 mM Tris, pH 8.3). The electrophoresis was carried out for 30 min at 5 V cm^{-1}. Images were scanned using Epson Perfection 4990 Photo scanner (Seiko Epson Corporation, Suwa, Japan).

2.4. Cell Cultures and Spheroid Production

Cell cultures of human hepatocarcinoma (HepG2) and human embryo kidney (HEK293) cells were obtained from the Russian collection of cell cultures (Institute of Cytology RAS, Saint Petersburg, Russia). The monolayers were cultured in IMDM (HepG2) or DMEM (HEK 293) media, containing 10% embryonic calf serum (Thermo Fisher Scientific, Waltham, MA, USA) and 100 u/mL of penicillin and streptomycin (Thermo Fisher Scientific, Waltham, MA, USA) in an atmosphere of 5% CO_2 at 37 °C.

To obtain spheroids (3D culture), Corning® spheroid microplates 96 well black/clear bottom round ULA (Ultra-Low Attachment surface) (CLS4515-5EA) (Corning, Corning, NY, USA) were used. Cells of the HepG2 and HEK 293 lines were seeded at a dose of 300 and 600 cells, correspondingly, per well. The spheroids were cultured for 7 days with daily imaging using a ZEISS Axiovert 200 m microscope (Carl Zeiss AG, Oberkochen, Germany), equipped with an AxioCam MRm camera (Carl Zeiss AG,

Oberkochen, Germany) and a CO_2 Incubator XL-3 (PeCon GmbH, Erbach, Germany). Measurements of spheroids were performed using AxioVision program.

2.5. Incubation of Cells and Spheroids with the NPs

Cells of the HepG2 and HEK293 lines were sown in Petri dishes (40 mm diameter, TPP Techno Plastic Products AG, Trasadingen, Switzerland), 10^5 cells per dish. After reaching 70% coverage, the monolayers were washed with a culture medium, and AuNPs or AuBSA-NPs, or AuPEI-NPs suspended in an IMDM (for HepG2) or DMEM (for HEK293) were added to cells. Final concentration of AuNPs in the medium was 1 nM.

The cells were incubated for 15 min, 30 min, 1, 2 and 4 h in a medium without serum. Then the cells were rinsed three times with PBS, removed with trypsin, sedimented by centrifugation (5 min at 3000 rpm), and fixed with 4% paraformaldehyde for TEM studies.

Seven-day spheroids of HepG2 and HEK 293 cells cultured in 96-well plates were washed with a culture medium. The AuNPs or AuBSA-NPs or AuPEI-NPs were added to spheroids in an IMDM (HepG2-spheroids) or DMEM (HEK293 spheroids); final concentration of AuNPs was 1 nM. The spheroids were incubated with NPs for 1, 2 and 4 h without serum, and then fixed with 4% paraformaldehyde.

2.6. TEM Studies of NPs

Suspension of AuNPs was adsorbed on formvar-coated copper grids for 1 min, then liquid excess was removed by a filter paper, and the grid was air dried. Suspensions of AuNPs-PEI and AuNPs-BSA also were adsorbed on a grid for 1 min, and after removing of liquid excess were contrasted with 2% phosphotungstic acid (EMS, Hatfield, PA, USA), pH 0.5. The samples were examined with a JEM 1400 TEM (JEOL, Japan) equipped with a Veleta digital camera (EM SIS, Muenster, Germany). iTEM program, version 5.2 (EM SIS, Muenster, Germany) was used for direct measurement of NPs sizes.

2.7. TEM studies of Cell Cultures and Spheroids

All reagents for microscopic studies were purchased from EMS (Hatfield, PA, USA).

Samples of fixed cell cultures and spheroids were washed from paraformaldehyde with Hank's balanced solution and were postfixed with 1% osmium tetraoxide solution for 1 h, dehydrated in ethanol and acetone according to the standard method, and then embedded in an epon-araldite mixture to obtain hard blocks.

Ultrathin and semithin sections were prepared on an ultramicrotome EM UC7 (Leica, Wetzlar, Germany) using a diamond knife (Diatome, Nidau, Switzerland). The semithin sections of spheroids were stained with Azur II and were examined in a Leica DM 2500 light microscope (Leica, Wetzlar, Germany) to choose an area for ultrathin sectioning. Ultrathin sections were contrasted with 2% water solutions of uranyl acetate and lead citrate and examined in a JEM 1400 TEM (JEOL, Japan). Digital images were collected using a Veleta side-mounted camera (EM SIS, Muenster, Germany).

2.8. Scanning Electron Microscopy

The seven-day spheroids of HepG2 and HEK 293 cells were fixed with a 4% paraformaldehyde at 4 °C for 24 h. Fixed spheroids were rinsed with PBS (Sigma-Aldrich, St. Louis, MO, USA), dehydrated using a graded ethanol series (50%, 70%, 80%, 90%, 96% and 100%) and then immersed to mixture of ethanol and hexamethyldisilazane (HMDS; Sigma-Aldrich, St. Louis, MO, USA) in a ratio 1:1 for 10 min, and then to 100% HMDS for 10 min. Spheroids were fixed on a sample stand using double-sided carbon tape and dried overnight in air. Spheroids were sputter coated with 10 nm gold/palladium and analyzed using a scanning electron microscope EVO 10 (Carl Zeiss AG, Oberkochen, Germany) at an accelerating voltage of 10 kV.

3. Results

3.1. Physicochemical Characteristics of the NPs

We prepared AuNPs and covered them with PEI or BSA for cell studies. Values of polydispersity indexes evidenced that NP preparations represent well dispersed aqueous suspensions (Table 1). Examination in TEM revealed spherical naked particles of high electron density (d = 12.0 ± 0.1 nm) in sample of AuNPs, and the same particles surrounded with "corona" of PEI or BSA having middle electron density, in the samples of AuPEI-NPs and AuBSA-NPs (Figure 1A).

Table 1. Physicochemical characteristics of AuNPs, AuPEI-NPs and AuBSA-NPs.

Sample	Zeta-Potential (mV)	Polydipersity Index	Hydrodynamic Diameter (nm)
AuNPs	−33.6 ± 2.0	0.145 ± 0.006	17.4 ± 0.4
AuMUA-NPs	−53.8 ± 3.4	0.288 ± 0.001	46.0 ± 2.2
AuMUA-PEI-NPs	39.9 ± 1.3	0.258 ± 0.008	125.9 ± 2.8
AuBSA-NPs	−35.7 ± 1.8	0.212 ± 0.008	35.9 ± 0.5

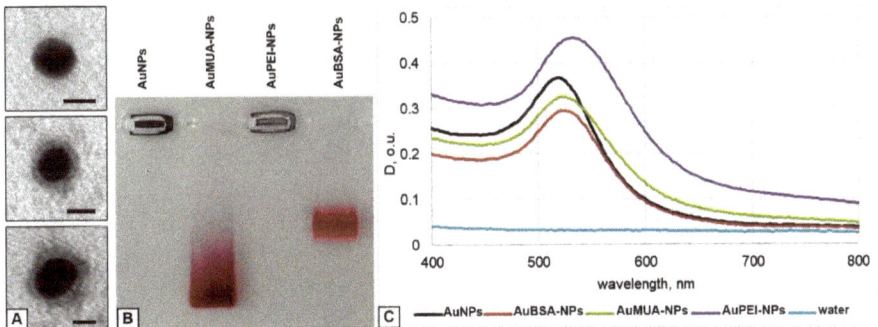

Figure 1. Physicochemical characterization of the NPs. (**A**) TEM images of AuNP (top), AuPEI-NP (middle) and AuBSA-NP (bottom). Negative staining with phosphotungstic acid. Bars correspond to 10 nm. (**B**) Image of the gel after electrophoretic analysis of AuNPs, AuMUA-NPs, AuPEI-NPs and AuBSA-NPs. (**C**) Optical extinction spectra of AuNPs, AuMUA-NPs, AuPEI-NPs and AuBSA-NPs in water. We used samples with different concentrations to separate the curve maximums for clear visualization.

To prepare AuPEI-NPs we modified previously described layer-by-layer method, which uses MUA for stabilization of AuNPs [31]. We introduced a step of AuNPs preliminary incubation with ON (anyone with length 20–30 n.) [29]. This ON layer allowed to increase colloid stability of the NPs at subsequent stages of interaction with MUA and PEI. The resulting AuPEI-NPs had a positive net charge, unlike AuNPs and AuBSA-NPs, which have a negative net charge (Zeta potential) (Table 1). Optical extinction spectra did not critically change after covering of AuNPs with PEI or BSA (Figure 1C).

Thus, we obtained three types of well dispersed NPs to study their interaction with cells: AuNPs, AuPEI-NPs and AuBSA-NPs, similar by size, and differing in the magnitude of net charge (Table 1, Figure 1B). Detailed presentation of physico-chemical properties of NPs, similar to studied in this work could be found in our previous studies [32,33]. Absence of noticeable cytotoxicity of all studied NPs was shown in our previous work using two different cell cultures [32].

3.2. Cell Experimental Models

3.2.1. Monolayer Cell Cultures

The well-differentiated hepatoma cell line HepG2, which has a wide set of properties inherent to human hepatocytes in vivo, has been actively used for about 40 years in various studies exploiting organ-specific features of the line [10,11,34–37]. Morphology of HepG2 cells was shown to keep main features of the hepatocytes: tight junctions separate apical and basolateral plasmalemma providing formation of bile capillaries and blood-biliary barrier; ultrastructural observations were supported by immunohistochemical and biochemical studies [38,39]. Based on current knowledge about the role of tight junctions in hepatic physiology and pathology, it is possible to claim that formation of these structures by HepG2 cells evidences for high levels of differentiation [40].

Our examination of HepG2 cells on ultrathin sections revealed formation of bile capillaries that carry microvilli on the surface and had tight junctions between the cells; desmosomes connecting cell lateral surfaces were occasionally observed (Figure 2A,B). The cells were filled with granular cytoplasm containing mitochondria and cisternae of endoplasmic reticulum covered with ribosomes. Relatively small Golgi apparatus usually was located in perinuclear region. Many cells contained lipid droplets of medium electron density. Basolateral cell surfaces were mostly flat, some small outgrowths of cytoplasm of various shapes were observed (Figure 2A,B). Our study clearly showed that monolayer HepG2 cells retain characteristics of hepatocyte unique polarity, which differ from those in other types of epithelia [39,41].

HEK 293 cell line also was used in various studies for about 40 years for examining molecular characteristics of different cellular processes, endocytosis, gene expression, for transfection and production of proteins and lentiviral vectors for pharmaceutical industry and science [42–44]. HEK293 cells were obtained from human embryo kidney [42] and have "columnar" polarity, which is typical for non-hepatic epithelia [39,41].

HEK293 cells in monolayer were arranged in a disordered manner, tight junctions were not observed (Figure 2C,D). Cell surface was covered with numerous outgrowths; some of them were long and evidenced for macropinocytosis. On the sections, extended areas of cell close contact were observed, the distance between cell surfaces was about 10 nm, however, no interdigitations and tight junctions were present, which indicates absence of cell integration into "epithelial" layer. The cytoplasm contained numerous polysomes; mitochondria and endoplasmic reticulum cisternae were scarce (Figure 2C,D). In contrast to HepG2 cells, HEK293 monolayer cells did not possess signs of organ specialization.

3.2.2. Spheroids of HepG2 and HEK293 Cells

Previously published studies showed changes in the shape and compactization of HepG2 spheroids during their development; early, middle and late stages of spheroid growth were identified, the duration of which varied in different works and mainly depended on the dose of cell seeding. Common recommendation was to work with HepG2 spheroids at middle stage (beginning from days 4–5 after cell seeding) which is characterized by active function of spheroid cells and absence of cell destruction [10,14,45]. Amount of published studies using HEK293 spheroids is incomparably less than studies with HepG2 spheroids; however, authors noted a very fast compactization of HEK293 cells on a non-adhesive surface and regular spherical shape of the spheroids [46,47].

To examine interaction of AuNPs, AuPEI-NPs and AuBSA-NPs with HepG2 and HEK293 cells in 3D-culture we used corresponding spheroids cultured for 7 days with daily monitoring and photographing. In the first three days after cell seeding HepG2 spheroids looked loose and had an irregular shape, while HEK293 spheroids became spherical within a day. The spheroids showed differences in shape and rate of growth (Figure 3A–D). HepG2 spheroids always had somewhat irregular shape and surface with various recesses and ledges, as it is clearly seen on SEM image (Figure 3E). In contrast, HEK293 spheroids had a shape very close to spherical and relatively smooth surface (Figure 3F). We did not set out to study the growth features of HepG2 and HEK293 spheroids, since they are sufficiently described in literature, and we present here brief information on the growth and "appearance" of spheroids only to confirm the adequacy of our 3D models with published data.

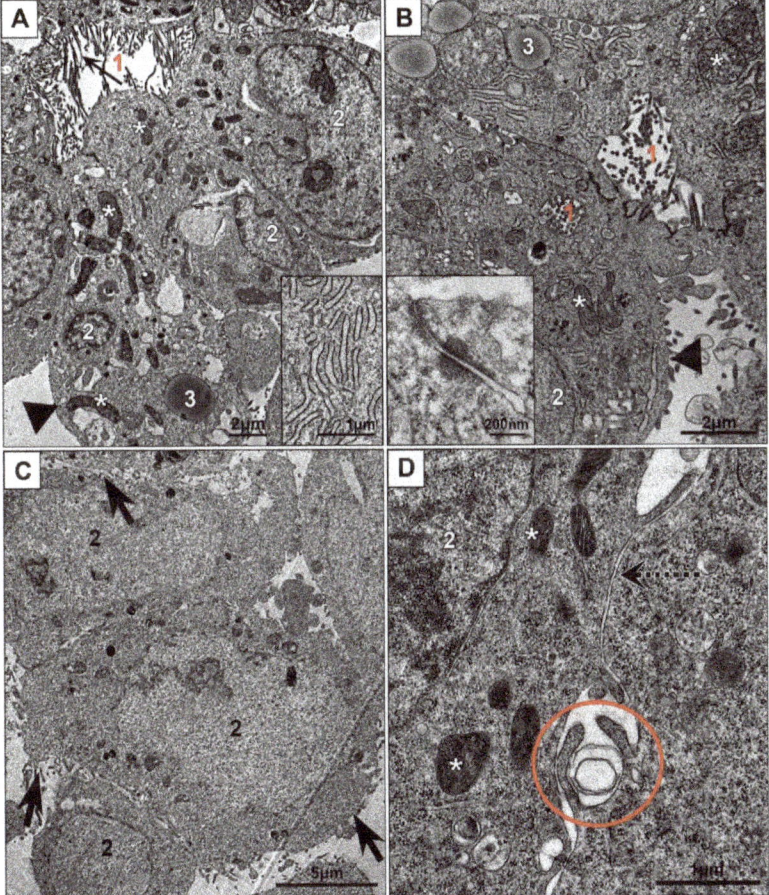

Figure 2. Cell cultures in monolayer: (**A,B**)—HepG2, (**C,D**)—HEK293. Inserts: (**A**) cisternae of endoplasmic reticulum; (**B**) tight junction and desmosome between cells at apical pole. 1—"bile capillaries", arrows show microvilli; 2—nucleus; 3—lipid droplet; asterisks show mitochondria; arrowheads show basolateral membranes; dotted arrow shows area of "simple" contact of two cells; oval shows site of macropinocytosis; tick arrows show cell surface with many outgrowths.

3.2.3. Electron Microscopic Features of HepG2 and HEK293 Spheroids

All published studies with HepG2 spheroids describe the "general appearance" of entire spheroids, noting the irregularity of shape and surface. Control of spheroids growth and analysis of their changes is carried out by means of light-optical observation of intravital characteristics as the perimeter length and square of spheroids, their roundness and compactness. Routine staining of paraffin sections mostly is used to show absence or presence of necrosis. Immunohistochemistry and fluorescence methods are increasingly introduced in recent years [11–15,45]. Published TEM data are scarce and usually present small portions of HepG2 cells [14,48]. Here we describe the ultrastructure of HepG2 spheroids with an emphasis on cell relationships and structure of spheroid outer surface and adjacent areas. We used a semithin section of each spheroid to choose a location for the pyramid, so we knew exactly which part of the spheroid was being explored in the TEM.

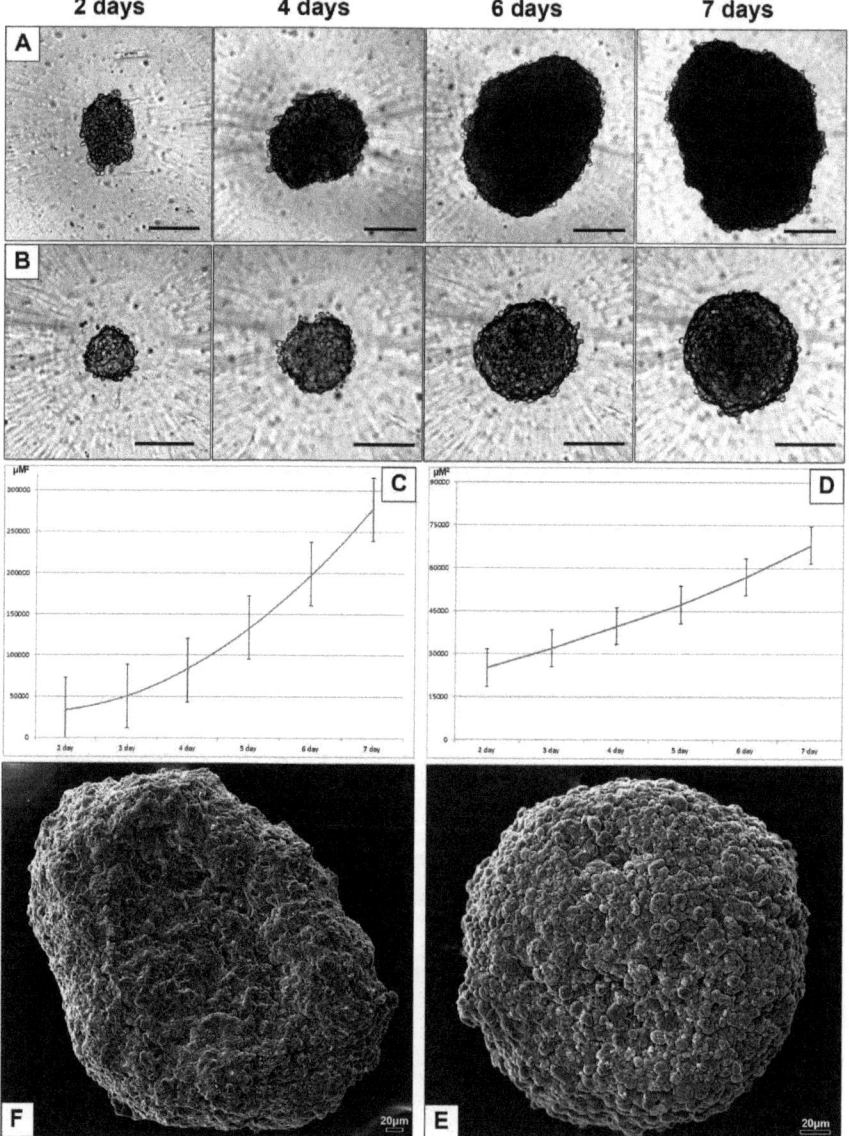

Figure 3. Characteristics of spheroids in culture. Representative light microscopic images of HepG2 spheroids (**A**) and HEK293 spheroids (**B**), days 2–7 after seeding. Bars correspond to 200 µm. Growth curves of spheroids square: (**C**) HepG2, (**D**) HEK293. Representative images of 7-day HepG2 (**E**) and HEK293 (**F**) spheroids obtained with SEM.

SEM examination of the HepG2 spheroids revealed an uneven surface resembling a "lunar landscape" with some bulging cells and "craters" extending into the interior of spheroid (Figure 4A).

"Craters" looked as openings between spheroid cells and were randomly located on spheroid surface. Surface of the cells was covered with many small outgrowths.

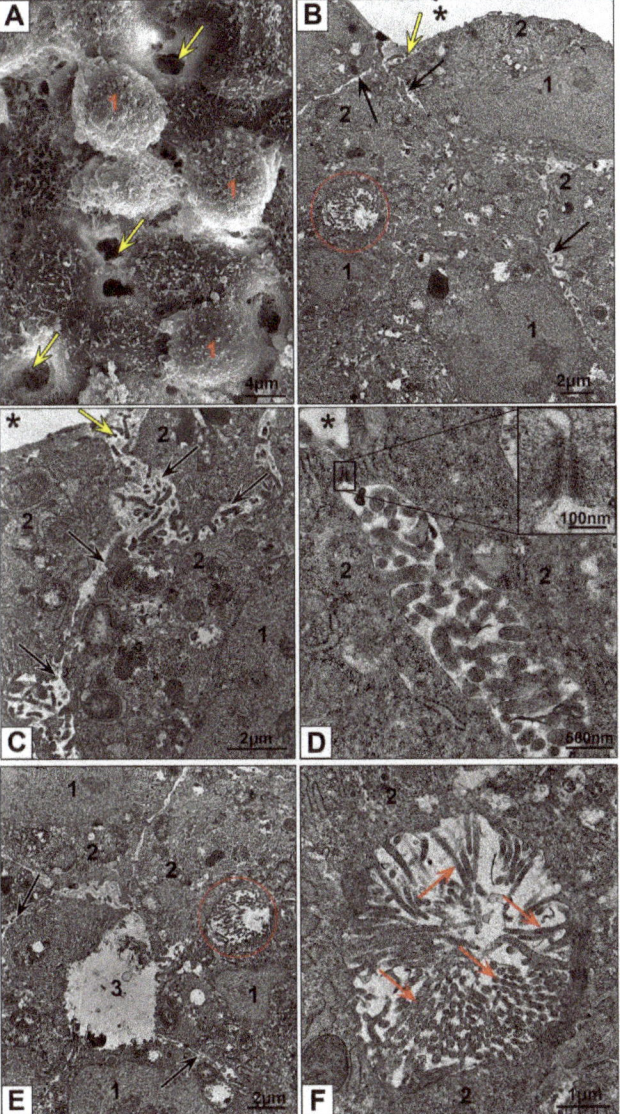

Figure 4. Ultrastructure of HepG2 spheroids. (**A**) Representative SEM image of spheroid surface. 1—bulging cells; arrows show openings on spheroid surface; (**B–D**) HepG2 spheroid periphery; (**E**) area at a distance of 50 μm from the surface; (**F**) bile capillary with microvilli. 1—nucleus; 2—cytoplasm; 3—lumen of cross-sectioned psedosinusoid; asterisks show external space; ovals show bile capillaries; yellow arrows show a space between hepatocytes (openings in SEM); black arrows show a space between lateral surfaces of neighboring cells; red arrows show microvilli; a frame shows desmosome between cells, and insert shows this desmosome at high magnification. (**B–F**) Ultrathin sections, TEM.

Analyzing the results obtained by light microscopy, SEM and TEM we found that the openings are expansions of the space between the lateral surfaces of neighboring cells, serving as an "entrance" into the spheroid (Figure 4B,C and Figure S1). This "entrance" continued in the form of a space expanded up to one µm between the lateral surfaces of cells, covered with cytoplasmic outgrowths of different lengths and shapes. It should be noted that these outgrowths were distinctly different from microvilli on the surface of bile capillaries (Figure 4C–F). The openings were not formed by all cells: the "entrance" between the lateral cell surfaces could be closed with desmosomes (Figure 4D). Observed patterns suggest that cell basal membranes form outer surface of HepG2 spheroids contacting with culture medium and receiving the nutrients and external influences. Presence of the "pores" on surface of HepG2 spheroids were noted in SEM and TEM earlier [48].

Hepatocytes are epithelial cells with unique type of polarization, which sets a direction of their morphology and function, determines formation of bile capillaries by the apical surface, and retrieval of metabolites and other substances from sinusoid blood by basolateral surfaces [11,49]. In the liver, sinusoids formed by endothelial cells provide blood flow that is cleared by hepatocytes. Inside the spheroids we observed empty spaces between HepG2 cells resembling the sinusoids up to 2–2.5 µm width (Figure 4E and Figure S2). This similarity allowed us to designate these spaces as "pseudosinusoids". It is unknown whether pseudosinusoids form a common network that permeates the spheroid; a special research is required to establish this.

Bile capillaries (bile canaliculi) formed by hepatocyte apical plasmalemma are bright morphological feature of hepatic tissue [11]. Bile capillaries are clearly visible in groups of HepG2 cells in monolayer (Figure 2A,B) and in ultrathin sections of HepG2 spheroids (Figure 4B,E,F and Figure S3). These structures are easily differentiated by the presence of microvilli on their surface, and could be found in various parts of spheroid, there are no visible ordering in their location. Analysis of the data obtained by TEM, SEM and light microscopy, clearly indicates that bile capillaries never come to the surface; they are "hidden" inside the spheroids. Correct identification of bile capillaries in HepG2 spheroids by TEM was reported in [14], and some published TEM studies of HEpG2 spheroids demonstrated pseudosinusoids instead bile capillaries [48,50].

Thus, the spheroids formed by HepG2 cells maintain typical for liver histology parameters: separation of the plasmalemma into apical and basolateral parts, formation of bile capillaries and pseudosinusoids. It is important that HepG2 spheroids face the environment with cell basal plasmalemma, which provides contact of hepatocytes with blood components in the liver. This feature of HepG2 spheroids should be taken into account when studying the effects of various preparations, including nanoparticles.

Examination of HEK293 spheroids in a SEM revealed a significantly flatter surface than those in HepG2 spheroids due to absence of "craters" (Figure 3E,F, 4A and 5A). Thin flat folds of plasmalemma indicating macropinocytosis were visible between bulging cell bodies. Small cytoplasm protrusions were present on cell surface in different amount, some cells had smooth surface (Figure 5A). Different appearance of cell surface could reflect different functional state of the cells in HEK293 spheroids.

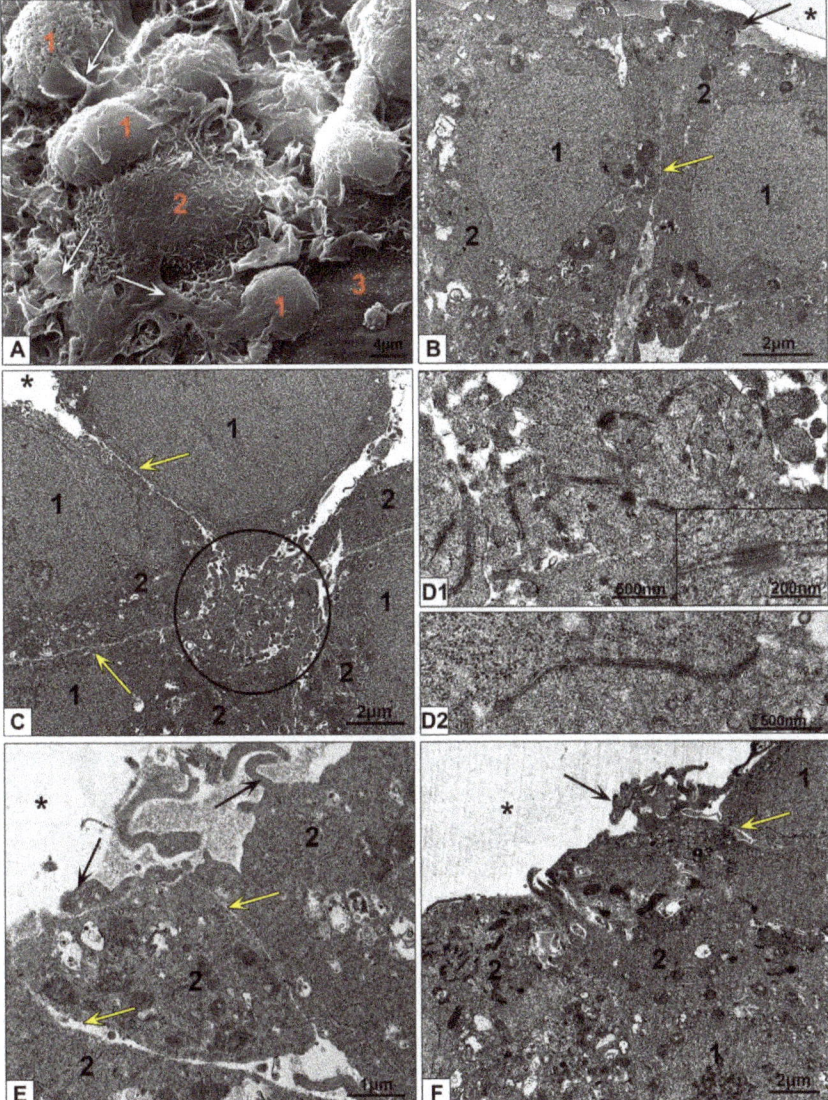

Figure 5. Ultrastructure of HEK293 spheroids. (**A**) Representative SEM image of spheroid surface. 1—cell body; 2—cell surface with small microvilli; 3—flat cell surface; white arrows show flat folds. (**B–F**) Cells at the periphery of spheroid, ultrathin sections. 1—nucleus; 2—cytoplasm; asterisks show external space; circle shows a conglomerate of apical outgrowths; arrows show outgrowths protruding in external space; yellow arrows show narrow space between lateral cell surfaces. (**D1**) Outgrowth conglomerate at higher magnification, the insert shows desmosomes; (**D2**) this photo presents a structure similar to apical tight junction.

HEK293 cell were isolated from human embryo kidney and transformed with sheared DNA of adenovirus type 5 [42]. The obtained cell line was considered as epithelial cells. Presence of morphologically visible tight junctions in HEK293 monolayer were not reported [51,52], although expression of markers of epithelial tight junctions (zonula occludens) including ZO-1 and occludins was detected [53]. We did not observe tight junctions in monolayer HEK293 cells (Figure 2C,D).

Ultrathin sections of HEK293 spheroids showed groups of pyramidal cells (Figure 5C,E) connected to each other with narrow apical parts, which formed a conglomerate of interlaced cytoplasmic outgrowths bound by desmosomes and structures similar to tight junctions (Figure 5(D1,D2)). The conglomerates were observed throughout entire thickness of spheroids, not only at the periphery. On the ultrathin sections, these conglomerates looked like a disheveled skein of ribbons with ends sticking out in different directions. The center of conglomerate looked solid; there were no signs of a lumen formation, as in bile capillaries or glandular acini. We propose that apical cytoplasmic conglomerates organize HEK293 cells into groups, reflecting non-complete (without a lumen) formation of epithelial tube, determined by "columnar" polarization typical for of non-hepatic epithelia [39,41]. Thus, it is clear that cultivation of HEK293 cells in the 3D system induced formation of typical for epithelia structures (tight junctions and desmosomes) that were absent in the monolayer of these cells.

Surface of HEK293 spheroids was formed by basal plasmalemma of the cells, which was flat or covered with small protrusions. Some cells showed large outgrowths protruding in external space usually located near cell lateral borders (Figure 5B,E,F). It is obvious that formation of these structures is associated with the ability of HEK293 cells to macropinocytosis, which we noted on a monolayer culture. Similar structures were not observed in cells of HepG2 spheroid.

The lateral surfaces of spheroid cells were usually smooth and separated by narrow gaps led deep into the spheroid, widening of these gaps were observed in area of apical conglomerates (Figure 5B,C,E). Lateral plasmalemma of neighboring cells did not form interdigitations.

The results we obtained showed that cultivation of HepG2 and HEK293 cells in non-adhesive conditions in full media and without scaffold provide formation of spheroids; their morphological characteristics reflect structural polarization of epithelium in maternal organ. While HepG2 cells form bile capillaries and pseudosinusoids, HEK293 cells in these conditions are unable create complete structural units of epithelium with "columnar" polarization. Interestingly, the cells of both cultures were exposed to the culture medium by their basal plasmalemma, and the apical parts of the cells were inside spheroids.

3.3. Interaction of AuNPs, AuPEI-NPs and AuBSA-NPs with HepG2 and HEK293 Cells

3.3.1. Ultrastructural Features of NPs Interaction with the Cells in Monolayer

Study of NPs uptake by HepG2 and HEK293 cells were performed in culture medium without serum during 4 h to prevent "corona" formation by serum proteins, because "corona" forms differently on differently charged NPs, and it can alter their behavior by unknown way [54,55].

First, we examined interaction of AuNPs with HepG2 cells and unexpectedly found that all AuNPs remained on cell surface, no signs of the NPs penetration into cells were observed during 4 h of incubation (Figure 6A). In contrast, HEK293 cells readily internalized the same AuNPs, which were observed in structures associated with endocytosis after 15 min of incubation, and accumulated in cells up to 4 h (Figure 6B). At the same time, HepG2 cells actively engulfed AuNPs covered with PEI or BSA, as HEK293 cells did (Figure 6C–F). The accumulation of AuBSA-NPs was detected later than AuPEI-NPs (first AuBSA-NPs were found in both cell cultures after 2 h of incubation, the particles were dispersed in endosomes, and this reflects endocytosis of single particles (Figure 6C,D). The cells are able to accumulate many AuBSA-NPs in late endosomes (Figure S4), and it is easy to imagine the huge amount of NPs accumulated inside the cell, remembering that one ultra-thin section is about 70 nm thick, and the cell diameter is more than 10 microns. Previously long-term flotation of AuBSA-NPs was observed on HeLa cells [32], what is similar to current observation and obviously associated with particle negative net charge (Table 1). Penetration of AuPEI-NPs into both cell lines visually was highest, and numerous particles were found in endosomes after 15 minutes of incubation (Figure 6 E,F), obviously due to their positive net charge (Table 1). It is interesting, that all kinds of the NPs had different behavior inside endosomes of HepG2 and HEK293 cells: AuNPs formed loose aggregations of various shape, AuBSA-NPs localized individually; and AuNP-PEI formed compact aggregations or were located separately (Figure 6).

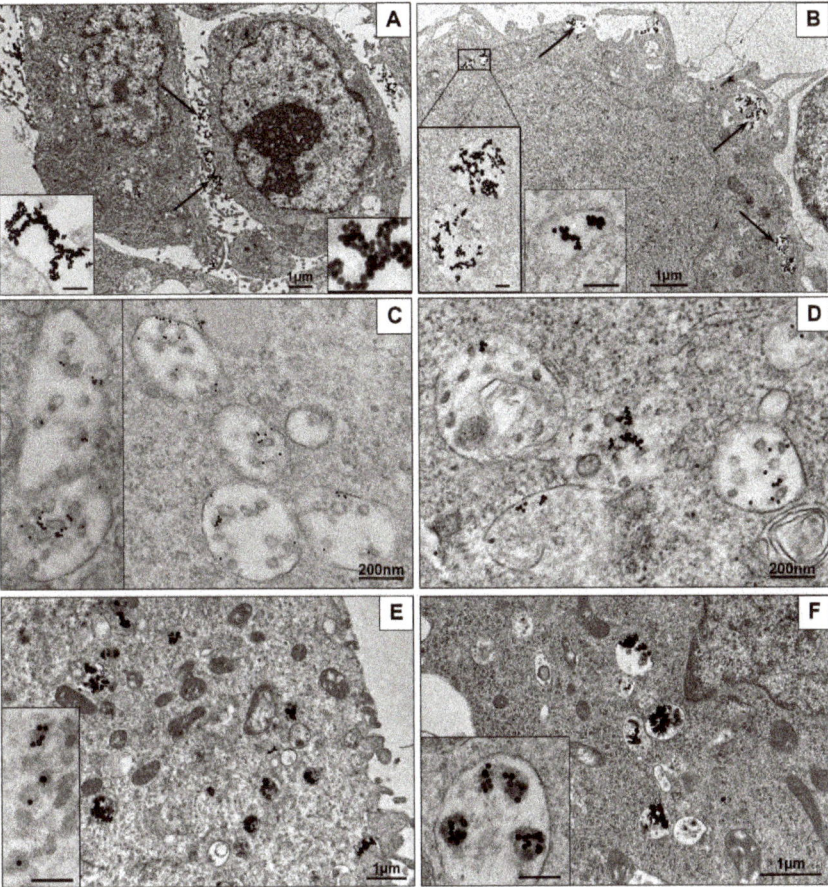

Figure 6. Representative TEM-images of NPs uptake by cells. (**A**) AuNPs on HepG2 cell surface are shown with arrows; inserts show AuNPs aggregations on plasmalemma at high magnification. 4 h incubation. (**B**) Penetration of AuNPs into HEK293 cells. Arrows show endocytosis-associated structures containing AuNPs; left insert shows two enlarged endosomes; right insert shows early endosome containing AuNPs. 30 min incubation. (**C**) AuBSA-NPs inside late endosomes of HepG2 cells. 4 h incubation. (**D**) AuBSA-NPs inside HEK293 cells. 4 h incubation. (**E**) AuPEI-NPs in endosomes of HepG2 cells; insert shows enlarged particles inside endosome, PEI looks as grey material around gold core. 1 h incubation. (**F**) AuPEI-NPs in endosomes of HEK293 cells; insert shows aggregates of AuPEI-NPs inside endosome. 1 h incubation. Bars in inserts correspond to 100 nm.

Undoubtedly, most interesting of our findings is absence of AuNPs uptake by HepG2 cells in contrast with active internalization of the same AuNPs covered with BSA or PEI. We did not find any study confirming or neglecting our results. Uptake of AuNPs (20 nm) by HepG2 cells was detected by inductively coupled plasma mass spectrometry [26], however, this method did not provide reliable results because it operates with a whole mass of the cells dissolved in 3% HNO3, so it is impossible say were AuNPs inside the cells or were they adsorbed on cell surface [25]. The TEM of ultrathin sections is the only method that unambiguously demonstrates the penetration of metal NPs into cells and allows identification of cell structures without a special labeling. Most published studies skip TEM examination of cell-NPs interaction. A number of studies provide images of the final stages of NPs accumulation in cells after several days of incubation; such data only confirm the presence of NPs in cells without bringing details of their penetration and interaction with cellular structures [22,23]. Meanwhile, understanding of the pathways of NPs internalization is necessary for biomedicine and nanotoxicology, current knowledge in the field is comprehensively analyzed in recent reviews, which noted advantages of TEM: possibility of direct and simultaneous visualization of NPs and cell structures on ultrathin sections [4,55,56].

Our examination of ultrathin sections in TEM revealed that clathrin-mediated endocytosis is main way to enter both HepG2 and HEK293 cells for all studied types of NPs. Figure 7 demonstrates sequential steps of clathrin-mediated endocytosis: adsorption, transfer by vesicle to early endosome and accumulation in late endosomes. All types of NPs were observed only in membrane-bound structures (endosomes and lysosomes); no signs of NPs cytoplasmic localization were detected during 4 h of incubation. Our previous studies showed that AuNPs stay inside late endosomes and lysosomes of HeLa cells at least for 72 h [32].

HEK293 cells also showed the signs of macrpinocytosis of all studied NPs, cells developed long outgrowths and macropinocytic cups (Figure 7J,K). Morphological signs of macropinocytosis in HEK293 cells were identical to earlier published TEM data on this type of endocytosis, the authors noted independence of macropinocytosis and clathrin-mediated endocytosis [57–59].

Clathrin-mediated endocytosis was examined in HepG2 cells incubated with AuNPs coated with human ferrotransferrin (8 nm) or asialoorosomucoid (20 nm) in TEM and the data showed all subsequent steps of the endocytosis [60], identical to our images, however, author did not study interaction of HepG2 cells with AuNPs.

3.3.2. Features of NPs Interaction with Spheroids Cells

Examination of ultrathin sections of HepG2 spheroids incubated with AuNPs showed inability of these cells to internalize these NPs, which were localized only on spheroid surface during 4 h (Figure 8A–C). At the same time, ultrathin sections of HEK293 spheroids showed signs of both clathrin-mediated endocytosis and macropinocytosis of AuNPs which were found mostly in late endosomes starting from 1 h of incubation (Figure 8D–H). HEK293 cells containing AuNPs were located in spheroid external zone (about 35–40 µm from the surface).

Thus, both HepG2 and HEK293 cultures in form of spheroid (3D-culture) kept the character of interaction with AuNPs observed in their monolayers. The same phenomenon occurred during incubation with AuBSA-NPs: ultrathin sections of both HepG2 and HEK293 spheroids showed adsorption of NPs on plasmalemma and presence of individual particles in late endosomes (Figure 9). The cells containing AuBSA-NPs were located in external zone (about 35–40 µm from the surface) of HepG2 and HEK293 spheroids.

AuPEI-NPs were observed on basal plasmalemma of cells forming outer surface of HepG2 and HEK293 spheroids, and in the spaces between lateral cell surfaces, and in pseudosinusoids of HepG2 spheroids (Figure 10A–D). As in the case of a monolayer, AuPEI-NPs more actively penetrated the cells than other studied NPs and accumulated in late endosomes of both HepG2 and HEK293 cells (Figure 10D,E). AuPEI-NPs visually were more abundant in a tissue of HepG2 and HEK293 spheroids than AuBSA-NPs, however, their penetration depth was similar: 35–40 µm. Thus, positive net charge of AuPEI-NPs did not influence the depth of NPs penetration into spheroids, although it increased their accumulation inside spheroids, as well as in monolayer HepG2 and HEK293 cells.

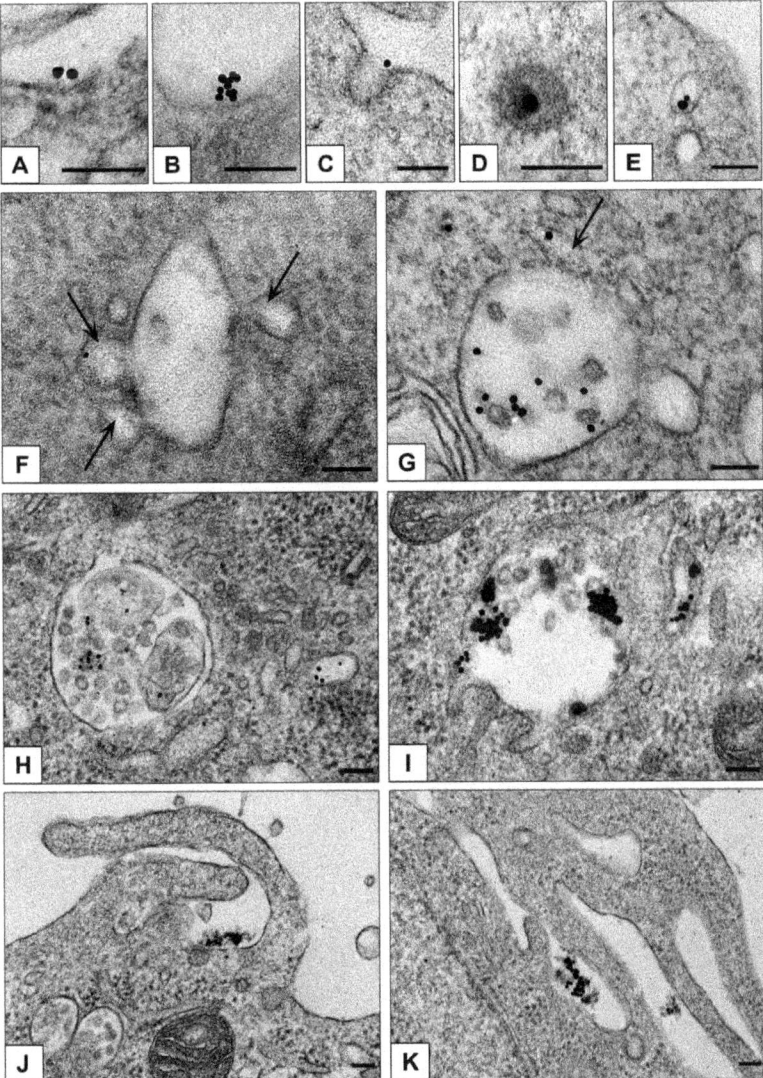

Figure 7. Representative images of NPs penetration into monolayer cells. Adsorption of single AuBSA-NP (**A**) and small cluster (**B**) of AuNPs on plasmalemma (HepG2); (**C**) coated pit containing AuNP and (**D**) coated vesicle containing AuPEI-NP (HEK293); (**E**) endocytotic vesicle containing AuBSA-NPs (HepG2). (**F**) Early endosome receives AuNP in vesicle; arrows show vesicles fusing with endosome body (HEK293). (**G**) AuNPs in endosome cavity, arrow shows NP in tubule (HEK293). (**H**) AuPEI-NPs in late endosome and a vesicle (HepG2). (**I**) AuNPs in late endosome (HEK293). (**J**,**K**) Macropinocytosis of AuPEI-NPs (HEK293). TEM, ultrathin sections. Bars correspond to 100 nm.

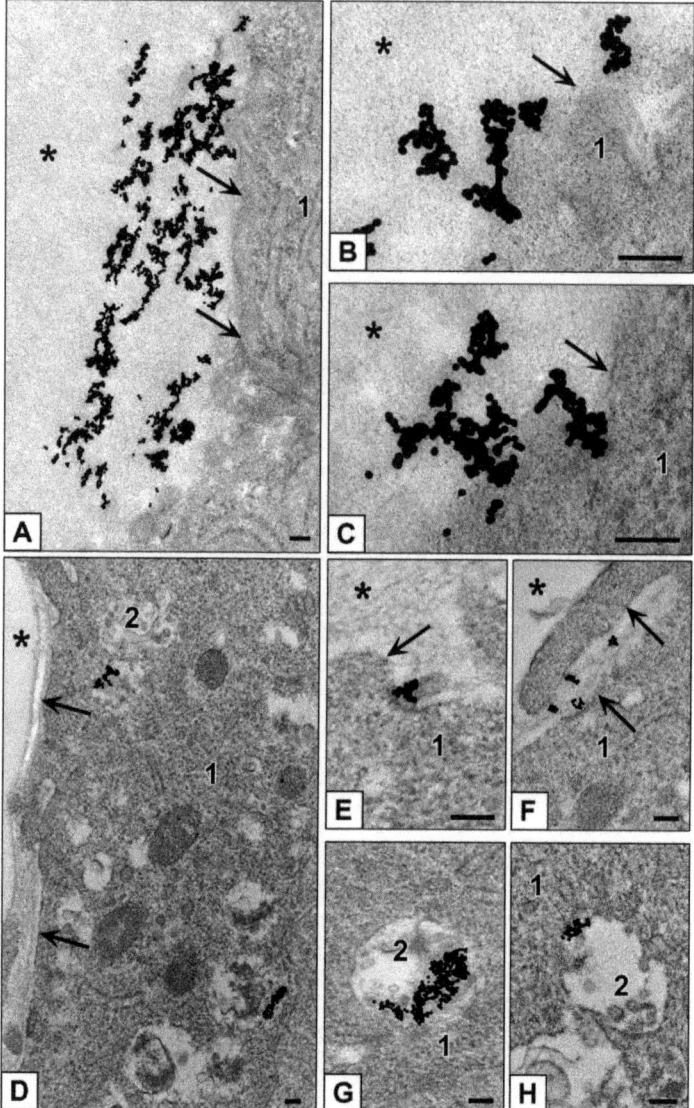

Figure 8. Interaction of AuNPs with cells of different spheroids. (**A–C**) adsorption of AuNPs on plasmalemma (HepG2 cells). (**D–H**) Penetration of AuNPs into HEK293 cells. (**E**) Adsorption of AuNPs on plasmalemma; (**F**) Macropinocytosis of AuNPs; (**G,H**) AuNPs in late endosomes. 1—cytoplasm; 2—late endosome; asterisks show external space and arrows show plasmalemma. Bars correspond to 100 nm.

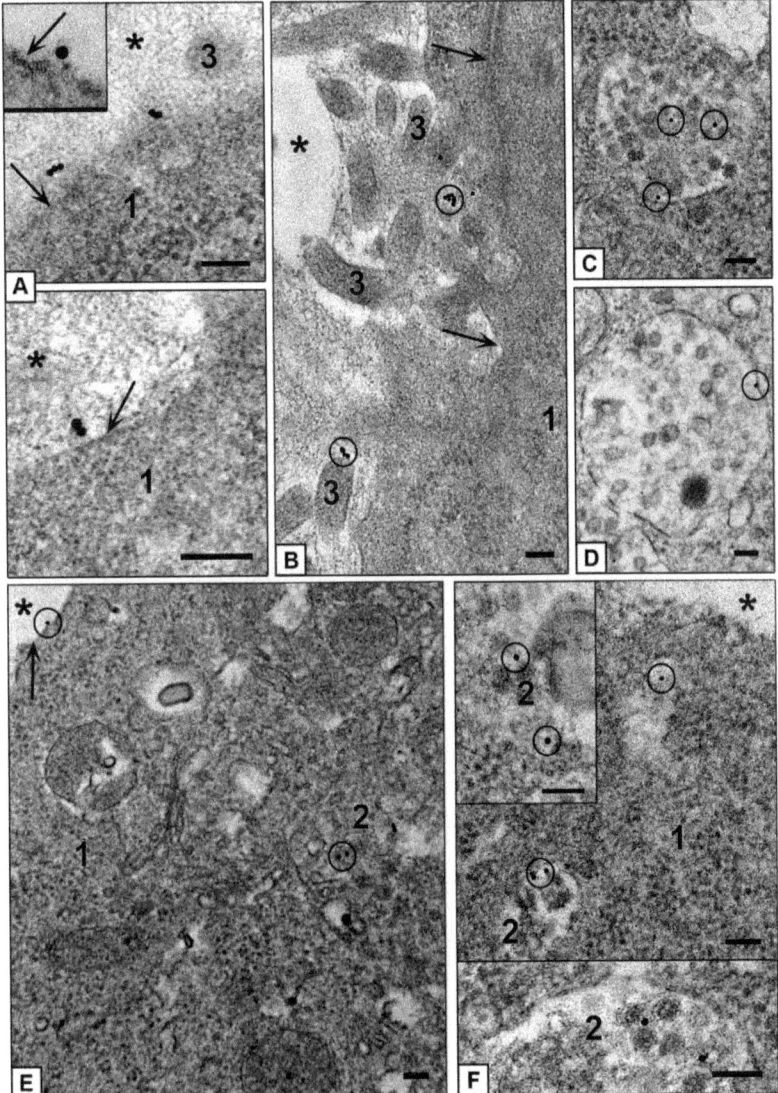

Figure 9. Interaction of AuBSA-NPs with cells of different spheroids. (**A–D**) Penetration of AuBSA-NPs into HepG2 cells. (**A,B**) adsorption of NPs on plasmalemma, insert shows NP adsorption at high magnification. (**C,D**) AuBSA-NPs in late endosomes. (**E,F**) Penetration of AuBSA-NPs into HEK293 cells. (**E**) NPs on plasmalemma and in late endosome. (**F**) AuBSA-NPs in late endosomes and in a vesicle. 1—cytoplasm; 2—late endosomes; 3—cell outgrowths; asterisks show external space and arrows show plasmalemma. Bars correspond to 100 nm.

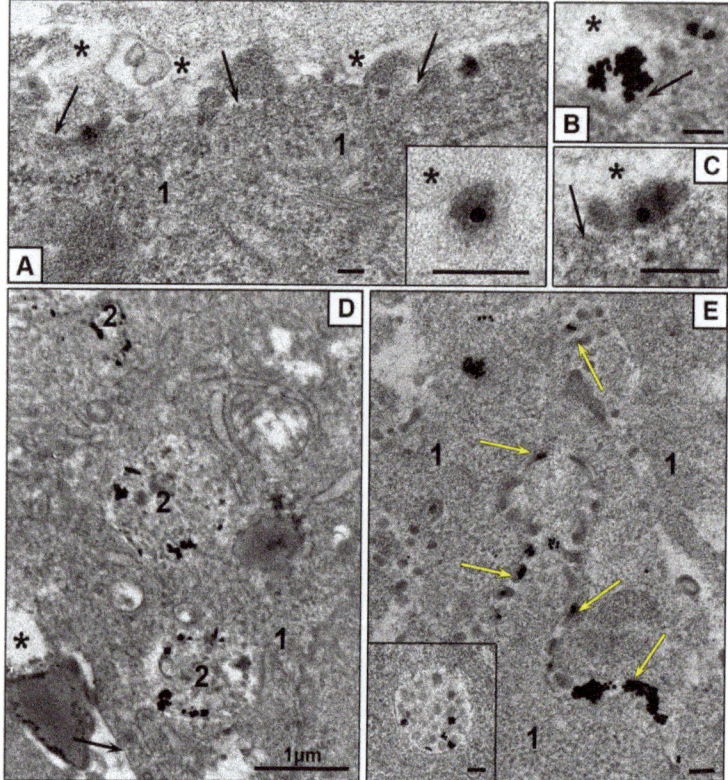

Figure 10. Interaction of AuPEI-NPs with cells of different spheroids. (**A**) Adsorption of AuPEI-NPs on HepG2 cell plasmalemma. Images in insert, (**B,C**) show NP adsorption at high magnification, HepG2 cells. (**D**) AuPEI-NPs in late endosomes of HepG2 cells. (**E**) Penetration of AuPEI-NPs into HEK293 cell, insert shows NPs in late endosome at high magnification, yellow arrows show NPs between spheroid cells. 1—cytoplasm; 2—late endosomes; asterisks show external space and arrows show plasmalemma. Bars correspond to 100 nm.

4. Discussion

HepG2 cells cultured in 2D- and 3D-forms are used as experimental model in various studies related with hepatic functions and pathology, drug delivery and safety, toxicology and others [11,12,14,15]. Such a wide range of applications is due to the unique properties of this cell line, which reproduces structural and functional features of the liver, in particular, in 3D-form (spheroids), which is reviewed in [7,9,11]. Liver hepatocytes and HepG2 cells possess unique structural and functional polarity, it was interesting to compare their features with another cell line, representing "standard columnar" polarity, and we used HEK293 cell line for that. Using the TEM, we compared not only morphology of HepG2 and HEK293 cells in monolayers and spheroids, but also their interaction with three types of gold NPs differing by a coating nature, hydrodynamic size, and net charge.

In monolayer, HepG2 cells formed bile capillaries with typical microvilli and tight junctions, thereby showing liver-specific features. In contrast, HEK293 cells did not show any tissue-specific signs. In spheroids, both HepG2 and HEK293 cells formed outer surface by basal plasma membrane, which contacts with exterior environment (culture medium), and this finding can be important for understanding of the mechanisms of experimental influences. Our data show that spheroids consist of structural blocks, formation of which is specified by bile capillaries in case of HepG2 cells, and conglomerates of cell apical parts in case of HEK293. In HepG2 spheroids, blocks are separated by pseudosinusoids and intercellular spaces formed by lateral membranes, but more research is needed to find out whether pseudosinusoids form a common network within the spheroid. More research is also needed to understand how the blocks interact with each other; nevertheless, at present we can definitely say that the cells do not form shaped layers in HepG2 and HEK293 spheroids.

AuNPs are considered a promising platform for development of targeted nanomedicines and are extensively explored; however, there are many unknown details in their interaction with a cell [1–6]. We examined internalization of positively charged AuPEI-NPs, and negatively charged AuNPs and AuBSA-NPs with HepG2 and HEK293 cells in monolayers and spheroids to learn more about the mechanisms of their internalization. To our surprise, AuNPs did not penetrate HepG2 cells either in the monolayer or in the spheroids. Published TEM studies of AuNPs penetration into HepG2 cells were conducted in presence of serum [23], which contains proteins forming corona and so change a pattern of AuNPs interaction with a cell. However, our data corresponded to published TEM data that AuNPs (10 nm) did not penetrate hepatocytes in mouse liver, their uptake was detected in Kuppfer and endothelial cells (in contrast to AgNPs which penetrated the hepatocytes [4]. More research is needed to explain why hepatocytes and HepG2 cells "ignore" AuNPs, but an important point following from this observation is that cells can possess a selectivity for at least one type of the NPs. In connection with the selectivity of cells, it is pertinent to note the known effect of the size of AuNPs on penetration into cells. Thus, size-dependent accumulation of AuNPs (2–15 nm) coated with tiopronin was shown for MCF-7 breast cancer cells and their multicellular spheroids, and tumors in mice [61]. Different penetration rates were also reported for AuNPs (50 and 100 nm) coated with thiopronine in the same experimental MCF-7 cell models [62].

Interest to penetration of a drug into spheroid tissue is related with known block of the diffusion in tissue of solid tumors in vivo influencing drug effect [63]. Published studies show that the penetration of various NPs into HepG2 and other spheroids is limited to a depth of 20–50 µm, despite a fairly long incubation (for 24–72 h) [10,15,64]. The same values of penetration into HepG2 spheroids were reported for sorafenib [14]. Examination of MCF-7 spheroids treated with doxorubicin, revealed a dependence of penetration on spheroid sizes and ability of the drug to completely penetrate into the small-size spheroids [65]. Ability of doxorubicin for complete penetration into C3-HepG2 spheroid during 24 h was shown using confocal microscopy [45]. Our study showed that all studied NPs penetrated to a depth of 30–40 µm into HepG2 and HEK293 spheroids during 4 h of incubation. Limited penetration of NPs into spheroids is a "good" feature when a research is devoted to antitumor drugs, however, it may influence the results of toxicological and other studies.

Obviously, the use of spheroids in NPs research will expand and the methods of their cultivation and study of experimental effects will be increasingly improved. Presently, direct visualization of a NP in a cell and identification of cell structures is possible only by TEM of ultrathin sections. Currently, electron microscopy is overshadowed by other methods, faster and sometimes simpler, however, do not allowing to see directly nanoparticles in cells. Application of TEM allowed us to obtain a new data about features of HepG2 and HEK293 morphology in monolayer and spheroids, and clarify details of AuNPs, AuBSA-NPs and AuPEI-NPs uptake by these cells.

5. Conclusions

We compared ultrastructure of epithelial cells, which possess hepatocyte-type of polarization (HepG2) and columnar polarization (HEK 293) cultured in 2D- and 3D-forms (monolayer and spheroids). Monolayer HepG2 cells showed hepatic epithelia-specific morphological features, while HEK293 cells in monolayer did not show signs of epithelial tissue.

Cultivation of HepG2 and HEK293 cells on non-adhesive conditions led to formation of spheroids, a common feature of which was formation of spheroid outer surface by basal cell plasma membrane. This finding should be taken in account in experiments on drug delivery.

To examine interaction of different NPs with cells in monolayer and spheroids, we synthesized AuNPs (12.0 ± 0.1 nm in diameter, TEM data) and covered them with BSA and PEI. Values of hydrodynamic diameter were 17.4 ± 0.4; 35.9 ± 0.5 and 125.9 ± 2.8 nm for AuNPs, AuBSA-NPs and AuPEI-NPs, and Z-potential (net charge) values were −33.6 ± 2.0; −35.7 ± 1.8 and 39.9 ± 1.3 mV, respectively.

TEM study revealed inability of AuNPs uptake by HepG2 cells both in monolayer and spheroid form, while AuPEI-NPs and AuBSA-NPs were actively internalized via clathrin-mediated endocytosis, and this is an evidence for selectivity of HepG2 cells in respect to different NPs. At the same time, AuNPs actively penetrated the HEK293 cells in monolayer and spheroids.

Our data showed that the presence of a protein or polymer corona affects the behavior of NPs in endosomes after their endocytosis: AuBSA-NPs remained dispersed, while AuPEI-NPs were fused and formed aggregates. These features could influence drug release from an endosome, and so deserve attention when studying efficacy of drug delivery.

We did not observe appreciable distinctions in mechanisms of all studied NPs interaction with HepG2 and HEK293 cells in monolayer and spheroids. This observation is important for planning of different experiments because allow choosing cell monolayers or spheroids as experimental model, depending on a task. Thus, to know a depth of drug penetration, only spheroids are suitable, and for studies of drug-cell interaction mechanisms monolayers can be used. Undoubtedly, the use of multicellular spheroids as a 3D model of tumors and organs provides additional and "useful" opportunities for studying nanomedicine preparations in comparison with the cell monolayer.

Supplementary Materials: The following are available online at http://www.mdpi.com/2079-4991/10/10/2040/s1, Figure S1: "Openings" on surface of HepG2 spheroids in SEM and semithin sections, Figure S2: Pseudosinusoids in ultrathin sections of HepG2 spheroids, Figure S3: Periphery of HepG2 spheroid, Figure S4: Accumulation of AuBSA-NPs in HepG2 cells.

Author Contributions: Conceptualization, E.R.; methodology, B.C. and A.T.; validation, I.P. and A.E.; investigation, B.C., J.P., A.E. and J.P.; data curation, E.R.; writing, E.R., B.C. and J.P.; original draft preparation, E.R.; writing—review and editing, E.R.; visualization, B.C., J.P. and A.T.; supervision, E.R.; project administration, I.P.; funding acquisition, E.R. All authors have read and agreed to the published version of the manuscript.

Funding: This research was funded by Russian Science Foundation, grant number 19-15-00217; preparation of the nanoparticles were funded by Russian State Funded Budget Project of ICBFM SB RAS # VI.62.1.4, 0309-2016-0004.

Conflicts of Interest: The authors declare no conflict of interest.

References

1. Capek, I. Polymer decorated gold nanoparticles in nanomedicine conjugates. *Adv. Colloid Interface Sci.* **2017**, *249*, 386–399. [CrossRef] [PubMed]
2. Durymanov, M.; Reineke, J. Non-viral Delivery of Nucleic Acids: Insight into mechanisms of overcoming intracellular barriers. *Front. Pharmacol.* **2018**, *9*, 971. [CrossRef] [PubMed]
3. Nunes, T.; Hamdan, D.; Leboeuf, C.; El Bouchtaoui, M.; Gapihan, G.; Nguyen, T.T.; Meles, S.; Angeli, E.; Ratajczak, P.; Lu, H.; et al. Targeting cancer stem cells to overcome chemoresistance. *Int. J. Mol. Sci.* **2018**, *19*, 4036. [CrossRef]
4. Panzarini, E.; Mariano, S.; Carata, E.; Mura, F.; Rossi, M.; Dini, L. Intracellular transport of silver and gold nanoparticles and biological responses: An update. *Int. J. Mol. Sci.* **2018**, *19*, 1305. [CrossRef]
5. Artiga, Á.; Serrano-Sevilla, I.; De Matteis, L.; Mitchell, S.G.; De La Fuente, J.M. Current status and future perspectives of gold nanoparticle vectors for siRNA delivery. *J. Mater. Chem. B* **2019**, *7*, 876–896. [CrossRef] [PubMed]
6. Peng, J.; Liang, X. Progress in research on gold nanoparticles in cancer management. *Medicine* **2019**, *98*, e15311. [CrossRef] [PubMed]
7. Lu, H.; Stenzel, M. Multicellular Tumor Spheroids (MCTS) as a 3D in vitro evaluation tool of nanoparticles. *Small* **2018**, *14*, e1702858. [CrossRef]

8. Lauschke, V.M.; Shafagh, R.Z.; Hendriks, D.F.G.; Ingelman-Sundberg, M. 3D primary hepatocyte culture systems for analyses of liver diseases, drug metabolism, and toxicity: Emerging culture paradigms and applications. *Biotechnol. J.* **2019**, *14*. [CrossRef] [PubMed]
9. Elje, E.; Mariussen, E.; Moriones, O.H.; Bastús, N.G.; Puntes, V.F.; Kohl, Y.; Dusinska, M.; Rundén-Pran, E. Hepato(Geno)Toxicity Assessment of nanoparticles in a HepG2 liver spheroid model. *Nanomaterials* **2020**, *10*, 545. [CrossRef] [PubMed]
10. Sobańska, Z.; Domeradzka-Gajda, K.; Szparaga, M.; Grobelny, J.; Tomaszewska, E.; Ranoszek-Soliwoda, K.; Celichowski, G.; Zapór, L.; Kowalczyk, K.; Stępnik, M. Comparative analysis of biological effects of molybdenum(IV) sulfide in the form of nano- and microparticles on human hepatoma HepG2 cells grown in 2D and 3D models. *Toxicol. Vitro* **2020**, *68*, 104931. [CrossRef]
11. Godoy, P.; Hewitt, N.J.; Albrecht, U.; Andersen, M.E.; Ansari, N.; Bhattacharya, S.; Bode, J.G.; Bolleyn, J.; Borner, C.; Böttger, J.; et al. Recent advances in 2D and 3D in vitro systems using primary hepatocytes, alternative hepatocyte sources and non-parenchymal liver cells and their use in investigating mechanisms of hepatotoxicity, cell signaling and ADME. *Arch. Toxicol.* **2013**, *87*, 1315–1530. [CrossRef] [PubMed]
12. Millard, M.; Yakavets, I.; Zorin, V.; Kulmukhamedova, A.; Marchal, S.; Bezdetnaya, L. Drug delivery to solid tumors: The predictive value of the multicellular tumor spheroid model for nanomedicine screening. *Int. J. Nanomed.* **2017**, *12*, 7993–8007. [CrossRef] [PubMed]
13. Brand, D.V.D.; Massuger, L.F.; Brock, R.; Verdurmen, W.P.R. Mimicking tumors: Toward more predictive in vitro models for peptide- and protein-conjugated drugs. *Bioconjugate Chem.* **2017**, *28*, 846–856. [CrossRef]
14. Eilenberger, C.; Rothbauer, M.; Ehmoser, E.-K.; Ertl, P.; Küpcü, S. Effect of spheroidal age on sorafenib diffusivity and toxicity in a 3D HepG2 spheroid model. *Sci. Rep.* **2019**, *9*, 4863. [CrossRef] [PubMed]
15. Fleddermann, J.; Susewind, J.; Peuschel, H.; Koch, M.; Tavernaro, I.; Kraegeloh, A. Distribution of sio2 nanoparticles in 3d liver microtissues. *Int. J. Nanomed.* **2019**, *14*, 1411–1431. [CrossRef]
16. Kyffin, J.A.; Sharma, P.; Leedale, J.A.; Colley, H.E.; Murdoch, C.; Mistry, P.; Webb, S. Impact of cell types and culture methods on the functionality of in vitro liver systems—A review of cell systems for hepatotoxicity assessment. *Toxicol. Vitro* **2018**, *48*, 262–275. [CrossRef]
17. Underhill, G.H.; Khetani, S.R. Bioengineered liver models for drug testing and cell differentiation studies. *Cell. Mol. Gastroenterol. Hepatol.* **2018**, *5*, 426–439.e1. [CrossRef]
18. Zhou, Y.; Shen, J.X.; Lauschke, V.M. Comprehensive evaluation of organotypic and microphysiological liver models for prediction of drug-induced liver injury. *Front. Pharmacol.* **2019**, *10*, 1093. [CrossRef]
19. Cao, J.; Ge, R.; Zhang, M.; Xia, J.; Han, S.; Lu, W.; Liang, Y.; Zhang, T.; Sun, Y. A triple modality BSA-coated dendritic nanoplatform for NIR imaging, enhanced tumor penetration and anticancer therapy. *Nanoscale* **2018**, *10*, 9021–9037. [CrossRef]
20. Goncalves, D.P.N.; Park, D.M.; Schmidt, T.-L.; Werner, C. Modular peptide-functionalized gold nanorods for effective glioblastoma multicellular tumor spheroid targeting. *Biomater. Sci.* **2018**, *6*, 1140–1146. [CrossRef]
21. Obinu, A.; Rassu, G.; Corona, P.; Maestri, M.; Riva, F.; Miele, D.; Giunchedi, P.; Gavini, E. Poly (ethyl 2-cyanoacrylate) nanoparticles (PECA-NPs) as possible agents in tumor treatment. *Coll. Surf. B Bioint.* **2019**, *177*, 520–528. [CrossRef]
22. Cebrián, V.; Martín-Saavedra, F.; Yagüe, C.; Arruebo, M.; Santamaría, J.; Vilaboa, N. Size-dependent transfection efficiency of PEI-coated gold nanoparticles. *Acta Biomater.* **2011**, *7*, 3645–3655. [CrossRef] [PubMed]
23. Fraga, S.; Faria, H.; Soares, M.E.; Duarte, J.A.; Soares, L.; Pereira, E.; Costa-Pereira, C.; Teixeira, J.P.; Bastos, M.D.L.; Carmo, H. Influence of the surface coating on the cytotoxicity, genotoxicity and uptake of gold nanoparticles in human HepG2 cells. *J. Appl. Toxicol.* **2013**, *33*, 1111–1119. [CrossRef] [PubMed]
24. Miyamoto, Y.; Koshidaka, Y.; Noguchi, H.; Oishi, K.; Saito, H.; Yukawa, H.; Kaji, N.; Ikeya, T.; Suzuki, S.; Iwata, H.; et al. Observation of positively charged magnetic nanoparticles inside hepg2 spheroids using electron microscopy. *Cell Med.* **2013**, *5*, 89–96. [CrossRef]
25. Cho, E.C.; Xie, J.; Wurm, P.A.; Xia, Y. Understanding the role of surface charges in cellular adsorption versus internalization by selectively removing gold nanoparticles on the cell surface with a i2/ki etchant. *Nano Lett.* **2009**, *9*, 1080–1084. [CrossRef]
26. Xia, Q.; Huang, J.; Feng, Q.; Chen, X.; Liu, X.; Li, X.; Zhang, T.; Xiao, S.; Li, H.; Zhong, Z.; et al. Size- and cell type-dependent cellular uptake, cytotoxicity and in vivo distribution of gold nanoparticles. *Int. J. Nanomed.* **2019**, *14*, 6957–6970. [CrossRef]

27. Frens, G. Controlled nucleation for the regulation of the particle size in monodisperse gold suspensions. *Nat. Phys. Sci.* **1973**, *241*, 20–22. [CrossRef]
28. Liu, X.; Atwater, M.; Wang, J.; Huo, Q. Extinction coefficient of gold nanoparticles with different sizes and different capping ligands. *Colloids Surfaces B Biointerfaces* **2007**, *58*, 3–7. [CrossRef]
29. Epanchintseva, A.V.; Vorobjev, P.; Pyshnyi, D.V.; Pyshnaya, I. Fast and strong adsorption of native oligonucleotides on citrate-coated gold nanoparticles. *Langmuir* **2017**, *34*, 164–172. [CrossRef]
30. Pramanik, S.; Banerjee, P.; Sarkar, A.; Bhattacharya, S.C. Size-dependent interaction of gold nanoparticles with transport protein: A spectroscopic study. *J. Lumin.* **2008**, *128*, 1969–1974. [CrossRef]
31. Elbakry, A.; Zaky, A.; Liebl, R.; Rachel, R.; Goepferich, A.; Breunig, M. Layer-by-layer assembled gold nanoparticles for sirna delivery. *Nano Lett.* **2009**, *9*, 2059–2064. [CrossRef]
32. Pyshnaya, I.A.; Razum, K.; Poletaeva, J.E.; Pyshnyi, D.V.; Zenkova, M.A.; Ryabchikova, E.I. Comparison of Behaviour in Different liquids and in cells of gold nanorods and spherical nanoparticles modified by linear polyethyleneimine and bovine serum albumin. *BioMed Res. Int.* **2014**, *2014*, 908175. [CrossRef]
33. Pyshnaya, I.A.; Razum, K.V.; Dolodoev, A.S.; Shashkova, V.V.; Ryabchikova, E.I. Surprises of electron microscopic imaging of proteins and polymers covering gold nanoparticles layer by layer. *Colloids Surf. B Biointerfaces* **2017**, *150*, 23–31. [CrossRef] [PubMed]
34. Alexander, J.J.; Bey, E.M.; Geddes, E.W.; Lecatsas, G. Establishment of a continuously growing cell line from primary carcinoma of the liver. *S. Afr. Med J.* **1976**, *50*, 2121–2128.
35. Chang, C.; Lin, Y.; O-Lee, T.W.; Chou, C.K.; Lee, T.S.; Liu, T.J.; P'Eng, F.K.; Chen, T.Y.; Hu, C.P. Induction of plasma protein secretion in a newly established human hepatoma cell line. *Mol. Cell. Biol.* **1983**, *3*, 1133–1137. [CrossRef]
36. Zheng, G.; Wang, M.; Ren, Q.; Han, T.; Li, Y.; Sun, S.; Li, X.; Feng, F. Experimental observation of mitochondrial oxidative damage of liver cells induced by isonicotinic acid hydrazide. *Exp. Ther. Med.* **2019**, *17*, 4289–4293. [CrossRef]
37. Męczyńska-Wielgosz, S.; Wojewódzka, M.; Matysiak-Kucharek, M.; Czajka, M.; Jodłowska-Jędrych, B.; Kruszewski, M.; Kapka-Skrzypczak, L. Susceptibility of HepG2 cells to silver nanoparticles in combination with other metal/metal oxide nanoparticles. *Materials* **2020**, *13*, 2221. [CrossRef]
38. Chiu, J.-H.; Hu, C.-P.; Lui, W.-Y.; Lo, S.J.; Chang, C. The formation of bile canaliculi in human hepatoma cell lines. *Hepatology* **1990**, *11*, 834–842. [CrossRef]
39. Gissen, P.; Arias, I.M. Structural and functional hepatocyte polarity and liver disease. *J. Hepatol.* **2015**, *63*, 1023–1037. [CrossRef]
40. Roehlen, N.; Suarez, A.A.R.; El Saghire, H.; Saviano, A.; Schuster, C.; Lupberger, J.; Baumert, T.F. Tight junction proteins and the biology of hepatobiliary disease. *Int. J. Mol. Sci.* **2020**, *21*, 825. [CrossRef]
41. Müsch, A. The unique polarity phenotype of hepatocytes. *Exp. Cell Res.* **2014**, *328*, 276–283. [CrossRef] [PubMed]
42. Graham, F.L.; Russell, W.C.; Smiley, J.; Nairn, R. Characteristics of a human cell line transformed by dna from human adenovirus type 5. *J. Gen. Virol.* **1977**, *36*, 59–72. [CrossRef] [PubMed]
43. Dumont, J.; Euwart, D.; Mei, B.; Estes, S.; Kshirsagar, R. Human cell lines for biopharmaceutical manufacturing: History, status, and future perspectives. *Crit. Rev. Biotechnol.* **2015**, *36*, 1110–1122. [CrossRef] [PubMed]
44. Minh, A.D.; Tran, M.Y.; Kamen, A.A. Lentiviral vector production in suspension culture using serum-free medium for the transduction of car-t cells. *Recent Results Cancer Res.* **2020**, *2086*, 77–83. [CrossRef]
45. Gaskell, H.; Sharma, P.; Colley, H.E.; Murdoch, C.; Williams, D.P.; Webb, S.D. Characterization of a functional C3A liver spheroid model. *Toxicol. Res.* **2016**, *5*, 1053–1065. [CrossRef]
46. Molla, A.; Couvet, M.; Coll, J.-L. Unsuccessful mitosis in multicellular tumour spheroids. *Oncotarget* **2017**, *8*, 28769–28784. [CrossRef]
47. Iuchi, K.; Oya, K.; Hosoya, K.; Sasaki, K.; Sakurada, Y.; Nakano, T.; Hisatomi, H. Different morphologies of human embryonic kidney 293T cells in various types of culture dishes. *Cytotechnology* **2019**, *72*, 131–140. [CrossRef]
48. Kelm, J.M.; Timmins, N.E.; Brown, C.J.; Fussenegger, M.; Nielsen, L.K. Method for generation of homogeneous multicellular tumor spheroids applicable to a wide variety of cell types. *Biotechnol. Bioeng.* **2003**, *83*, 173–180. [CrossRef]
49. Slim, C.L.; Van Ijzendoorn, S.C.D.; Lázaro-Diéguez, F.; Müsch, A. The special case of hepatocytes. *BioArchitecture* **2014**, *4*, 47–52. [CrossRef]

50. Sharma, V.R.; Shrivastava, A.; Gallet, B.; Karepina, E.; Charbonnier, P.; Chevallet, M.; Jouneau, P.-H.; Deniaud, A. Canalicular domain structure and function in matrix-free hepatic spheroids. *Biomater. Sci.* **2020**, *8*, 485–496. [CrossRef]
51. Cording, J.; Berg, J.; Käding, N.; Bellmann, C.; Tscheik, C.; Westphal, J.K.; Milatz, S.; Günzel, R.; Wolburg, H.; Piontek, J.; et al. In tight junctions, claudins regulate the interactions between occludin, tricellulin and marveld3, which, inversely, modulate claudin oligomerization. *J. Cell Sci.* **2012**, *126*, 554–564. [CrossRef]
52. Beutel, O.; Maraspini, R.; Pombo-García, K.; Martin-Lemaitre, C.; Honigmann, A. Phase separation of zonula occludens proteins drives formation of tight junctions. *Cell* **2019**, *179*, 923–936. [CrossRef] [PubMed]
53. Inada, M.; Izawa, G.; Kobayashi, W.; Ozawa, M. 293 cells express both epithelial as well as mesenchymal cell adhesion molecules. *Int. J. Mol. Med.* **2016**, *37*, 1521–1527. [CrossRef] [PubMed]
54. Fleischer, C.C.; Payne, C.K. Nanoparticle–cell interactions: Molecular structure of the protein corona and cellular outcomes. *Accounts Chem. Res.* **2014**, *47*, 2651–2659. [CrossRef] [PubMed]
55. Francia, V.; Montizaan, D.; Salvati, A. Interactions at the cell membrane and pathways of internalization of nano-sized materials for nanomedicine. *Beilstein J. Nanotechnol.* **2020**, *11*, 338–353. [CrossRef] [PubMed]
56. Patel, S.; Kim, J.; Herrera, M.; Mukherjee, A.; Kabanov, A.V.; Sahay, G. Brief update on endocytosis of nanomedicines. *Adv. Drug Deliv. Rev.* **2019**, *144*, 90–111. [CrossRef]
57. Kerr, M.C.; Teasdale, R.D. Defining macropinocytosis. *Traffic* **2009**, *10*, 364–371. [CrossRef]
58. Poussin, C.; Foti, M.; Carpentier, J.-L.; Pugin, J. CD14-dependent endotoxin internalization via a macropinocytic pathway. *J. Biol. Chem.* **1998**, *273*, 20285–20291. [CrossRef]
59. Stow, J.L.; Hung, Y.; Wall, A.A. Macropinocytosis: Insights from immunology and cancer. *Curr. Opin. Cell Biol.* **2020**, *65*, 131–140. [CrossRef]
60. Neutra, M.R.; Ciechanover, A.; Owen, L.S.; Lodish, H.F. Intracellular transport of transferrin- and asialoorosomucoid-colloidal gold conjugates to lysosomes after receptor-mediated endocytosis. *J. Histochem. Cytochem.* **1985**, *33*, 1134–1144. [CrossRef]
61. Huang, K.; Ma, H.; Liu, J.; Huo, S.; Kumar, A.; Wei, T.; Zhang, X.; Jin, S.; Gan, Y.; Wang, P.C.; et al. Size-Dependent Localization and Penetration of Ultrasmall Gold Nanoparticles in Cancer Cells, Multicellular Spheroids, and Tumors in Vivo. *ACS Nano* **2012**, *6*, 4483–4493. [CrossRef] [PubMed]
62. Huo, S.; Ma, H.; Huang, K.; Liu, J.; Wei, T.; Jin, S.; Zhang, J.; He, S.; Liang, X.-J. Superior penetration and retention behavior of 50 nm gold nanoparticles in tumors. *Cancer Res.* **2012**, *73*, 319–330. [CrossRef] [PubMed]
63. Minchinton, A.I.; Tannock, I.F. Drug penetration in solid tumours. *Nat. Rev. Cancer* **2006**, *6*, 583–592. [CrossRef] [PubMed]
64. Sujai, P.T.; Joseph, M.M.; Saranya, G.; Nair, J.B.; Murali, V.P.; Maiti, K.K.; T, S.P. Surface charge modulates the internalization vs. penetration of gold nanoparticles: Comprehensive scrutiny on monolayer cancer cells, multicellular spheroids and solid tumors by SERS modality. *Nanoscale* **2020**, *12*, 6971–6975. [CrossRef]
65. Gong, X.; Lin, C.; Cheng, J.; Su, J.; Zhao, H.; Liu, T.; Wen, X.; Zhao, P. Generation of multicellular tumor spheroids with microwell-based agarose scaffolds for drug testing. *PLoS ONE* **2015**, *10*, e0130348. [CrossRef] [PubMed]

Publisher's Note: MDPI stays neutral with regard to jurisdictional claims in published maps and institutional affiliations.

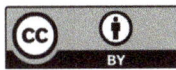

© 2020 by the authors. Licensee MDPI, Basel, Switzerland. This article is an open access article distributed under the terms and conditions of the Creative Commons Attribution (CC BY) license (http://creativecommons.org/licenses/by/4.0/).

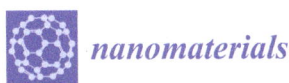

Article

Assessment of the Theranostic Potential of Gold Nanostars—A Multimodal Imaging and Photothermal Treatment Study

Antoine D'Hollander [1,2,3], Greetje Vande Velde [1,2], Hilde Jans [3], Bram Vanspauwen [3], Elien Vermeersch [1,2], Jithin Jose [4], Tom Struys [5], Tim Stakenborg [3], Liesbet Lagae [3,6] and Uwe Himmelreich [1,2,*]

1. Biomedical MRI, Department of Imaging and Pathology, Faculty of Medicine, KU Leuven, Herestraat 49, 3000 Leuven, Belgium; antoinedhollander@hotmail.com (A.D.); greetje.vandevelde@kuleuven.be (G.V.V.); elien.vermeersch@kuleuven.be (E.V.)
2. Molecular Small Animal Imaging Center (MoSAIC), KU Leuven, Herestraat 49, 3000 Leuven, Belgium
3. Department of Life Science Technology, IMEC, Kapeldreef 75, 3001 Leuven, Belgium; Hilde.Jans@imec.be (H.J.); brmvanspauwen@gmail.com (B.V.); Tim.Stakenborg@imec.be (T.S.); liesbet.lagae@imec.be (L.L.)
4. Fujifilm Visualsonics, Joop Geesinkweg140, 1114 AB Amsterdam, The Netherlands; jithin.jose@fujifilm.com
5. Lab of Histology, Biomedical Research Institute, Hasselt University, Agora Laan Gebouw C, 3590 Diepenbeek, Belgium; tom.struys@sprofit.com
6. Department of Physics, Faculty of Sciences, Laboratory of Soft Matter and Biophysics, KU Leuven, Celestijnenlaan 200D, 3001 Leuven, Belgium
* Correspondence: uwe.himmelreich@kuleuven.be; Tel.: +32-16-330925

Received: 31 August 2020; Accepted: 21 October 2020; Published: 23 October 2020

Abstract: Gold nanoparticles offer the possibility to combine both imaging and therapy of otherwise difficult to treat tumors. To validate and further improve their potential, we describe the use of gold nanostars that were functionalized with a polyethyleneglycol-maleimide coating for in vitro and in vivo photoacoustic imaging (PAI), computed tomography (CT), as well as photothermal therapy (PTT) of cancer cells and tumor masses, respectively. Nanostar shaped particles show a high absorption coefficient in the near infrared region and have a hydrodynamic size in biological medium around 100 nm, which allows optimal intra-tumoral retention. Using these nanostars for in vitro labeling of tumor cells, high intracellular nanostar concentrations could be achieved, resulting in high PAI and CT contrast and effective PTT. By injecting the nanostars intratumorally, high contrast could be generated in vivo using PAI and CT, which allowed successful multi-modal tumor imaging. PTT was successfully induced, resulting in tumor cell death and subsequent inhibition of tumor growth. Therefore, gold nanostars are versatile theranostic agents for tumor therapy.

Keywords: gold nanostars; photothermal therapy; photoacoustic imaging; computed tomography; nanoparticles; cancer; theranostic agents

---

1. Introduction

'Nanotheranostics'—referring to the use of nanotechnology for combined imaging and treatment of diseases—is currently an active research field as combining diagnosis with therapy has several advantages. The knowledge of the biodistribution of therapeutic agents through imaging can improve the guidance and initiation of cancer therapy. This can, for example, help to decide on the best time point for applying photothermal therapy. In addition, therapy success can be assessed at earlier time points and follow-up of therapy efficiency can be improved drastically. In the clinic, this will ultimately result in earlier intervention, better patient management, and improved prognosis [1]. Within the field of nanotheranostics, especially gold nanoparticles (AuNPs) that show a localized surface plasmon resonance (LSPR) can have a significant impact, as the LSPR effect can be used for both imaging and therapy [2]. The LSPR effect can be explained by the collective oscillation of the conduction band electrons due to light. This collective oscillation induces an enhanced absorption and scattering of the light [3]. The scattering properties of the light can be exploited by several imaging techniques including surface enhanced Raman scattering [4,5] and darkfield microscopy [2]. The light energy that is not scattered by the particles but absorbed, is converted into heat. This specific heat generation is the basis for both photoacoustic imaging (PAI) and photothermal therapy (PTT) [6,7].

PAI is based on the acoustic waves generated by the thermo-elastic expansion that occurs when a specific compound absorbs a pulsed electromagnetic wave [8]. Exogenous contrast (e.g., carbon nanotubes, AuNPs) have shown to generate higher PAI contrast compared to endogenous molecules (e.g., hemoglobin) [9]. Due to the negligible scattering of ultrasound in tissue compared to light, a relatively high imaging depth of approximately 5 cm is possible with PAI [10]. PTT on the other hand is also based on the heat conversion of AuNPs during irradiation with a continuous laser [11]. Since cancer cells are more sensitive to heat than other cell types, a temperature increase above 43 °C is lethal due to the inability to remove the heat in poorly vascularized tumor tissue [12].

For PAI and PTT, the ratio between the light scattering and absorption properties per AuNP is crucial. Hereto, several shapes of AuNPs have been studied ranging from nanorods, nanoshells, nanocages to nanostars [8]. Usually, nanostars have higher absorption vs. scattering coefficients compared to nanorods and nanoshells, but similar to nanocages [11,13]. This higher absorption coefficient is the crucial parameter for efficient heat conversion, important for PAI and PTT. Several studies have examined the use of gold nanorods as a contrast agent for PAI in tumors [14–18]. For nanostar-shaped AuNPs, mainly non-quantitative in vitro data [19] and in vivo mapping of the lymphatic system and first results on tumor imaging have been shown [20,21]. We have recently demonstrated their tumor-targeting ability using PAI [22]. For PTT of tumors, several groups have reported on nanostars as an effective in vitro PTT agent [13,19,21,23,24], but many questions remain regarding the PTT efficiency using these nanostars in vivo [23,25].

Alternatively, AuNPs can also be imaged with computed tomography (CT), since they absorb X-rays more efficiently compared to frequently used contrast agents such as iodine-based compounds [26,27]. In general, heavy atoms are frequently used as a contrast agent for X-ray based CT for diagnostic imaging in the clinic and for preclinical research [26]. Nonetheless, relatively high local AuNP concentrations are needed to generate sufficient contrast for CT, in particular for small voxel sizes as required for preclinical imaging applications [28]. AuNPs, such as nanorods or spheres, have shown their effectiveness as blood-pool and tumor-targeting contrast agent using CT [26,29]. However, for nanostars, quantitative in vitro and in vivo studies regarding their potential as contrast agents for CT are lacking [19].

Several routes have been explored to administer AuNPs as a theranostic agent against cancer, but many questions remain. Intratumoral administration is the most straight forward way for theranostic application, while i.v. injection has shown mixed results in terms of tumor accumulation [30,31]. Few reports showed reasonable tumor accumulation where the charge of the nanoparticles played a crucial role for tumor targeting [26,32]. Even functionalizing the nanoparticles with biological ligands gave different outcomes in terms of intra-tumor accumulation [33,34]. Active targeting, suggested to overcome problems with low intra-tumor accumulation after intravenous delivery, may have no influence on tumor uptake but does on the distribution within the tumor [33]. To improve biocompatibility and active targeting, AuNPs are frequently coated through an Au-S-bond. These non-covalent bonds are subject to potential thermal instability, releasing part of the coating material [35].

AuNPs have to fulfill some essential requirements to be applicable for in vivo theranostic photothermal approaches. First, the absorption band of the AuNP must be tuned to the near infrared region (NIR) frequency range for having maximal contrast generation and therapy efficiency due to its relative high depth penetration [36]. Second, the diameter of the AuNPs has to be around or below 100 nm to cross leaky blood vessels and being retained in the tumor. Third, charged particles are favored since such particles show better retention after intra-tumor injection because of immediate interaction with the tumor cells [37].

Exploiting the advantage of the specific high absorption capacity of nanostars, we have studied the potential of nanostars for PAI/CT and PTT in vitro and in vivo. In this study, we first optimized the synthesis and functionalization of nanostars for efficient uptake by tumor cells and assessed their PAI and PTT capabilities in vitro using an ovarian cancer cell line (SKOV3). For in vivo validation, gold nanostars were intratumorally injected in a xenograft mouse model and their local distribution in the tumor assessed with CT and PAI. Finally, photothermal therapy was performed and evaluated using bioluminescence imaging (BLI), magnetic resonance imaging (MRI), and histology.

2. Materials and Methods

2.1. Synthesis and Chemical Functionalization of Nanostars

Gold nanostars were prepared based on the procedure described by Hao et al. [38] and further optimized by Van de Broek et al. [39]. In brief, 2 mg bis(psulfonatophenyl) phenylphosphine dihydrate dipotassium (BSPP; Strem Chemicals, Newburyport, MA, USA) and 100 μL H_2O_2 (30% v/v, Air Products, Vilvoorde, Belgium) were added to 50 mL of a 6.8×10^{-3} M aqueous sodium citrate solution (Acros Organics, Geel, Belgium). In a next step, 100 μL of 0.075 M $HAuCl_4$ (Acros Organics) was added slowly under constant stirring at room temperature. By using an Atlas Syringe Pump (Syrris, Ruisbroek, Belgium) a slower addition rate of 12.5 μL/min was used in comparison to previously published articles in order to achieve the desired shape and size [36]. The 50 mL AuNP suspension was centrifuged at 4500 rpm for 1 h and the pellet was re-suspended in 10 mL of water. The star-shape of the AuNPs was stabilized using a disulfide molecule, according to Lin et al. [40]. Hereby, 1 mL of an 1.2 mM disulfide $(S-(CH_2)_{11}-(O-CH_2-CH_2)_6-O-CH_2-CO-NH-(CH_2)_2$-maleimide$)_2$ (Prochimia, Sopot, Poland) solution was added to 10 mL of the AuNP suspension mixed with 100 μL 0.5 M NaOH (Merck, Overijse, Belgium). After 90 min of shaking, the mixture was centrifuged at 4000 rpm for 60 min and re-suspended in water resulting in an optical density of ~1 at their maximum plasmon band. These nanostars were characterized in water and cell culture medium using UV-Vis absorption spectroscopy (Shimadzu UV-1601PC, Brussels, Belgium), dynamic light scattering (DLS; Malvern Nanosizer, WR, United Kingdom) and transmission electron microscopy (TEM; Tecnai F30, FEI company, Eindhoven, The Netherlands). A terminal maleimide group was chosen for future functionalization with anti/nanobodies and targeting of specific cell types as described [22].

2.2. Dynamic Light Scattering and Zeta Protocol

For dynamic light scattering (DLS), the hydrodynamic diameters of the nanostars under investigation were measured using a Zetasizer Nano ZS90 DLS system equipped with a red (633 nm) laser and an Avalanche photodiode detector (APD) (quantum efficiency > 50% at 633 nm) (Malvern Instruments Ltd., Malvern, UK). Hydrodynamic diameters represent estimates of average diameters as the Zetasizer Nano ZS90 DLS system is optimized for spherical nanoparticles and not nanostars. A 1.5 mL semi-micro cuvette was used as sample container. The 'DTS applications 5.10' software was used to analyze the data. All sizes reported here were based on intensity average where the intensity was observed using a non-negative least squares (NNLS) analysis method. For each sample, two DLS measurements were conducted with a fixed 15 runs and each run lasts 10 s. A detection angle of 173° was chosen for the size measurement.

For determining the zeta potential, an average was taken on three distinct measurements where the nanostars were dissolved in water. A u-shaped polycarbonate flow cell with embedded electrodes at either end, referred to as 'clear disposable zeta cell', was used during these measurements. As with the size experiments the 'DTS applications 5.10' software was used to process the data.

2.3. Transmission Electron Microscopy

We used a transmission electron microscopy (TEM) protocol as previously described [41]. In more detail, tumor tissue was collected after sacrificing the animals. Tissue was cut into cubes of 2 mm^3 and fixed overnight in 2% glutaraldehyde and 0.05 M sodium cacodylate buffer (pH 7.3) at 4 °C. Tissue samples were post-fixed in 2% OsO$_4$ in 0.05 M sodium cacodylate buffer (pH 7.3) for 1 h and stained with 2% uranyl acetate in 10% acetone for 20 min. Next, samples were dehydrated in graded concentrations of acetone and were embedded in epoxyresin (Araldite). Semi-thin slices (500 nm) were cut, stained with toluidine-blue and used for selecting regions of interest. Ultra-thin sections were mounted on 0.7% formvar coated grids, contrasted with uranyl acetate followed by lead citrate and examined with a Philips EM 208 transmission electron microscope operated at 80 kV. Digital images were taken with the MORADA 10/12 camera (Olympus, Hamburg, Germany). TEM analysis was performed with a Philips EM 208 S electron microscope (Philips, Eindhoven, The Netherlands). The microscope was provided with a Morada Soft Imaging System camera to acquire high resolution images of the evaluated samples. The images were processed digitally with the iTEM-FEI software (Olympus SIS, Münster, Germany).

2.4. Cell Culture

SKOV3 cells (ATCC® HTB77, Cedex, France) were cultured in Roswell Park Memorial Institute medium (RPMI) 1640 medium supplemented with 10% fetal calf serum, 50 units/L penicillin, 50 μg/mL streptomycin, and 2 mM L-glutamine. Cells were incubated at 37 °C in a 5% CO$_2$ environment. All cell culture reagents were obtained from Life Technologies (Gent, Belgium). The SKOV3 cells were transduced with a lentiviral vector (LV-CMV-eGFP-T2A-fLuc) to stably express eGFP and firefly luciferase [42].

2.5. Inductively Coupled Plasma Optical Emission Spectroscopy (ICP-OES)

For uptake confirmation, 100,000 cells per well were seeded in a 12-well plate. After 24 h, nanostars (2.3×10^{10} particles in 1 mL) were added to the cells and incubation continued for different time periods (1, 3, 6, 12 and 24 h). Next, cells were washed with PBS and again incubated overnight with fresh medium. After trypsinization, 100,000 cells were acid-digested with Kingswater (HCl/HNO$_3$) with a ratio of 3:1) and diluted with de-ionized water to a volume of 10 mL for inductively coupled plasma optical emission spectroscopy (ICP-OES) (3300 DV, Perkin-Elmer, Waltham, MA, USA). Reference standards were prepared by dissolving HAuCl$_4$ to final concentrations between 0.1 and 2 ppm.

2.6. In Vivo Xenograft Model and Nanostar Administration

Female Hsd:Athymic *Nude-Foxn1^{nu}* mice were used (8 weeks, Harlan, Horst, The Netherlands) during these experiments. All animal experiments were approved by the local animal ethics committee of the KU Leuven and were performed according to the national and European regulations. Animals were kept in individually ventilated cages with food and water ad libitum. A total number of 1×10^7 SKOV3 tumor cells suspended in 100 μL were injected into each hind limb of the mice and left for two weeks to grow into solid tumors [22].

After formation of tumors (size > 200 μm^3), 100 μL containing 9.2×10^{11} NPs/mL were injected into the tumor on the left hind limb. For controls, 100 μL PBS was injected into the right tumor in all animals (sham control). During all imaging experiments, tumor cell and nanostar injections, the animals were anesthetized with 1.5% isoflurane in 100% O$_2$. The body temperature and respiration rate were monitored and maintained at 37 °C and 80–120 min^{-1}, respectively. For the imaging experiments, three mice were used per condition while for the therapy experiments, six animals were used per condition.

2.7. Photoacoustic Imaging (PAI)

PAI was performed with a Vevo® Lazer 2000 (Fujifilms Visualsonics, Amsterdam, The Netherlands) using a 10 ns pulse laser (680–900 nm) with an energy fluence of 20 mJ/cm^2 and 21 MHz central frequency. These conditions were maintained for the in vitro and in vivo experiments. For in vitro PAI, 200,000 cells were suspended in 100 µL PBS and mixed with 100 µL warm agar (Sigma, Diegem, Belgium). This solution was added and solidified in a bigger agar block. During in vivo PAI, ultrasound imaging is used to determine the tumor location, after which PAI was performed to validate nanostar injection.

2.8. Computed Tomography (CT)

In vivo and in vitro CT images were acquired using an in vivo microCT scanner (Skyscan 1076, Bruker microCT, Kontich, Belgium) with the following settings: 50 kV X-ray source, 200 µA source current, 0.5 mm Al filter, 120 ms exposure time, 22 × 29 mm field of view, 0.7° rotation step over a total angel of 180°, which results in a tomographic dataset with a 35 µm isotropic resolution. The data has been processed using software from the manufacturer (NRecon, Dataviewer, CTvox and CTan). Sample preparation was similar for CT as for PAI.

2.9. Photothermal Therapy (PTT)

In vitro and in vivo PTT experiments were performed using a home-built laser setup [12]. For in vitro PTT, nanostars (2.3×10^{10} particles in 1 mL) were added to a 12-well plate containing 100,000 cells/well that were pre-incubated overnight. Nanostar concentrations were calculated as previously described in the supplementary methods section of [13]. The cells were then incubated with the nanostars for 24 h or with fresh medium as a control sample and washed twice with PBS. Next, the incubated cells were exposed to laser irradiation (690 nm, 20 W/cm^2, 5 min) and incubated for an additional 2 h at 37 °C. Afterwards, the cells were washed with PBS. The cell viability was assessed using a live/dead staining (Calcein AM/Hoechst; Life Technologies Europe B.V., Gent, Belgium). After staining, the cells were imaged using a fluorescence microscope with 5× objective (CellR system, Olympus, Aartselaar, Belgium). During the in vivo experiments, the mice were irradiated for five minutes with a laser (λ = 690 nm; 2 W/cm^2), inducing PTT one day after nanostar administration. During this laser treatment, the mice were anesthetized with ketamine/domitor [43].

2.10. Magnetic Resonance Imaging (MRI)

MRI data acquisition and processing was similar to previous reports [44]. In brief, in vivo MRI was performed using a 9.4 T small animal MRI system (BioSpec, Bruker Biospin, Ettlingen, Germany) equipped with a gradient insert with a maximum gradient strength of 600 mT m^{-1}. A quadrature transmit-receive coil (Bruker Biospin) with an inner diameter of 7 cm was used for data acquisition. The MRI protocol included a spin echo sequence with TR = 6000 ms, TE = 15.8 ms, matrix = 200 × 200 mm, field of view 40 × 40 mm, slice thickness = 0.5 µm and 40 slices.

2.11. Bioluminescence Imaging (BLI)

BLI experiments were performed with an IVIS 100 imaging system (Perkin Elmer, Massachusetts, United States). The mice were injected intra-venously (i.v.) with D-luciferin (126 mg/kg body weight, Promega) dissolved in PBS (15 mg/kg). Afterwards, they were placed in the IVIS 100 imaging system and one image frame per second was acquired until a signal intensity plateau was reached. The following settings were used: 1 s exposure time, FOV of 10 cm, binning of 4, and an f/stop of 8. For in vivo quantification of fLuc reporter gene activity, the data were analyzed as photon flux per second (p/s) from a 1 cm^2 circular ROI located on the tumor using the Living Image software (version 2.50.1, Perkin Elmer). The signal intensity values at different time points (day 0, 1, 5, 8 and 15) were presented relative to the BLI signal of the same mouse at day 0.

2.12. Histopathology

Mice were sacrificed and transcardially perfused with 4% paraformaldehyde (PFA) in PBS 15 days after treatment. The tumors were dissected and post fixed overnight in 4% PFA. The tumor tissue was embedded in paraffin and sectioned into 5 μm slices, stained with hematoxylin and eosin (H&E) and visualized with a Mirax desk scanner (Zeiss, Jena, Germany). In addition to histopathology, TEM analysis was performed on the tumor tissue following the protocol supplied in the supplementary information of Trekker et al. [45].

2.13. Data Analysis

For quantification of CT and PAI data, contrast to noise ratios (CNR = $(SI_0 - SI_1)/\sigma(noise)$) were calculated. Statistical analyses were executed on the quantitative data using a paired t-test where the degree of significance is indicated with * $p < 0.05$; ** $p < 0.01$; *** $p < 0.001$.

3. Results

3.1. Synthesis and Functionalization of Nanostar-Shaped AuNPs Optimized for In Vivo Use

To be able to use nanostars as a theranostic agent in vivo, they need to be stable under physiological conditions, preferably absorb the light in the NIR-range and have a size around 100 nm for optimal retention in tumors. To meet these requirements, we optimized a two-step method by changing the flow rate of the HAuCl$_4$ to 12.5 μL/min during synthesis and by functionalizing them with a self-assembled monolayer to stabilize their specific shape (Figure 1) [13]. The resulting nanostars showed an improved plasmon absorption band around 670 nm and 679 nm (Supplementary Figure S1). This red shift indicated a successful chemical functionalization with the disulfide, resulting from a local refractive index change due to the chemisorption of the disulfide onto the nanostars. These results were confirmed by DLS, showing an average diameter of 66.3 ± 7.8 nm for the synthesized nanostars and 75.0 nm ± 5.6 nm for the further functionalized nanostars. After functionalization with disulfide-PEG-maleimide, the zeta potential was −41.3 ± 1.2 mV, indicating negatively charged nanostars (Supplementary Figure S2). The branched shape of the nanostars was confirmed using TEM (Figure 1). Incubating the nanostars in biological medium for one week at 37 °C did not show any indication of instability, confirmed by the absence of peak broadening of the LSPR band or increase in diameter of the nanostars over time (Supplementary Figure S2). Still, an increase of the diameter to 100.6 ± 1.8 nm was seen immediately after incubation in cell culture medium due to the formation of a protein corona. As a consequence, these optimized nanostars are suitable for in vitro and in vivo theranostic applications.

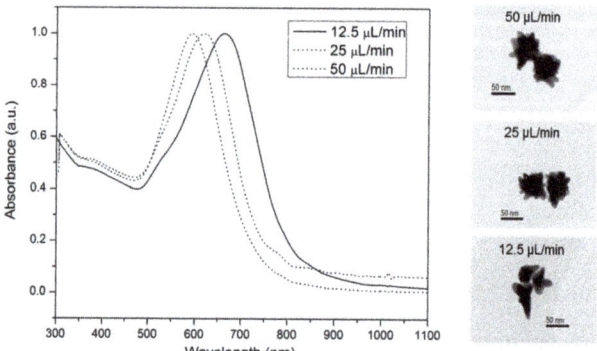

Figure 1. UV-Vis absorption spectroscopy of nanostars using different flow rates for the gold salt. Note the shift to the near infrared region (NIR) region with lower flow rates. TEM images of the nanostars that were generated with flow rates of 50 μL/min, 25 μL/min and 12.5 μL/min (from top to bottom). These images suggest that the amount and length of spikes change with different flow rates. The diameter of the nanostars did not significantly change as confirmed by dynamic light scattering (DLS) where no significant increase was noticed with lower flow rates (50 μL/min: 66.0 ± 1.5 nm; 25 μL/min: 67.5 ± 2.7 nm: 12.5 μL/min: 66.3 ± 7.8 nm; data not shown).

After functionalization, the capability of the nanostars to generate image contrast was studied in water using a concentration of 1.55 mg Au/mL. A PAI signal of 0.33 ± 0.04 a.u. was measured for the nanostars while water shows a signal of 0.13 ± 0.01 a.u. (Figure 2). For CT, a signal of 175.67 ± 2.74 and 57.33 ± 0.17 for the nanostars and water was measured, respectively. As a consequence, both imaging modalities showed almost an identical CNR of 32.85 for PAI and 32.53 for CT, respectively.

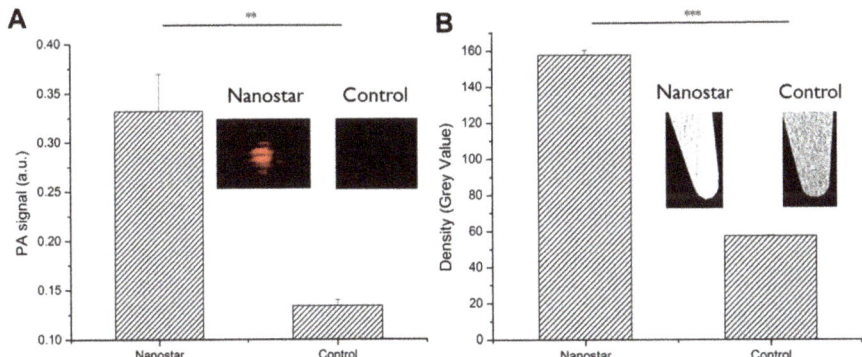

Figure 2. (**A**) Photoacoustic images of nanostars and water in tubes, which were quantified by plotting the signal amplitudes. (**B**) Computed tomography (CT) images of microcentrifuge tubes either filled with water or nanostars suspension. The corresponding signal amplitudes were used for quantification. (Error bars represent SD of triplicate samples; * $p < 0.05$, ** $p < 0.01$, *** $p < 0.001$).

3.2. PAI and CT Confirm Efficient Nanostar Uptake by Tumor Cells

In order to test whether tumor cells efficiently take up the nanostars, SKOV3 cells were incubated with these NPs for different time periods (1, 3, 6, 12, and 24 h). Their uptake was examined by using ICP-OES, CT and PAI. ICP-OES measurements showed for the first incubation time points an almost linear increase of intracellular gold concentration while over time this seemed to change into a plateau phase as visualized by the fitting curve in Supplementary Figure S3. After 24 h, an intracellular gold amount of 11.28 ± 0.82 pg Au/cell was observed. TEM confirmed intracellular uptake of the nanostars as they were found inside vesicular structures of the cells but not at the cell membrane.

Furthermore, we evaluated whether this uptake was sufficiently high to be visualized by PAI and CT. Hereby, the tumor cells labeled with different amounts of gold nanostars were homogenously suspended in an agar phantom at 1000 cells/µL. PA images shown in Figure 3 indicated an increased PA signal (red pixels) over incubation time, where an exponential correlation was found between the PA signal and intracellular gold concentration. After 24 h, a PAI signal 1.93 ± 0.42 a.u. was measured compared to a PA signal of 0.19 ± 0.02 a.u. for the unlabeled cells. This successful nanostar-labeling resulted in an CNR of 180.73 for PAI and a limit of detection (LOD) of 3.5 pg Au/cell (17 µM).

For CT, the contrast visualized on a grey intensity scale is shown in Figure 4 where an increase of density was noticed over time. When plotting these density values over the different intracellular gold concentrations, an exponential fit was deducted. After 24 h, a CT signal of 161.33 ± 1.42 was measured for cells labeled for 24 h with nanostars compared to 130.28 ± 3.25 for unlabeled cells. The CT imaging capabilities results in a CNR of 7.36 for CT and a LOD of 5.5 pg Au/cell (28 µM).

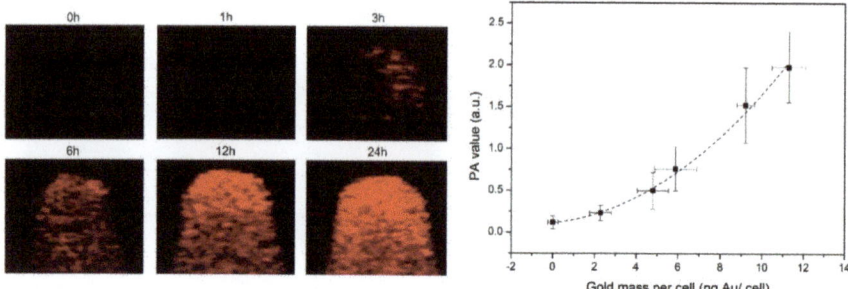

Figure 3. Left: PA images of a phantom loaded with tumor cells (n = 3) incubated for different time slots with the nanostars. **Right**: PA signal plotted for the different gold masses per cell, where the dotted line suggests an exponential relation between those 2 variables.

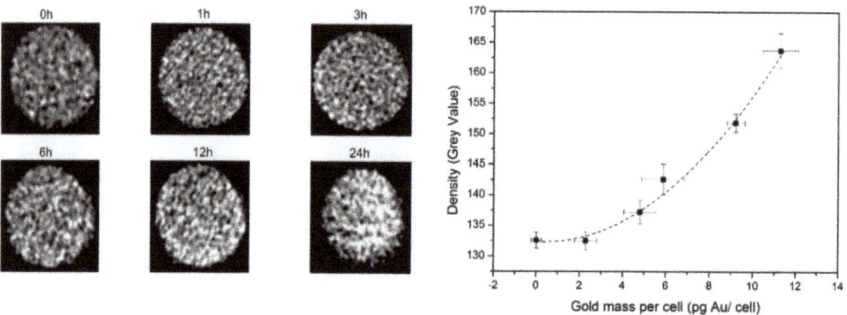

Figure 4. Left: CT images of an agar phantom loaded with tumor cells (n = 3) incubated for different time points with the nanostars. **Right**: CT signal quantified as density (grey values) plotted for the different gold masses per cell, where the dotted line suggests an exponential relation between those 2 variables.

3.3. Effective In Vitro Photothermal Tumor Cell Ablation Using Gold Nanostars

Since tumor cells were effectively labeled with nanostars, we investigated if the in vitro uptake was sufficient to eradicate tumor cells by PTT. First, the potential of nanostars for heat generation necessary for PTT was investigated using a glass capillary filled with either 4.6×10^{10} nanostars/mL or water as a negative control. When irradiating the sample with a 690 nm laser (7 W/cm^2), a temperature increase of 25 °C was observed for the nanostar suspension, while no temperature increase was measured for the water filled capillary (Supplementary Figure S4).

A crucial parameter for determining the effectiveness of PTT is to calculate the cell killing capacity (IC50 value). To determine this value, the tumor cells were labeled with the nanostars using the same conditions as for the imaging experiments. After PTT, cell death was visualized by calcein AM living cells staining and quantified by calculating the total green pixels. As visualized by fluorescence microscopy a radius increase of non-viable cells at the laser spot indicates a higher PTT effectiveness with an increasing intracellular gold concentration (Figure 5). By plotting the relative green fluorescence signal compared to the fluorescence signal of the control cells, a sigmoidal curve was fitted where an IC50 of 4.8 pg Au/cell (23 µM) was calculated.

3.4. In Vivo CT and PAI Confirms Nanostar Delivery into Tumors

We evaluated if nanostars injected into tumors can be visualized by in vivo imaging. Tumor-bearing mice (n = 3) were imaged with CT and PAI before and one day after gold nanostar injection into the tumor. Before injection, only the contrast between the skeleton and the soft tissue was visible using CT (Figure 6A). After injection of the nanostars, an intense contrast of 94.63 ± 6.77 was observed at the left side of the tumor, corresponding to the place of the tumor (Figure 6A, right). No significant change in contrast was generated in the PBS-injected control tumor with a signal of 74.11 ± 1.43 (Figure 6A, left). A CNR increase of 25.31 was calculated after intratumoral injection of gold nanostars, indicating that intratumoral delivery of nanostars can be monitored with CT in vivo.

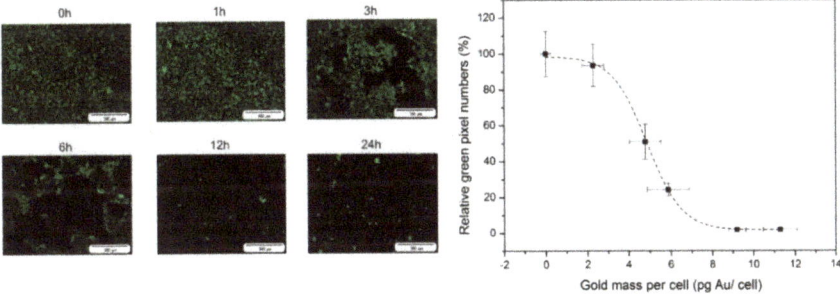

Figure 5. **Left**: Fluorescence images of the living cells after photothermal therapy (PTT) using calcein AM staining for tumor cells (n = 3) incubated for different time periods with the nanostars. **Right**: Relative green pixel numbers plotted against the gold mass per cell. Fluorescence signal intensity is expressed relative to the unlabeled control cells (0 h).

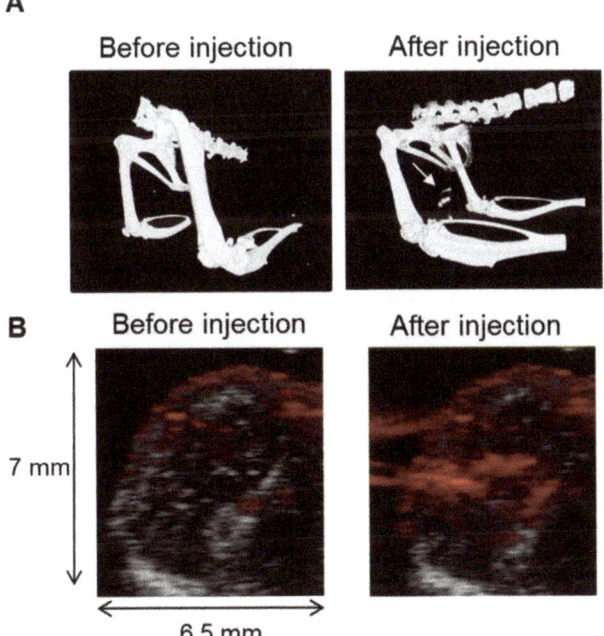

Figure 6. (**A**) CT images before and after injection of gold nanostars into the tumor. An increased contrast was noticed at the tumor site after gold nanostars injection as indicated by the arrow; (**B**) In vivo PA images before and 24 h after nanostar injection. The photoacoustic imaging (PAI) signal (red pixels) is overlaid over the anatomical ultrasound images (grey pixels).

Alternatively, we evaluated whether intratumoral nanostar delivery can also be followed up with PAI. Hereby, both ultrasound and photoacoustic images were overlaid as shown in Figure 6B. The ultrasound image was used for localizing and visualizing the tumor. Although some background photoacoustic contrast due to hemoglobin is present before nanostar injection, PAI could be used to visualize the nanostars as indicated by a significant increase in signal intensity compared to the background (1.20 ± 0.17 a.u. compared to the control 0.44 ± 0.05 a.u.) with a CNR of 80.31.

3.5. Gold Nanostars Mediate In Vivo Photothermal Therapy

The effectiveness of nanostars to mediate PTT was studied in a xenograft mouse model (n = 6). The left tumor was used for injection with gold nanostars, while the right tumor acted as control after sham injection with PBS. 24 h after nanostar injection, both tumors were irradiated with a continuous laser (5 min, 690 nm and 2 W/cm^2). Therapy efficacy was assessed in vivo by using MRI and BLI to evaluate tumor regression and viability. For quantification of the tumor cell viability, the BLI signal was monitored one day before and 0, 1, 5, 8 and 15 days after PTT. The day before PTT and after imaging, nanostars/PBS were injected into the tumors. A decrease in BLI signal intensity was detected for the nanostar-injected tumor at day 0, which was not observed for the PBS injected tumor (Supplementary Figure S5). This is explained by the nanostars absorbing/scattering a part of the BLI signal. This time point was used as baseline for assessment of PTT. One day after PTT, a significant decrease in relative BLI signal intensity to 10.13 ± 1.41% was observed for the nanostar-injected tumor compared to the tumor at day 0, indicating a decrease in viable tumor cells or vessel patency (Figure 7). After 5 days, an increase of the BLI signal intensity was noticed to a relative value of 45.78 ± 10.02%, which indicates partial re-growth of the PTT treated tumor as probably not all tumor cells were photothermally ablated. Although, a significant difference in signal intensity was maintained when compared to the tumor at baseline. In contrast, the right control tumor showed a constant increase in BLI signal intensity over time until a relative BLI signal of 440.24 ± 51.14% after 15 days, confirming that the viability of the control tumor was not affected by laser irradiation. When comparing the nanostar-injected with the control tumor, a significant difference in BLI signal intensity was detected at day 1, 5, and 8, indicating a significant inhibition of tumor growth by PTT.

For providing more information on the therapeutic effect, MR images were acquired on day 0, 1, 8 and 15 to monitor tumor size, anatomy, and heterogeneity. After 8 and 15 days, a relative tumor volume of 68.64 ± 18.45% and 55.25 ± 30.1% was observed for the left tumor compared to day 0, indicating effective PTT (Figure 7B). This was confirmed by the significant difference between this volume and the volume of the control tumor (PBS injection), where a relative tumor volume of 142.27 ± 28.49% at day 5 and 184.12 ± 39.13% at day 8 was measured, respectively. MRI also indicate that the nanostar-injected tumors were not affected evenly by PTT over the whole tumor volume, indicating local differences due to inhomogeneous distribution of the nanostars (Figure 7B).

For validation, mice (n = 3) were sacrificed after the first (day 1) and last (day 15) imaging time point following PTT. Tumors were resected and histologically examined. After one day, a distinct blue color was seen on these histological slices originating from the nanostars with an LSPR band of 679 nm, which were visible in the tumor. These nanostars were only noticed in the tumor region where also necrotic cells were visible (Supplementary Figure S6). As can be seen on the H&E stained images, the nuclei were either defragmented or darkened in comparison to the healthy cells (Figure 8). For the PBS-injected control tumors, the blue color due to the nanostars was absent and the majority of cells appeared healthy. At the last imaging time point, no necrotic cells were visible on the histology sections for both the PBS- and nanostar-injected tumors (Supplementary Figure S6).

Using TEM, the presence of nanostar clusters inside vesicles of the cells was confirmed (Figure 8). At the ultrastructural level, tumor cells were identified based on their pleomorphic aspects, increased nuclear/cytoplasmic ratio and distinct anaplasia. The latter was typically represented by nuclear hyperchromatism, thereby confirming that the tumor cells took up the nanostars. These nanostars were present in the cytoplasm and typically stored in membrane-bound compartments (endosomes, arrows in Figure 8B). As the endosomes were packed with nanostars, it was difficult to identify single nanostars, demonstrating efficient intracellular uptake in vivo upon intra-tumoral injection.

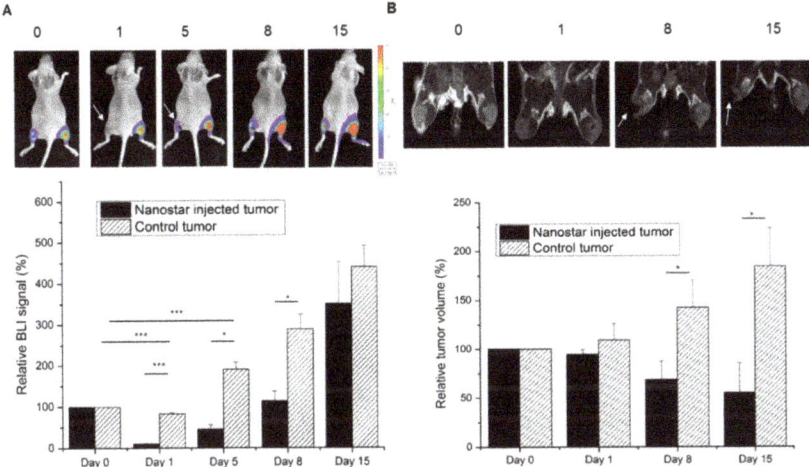

Figure 7. (**A**) In vivo bioluminescence imaging (BLI) before (day 0) and after PTT (days 1, 5, 8) illustrated in a color-coded intensity map. A quantification of the BLI signal intensity relative to day 0 (set to 100% for each mouse) is plotted for both nanostar-injected and control (PBS-injected) tumors (RT); (**B**) MR images of the tumor-bearing hind limbs taken at corresponding time points (days) after nanostar- or PBS-injection. The white arrow indicates the tumor damage (hypointense area) after PTT at the nanostar-injected tumor. The relative mass volumes were quantified relative to day 0 (set at 100% per mice). For both BLI and magnetic resonance imaging (MRI) graphs, the error bars represent SD; n = 6; * $p < 0.05$, ** $p < 0.01$, *** $p < 0.001$.

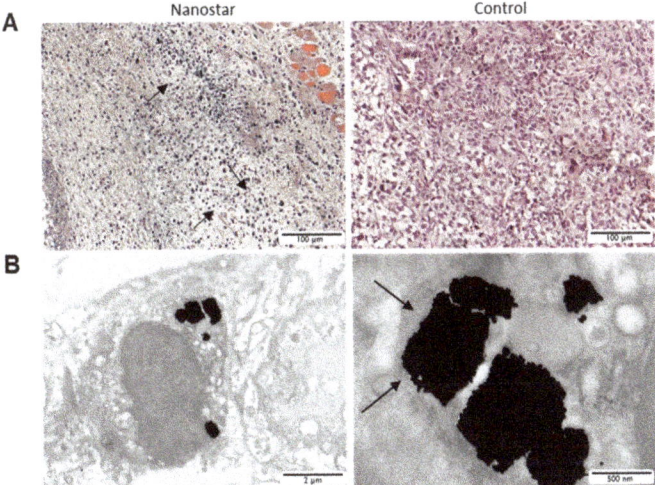

Figure 8. (**A**) Bright field microscopy images of control (right) and nanostar (left) injected hematoxylin and eosin (H&E) stained tumor sections. Defragmented nuclei of the tumor cells could be visualized after therapy. (**B**) Ex vivo TEM images of tumor cells that indicate the presence of NP clusters in endosomes. The right panel shows a zoomed section of these endosomes with vesicular structures visible.

4. Discussion

We report the use of gold nanostars as theranostic agent against cancer using their photoacoustic and CT imaging capabilities to guide PTT after intratumoral injection. This strategy has clinical potential for the ablation of superficially localized tumor masses, or for aiming at complete tumor cell eradication during tumor resection surgery. The clinical potential for a similar approach was demonstrated before, using magnetic nanoparticles [31,46].

Hereby, the efficient cellular uptake of nanostars into tumor cells is important for later in vivo applications. A first criterion is the size where two processes need to be considered: (1) optimal NP/cell interaction and (2) optimal tumor retention [47,48]. Nanoparticles having a hydrodynamic diameter above 100 nm are shown to have better tumor retention after intra-tumoral injection compared to smaller sized particles. In vitro studies, on the other hand, have shown that nanoparticles of around 50 nm diameter have the ideal size for cell interaction, while the cell uptake is less efficient for larger nanoparticles [47]. We have optimized nanostars to have a hydrodynamic diameter of around 100 nm in serum, which is the cutoff-value for optimal tumor retention and efficient tumor cell interaction. Second, the protrusions of the nanostars with a small curvature potentially increase cellular uptake by increasing their membrane interaction [48]. Third, the anionic particles used in this and previous studies show a much higher stability compared to previously described cationic particles and still result in high cellular accumulation due to electrostatic interactions with the cell membrane [47]. Consequently, we were able to show that nanostars were taken up reaching a gold concentration 11.28 ± 0.82 pg Au/cell after 24 h incubation, indicating that they are suitable for efficient passive labeling of tumor cells.

Given their favorable properties for tumor cell uptake, we demonstrated that nanostars can be used as an in vitro and in vivo theranostic agent combining both dual-modality imaging (PAI and CT) and PTT. Pure nanostar suspensions resulted in an almost equally high CNR for both imaging modalities. This is different for in vitro cell experiments, where a higher CNR for PAI is measured compared to CT. This is due to the lower background signal of PAI compared to CT. Effective PTT was possible for nanostar labeled tumor cells in vitro. In contrast, unlabeled cells remained unaffected by laser treatment. For comparing the PTT effectiveness of different nanoparticles, the irradiation power that is needed to cause cell death is used as an indicator. The radiation power of 7 W/cm^2 used in our study is in the same range or lower as in similar experiments that were performed with nanorods (10 W/cm^2) [49], nanoshells (35 W/cm^2) [50], and nanocages (5 W/cm^2) [51]. The relatively low radiation power used for our nanostars indicates their efficiency when compared with many nanostars reported in the literature (15 W/cm^2, 38 W/cm^2 and 0.2 W/cm^2) [13,19,21]. The maximum absorption of the nanostars used in our study is just outside the preferred window of 750–900 nm. Here, we had to find a compromise between the reduced size to enable possible delivery through leaky blood vessels and tumor cell uptake on one side and a red-shifted absorption band which would have resulted in larger nanostars [39]. In addition to inherent characteristics of the nanoparticles (absorption coefficient, size, and wavelength), other factors like cellular labeling conditions, chemical coatings, biofunctionalization of the AuNPs, cellular properties, and location of the AuNPs in the cells are equally important when comparing AuNPs regarding the irradiation power for PTT [35,48,52,53]. Consequently, there is a need for more in-depth and standardized studies for comparing different shapes of AuNPs and their theranostic potential as well as the stability of coating material at temperatures of 37 °C and above [35]. Although, we did not see any adverse effects on cell biology after incubation of cells with PEGylated Au-nanostars in a previous study [22], it cannot be excluded that the non-covalent Au-S-bond shows instability at elevated temperatures [35].

In addition to in vitro experiments, we evaluated the use of in vivo imaging modalities (CT and PAI) to monitor intra-tumor nanostar delivery and their corresponding contrast generating capabilities. With nanostars having optimal dimensions for intra-tumoral delivery, efficient nanostar accumulation in the tumor 24 h after injection was confirmed by PAI and CT in vivo and ex vivo TEM. These nanostars were densely packed in endosomes, as visualized by TEM. Concerning the contrast generation of these nanostars in vivo, for PAI a significantly higher CNR (approx. 80) was observed compared to CT (approx. 25). The high sensitivity of PAI could potentially be further improved by coating the nanostars with a silica shell [54]. An additional advantage of PAI over CT is its high temporal resolution, while CT provides additional anatomical information. We were able to demonstrate that both imaging techniques can be used for intra-tumoral nanostar detection if high local concentrations can be achieved. By combining CT and PAI in a dual-modality approach using highly sensitive gold nanostars, PAI could provide rapid and detailed information on local nanostar distribution and their temporal changes, while CT could provide a full body scan with more detailed anatomical information. Compared to dual contrast agents that use radio-nuclei labeling like for PET-MRI [55,56], the combination of CT and PAI provides long-lasting contrast.

We have also confirmed the efficiency of the nanostars for PTT. Due to their star shape, they have a high absorption coefficient resulting in a large temperature increase of $\Delta 25\,°C$ when irradiated with a laser power of only 2 W/cm^2. Reaching a local temperature higher than 43 °C will result in necrosis of tumor cells [28,57]. In vivo necrosis was confirmed in this study after tumor irradiation (2 W/cm^2), while the control tumors did not show any side effects of laser irradiation. Using laser powers higher than the prescribed laser norm of 0.2 W/cm^2 defined by the American Laser Institute did not damage tissue when irradiating the control sample as confirmed by histology (Figure 7) [58]. Compared to nanoshells (4 W/cm^2) [50] and nanorods (2 W/cm^2) [30], the nanostars require the same magnitude of laser power to induce ablation after intratumoral injection. However, comparisons between different nanoparticles to assess their therapeutic efficiency are difficult due to the different experimental conditions used and incomplete or limited information available.

The in vivo efficiency of PTT was shown in detail using BLI, MRI, and histology (Figure 6). The BLI signal intensity decrease one day after irradiation was either caused by a decrease in tumor cell viability, destroyed tissue, vessel patency or a combination of them. As a significant decrease in tumor volume is noticed by MRI from day 8 onwards, the decrease in BLI signal is most likely caused by tumor cell death. The large number of necrotic cells seen in H&E staining of the nanostar-injected tumors confirmed this hypothesis. Regrowth of the tumor after PTT treatment was observed by BLI after day 8. This is most likely due to an incomplete delivery of gold nanostars to all tumor cells so that some residual tumor tissue/cells remain as also confirmed by MRI and histology after 15 days. As local injections of nanostars will result in an inhomogeneous distribution within the tumor, applying multiple injections and irradiations will most likely improve outcome [23]. Hereby, the combination with imaging techniques that provide information on the nanostar distribution and therapy outcome is of utmost importance. Additional treatment options to improve outcome are a combination of PTT with chemotherapy, photodynamic therapy, or the introduction of tumor-targeting moieties to the nanostars [59,60].

5. Conclusions

We have demonstrated an optimized synthesis and application of gold nanostars as a theranostic agent for combined multimodal imaging using CT, PAI and photothermal therapy. Due to the red shift of the LSPR band and the high absorption coefficient, these nanostars could have a better theranostic outcome compared to other shaped nanoparticles. The gold nanostars created significant contrast in both CT and PAI and proved to be an effective therapeutic agent for PTT, due to a successful passive uptake by the tumor cells. Future work should focus on the intravenous delivery of gold nanostars (passively or actively) leading most likely to further improvements in the nanotheranostics field, aiming for imaging and therapy of specific tumor types, which also has the potential to target and treat tumor metastases.

Supplementary Materials: The following are available online at http://www.mdpi.com/2079-4991/10/11/2112/s1, Figure S1: UV-Vis absorption spectroscopy of nanostars. Figure S2: UV-Vis absorption spectroscopy, DLS intensity plots and zeta-potential measurements of nanostars. Figure S3: Intracellular gold concentration using ICP-OES. Figure S4: Temperature profile, fluorescence and bright field microscopy of gold nanostars and irradiated tumor tissue. Figure S5: In vivo BLI before and after nanostar injection. Figure S6: Bright field microscopy images and histology of control and nanostar-injected tumors.

Author Contributions: Conceptualization, A.D., L.L. and U.H.; methodology, A.D., G.V.V., H.J., B.V., E.V., J.J., T.S. (Tim Stakenborg) and T.S. (Tom Struys); data analysis, A.D., T.S. (Tim Stakenborg), H.J. and E.V.; validation, T.S. (Tim Stakenborg), H.J., A.D., L.L. and U.H.; investigation, A.D., H.J., B.V. and T.S. (Tom Struys); resources, J.J., T.S. (Tim Stakenborg), L.L. and U.H.; data curation, A.D., L.L. and U.H.; writing—original draft preparation, A.D., L.L. and U.H.; writing—review and editing, all authors; supervision, G.V.V., H.J., L.L. and U.H.; funding acquisition, L.L. and U.H. All authors have read and agreed to the published version of the manuscript.

Funding: This research was funded by the Flemish foundation for Innovation, Science and Technology for the IWT SBO 'Imagine' (080017) and IWT SBO 'NanoCoMIT' (140061), the European Commission under the 'PANA' project, Call H2020-NMP-2015-two-stage (grant 686009), and by the University of Leuven for program financing PF IMIR (10/017).

Acknowledgments: We are grateful for technical assistance by Jesse Trekker (IMEC, KULeuven) for particle characterization, Marc Jans (Lab of Histology, UHasselt) for ex vivo TEM measurement, Tom Dresselaers (Biomedical MRI, KULeuven) for help with MRI experiments and Joris Deconinck (IMEC) for ICP-OES experiments is highly appreciated. We would also like to thank Visualsonics for their guidance and help with photoacoustic imaging experimentation.

Conflicts of Interest: Jithin Jose is an employee of VisualSonics. All other authors declare no conflict of interest.

References

1. Janib, S.M.; Moses, A.S.; MacKay, J.A. Imaging and drug delivery using theranostic nanoparticles. *Adv. Drug Deliv. Rev.* **2010**, *62*, 1052–1063. [CrossRef]
2. Jain, P.K.; Huang, X.; El-Sayed, I.H.; El-Sayed, M.A. Noble metals on the nanoscale: Optical and photothermal properties and some applications in imaging, sensing, biology, and medicine. *Acc. Chem. Res.* **2008**, *41*, 1578–1586. [CrossRef]
3. Cho, E.C.; Glaus, C.; Chen, J.; Welch, M.J.; Xia, Y. Inorganic nanoparticle-based contrast agents for molecular imaging. *Trends Mol. Med.* **2010**, *16*, 561–573. [CrossRef]
4. Qian, X.; Peng, X.-H.; Ansari, D.O.; Yin-Goen, Q.; Chen, G.Z.; Shin, D.M.; Yang, L.; Young, A.N.; Wang, M.D.; Nie, S. In Vivo tumor targeting and spectroscopic detection with surface-enhanced Raman nanoparticle tags. *Nat. Biotechnol.* **2008**, *26*, 83–90. [CrossRef]
5. D'Hollander, A.; Mathieu, E.; Jans, H.; Velde, G.V.; Stakenborg, T.; van Dorpe, P.; Himmelreich, U.L. Lagae: Development of nanostars as a biocompatible tumor contrast agent: Towards in vivo SERS. *Int. J. Nanomed.* **2016**, *11*, 3703–3714. [CrossRef]
6. Sheng, Y.; De Liao, L.; Thakor, N.V.; Tan, M.C. Nanoparticles for Molecular Imaging. *J. Biomed. Nanotechnol.* **2014**, *10*, 2641–2676. [CrossRef]
7. Jokerst, J.V.; Gambhir, S.S. Molecular imaging with theranostic nanoparticles. *Acc. Chem. Res.* **2011**, *44*, 1050–1060. [CrossRef]
8. Li, C.; Wang, L.V. Photoacoustic tomography and sensing in biomedicine. *Phys. Med. Biol.* **2009**, *54*, R59. [CrossRef]
9. Hu, M.; Chen, J.; Li, Z.-Y.; Au, L.; Hartland, G.V.; Li, X.; Marquez, M.; Xia, Y. Gold nanostructures: Engineering their plasmonic properties for biomedical applications. *Chem. Soc. Rev.* **2006**, *35*, 1084–1094. [CrossRef]
10. Wang, L.V. Multiscale photoacoustic microscopy and computed tomography. *Nat. Photonics* **2010**, *3*, 503–509. [CrossRef]
11. Yang, X.; Stein, E.W.; Ashkenazi, S.; Wang, L.V. Nanoparticles for photoacoustic imaging. *Wiley Interdiscip. Rev. Nanomed. Nanobiotechnol.* **2009**, *1*, 360–368. [CrossRef]
12. Song, C.W. Effect of Local Hyperthermia on Blood Flow and Microenvironment: A Review Effect of Local Hyperthermiaon BloodFlow and Microenvironment. *Cancer Res.* **1984**, *44*, 4721–4730.
13. Van de Broek, B.; Devoogdt, N.; D'Hollander, A.; Gijs, H.-L.; Jans, K.; Lagae, L.; Muyldermans, S.; Maes, G.; Borghs, G. Specific cell targeting with nanobody conjugated branched gold nanoparticles for photothermal therapy. *ACS Nano* **2011**, *5*, 4319–4328. [CrossRef] [PubMed]
14. Bayer, C.L.; Chen, Y.-S.; Kim, S.; Mallidi, S.; Sokolov, K.; Emelianov, S. Multiplex photoacoustic molecular imaging using targeted silica-coated gold nanorods. *Biomed. Opt. Express* **2011**, *2*, 1828–1835. [CrossRef] [PubMed]
15. Joshi, P.P.; Yoon, S.J.; Hardin, W.G.; Emelianov, S.; Sokolov, K.V. Conjugation of antibodies to gold nanorods through Fc portion: Synthesis and molecular specific imaging. *Bioconjug. Chem.* **2013**, *24*, 878–888. [CrossRef] [PubMed]

16. Jokerst, J.V.; Cole, A.J.; Van de Sompel, D.; Gambhir, S.S. Gold nanorods for ovarian cancer detection with photoacoustic imaging and resection guidance via Raman imaging in living mice. *ACS Nano* **2012**, *6*, 10366–10377. [CrossRef]
17. Agarwal, A.; Huang, S.W.; O'Donnell, M.; Day, K.C.; Day, M.; Kotov, N.; Ashkenazi, S. Targeted gold nanorod contrast agent for prostate cancer detection by photoacoustic imaging. *J. Appl. Phys.* **2007**, *102*, 064701. [CrossRef]
18. Li, P.-C.; Wang, C.-R.C.; Shieh, D.-B.; Wei, C.-W.; Liao, C.-K.; Poe, C.; Jhan, S.; Ding, A.-A.; Wu, Y.-N. In Vivo photoacoustic molecular imaging with simultaneous multiple selective targeting using antibody-conjugated gold nanorods. *Opt. Express* **2008**, *16*, 18605–18615. [CrossRef]
19. Liu, Y.; Chang, Z.; Yuan, H.; Fales, A.M.; Vo-Dinh, T. Quintuple-modality (SERS-MRI-CT-TPL-PTT) plasmonic nanoprobe for theranostics. *Nanoscale* **2013**, *5*, 12126–12131. [CrossRef]
20. Kim, C.; Song, H.-M.; Cai, X.; Yao, J.; Wei, A.; Wang, L.V. In Vivo photoacoustic mapping of lymphatic systems with plasmon-resonant nanostars. *J. Mater. Chem.* **2011**, *21*, 2841–2844. [CrossRef]
21. Raghavan, V.; O'Flatharta, C.; Dwyer, R.; Breathnach, A.; Zafar, H.; Dockery, P.; Wheatley, A.; Keogh, I.; Leahy, M.; Olivio, M. Dual plosmonic gold nanostars for photoacoustic imaging and photothermal therapy. *Nanomedicine* **2017**, *12*, 457–471.
22. D'Hollander, A.; Jans, H.; Velde, G.V.; Verstraete, C.; Masa, S.; Devoogdt, N.; Stakenborg, T.; Muyldermans, S.; Lagae, L.; Himmelreich, U. Limiting the protein corona: A successful strategy for in vivo active targeting of anti-HER2 nanobody-functionalized nanostars. *Biomaterials* **2017**, *123*, 15–23. [CrossRef]
23. Yuan, H.; Khoury, C.G.; Wilson, C.M.; Grant, G.A.; Bennett, A.J.; Vo-Dinh, T. In Vivo particle tracking and photothermal ablation using plasmon-resonant gold nanostars. *Nanomedicine* **2012**, *8*, 1355–1363. [CrossRef]
24. Depciuch, J.; Stec, M.; Maximenko, A.; Pawlyta, M.; Baran, J.; Parlinska-Wojtan, M. Control of arms of Au stars size and its Dependent cytotoxicity and photosensitizer effects in photothermal anticancer therapy. *Int. J. Mol. Sci.* **2019**, *20*, 5011. [CrossRef]
25. Chen, H.; Zhang, X.; Dai, S.; Ma, Y.; Cui, S.; Achilefu, S.; Gu, Y. Multifunctional gold nanostar conjugates for tumor imaging and combined photothermal and chemo-therapy. *Theranostics* **2013**, *3*, 633–649.
26. von Maltzahn, G.; Park, J.-H.; Agrawal, A.; Bandaru, N.K.; Das, S.K.; Sailor, M.J.; Bhatia, S.N. Computationally guided photothermal tumor therapy using long-circulating gold nanorod antennas. *Cancer Res.* **2009**, *69*, 3892–3900.
27. Hainfeld, J.F.; Slatkin, D.N.; Focella, T.M.; Smilowitz, H.M. Gold nanoparticles: A new X-ray contrast agent. *Br. J. Radiol.* **2006**, *79*, 248–253. [CrossRef] [PubMed]
28. Xiao, M.; Nyagilo, J.; Arora, V.; Kulkarni, P.; Xu, D.; Sun, X.; Davé, D.P. Gold nanotags for combined multi-colored Raman spectroscopy and x-ray computed tomography. *Nanotechnology* **2010**, *21*, 035101.
29. Reuveni, T.; Motiei, M.; Romman, Z.; Popovtzer, A.; Popovtzer, R. Targeted gold nanoparticles enable molecular CT imaging of cancer: An in vivo study. *Int. J. Nanomed.* **2011**, *6*, 2859–2864.
30. Dickerson, E.B.; Dreaden, E.C.; Huang, X.; El-Sayed, I.H.; Chu, H.; Pushpanketh, S.; McDonald, J.F.; El-Sayed, M.A. Gold nanorod assisted near-infrared plasmonic photothermal therapy (PPTT) of squamous cell carcinoma in mice. *Cancer Lett.* **2008**, *269*, 57–66. [CrossRef]
31. Maier-Hauff, K.; Ulrich, F.; Nestler, D.; Niehoff, H.; Wust, P.; Thiesen, B.; Orawa, H.; Budach, V.; Jordan, A. Efficacy and safety of intratumoral thermotherapy using magnetic iron-oxide nanoparticles combined with external beam radiotherapy on patients with recurrent glioblastoma multiforme. *J. Neurooncol.* **2011**, *103*, 317–324. [CrossRef] [PubMed]
32. Ernsting, M.J.; Murakami, M.; Roy, A.; Li, S.-D. Factors controlling the pharmacokinetics, biodistribution and intratumoral penetration of nanoparticles. *J. Control. Release* **2013**, *172*, 782–794. [CrossRef] [PubMed]
33. Huang, X.; Peng, X.; Wang, Y.; Wang, Y.; Shin, D.M.; El-Sayed, M.A.; Nie, S. A Reexamination of Active and Passive Tumor Targeting by Using Rod-Shaped. *ACS Nano* **2010**, *4*, 5887–5896. [CrossRef]
34. Kunjachan, S.; Pola, R.; Gremse, F.; Theek, B.; Ehling, J.; Moeckel, D.; Hermanns-Sachweh, B.; Pechar, M.; Ulbrich, K.; Hennink, W.E.; et al. Passive versus active tumor targeting using RGD- and NGR-modified polymeric nanomedicines. *Nano Lett.* **2014**, *14*, 972–981. [CrossRef]
35. Borzenkov, M.; Chirico, G.; D'Alfonso, L.; Sironi, L.; Collini, M.; Cabrini, E.; Dacarro, G.; Milanese, C.; Pallavicini, P.; Taglietti, A.; et al. Thermal and chemical stability of thiol bonding on gold nanostars. *Langmuir* **2015**, *31*, 8081–8091. [CrossRef]
36. Weissleder, R. A clearer vision for in vivo imaging. *Nat. Biotechnol.* **2001**, *19*, 316–317. [CrossRef]

37. Nomura, T.; Koreeda, N.; Yamashita, F.; Takakura, Y.; Hashida, M. Effect of particle size and charge on the disposition of lipid carriers after intratumoral injection in to tissue-isolated tumors. *Pharm. Res.* **1998**, *15*, 128–132. [CrossRef]
38. Hao, E.; Bailey, R.C.; Schatz, G.C.; Hupp, J.T.; Li, S. Synthesis and Optical Properties of "Branched" Gold Nanocrystals. *Nano Lett.* **2004**, *4*, 327–330. [CrossRef]
39. Van de Broek, B.; Frederix, F.; Bonroy, K.; Jans, H.; Jans, K.; Borghs, G.; Maes, G. Shape-controlled synthesis of NIR absorbing branched gold nanoparticles and morphology stabilization with alkanethiols. *Nanotechnology* **2011**, *22*, 015601. [CrossRef]
40. Lin, S.-Y.; Tsai, Y.-T.; Chen, C.-C.; Lin, C.-M.; Chen, C. Two-Step Functionalization of Neutral and Positively Charged Thiols onto Citrate-Stabilized Au Nanoparticles. *J. Phys. Chem. B* **2004**, *108*, 2134–2139. [CrossRef]
41. Ketkar-Atre, A.; Struys, T.; Dresselaers, T.; Hodenius, M.; Mannaerts, I.; Ni, Y.; Lambrichts, I.; Van Grunsven, L.A.; De Cuyper, M.; Himmelreich, U. In Vivo hepatocyte MR imaging using lactose functionalized magnetoliposomes. *Biomaterials* **2014**, *35*, 1015–1024. [CrossRef]
42. Gijsbers, R.; Ronen, K.; Vets, S.; Malani, N.; De Rijck, J.; McNeely, M.; Bushman, F.D.; Debyser, Z. LEDGF hybrids efficiently retarget lentiviral integration into heterochromatin. *Mol. Ther.* **2010**, *18*, 552–560. [CrossRef]
43. Vande Velde, G.; Kucharíková, S.; Schrevens, S.; Himmelreich, U.; Van Dijck, P. Towards non-invasive monitoring of pathogen-host interactions during Candida albicans biofilm formation using in vivo bioluminescence. *Cell. Microbiol.* **2013**, *16*, 115–130. [CrossRef] [PubMed]
44. Soenen, S.J.; De Meyer, S.F.; Dresselaers, T.; Vande Velde, G.; Pareyn, I.M.; Braeckmans, K.; De Cuyper, M.; Himmelreich, U.; Vanhoorelbeke, K.I. MRI assessment of blood outgrowth endothelial cell homing using cationic magnetoliposomes. *Biomaterials* **2011**, *32*, 4140–4150. [CrossRef]
45. Trekker, J.; Leten, C.; Struys, T.; Lazenka, V.V.; Argibay, B.; Micholt, L.; Lambrichts, I.; Van Roy, W.; Lagae, L.; Himmelreich, U. Sensitive in vivo cell detection using size-optimized superparamagnetic nanoparticles. *Biomaterials* **2014**, *35*, 1627–1635. [CrossRef]
46. Thiesen, B.; Jordan, A. Clinical applications of magnetic nanoparticles for hyperthermia. *Int. J. Hyperth.* **2008**, *24*, 467–474. [CrossRef] [PubMed]
47. Verma, A.; Stellacci, F. Effect of surface properties on nanoparticle-cell interactions. *Small* **2010**, *6*, 12–21. [CrossRef]
48. Nel, A.E.; Mädler, L.; Velegol, D.; Xia, T.; Hoek, E.M.V.; Somasundaran, P.; Klaessig, F.; Castranova, V.; Thompson, M. Understanding biophysicochemical interactions at the nano-bio interface. *Nat. Mater.* **2009**, *8*, 543–557. [CrossRef]
49. Huang, X.; El-Sayed, I.H.; Qian, W.; El-Sayed, M.A. Cancer cell imaging and photothermal therapy in the near-infrared region by using gold nanorods. *J. Am. Chem. Soc.* **2006**, *128*, 2115–2120. [CrossRef] [PubMed]
50. Hirsch, L.R.; Stafford, R.J.; Bankson, J.A.; Sershen, S.R.; Rivera, B.; Price, R.E.; Hazle, J.D.; Halas, N.J.; West, J.L. Nanoshell-mediated near-infrared thermal therapy of tumors under magnetic resonance guidance. *Proc. Natl. Acad. Sci. USA* **2003**, *100*, 13549–13554. [CrossRef]
51. Chen, J.; Wang, D.; Xi, J.; Au, L.; Siekkinen, A.; Warsen, A.; Li, Z.-Y.; Zhang, H.; Xia, Y.; Li, X. Immuno gold nanocages with tailored optical properties for targeted photothermal destruction of cancer cells. *Nano Lett.* **2007**, *7*, 1318–1322. [CrossRef] [PubMed]
52. Bai, Y.-Y.; Zheng, S.; Zhang, L.; Xia, K.; Gao, X.; Li, Z.-H.; Li, C.; He, N.; Ju, S. Non-Invasively Evaluating Therapeutic Response of Nanorod-Mediated Photothermal Therapy on Tumor Angiogenesis. *J. Biomed. Nanotechnol.* **2014**, *10*, 3351–3360. [CrossRef]
53. Singh, R.; Nalwa, H.S. Medical Applications of Nanoparticles in Biological Imaging, Cell Labeling, Antimicrobial Agents, and Anticancer Nanodrugs. *J. Biomed. Nanotechnol.* **2011**, *7*, 489–503.
54. Chen, Y.-S.; Frey, W.; Kim, S.; Kruizinga, P.; Homan, K.; Emelianov, S. Silica-coated gold nanorods as photoacoustic signal nanoamplifiers. *Nano Lett.* **2011**, *11*, 348–354. [CrossRef] [PubMed]
55. Gómez, M.A.G.; Belderbos, S.; Vilar, S.Y.; Redondo, Y.P.; Cleeren, F.; Bormans, G.; Deroose, C.M.; Gsell, W.; Himmelreich, U.; Rivas, J. Development of superparamagnetic nanoparticles coated with polyacrylic acid and aluminum hydroxide as an efficient contrast agent for multimode imaging. *Nanomaterials* **2019**, *9*, 1626.
56. Belderbos, S.; González-Gómez, M.A.; Cleeren, F.; Wouters, J.; Piñeiro, Y.; Deroose, C.M.; Coosemans, A.; Gsell, W.; Bormans, G.; Rivas, J.; et al. Simultaneous in vivo PET/MRI using fluorine-18 labeled Fe_3O_4@Al(OH)$_3$ nanoparticles: Comparison of nanoparticle and nanoparticle-labeled stem cell distribution. *Eur. J. Nucl. Med. Mol. Imag. Res.* **2020**, *10*, 73.

57. Huang, X.; Jain, P.K.; El-Sayed, I.H.; El-Sayed, M.A. Plasmonic photothermal therapy (PPTT) using gold nanoparticles. *Lasers Med. Sci.* **2008**, *23*, 217–228.
58. American National Standards Institute. *American National Standard for Safe Use of Lasers*; Laser Institute of America: Orlando, FL, USA, 2007.
59. You, J.; Zhang, G.; Chun, L. Exceptionally High Payload of doxorubicin in hollow gold nanospheres for near-infrared light-triggered drug release. *ACS Nano* **2010**, *4*, 1033–1041. [CrossRef]
60. Cho, S.K.; Emoto, K.; Su, L.-J.; Yang, X.; Flaig, T.W.; Park, W. Functionalized Gold Nanorods for Thermal Ablation Treatment of Bladder Cancer. *J. Biomed. Nanotechnol.* **2014**, *10*, 1267–1276.

Publisher's Note: MDPI stays neutral with regard to jurisdictional claims in published maps and institutional affiliations.

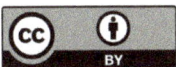 © 2020 by the authors. Licensee MDPI, Basel, Switzerland. This article is an open access article distributed under the terms and conditions of the Creative Commons Attribution (CC BY) license (http://creativecommons.org/licenses/by/4.0/).

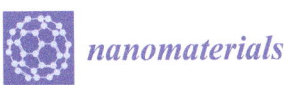

Communication

Magnetoliposomes Incorporated in Peptide-Based Hydrogels: Towards Development of Magnetolipogels

Sérgio R. S. Veloso [1], Raquel G. D. Andrade [1], Beatriz C. Ribeiro [1], André V. F. Fernandes [1], A. Rita O. Rodrigues [1], J. A. Martins [2], Paula M. T. Ferreira [2], Paulo J. G. Coutinho [1] and Elisabete M. S. Castanheira [1,*]

1. Centre of Physics (CFUM), University of Minho, Campus de Gualtar, 4710-057 Braga, Portugal; sergioveloso96@gmail.com (S.R.S.V.); raquel.gau@gmail.com (R.G.D.A.); pg37976@alunos.uminho.pt (B.C.R.); pg38822@alunos.uminho.pt (A.V.F.F.); ritarodrigues@fisica.uminho.pt (A.R.O.R.); pcoutinho@fisica.uminho.pt (P.J.G.C.)
2. Centre of Chemistry (CQUM), University of Minho, Campus de Gualtar, 4710-057 Braga, Portugal; jmartins@quimica.uminho.pt (J.A.M.); pmf@quimica.uminho.pt (P.M.T.F.)
* Correspondence: ecoutinho@fisica.uminho.pt; Tel.: +351-253-604-320

Received: 11 July 2020; Accepted: 27 August 2020; Published: 29 August 2020

Abstract: A major problem with magnetogels is the encapsulation of hydrophobic drugs. Magnetoliposomes not only provide these domains but also improve drug stability and avert the aggregation of the magnetic nanoparticles. In this work, two magnetoliposome architectures, solid and aqueous, were combined with supramolecular peptide-based hydrogels, which are of biomedical interest owing to their biocompatibility, easy tunability, and wide array of applications. This proof-of-concept was carried out through combination of magnetoliposomes (loaded with the model drug curcumin and the lipid probe Nile Red) with the hydrogels prior to pH triggered gelation, and fluorescence spectroscopy was used to assess the dynamics of the encapsulated molecules. These systems allow for the encapsulation of a wider array of drugs. Further, the local environment of the encapsulated molecules after gelation is unaffected by the used magnetoliposome architecture. This system design is promising for future developments on drug delivery as it provides a means to independently modify the components and adapt and optimize the design according to the required conditions.

Keywords: magnetoliposomes; hydrogels; magnetolipogels; self-assembly; fluorescence; Förster resonance energy transfer

1. Introduction

Nanomedicine has provided many tools to reduce invasiveness and many acute and chronic side effects associated with chemotherapy while improving patients' quality of life [1]. The development of new nanosystems has clearly contributed to these advancements. A recent strategy is the combination of liposomes and hydrogels, that might provide better drug formulation stability and drug administration routes [2]. A more robust soft material is attained with the incorporation of magnetic nanoparticles. Such can be obtained, for example, through the combination with magnetoliposomes [3,4]. A different concept is the separate embedding of both nanoparticles and liposomes in the hydrogel matrix [3]. These strategies offer a means of developing multifunctional smart materials that can host membrane-bound enzymes/glycolipids, besides the targeting with a magnetic field gradient and the stimuli-responsiveness through the application of an alternating magnetic field [5]. The on-demand release from stimuli-responsive liposomes enables the use of more potent drugs [6], while the hydrogel immobilizes the components and provides the local environment required to support cell growth [7]. Further, all the components can be independently adjusted, which allows, for example, for the evaluation of which hydrogel is better fitted for a certain composite and application [2]. However, the majority of the developed magnetic liposome-hydrogel complexes have been restricted to the use of polymeric matrices, mainly alginate, and no attention has been given to supramolecular hydrogels.

The self-assembly of supramolecular hydrogelators is driven towards a kinetically trapped intertwined fibrillar structure encompassing solvent pocket microdomains through the cooperative effect of different non-covalent intermolecular interactions [8,9]. The variety of non-covalent intermolecular interactions, both of liposomes and supramolecular hydrogels, might lead to complex behavior and less straightforward magnetic liposome-hydrogel formulation. Hereby, in this work three different hydrogelators (Figure 1A) known to be adequate for drug delivery [10,11] were evaluated as carrying matrixes of magnetoliposomes. Two different types of magnetoliposomes were developed, solid and aqueous, which are schematically represented in Figure 1B. The strategy employed to evaluate this proof-of-concept consisted in preparing the magnetoliposomes, confirming their formation and posterior gelation of the supramolecular hydrogel under the presence of a dilute solution of magnetoliposomes, thus ensuring that the dominant observed effects are exerted by the hydrogel network (or hydrogelator) over the magnetoliposomes membrane (Figure 1C).

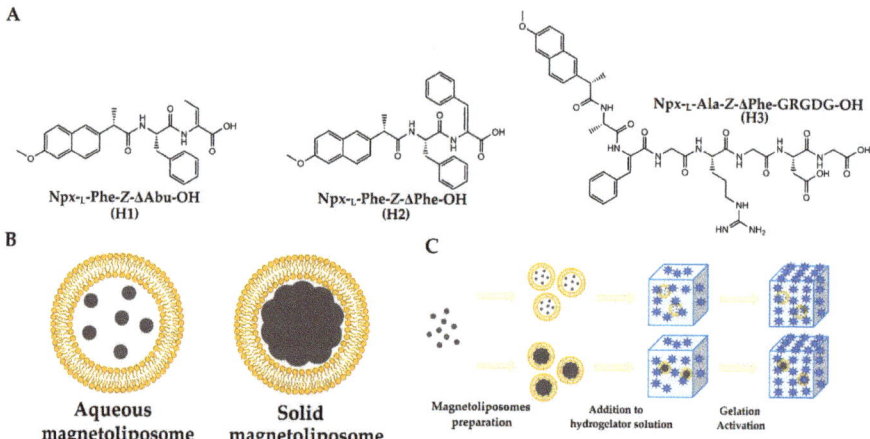

Figure 1. (**A**) Hydrogelator molecules used in this work. Legend: Npx: naproxen; Phe: phenylalanine; Ala: alanine; G: glycine; R: arginine; D: aspartate; ΔAbu: dehydroaminobutyric acid; ΔPhe: Dehydrophenylalanine. (**B**) Schematic representation of the aqueous and solid magnetoliposomes. (**C**) Schematic representation of the strategy used for the development of the supramolecular magnetic liposome-hydrogel complexes.

2. Materials and Methods

All the solutions were prepared using spectroscopic grade solvents and ultrapure water of Milli-Q grade (MilliporeSigma, St. Louis, MO, USA).

2.1. Preparation of Manganese Ferrite Nanoparticles

Manganese ferrite nanoparticles were synthesized by the co-precipitation method, as described in previous works [8,9,12]. Briefly, a mixture of 500 µL of $MnSO_4 \cdot H_2O$ 0.5 M aqueous solution and 500 µL of $FeCl_3 \cdot 6H_2O$ 1 M was prepared and added, drop by drop, to a 4 mL NaOH 3.4 M aqueous solution at 90 °C, with constant magnetic stirring. After 2 h, nanoparticles purification was carried out by repeated centrifugations, dispersion in deionized water, and drying at 100 °C. The stability of nanoparticles dispersions in PBS medium (pH = 7.0) (with the same nanoparticle concentration used in the preparation of magnetoliposomes) was evaluated by following the UV/Visible absorption for one hour.

2.2. Preparation of Magnetoliposomes

For magnetoliposomes preparation, the lipid 1,2-dipalmitoyl-*sn*-glycero-3-phosphatidylcholine (DPPC) (from Sigma-Aldrich, St. Louis, MO, USA), was used. The aqueous magnetoliposomes (AMLs) were developed through the ethanolic injection method [12,13]. Briefly, a 10 mM lipid solution in ethanol was injected, under vigorous agitation, to an aqueous dispersion of magnetic nanoparticles, above the melting transition temperature of DPPC (41 °C) [14]. The mixture was washed with water and purified by magnetic decantation to remove non-encapsulated nanoparticles, as previously reported [15].

Solid magnetoliposomes (SMLs) were developed by a reported method for manganese ferrite nanoparticles [12]. First, 10 µl of a nanoparticle solution (0.02 mg/mL), previously dispersed by sonication at 180 W for one minute, was added to 3 mL of chloroform. After brief sonication and under vigorous agitation, 150 µL of a DPPC 20 mM methanolic solution was added to form the first lipid layer. The first layer-coated nanoparticles were thoroughly washed with water to remove the lipids not attached to the nanoparticles' surfaces. The nanoparticles were dispersed in 3 mL of water and, under strong agitation, 150 µL of DPPC 20 mM methanolic solution was injected to form the second layer. The resulting solid magnetoliposomes were then washed and purified with ultrapure water by magnetic decantation [12,13].

Curcumin and Nile Red were loaded in AMLs through the co-injection method, while in SMLs they were incorporated through the injection of an ethanolic solution upon formation of the second lipid layer [12,13].

2.3. Spectroscopic and Characterization Measurements

Fluorescence measurements were carried out using a Fluorolog 3 spectrofluorimeter (HORIBA Jobin Yvon IBH Ltd., Glasgow, UK), having double monochromators in excitation and emission, a temperature-controlled cuvette holder and Glan-Thompson polarizers. All fluorescence spectra were corrected for the instrumental response of the system. Absorption spectra were recorded in a Shimadzu UV-3600 Plus UV–Vis–NIR spectrophotometer (Shimadzu Corporation, Kyoto, Japan).

The mean hydrodynamic diameter, zeta potential and polydispersity index of aqueous and solid magnetoliposomes (lipid concentration: 1 mM) were measured using a NANO ZS Malvern Zetasizer (Malvern Panalytical Ltd., Malvern, UK) dynamic light scattering (DLS) equipment at 25 °C, using a He-Ne laser of λ = 632.8 nm and a detector angle of 173°. Five independent measurements were performed for each sample. High-resolution transmission electron microscopy (HR-TEM) images were obtained in a JEOL JEM 2010F microscope operating at 200 kV (JEOL Ltd., Tokyo, Japan) at C.A.C.T.I (Centro de Apoio Científico e Tecnolóxico á Investigación), Vigo, Spain. A conventional PAN'alytical X'Pert PRO (Malvern Panalytical Ltd., Malvern, UK) diffractometer was used for X-ray diffraction (XRD) analyses, operating with CuK_α radiation, in a Bragg–Brentano configuration. Magnetic measurements were performed at room temperature in a Superconducting Quantum Interference Device (SQUID) magnetometer (Quantum Design Inc., San Diego, CA, USA), using applied magnetic fields up to 5.5 T.

2.4. Incorporation of the Magnetoliposomes in Hydrogels

All the used hydrogels were prepared for a final concentration of 0.4 wt% (4 mg/mL). Hereby, 1.2 mg of each compound was added to 150 µL of an aqueous solution 2 *v/v*% NaOH 1M and dissolved through agitation. After the compound dissolution, the hydrogel solution was taken out of the water bath and mixed with 150 µL of the prepared magnetoliposomes solution. To each mixture, 0.4 wt% of glucono-δ-lactone (GdL) was added under agitation, which led to a final pH of ~6–7. The mixture was deployed in a fluorescence microcuvette and left cooling at room temperature, until the hydrogel was formed.

The curcumin release from hydrogels and magnetolipogels (300 µL) loaded with 0.05 mM curcumin was also assessed. The gels containing curcumin were prepared and left stabilizing overnight in Amicon® Ultra-0.5 mL centrifugal filters (MilliporeSigma, St. Louis, MO, USA) with 0.1 µm pore size. Then, pH = 7.0 buffer (800 µL) was added, and the filter tube was immersed and left standing at room temperature. Aliquots were taken after 7 h and fluorescence was measured to determine the concentration. The assays were performed in triplicate.

3. Results and Discussion

Manganese ferrite nanoparticles were used for magnetoliposomes development considering their well described synthesis and preparation in the literature [8,9,12,13,16]. The XRD profile is displayed in Figure 2A and confirms the synthesis of a pure crystalline phase of manganese ferrite, as well as presenting all its characteristic peaks, marked by their indices, corresponding to CIF file 2,300,618 (space group Fd-3m:2). The use of a degree of inversion of 0.60, $O_{x,y,z}$ = 0.257 and the micro-absorption correction resulted into a good fitting quality with R_f = 3.27 and χ^2 = 1.19, which is in agreement with the results of manganese ferrite nanoparticles obtained by co-precipitation reported in [16]. An average crystallite size estimate of 12.1 nm was obtained, which is also in close agreement with the sizes reported by Rodrigues et al. of 16.5 nm [12], and 13.3 nm [16], obtained by the same method used in this work. The magnetization hysteresis loop (Figure 2B) displays a saturation magnetization of 55 emu/g, a coercivity of 38.83 Oe, and an M_r/M_s ratio of 0.06, which indicates that the nanoparticles present a superparamagnetic behavior at room temperature, and is in agreement with previously reported values for manganese ferrite nanoparticles obtained through co-precipitation [12,13]. From the TEM measurements (Figure 2C) an average size of 24.2 ± 6.9 nm was obtained, which is also in accordance with previously reported values [9,12].

The stability of nanoparticle dispersions, with and without sonication, was also evaluated. From the UV–Visible absorption measurements over time (Figure S1 in Supplementary Material), it can be observed that nanoparticle dispersions are stable for one hour, with no significant sedimentation and the behavior is similar for nanoparticles with and without sonication. The zeta potential value of the magnetic nanoparticles is negative (−14.1 ± 1.2 mV), preventing their aggregation, as previously reported [9].

The nanoparticles were incorporated into aqueous magnetoliposomes (AMLs), which consist in nanoparticles embedded in the aqueous compartment enclosed by the lipid bilayer, obtained through ethanolic injection of lipids in a well dispersed nanoparticle aqueous solution. The solid magnetoliposomes (SMLs) were obtained as described in previous works, covering a cluster of magnetic nanoparticles with a lipid membrane through a layer-by-layer method [12,13,16]. A Scanning Electron Microscopy (SEM) image of SMLs is exhibited in Figure S2 of the Supplementary Materials. UV–Visible absorbance variations overtime are very low for both AMLs and SMLs (Figure S1 in Supplementary Material), indicating negligible short-time sedimentation. Dynamic light scattering (DLS) results are displayed in Table 1. The aqueous magnetoliposomes of DPPC with entrapped manganese ferrite nanoparticles have diameters of 113.5 ± 10 nm, which is in accordance with those previously reported [12], while DPPC solid magnetoliposomes with sizes around 160 nm were also formerly observed [13]. After one week of storage, the magnetoliposomes remain stable in terms of diameter and surface charge, as inferred from hydrodynamic size and zeta potential values (Table 1), proving the long-term stability of the nanosystems.

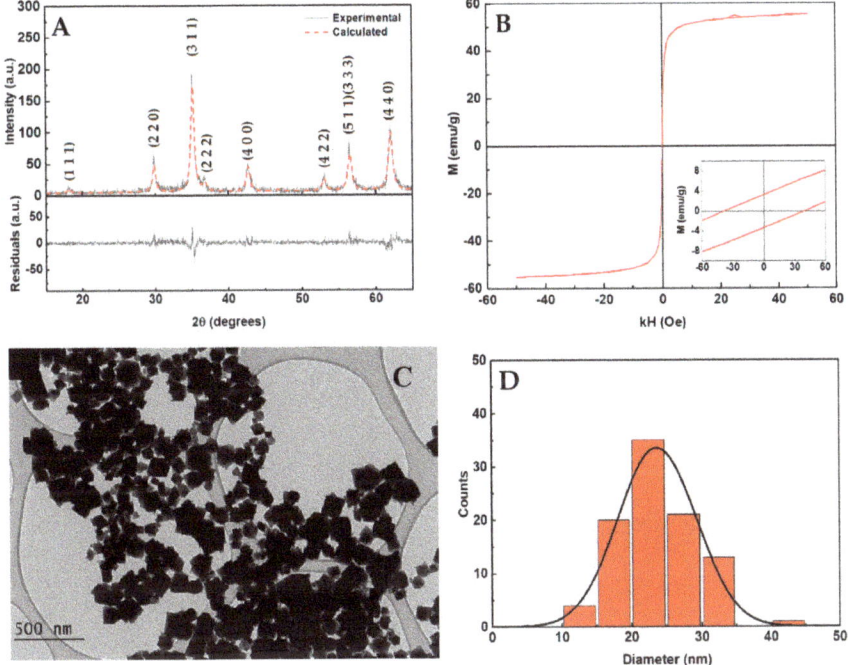

Figure 2. (**A**) X-ray diffraction pattern of manganese ferrite nanoparticles. Grey line: experimental pattern; red line: fitted pattern. (**B**) Magnetization hysteresis loop of the manganese ferrite nanoparticles at room temperature (T = 300 K). Inset: Enlargement of the loop in the low field region. (**C**) Transmission electron microscopy image of the synthesized manganese ferrite nanoparticles. (**D**) Size histogram of the synthesized nanoparticles obtained from TEM.

Table 1. Hydrodynamic size, zeta potential and polydispersity index values of aqueous and solid magnetoliposomes based on manganese ferrite nanoparticles, immediately after preparation and after one week of storage (SD: standard deviation; PDI: Polydispersity index).

	Size ± SD (nm)		PDI ± SD		Zeta Potential ± SD (mV)	
	After Preparation	1 Week After	After Preparation	1 Week After	After Preparation	1 Week After
AMLs	113.5 ± 10	98.7 ± 17	0.23 ± 0.04	0.22 ± 0.08	−15.3 ± 2	−16.1 ± 4
SMLs	156.3 ± 16	132.2 ± 21	0.25 ± 0.03	0.21 ± 0.07	−21.4 ± 4	−19.7 ± 3

The encapsulation efficiency of magnetic nanoparticles in AMLs was determined from the spectrophotometric determination of iron (III) content, through the formation of a phenylfluorone complex sensitized with Triton X-100 (Merck-Sigma, St. Louis, MO, USA), as previously described for other ferrites [15,17]. An encapsulation efficiency of EE(%) ± SD(%) = 74.5 ± 3.5 (from a triplicate assay) compares well with the value previously reported for calcium ferrite (around 70%) [15], being higher than the estimated for iron oxide nanoparticles (EE = 47% ± 15%) [17].

Curcumin was incorporated in AMLs as a model of hydrophobic drugs. Curcumin is a natural polyphenolic compound with various biological activity properties, such as anti-inflammatory, antioxidant and anti-cancer properties, and has been reported to be well encapsulated in magnetoliposomes by Cardoso et al. [14]. Curcumin has also been described to be fluorescent in different polar and non-polar solvents [11,14], and its photophysical behavior is associated with the enol-keto tautomerism of the diketo group, the properties of which are mostly dictated by the enol form (since it is the predominant form in most solvents) [18]. Yet, it has been demonstrated that water stabilizes the diketo form through the formation of stable complexes [19,20]. Fluorescence emission in polar medium is characterized by a large red shift, band enlargement and loss of vibrational structure [14,21].

The fluorescence emission spectrum of curcumin in magnetoliposomes is displayed in Figure 3A and compared with the emission in DPPC liposomes. The observed quenching effect in magnetoliposomes may result from an electronic energy transfer to the nanoparticles, as they absorb in a wide energy range [9], as well as due to the heavy-atoms effect, which enhances the efficiency of the intersystem crossing process [22]. The strong fluorescence emission of curcumin is an indication of its presence in the lipid membranes, as it is very weakly emissive in water [11,14]. It has also been reported that curcumin inserts into lipid bilayers in a hydrated environment [23]. Further, the same emission maximum in both liposomes and AMLs (503 nm) indicates that nanoparticles do not affect the membranes.

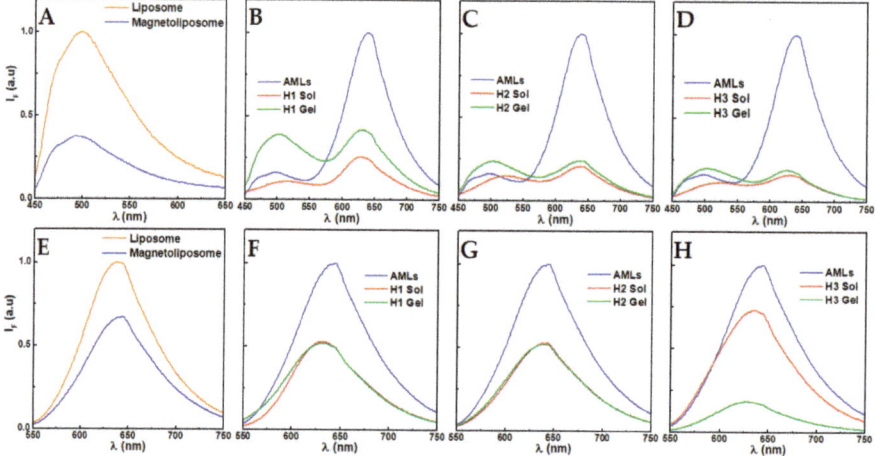

Figure 3. (**A**) Fluorescence emission spectra of curcumin in aqueous magnetoliposomes and liposomes of DPPC (λ_{exc} = 420 nm, [curcumin] = 1 × 10^{-6} M). (**B–D**) Fluorescence emission spectra of aqueous magnetoliposomes of DPPC containing curcumin and Nile Red (λ_{exc} = 420 nm, [curcumin] = 1 × 10^{-6} M, [Nile Red] = 1 × 10^{-6} M) in solution of AMLs (AMLs), in a pre-gelation solution (pH ≈ 12, Sol) and hydrogel state (Gel) of the compounds H1, H2 and H3. (**E**) Fluorescence emission spectra of Nile Red in aqueous magnetoliposomes and liposomes of DPPC (λ_{exc} = 520 nm, [Nile Red] = 1 × 10^{-6} M) and (**F–H**) in solution of AMLs, in a pre-gelation solution (pH ≈ 12, Sol) and hydrogel state (Gel) of the compounds H1, H2 and H3.

The hydrogelators used in this work were chosen based on their molecular differences. The hydrogelators H1 and H2 differ in the presence of the aromatic ring in the dehydroamino acid moiety, displaying fibers with an average width of 10 nm (pH ≈ 6) and 14 nm (pH ≈ 8), respectively [10]. The hydrogelator H3 is a linear pentapeptide, with both negative and positive charged groups, and self-assembles into thicker fibers, of 23 nm (pH ≈ 6) width [11].

The lipophilic and solvatochromic probe Nile Red was also included in the aqueous magnetoliposomes to assess any major change in the membrane stability. Its emission blueshifts with the reduction in polarity and is negligible in water, but intensely emits in non-polar environments [24–27]. Furthermore, the fluorescence risetime is sensitive to viscosity, owing to an activation barrier required for the formation of a twisted intramolecular charge transfer state (TICT) [28,29].

The Förster resonance energy transfer (FRET) process between curcumin (energy donor) and Nile Red (energy acceptor) that has been used in different works as the spectral overlap between the Nile Red absorption and curcumin fluorescence is significant [9,11,30]. Figure 3B–D display the FRET process between curcumin and Nile Red, as evidenced by the strong fluorescence emission of Nile Red, while exciting the curcumin dye (λ_{exc} = 420 nm). Before mixing the AMLs and hydrogelator solutions, curcumin displays its maximum around 500 nm, indicating an environment similar to chloroform [11], and characteristic of its incorporation in DPPC membranes (i.e., Nile Red co-encapsulation did not affect curcumin microenvironment) [31], while the Nile Red maximum is at ~638 nm. After the addition of the AMLs to the hydrogelator solutions, and before inducing gelation (2 v/v% NaOH 1 M), a decrease in the fluorescence emission and FRET efficiency is clearly observed. Besides the scattering associated with the presence of the hydrogelator micelles, such can also be a consequence of the deprotonation of curcumin. The formation of spherical or worm-like micelles by N-capped dipeptides at high pH has been reported by Cardoso et al. [32]. The curcumin deprotonation is further evidenced by the red-shift to λ ~ 530 nm. The high pH induces the deprotonation of the three hydroxyl groups of curcumin (pK_a values are 8.38, 9.88 and 10.51) and, consequently, its solubility is slightly improved [33,34]. Furthermore, while the neutral form is preferentially located in the hydrophobic phase, at basic pH it accumulates in the surface of the lipid bilayer [35]. Thus, while some curcumin is expected to remain in the inner cavity or membrane of the AMLs, some might relocate to the outer surface when the pH is increased, which leads to its release towards the aqueous phase and a larger distance from Nile Red. This potential outcome is also evidenced by the reduction in FRET efficiency upon pH decrease when the gel state is attained. In this state, a blue-shift of curcumin fluorescence emission is associated with its protonation and relocation or adsorption to hydrophobic cavities, both in the hydrogel matrix and hydrophobic phase of the liposomes, as suggested by both the reduced FRET efficiency and a slight increase in Nile Red emission.

The direct excitation of Nile Red provides further information on the membrane dynamics. Overall, a decrease in fluorescence intensity is observed in the concentrated hydrogelator solutions containing the AMLs. The decrease is similar in the gels of compounds H1 and H2, which remains unchanged after gelation, while the H3 gel displays a strong fluorescence decrease after gelation. Furthermore, in the gels H1 and H3, a slight blue-shift occurs from 640 nm to 631 nm and 628 nm, respectively. This suggests an interaction between the dehydrodipeptides and the AMLs membrane, leading to a higher hydrophobicity of the membrane region where Nile Red is localized. The stronger decrease in the H3 gel after gelation can be associated with the larger diameter of the fibers increasing the inner filter effect, considering that the solution changed from a translucid solution to a turbid gel.

The scheme in Figure 4 summarizes the observed behavior and the expected mechanism of encapsulation of hydrophobic drugs (e.g., curcumin, and Nile Red as a lipid probe), upon the preparation of magnetic lipogels bearing AMLs, though it is pointed out that curcumin becomes more hydrophilic at high pH [20]. Further, considering the AMLs membranes as mimetics of the biological membranes, it is expected that the in situ gelation of supramolecular gels will not lead to membrane disruption. Nonetheless, it cannot be ignored that the observed partition may result from a potential membrane perturbation by the encapsulated molecules. Curcumin is known to modify the lipid bilayer properties, such as bilayer stiffness, thickness, elasticity moduli, and curvature [36–38]. For instance, it was reported to decrease the membrane stiffness in the absence of cholesterol [39]. The increase in membrane flaccidity might also favor the redistribution of both curcumin and Nile Red between the membranes and the hydrogel fibers.

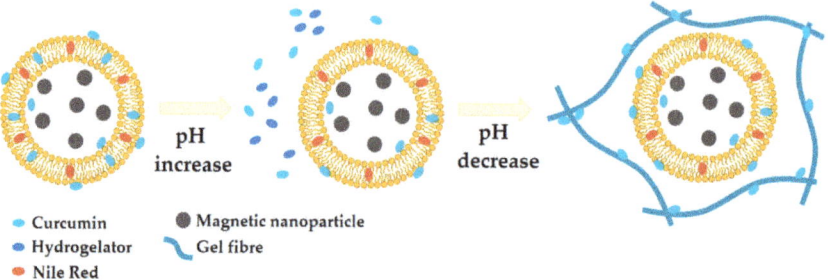

Figure 4. Scheme of the proposed process of incorporation of AMLs containing curcumin (that becomes more water soluble at high pH) and Nile Red in a supramolecular dehydrodipeptide hydrogel activated through GdL-induced slow pH decrease. As the pH is increased, some of the curcumin molecules are dissolved and, once the pH is decreased, it adsorbs and relocates to the hydrophobic cavities of both the hydrogel fibers and AMLs membranes.

Solid magnetoliposomes (SMLs) were prepared with the co-encapsulation of both curcumin and Nile Red, where the former was demonstrated in previous works to be finely encapsulated in these systems [14,21]. The fluorescence emission spectra of the aqueous solution of SMLs, after addition to the concentrated basic hydrogelator solutions and gelation, are displayed in Figure 5. The strong fluorescence quenching is a consequence of the proximity of both molecules to the cluster of magnetic nanoparticles. Both curcumin (maximum around 500 nm—i.e., similar microenvironment to liposomes and AMLs) and Nile Red (at 631 nm) fluorescence emission maxima are associated with their location in the membranes. Upon addition of the SMLs to the concentrated hydrogelator solution, a strong enhancement of curcumin emission is observed, which might be a result of the localization of curcumin from the SMLs membranes towards the hydrogelator micelles that display a more hydrated environment, as suggested by the red-shift (H1: 521 nm; H2: 524 nm; H3: 526 nm). Upon pH decrease, similar to what was described in the AMLs incorporation, curcumin accumulated either in the hydrogel fibers or in the SMLs membranes.

In H1 (510 nm) and H3 (511 nm) systems, curcumin is localized in an environment with a polarity similar to chloroform, while in H2 (521 nm) the emission is only slightly blue-shifted, indicative of an environment with a polarity similar to acetonitrile [11]. The fluorescence quenching of H1 suggests its proximity to the SMLs. The localization of curcumin in a hydrophobic environment has been reported in a previous work with magnetic gels [9]. Yet, the presence of membranes favored the location of curcumin to a more hydrophobic environment in the H3 gel, as opposed to the previously reported environment similar to acetonitrile in the magnetic gels. Further, after gelation, an increase around 630 nm is observed, which is associated with the occurrence of FRET between curcumin and Nile Red.

Similar to curcumin behavior, Nile Red fluorescence emission is unquenched and some changes in the environment occur upon mixture with the hydrogelator solutions (Figure 5). In the H1 gel, a redshift to 620 nm was obtained, while in H2 and H3 the maximum wavelength remained centered around 631 nm. The enhancement of Nile Red and curcumin fluorescence after gelation suggests that more hydrophobic cavities are made available to accommodate the molecules from the previously highly saturated magnetoliposomes—i.e., the curcumin and Nile Red release from the SMLs towards the hydrogels was favored.

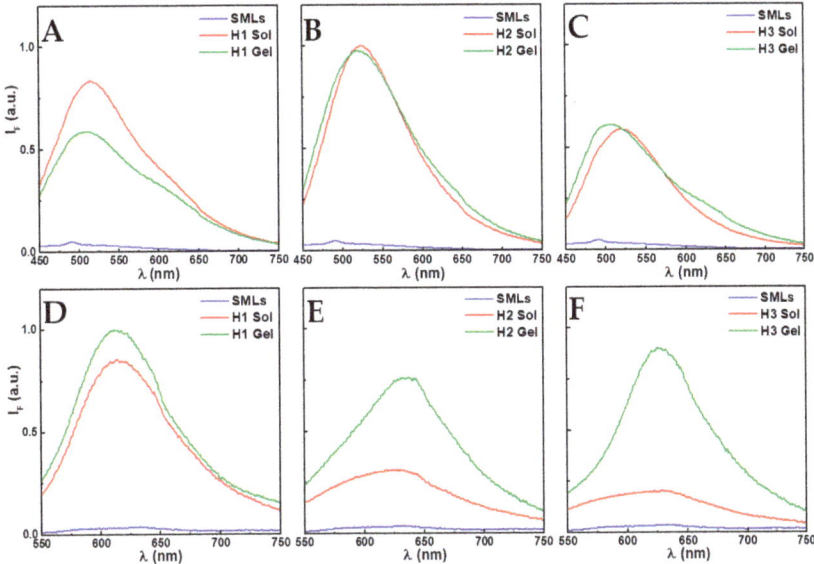

Figure 5. (**A–C**) Fluorescence emission spectra of curcumin and Nile Red in solid magnetoliposomes of DPPC (λ_{exc} = 420 nm, [curcumin] = 2 × 10^{-6} M, [Nile Red] = 2 × 10^{-6} M) in solution of SMLs (SMLs), in a pre-gelation solution (pH ≈ 12, Sol) and hydrogel state (Gel) of the compounds H1, H2 and H3. (**D–F**) Fluorescence emission spectra of Nile Red (λ_{exc} = 520 nm, [Nile Red] = 2 × 10^{-6} M) in solid magnetoliposomes in an aqueous solution (SMLs), in a pre-gelation solution (pH ≈ 12, Sol) and hydrogel state (Gel) of the compounds H1, H2 and H3.

The scheme included in Figure 6 summarizes the discussed process and the expected behavior of hydrophobic drugs (curcumin is sensitive to pH variations) encapsulated in SMLs upon the preparation of supramolecular magnetic lipogels through slow pH decrease by GdL. The observed behavior provides a means to ensure that no premature release of the administered drugs from the SMLs occurs, as they are retained by the hydrogel matrix or micelles. Moreover, it makes the co-delivery or incorporation of larger amounts of hydrophobic drugs possible, as the hydrogel matrix develops hydrophobic cavities capable of accommodating the excessive amount from the saturated SMLs. For instance, a lower percentage of curcumin release after 7 h of incubation with pH = 7.0 buffer was obtained in both magnetolipogels (Figure S3 in Supplementary Material). These results point out that the presence of magnetoliposomes in the hydrogel matrix can reduce the release of curcumin.

Steady-state fluorescence anisotropy measurements were carried out to evaluate the effect of the hydrogel on the microviscosity of Nile Red local environment. Table 2 displays the obtained values for both AMLs and SMLs before and after gelation through the pH trigger.

Table 2. Steady-state fluorescence anisotropy (r) values of Nile Red for gels with the incorporated AMLs or SMLs. Values in neat magnetoliposomes (MLs) are shown for comparison.

System	MLs	H1 Sol	H1 Gel	H2 Sol	H2 Gel	H3 Sol	H3 Gel
AMLs	0.20	0.17	0.26	0.27	0.28	0.22	0.26
SMLs	0.06	0.22	0.24	0.16	0.25	0.15	0.26

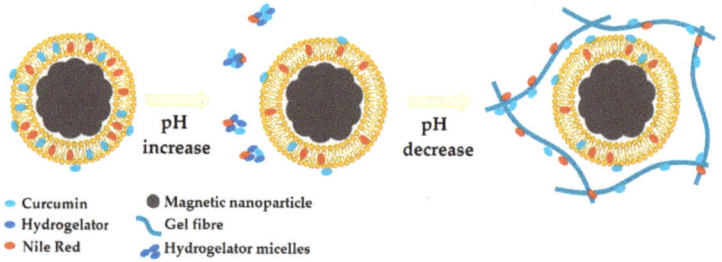

Figure 6. Scheme of the proposed process of incorporation of SMLs containing curcumin (that becomes more water soluble at high pH) and Nile Red in a supramolecular dehydrodipeptide hydrogel activated through GdL-induced slow pH decrease. Upon combination of the SMLs with the basic pH hydrogelator solution, both curcumin and Nile Red are released and accumulate in the hydrophobic cavities of the hydrogelator micelles. As the pH is lowered, both molecules can accumulate in both the hydrophobic cavities of the hydrogel matrix and the SMLs membrane.

In all systems, the fluorescence anisotropy (and, thus, the local microviscosity) increases when compared to the neat magnetoliposomes (Table 2). Further, the anisotropy converges to close values in both systems, which suggests that similar interactions are established between the hydrogel matrix and both magnetoliposome architectures. This convergence on microviscosity offers the possibility of exploring different systems to optimize therapeutic strategies, as the distribution and behavior of amphipathic and hydrophobic drugs are expected to be similar to the distribution of the molecules here discussed. For instance, the presence of AMLs allows for the delivery of hydrophilic drugs in the aqueous cavity, besides the delivery of hydrophobic drugs in the membrane and amphipathic drugs distributed along both the hydrogel matrix and the magnetoliposome, while the incorporation of SMLs allows for the delivery of hydrophobic and amphipathic drugs at higher concentrations than the single use of SMLs, without severely affecting the magnetization (and, consequently, hyperthermia) of the magnetic nanoparticles, as the amount of diamagnetic mass is reduced.

4. Conclusions

In this work, the incorporation of solid and aqueous magnetoliposomes in supramolecular hydrogels was assessed in three different gels through a pH trigger. It was demonstrated that, upon the incorporation of the magnetoliposomes, the encapsulated molecules distributed to a similar environment independently of the magnetoliposome architecture. Further, magnetoliposomes can be saturated with the required drug, as the hydrogel displays hydrophobic cavities that accommodate the excessive drug amount, which can be explored as a way to avert the premature release of the administered drug. This system design approach provides a useful strategy to increase the array of drugs that can be encapsulated compared to magnetic gels and magnetoliposomes alone. Concerning the discussed findings in this communication, research is being carried out to assess the influence of the different magnetic lipogel architectures on drug delivery control and tunability, as well as to evaluate its impact on hyperthermia capability.

Supplementary Materials: The following are available online at http://www.mdpi.com/2079-4991/10/9/1702/s1, Figure S1: Stability of Nanoparticles and Magnetoliposomes Dispersions, Figure S2: SEM Image of Solid Magnetoliposomes, Figure S3: Curcumin Release Assay.

Author Contributions: Conceptualization, S.R.S.V. and E.M.S.C.; methodology, P.M.T.F., J.A.M., P.J.G.C. and E.M.S.C., validation, A.R.O.R., J.A.M., P.M.T.F. and E.M.S.C.; formal analysis, S.R.S.V., R.G.D.A., A.R.O.R. and E.M.S.C.; investigation, S.R.S.V., R.G.D.A., B.C.R. and A.V.F.F.; writing—original draft preparation, S.R.S.V. and E.M.S.C.; writing—review and editing, P.J.G.C. and E.M.S.C.; supervision, P.M.T.F. and E.M.S.C.; project administration, P.J.G.C. and P.M.T.F. All authors have read and approved the final version of the manuscript.

Funding: This work was supported by the Portuguese Foundation for Science and Technology (FCT) in the framework of the Strategic Funding of CF-UM-UP (UIDB/04650/2020) and CQUM (UIDB/00686/2020). FCT, FEDER, PORTUGAL2020 and COMPETE2020 are also acknowledged for funding under research projects PTDC/QUI-QFI/28020/2017 (POCI-01-0145-FEDER-028020) and PTDC/QUI-QOR/29015/2017 (POCI-01-0145-FEDER-029015). S.R.S.V. acknowledges FCT for a PhD grant (SFRH/BD/144017/2019) and MAP-Fis PhD program for support.

Conflicts of Interest: The authors declare no conflict of interest.

References

1. Gogoi, M.; Jaiswal, M.K.; Banerjee, R.; Bahadur, D. Magnetic liposomes and hydrogels towards cancer therapy. In *Magnetic Nanoparticles: From Fabrication to Clinical Applications*, 1st ed.; Thanh, N.T.K., Ed.; CRC Press: Boca Raton, FL, USA, 2012; pp. 479–487.
2. Grijalvo, S.; Mayr, J.; Eritja, R.; Díaz, D. Biodegradable liposome-encapsulated hydrogels for biomedical applications: A marriage of convenience. *Biomater. Sci.* **2016**, *4*, 555–574. [CrossRef]
3. Hanuš, J.; Ullrich, M.; Dohnal, J.; Singh, M.; Štěpánek, F. Remotely controlled diffusion from magnetic liposome microgels. *Langmuir* **2013**, *29*, 4381–4387. [CrossRef] [PubMed]
4. De Cogan, F.; Booth, A.; Gough, J.; Webb, S. Spatially controlled apoptosis induced by released nickel(ii) within a magnetically responsive nanostructured biomaterial. *Soft Matter* **2013**, *9*, 2245. [CrossRef]
5. Mart, R.; Liem, K.; Webb, S. Magnetically-controlled release from hydrogel-supported vesicle assemblies. *Chem. Commun.* **2009**, *17*, 2287. [CrossRef] [PubMed]
6. Reimhult, E. Nanoparticle-triggered release from lipid membrane vesicles. *New Biotechnol.* **2015**, *32*, 665–672. [CrossRef]
7. Leng, F.; Gough, J.; Webb, S. Enhancing cell culture in magnetic vesicle gels. *MRS Proc.* **2010**, *1272*. [CrossRef]
8. Veloso, S.R.S.; Martins, J.A.; Hilliou, L.; Amorim, C.O.; Amaral, V.S.; Almeida, B.G.; Jervis, P.J.; Moreira, R.; Pereira, D.M.; Coutinho, P.J.G.; et al. Dehydropeptide-based plasmonic magnetogels: A supramolecular composite nanosystem for multimodal cancer therapy. *J. Mater. Chem. B* **2020**, *8*, 45–64. [CrossRef]
9. Veloso, S.R.S.; Magalhães, C.A.B.; Rodrigues, A.R.O.; Vilaça, H.; Queiroz, M.J.R.P.; Martins, J.A.; Coutinho, P.J.G.; Ferreira, P.M.T.; Castanheira, E.M.S. Novel dehydropeptide-based magnetogels containing manganese ferrite nanoparticles as antitumor drug nanocarriers. *Phys. Chem. Chem. Phys.* **2019**, *21*, 10377–10390. [CrossRef] [PubMed]
10. Vilaça, H.; Pereira, G.; Castro, T.G.; Hermenegildo, B.F.; Shi, J.; Faria, T.Q.; Micaêlo, N.; Brito, R.M.N.; Xu, B.; Castanheira, E.M.S.; et al. New self-assembled supramolecular hydrogels based on dehydropeptides. *J. Mater. Chem. B* **2015**, *3*, 6355–6367. [CrossRef]
11. Vilaça, H.; Castro, T.; Costa, F.M.G.; Melle-Franco, M.; Hilliou, L.; Hamley, I.W.; Castanheira, E.M.S.; Martins, J.A.; Ferreira, P.M.T. Self-assembled RGD dehydropeptide hydrogels for drug delivery applications. *J. Mater. Chem. B* **2017**, *5*, 8607–8617. [CrossRef]
12. Rodrigues, A.R.O.; Ramos, J.M.F.; Gomes, I.T.; Almeida, B.G.; Araújo, J.P.; Queiroz, M.J.R.P.; Coutinho, P.J.G.; Castanheira, E.M.S. Magnetoliposomes based on manganese ferrite nanoparticles as nanocarriers for antitumor drugs. *RSC Adv.* **2016**, *6*, 17302–17313. [CrossRef]
13. Rodrigues, A.R.O.; Almeida, B.G.; Rodrigues, J.M.; Queiroz, M.J.R.P.; Calhelha, R.C.; Ferreira, I.C.F.R.; Pires, A.; Pereira, A.M.; Araújo, J.P.; Coutinho, P.J.G.; et al. Magnetoliposomes as carriers for promising antitumor thieno[3,2-b]pyridin-7-arylamines: Photophysical and biological studies. *RSC Adv.* **2017**, *7*, 15352–15361. [CrossRef]
14. Cardoso, B.D.; Rio, I.S.R.; Rodrigues, A.R.O.; Fernandes, F.C.T.; Almeida, B.G.; Pires, A.; Pereira, A.M.; Araújo, J.P.; Castanheira, E.M.S.; Coutinho, P.J.G. Magnetoliposomes containing magnesium ferrite nanoparticles as nanocarriers for the model drug curcumin. *R. Soc. Open Sci.* **2018**, *5*, 181017. [CrossRef] [PubMed]
15. Pereira, D.S.M.; Cardoso, B.D.; Rodrigues, A.R.O.; Amorim, C.O.; Amaral, V.S.; Almeida, B.G.; Queiroz, M.J.R.P.; Martinho, O.; Baltazar, F.; Calhelha, R.C.; et al. Magnetoliposomes containing calcium ferrite nanoparticles for applications in breast cancer therapy. *Pharmaceutics* **2019**, *11*, 477. [CrossRef] [PubMed]

16. Rodrigues, A.R.O.; Matos, J.O.G.; Dias, A.M.N.; Almeida, B.G.; Pires, A.; Pereira, A.M.; Araújo, J.P.; Queiroz, M.J.R.P.; Castanheira, E.M.S.; Coutinho, P.J.G. Development of multifunctional liposomes containing magnetic/plasmonic $MnFe_2O_4$/Au core/shell nanoparticles. *Pharmaceutics* **2018**, *11*, 10. [CrossRef] [PubMed]
17. Rodrigues, A.R.O.; Mendes, P.M.F.; Silva, P.M.L.; Machado, V.A.; Almeida, B.G.; Araújo, J.P.; Queiroz, M.J.R.P.; Castanheira, E.M.S.; Coutinho, P.J.G. Solid and aqueous magnetoliposomes as nanocarriers for a new potential drug active against breast cancer. *Colloids Surf. B* **2017**, *158*, 460–468. [CrossRef]
18. Khopde, S.; Indira Priyadarsini, K.; Palit, D.; Mukherjee, T. Effect of solvent on the excited-state photophysical properties of curcumin. *Photochem. Photobiol.* **2007**, *72*, 625–631. [CrossRef]
19. Manolova, Y.; Deneva, V.; Antonov, L.; Drakalska, E.; Momekova, D.; Lambov, N. The effect of the water on the curcumin tautomerism: A quantitative approach. *Spectrochim. Acta Part A* **2014**, *132*, 815–820. [CrossRef]
20. Priyadarsini, K. The chemistry of curcumin: From extraction to therapeutic agent. *Molecules* **2014**, *19*, 20091–20112. [CrossRef]
21. Cardoso, B.D.; Rodrigues, A.R.O.; Almeida, B.G.; Amorim, C.O.; Amaral, V.S.; Castanheira, E.M.S.; Coutinho, P.J.G. Stealth Magnetoliposomes based on calcium-substituted magnesium ferrite nanoparticles for curcumin transport and release. *Int. J. Mol. Sci.* **2020**, *21*, 3641. [CrossRef]
22. Valeur, B. *Molecular fluorescence—Principles and Applications*, 1st ed.; Wiley-VCH: Weinheim, Germany, 2001.
23. Alsop, R.; Dhaliwal, A.; Rheinstädter, M. Curcumin protects membranes through a carpet or insertion model depending on hydration. *Langmuir* **2017**, *33*, 8516–8524. [CrossRef] [PubMed]
24. Greenspan, P.; Fowler, S. Spectrofluorometric studies of the lipid probe Nile Red. *J. Lipid Res.* **1985**, *26*, 781–789. [PubMed]
25. Krishnamoorthy, I.G. Probing the link between proton transport and water content in lipid membranes. *J. Phys. Chem. B* **2001**, *105*, 1484–1488.
26. Coutinho, P.J.G.; Castanheira, E.M.S.; Rei, M.C.; Oliveira, M.E.C.D.R. Nile Red and DCM fluorescence anisotropy studies in $C_{12}E_7$/DPPC mixed systems. *J. Phys. Chem. B* **2002**, *106*, 12841–12846. [CrossRef]
27. Hungerford, G.; Castanheira, E.M.S.; Real Oliveira, M.E.C.D.; Miguel, M.G.; Burrows, H. Monitoring ternary systems of $C_{12}E_5$/water/tetradecane via the fluorescence of solvato-chromic probes. *J. Phys. Chem. B* **2002**, *106*, 4061–4069. [CrossRef]
28. Swain, J.; Mishra, A. Nile red fluorescence for quantitative monitoring of micropolarity and microviscosity of pluronic F127 in aqueous media. *Photochem. Photobiol. Sci.* **2016**, *15*, 1400–1407. [CrossRef]
29. Swain, J.; Mishra, J.; Ghosh, G.; Mishra, A. Quantification of micropolarity and microviscosity of aggregation and salt-induced gelation of sodium deoxycholate (NaDC) using Nile red fluorescence. *Photochem. Photobiol. Sci.* **2019**, *18*, 2773–2781. [CrossRef]
30. Saxena, S.; Pradeep, A.; Jayakannan, M. Enzyme-responsive theranostic FRET probe based on l-aspartic amphiphilic polyester nanoassemblies for intracellular bioimaging in cancer cells. *ACS Appl. Biol. Mater.* **2019**, *2*, 5245–5262. [CrossRef]
31. El Khoury, E.; Patra, D. Length of hydrocarbon chain influences location of curcumin in liposomes: Curcumin as a molecular probe to study ethanol induced interdigitation of liposomes. *J. Photochem. Photobiol. B Biol.* **2016**, *158*, 49–54. [CrossRef]
32. Cardoso, A.; Mears, L.; Cattoz, B.; Griffiths, P.; Schweins, R.; Adams, D. Linking micellar structures to hydrogelation for salt-triggered dipeptide gelators. *Soft Matter* **2016**, *12*, 3612–3621. [CrossRef]
33. Moussa, Z.; Chebl, M.; Patra, D. Fluorescence of tautomeric forms of curcumin in different pH and biosurfactant rhamnolipids systems: Application towards on-off ratiometric fluorescence temperature sensing. *J. Photochem. Photobiol. B Biol.* **2017**, *173*, 307–317. [CrossRef] [PubMed]
34. Lee, W.; Loo, C.; Bebawy, M.; Luk, F.; Mason, R.; Rohanizadeh, R. Curcumin and its derivatives: Their application in neuropharmacology and neuroscience in the 21st century. *Curr. Neuropharmacol.* **2013**, *11*, 338–378. [CrossRef] [PubMed]
35. Priyadarsini, K. Photophysics, photochemistry and photobiology of curcumin: Studies from organic solutions, bio-mimetics and living cells. *J. Photochem. Photobiol. C Photochem. Rev.* **2009**, *10*, 81–95. [CrossRef]
36. Ingolfsson, H.I.; Koeppe, R.E.; Andersen, O.S. Curcumin is a modulator of bilayer material properties. *Biochemistry* **2007**, *46*, 10384–10391. [CrossRef]
37. Hung, W.-C.; Chen, F.-Y.; Lee, C.-C.; Sun, Y.; Lee, M.-T.; Huang, H.W. Membrane-thinning effect of curcumin. *Biophys. J.* **2008**, *94*, 4331–4338. [CrossRef] [PubMed]

38. Barry, J.; Fritz, M.; Brender, J.R.; Smith, P.E.; Lee, D.K.; Ramamoorthy, A. Determining the effects of lipophilic drugs on membrane structure by solid-state NMR spectroscopy: The case of the antioxidant curcumin. *J. Am. Chem. Soc.* **2009**, *131*, 4490–4498. [CrossRef]
39. Leite, N.B.; Martins, D.B.; Fazani, V.E.; Vieira, M.R.; Dos Santos Cabrera, M.P. Cholesterol modulates curcumin partitioning and membrane effects. *Biochim. Biophys. Acta Biomembr.* **2018**, *1860*, 2320–2328. [CrossRef]

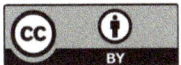

© 2020 by the authors. Licensee MDPI, Basel, Switzerland. This article is an open access article distributed under the terms and conditions of the Creative Commons Attribution (CC BY) license (http://creativecommons.org/licenses/by/4.0/).

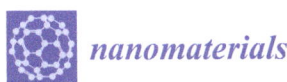

Article

Effects of Two Kinds of Iron Nanoparticles as Reactive Oxygen Species Inducer and Scavenger on the Transcriptomic Profiles of Two Human Leukemia Cells with Different Stemness

Tao Luo, Jinliang Gao, Na Lin and Jinke Wang *

State Key Laboratory of Bioelectronics, Southeast University, Nanjing 210096, China; luotao@seu.edu.cn (T.L.); jlgao880325@163.com (J.G.); yywymail@126.com (N.L.)
* Correspondence: wangjinke@seu.edu.cn

Received: 22 August 2020; Accepted: 28 September 2020; Published: 30 September 2020

Abstract: Leukemia is a common and lethal disease. In recent years, iron-based nanomedicines have been developed as a new ferroptosis inducer to leukemia. However, the cytotoxicity of iron nanoparticles to leukemia cells at the transcriptomic level remains unclear. This study investigated the effects of two kinds of iron nanoparticles, 2,3-Dimercaptosuccinic acid (DMSA)-coated Fe_3O_4 nanoparticles (FeNPs) as a reactive oxygen species (ROS) inducer and Prussian blue nanoparticles (PBNPs) as an ROS scavenger, on the transcriptomic profiles of two leukemia cells (KG1a and HL60) by RNA-Seq. As a result, 470 and 1690 differentially expressed genes (DEGs) were identified in the FeNP-treated HL60 and KG1a cells, respectively, and 2008 and 2504 DEGs were found in the PBNP-treated HL60 and KG1a cells, respectively. Among them, 14 common upregulated and 4 common downregulated DEGs were found, these genes were representative genes that play key roles in lipid metabolism (GBA and ABCA1), iron metabolism (FTL, DNM1, and TRFC), antioxidation (NQO1, GCLM, and SLC7A11), vesicle traffic (MCTP2, DNM1, STX3, and BIN2), and innate immune response (TLR6, ADGRG3, and DDX24). The gene ontology revealed that the mineral absorption pathway was significantly regulated by PBNPs in two cells, whereas the lipid metabolism and HIF-1 signaling pathways were significantly regulated by FeNPs in two cells. This study established the gene signatures of two kinds of nanoparticles in two leukemia cells, which revealed the main biological processes regulated by the two kinds of iron nanoparticles. These data shed new insights into the cytotoxicity of iron nanoparticles that differently regulate ROS in leukemia cells with variant stemness.

Keywords: leukemia; iron nanoparticles; RNA-Seq; cytotoxicity

---

1. Introduction

Leukemia, especially acute myeloid leukemia (AML), is a lethal disease characterized by the accumulation of DNA-damaged immature myeloid precursors [1]. Only around 20% of adult cases are expected to survive past 5 years after diagnosis, and it is a leading cause of cancer death in young adults [2]. Although conventional chemotherapy is highly offensive against the bulk of leukemic cells, chemotherapy resistance in the refractory of AML is still a serious and common problem [2,3]. Thus, the development of new and specific therapeutic strategies that can overcome conventional drug resistance is still in demand.

In recent years, the development of nanomedicines as ferroptosis inducer in cancer cells has become a new promising approach to leukemia [4–6]. Ferroptosis is an iron-dependent, unique type of cell death due to excessive accumulation of toxic lipid reactive oxygen species (ROS) [7]. Ferroptosis can be stimulated by the GPX4 inhibitors (erastin, sorafenib, altretamine, etc.) and reagents that cause cellar iron overload (FeCl$_2$, salinomycin, and hemoglobin), which leads to fueled ROS production and inhibition of tumor growth [8–11]. However, these compounds have already been challenged by the same resistance problem as that of traditional cancer drugs [12]. Iron nanoparticles are an emerging new ferroptosis inducer because it has the ability to increase iron levels and ROS. For example, a Fe$_3$O$_4$-based nanoparticle fabricated through self-assembly mechanism can generate ROS and can induce intracellular oxidative stress [6]. A Fenton-reaction-accelerable magnetic nanoparticle can be prepared to simultaneously enhance the local concentrations of Fe^{2+}, Fe^{3+}, and H$_2$O$_2$ to kill cancer cells [13]. Recently, a nanoparticle iron supplement, ferumoxytol, was found to have an antileukemia effect in vitro and in vivo in leukemia cells with a low level of ferroportin (FPN) by inducing ferroptosis [14].

However, as a new promising ferroptosis inducer, iron nanoparticle-induced cytotoxicity to leukemia cells at the transcriptomic level still remains unclear. This study thus investigated the effects of two kinds of iron nanoparticles, 2,3-Dimercaptosuccinic acid (DMSA)-coated Fe$_3$O$_4$ nanoparticles (FeNPs) and Prussian blue nanoparticles (PBNPs), on transcriptomic profiles of two leukemia cells (KG1a and HL60) by RNA-Seq. FeNPs can induce ROS generation through Fenton reactions, while PBNPs is an effective ROS scavenger with peroxidase (POD)-, catalase (CAT)-, and superoxide dismutase (SOD)-like activities [15]. HL60 is an AML cell with promyelocytic differentiation, while KG1a is a stem-like AML cell line that is resistant to chemotherapy and double negative T cell (DNT)-mediated cytotoxicity [2]. For example, fucoidan, a natural component of seaweeds with immunomodulatory and antitumor effects, was investigated in human AML cells. It can significantly increase apoptosis in HL60, but undifferentiated KG1a was resistant to the tumor inhibitory function of fucoidan [16].

2. Materials and Methods

2.1. Cell Lines and Reagents

The human acute myelogenous leukemia (AML) cell KG1a and the human acute promyelocytic leukemia (APL) cell HL60 were obtained by the China Center for Type Culture Collection (Shanghai, China). Dulbecco Modified Eagle Medium (DMEM) and fetal bovine serum (FBS) were acquired from Invitrogen Gibco (Carlsbad, CA, USA). Double antibiotics (penicillin plus streptomycin) were purchased from Beyotime Biotech (Shanghai, China). Counting Kit-8 and phosphate buffer saline were purchased from Sangon Biotech Co., Ltd. (Shanghai, China). The FeNPs and PBNPs were supplied by the Biological and Biomedical Nanotechnology Group of the State Key Lab of Bioelectronics, Southeast University (Nanjing, China) [15,17]. The size and potential of nanoparticles were measured again with a Malvern Particle size analyzer, Zetasizer Nano (Malvern Instruments, Malvern, UK).

2.2. Cell Viability, Iron Content, and ROS Measurement

The cell viability was measured with the CCK-8 assay (Cell Counting Kit-8; BS350B, Biosharp). The iron content was measured using a colorimetric assay. Briefly, cells were counted and then suspended in 5 M HCl. After incubation at 60 °C for 4 h, the cells were centrifuged and the supernatant was transferred. The supernatant was added with the freshly prepared detection reagent (0.08% K$_2$S$_2$O$_8$, 8% KSCN, and 3.6% HCl) and incubated at room temperature for 10 min. The absorbance at 490 nm was measured using an absorption reader (BioTek, Winooski, VT, USA). The iron content was determined according to a standard curve generated with FeCl$_3$ solution. The iron content was calculated as micrograms per cell. ROS was measured by the flow cytometer method. In brief, the cells were stained with 2′,7′-dichlorodihydrofluorescein diacetate (DCFH-DA) using Reactive Oxygen Species Assay Kit (Beyotime, Nantong, China) according to the manufacturer's instructions. ROS changes indicated by fluorescence shift was analyzed on a CytoFLEX LX Flow Cytometer (Beckman, Brea, CA, USA).

2.3. Cell Culture and Processing

The KG1a and HL60 cells were cultured in DMEM supplemented with 10% fetal bovine serum (FBS), 100 units/mL penicillin, and 100 µg/mL streptomycin. All iron nanoparticles were filtered through a 0.22-µm membrane. The KG1a and HL60 cells were exposed to 50 µg/mL of PBNPs or FeNPs for 72 h. To detect cell viability, the KG1a and HL60 cells were seeded in 96-well microplate (10^4 cells/well). After incubation with iron nanoparticles for 72 h, 10 µL of CCK-8 solution was dropped to each well and incubated in cell culture incubator for 2 h. Finally, the absorbance at 450 nm was measured.

2.4. RNA-Seq Analysis

RNA sequencing (RNA-Seq) was conducted in collaboration with the Decode Genomics (Nanjing, China). Two biological replicate cell treatments were performed for each cell and nanoparticle. Totally, 12 RNA samples (two independent RNA samples of blank HL60 and KG1a, FeNP-treated HL60 and KG1a, and PBNP-treated HL60 and KG1a) were used to perform RNA-Seq analysis. The total RNA was isolated using the TRIzol® Reagent Kit (Thermo Fisher Scientific, Waltham, MA, USA) following the manufacturer's instructions. The degradation and contamination status of RNA were analyzed by 1% agarose gel electrophoresis, and the RNA purity was evaluated by Nanodrop 2000 according to the ratio of OD_{260nm}/OD_{280nm} (around 1.8–2.2). The RNA concentration was accurately quantified by Qubit ($\geq$500 ng/µL), and the insert size of the library was assessed with Agilent 2100 to judge RNA integrity. After the library quality control was qualified, Illumina sequencing was performed using a paired end 150 bp (paired end, PE150) strategy. To ensure the quality of information analysis and clean reads, the raw reads obtained by sequencing were filtered to remove dirty reads that contained adapters, excessive N ($\geq$10%, N: bases information cannot be determined), and a large number of low-quality bases. Subsequent analysis was based on clean reads. The HISAT2 software was used to align clean reads with the reference genome.

2.5. GO and KEGG Analysis of Differentially Expressed Genes (DEGs)

Based on the HISAT2 results, HTSeq software was used to calculate the expression level of each mRNA gene in samples. The differentially expressed genes (DEGs, $p < 0.05$) were identified using the DESeq R package and are displayed in the Supplementary Materials File S1. DEGs with a false discovery rate (FDR) < 0.05 and absolute value of fold change $\geq$ 1.5 were used to perform the Gene Ontology (GO) and Kyoto Encyclopedia of Genes and Genomes (KEGG) analyses. The GO functional enrichment of DEGs was analyzed using Metascape software [18]. The signaling pathway annotations was mapped in the KEGG database. The key KEGG signaling pathway was draught by the Pathview [19].

2.6. RT-qPCR Analysis

The total RNA was extracted from cells using TRIzol Regent (Invitrogen, CA, USA) and purified by a treatment of DNase I (Thermo Fisher Scientific, Waltham, MA, USA). The high-quality RNA samples were used to generate the complimentary DNA (cDNA) using the PrimeScript™ RT reagent Kit (TaKaRa, Japan). The PCR primers were designed by NCBI Primer BLAST (https://www.ncbi.nlm.nih.gov/tools/primer-blast/) and synthesized by Genscript Biotechnology (Nanjing, China) (Table S1). The Real-Time quantitative PCR (RT-qPCR) detection was performed using the SYBR Green master mix (Thermo Fisher Scientific, Waltham, MA, USA) according to manufacturer's instruction. Each PCR detection was performed with three biological and technical replicates. The gene expression values were normalized to an internal control (glyceraldehyde-3-phosphate dehydrogenase, GAPDH). The relative gene expression level was calculated as the relative quantification (RQ) using the $2^{-\Delta\Delta Ct}$ method.

2.7. Statistical Analysis

All detection results were presented as mean ± standard deviation (SD). All data analysis were performed and plotted by the GraphPad Prism 8, in which the statistical significance was detected by the Student's *t*-test. *p*-values < 0.05 were considered statistically significant.

3. Results and Discussion

3.1. Characterization of Nanoparticles and Their Effects on Cell Viability, Iron Content, and ROS

Two kinds of iron nanoparticles were used in this study: one was PBNPs, and the other was FeNPs. The former was in blue color, and the latter was in brown color (Figure 1A,B). The PBNPs were at sizes of 152 nm and had potentials of −1.94, while the FeNPs were at sizes of 20 nm and had potentials of −20.9 (Figure 1A,B). The CCK8 assay showed that only the cell viability of HL60 was significantly reduced by FeNP treatment (Figure 1C). The cell viability of KG1a was not significantly reduced by all treatments (Figure 1C), indicating that KG1a was more resistant to iron nanoparticles. The intracellular iron content measurement revealed that the treatment of both iron nanoparticles significantly increased the intracellular iron content of two cell lines; however, the FeNP treatment more significantly increased the intracellular iron content of two cell lines (Figure 1D). Additionally, treatment of both iron nanoparticles more significantly increased the intracellular iron content of HL60 than KG1a (Figure 1D). The qPCR detection of the expressions of two leukemia stem cell (LSC) marker genes, CD34 and CD38, indicated that CD34 was only highly expressed in KG1a and that CD38 was expressed in two cells at low levels (Figure 1E). This demonstrated that KG1a had higher stemness than HL60. When treated with two kinds of nanoparticles, CD34 expression in KG1a was slightly downregulated by FeNPs but upregulated by PBNPs, whereas CD38 was significantly downregulated by PBNPs in two cells and by FeNPs in HL60 (Figure 1E). The ROS measurement indicated that the FeNP treatment increased the ROS level in both cell lines but that the PBNP treatment decreased the ROS level in the two cell lines (Figure 1F). Altogether, these data indicated the difference between two leukemia and two kinds of iron nanoparticles.

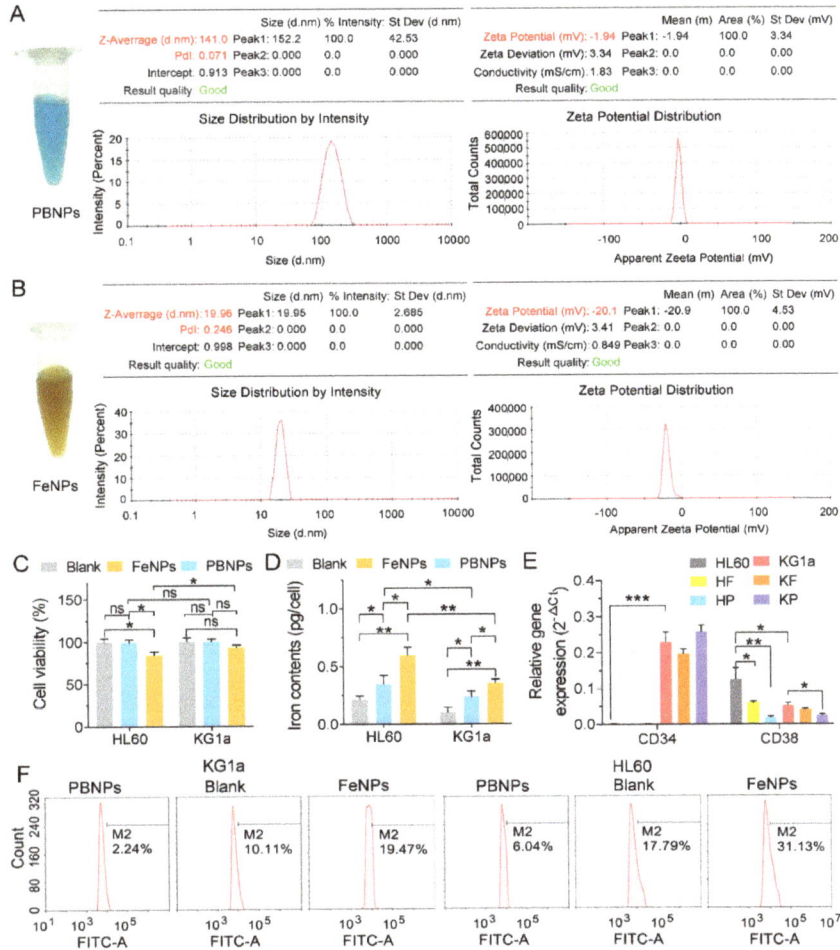

Figure 1. The characterization of two kinds of iron nanoparticles and their effects on KG1a and HL60: (**A**,**B**) hydrated particle size and zeta potential of Prussian blue nanoparticles (PBNPs) (**A**) and Fe_3O_4 nanoparticles (FeNPs) (**B**), (**C**) cell viability of the PBNP- and FeNP-treated HL60 and KG1a cells, (**D**) cellular iron contents of the PBNP- and FeNP-treated HL60 and KG1a cells, and (**E**) QPCR detection of CD34 and CD38 expression in two cells. HF, FeNP-treated HL60; HP, PBNP-treated HL60; KF, FeNP-treated KG1a; KP, PBNP-treated KG1a. ns, no significance; *, $p < 0.05$; **, $p < 0.01$; ***, $p < 0.001$. (**F**) ROS levels of the PBNP- and FeNP-treated HL60 and KG1a cells.

3.2. RNA-Seq and de Novo Transcriptome Assembly

To investigate the transcriptome modulation that occurred during exposure to iron nanoparticles, the KG1a and HL60 cells were treated with 50 μg/mL of FeNPs and PBNPs for 72 h, respectively. To obtain reliable global gene expression profiles, RNA-Seq was performed with as many as 12 samples, which consisted of two biological replicates of each treatment. Following the removal of adapters and low-quality reads, total mapped reads, unique mapped reads, and multiple reads were summarized and are presented in Table S2. The statistics of distribution of clean reads in different regions of the genome are shown in Figure S1. After alignment with the reference genome, the statistical results of mRNA peak insert size distribution were shown in Table S3. The correlation analysis of expression levels among samples and the density map of gene expression level of all samples were further calculated to demonstrate reliability of the experiment and rationality of the sample selection (Figures S2 and S3).

3.3. Identification of DEGs

To discover the effects of iron nanoparticles (FeNPs and PBNPs) on the gene expression profiles of HL60 and KG1a cells, a large number of DEGs ($p < 0.05$) were identified using the FPKM (Fragments Per Kilobase of transcript per Million mapped reads) method [20]. Totally, there were 470 (260 upregulated and 210 downregulated) and 1690 (720 upregulated and 970 downregulated) DEGs in the FeNP-treated HL60 and KG1a cells, respectively, and 2008 (1015 upregulated and 993 downregulated) and 2504 (986 upregulated and 1518 downregulated) DEGs in the PBNP-treated HL60 and KG1a cells, respectively. The detailed information of these DEGs is shown in File S1 (Supplementary Materials). The results showed that KG1a had more DEGs than HL60 after the treatment of iron nanoparticles. Especially, after the treatment of FeNPs, KG1a had 3.59 times more DEGs than HL60. These data indicated that KG1a that had higher stemness than HL60 could resist iron nanoparticle-induced ferroptosis by regulating much more genes than HL60, especially encountering FeNPs, a ROS inducer. This is in agreement with the observation that FeNPs induced the significant decrease of cell viability of HL60 but had no significant effect on cell viability of KG1a (Figure 1C).

A four-way Venn analysis displayed the numbers of unique and common DEGs in two cells treated by two kinds of nanoparticles (Figure 2A). It was found that each cell had many unique DEGs under the treatment of two kinds of nanoparticles. Besides those unique DEGs, two kinds of nanoparticles induced some common DEGs in two cells. In comparison, two different nanoparticles induced more common DEGs in a same cell line whereas a same nanoparticle induced less common DEGs in two different cells. There were limited numbers of common DEGs in two cells treated by two kinds of nanoparticles. To provide more detailed information on common DEGs, the common genes (fold change >1.5) regulated by two kinds of nanoparticles in a same cell (Figure 2B) and a nanoparticle in two cells (Figure 2C) were identified. Totally, 52 and 42 genes were commonly regulated by two kinds of nanoparticles in HL60 and KG1a cells, respectively (Figure 2B). In contrast, only 19 genes (fold change > 1.5) were commonly regulated by PBNPs in two cells (Figure 2C) and only 11 genes (fold change > 1.5) were commonly regulated by FeNPs in two cells (Figure 2C). These genes demonstrated the obvious cell- and nanoparticle-specific features in gene expression regulation. Finally, the most important genes that were commonly regulated in two cells treated by two kinds of nanoparticles were identified (Figure 2D). It was found that 14 genes were commonly upregulated in two cells by two kinds of nanoparticles (Figure 2D) and that only 4 genes were commonly downregulated in two cells by two kinds of nanoparticles (Figure 2D). These genes should have a close relationship with the common chemical essence of two kinds of nanoparticles: iron. These genes were closely related with five biological processes, including iron metabolism, antioxidation, lipid metabolism (lysosome dysfunction), vesicle traffic (exocytosis, endocytosis, and phagocytosis), innate immune system, and cytoskeleton. These processes typically reflect what commonly happens in cells when cells are treated by iron nanoparticles no matter their modification and structure.

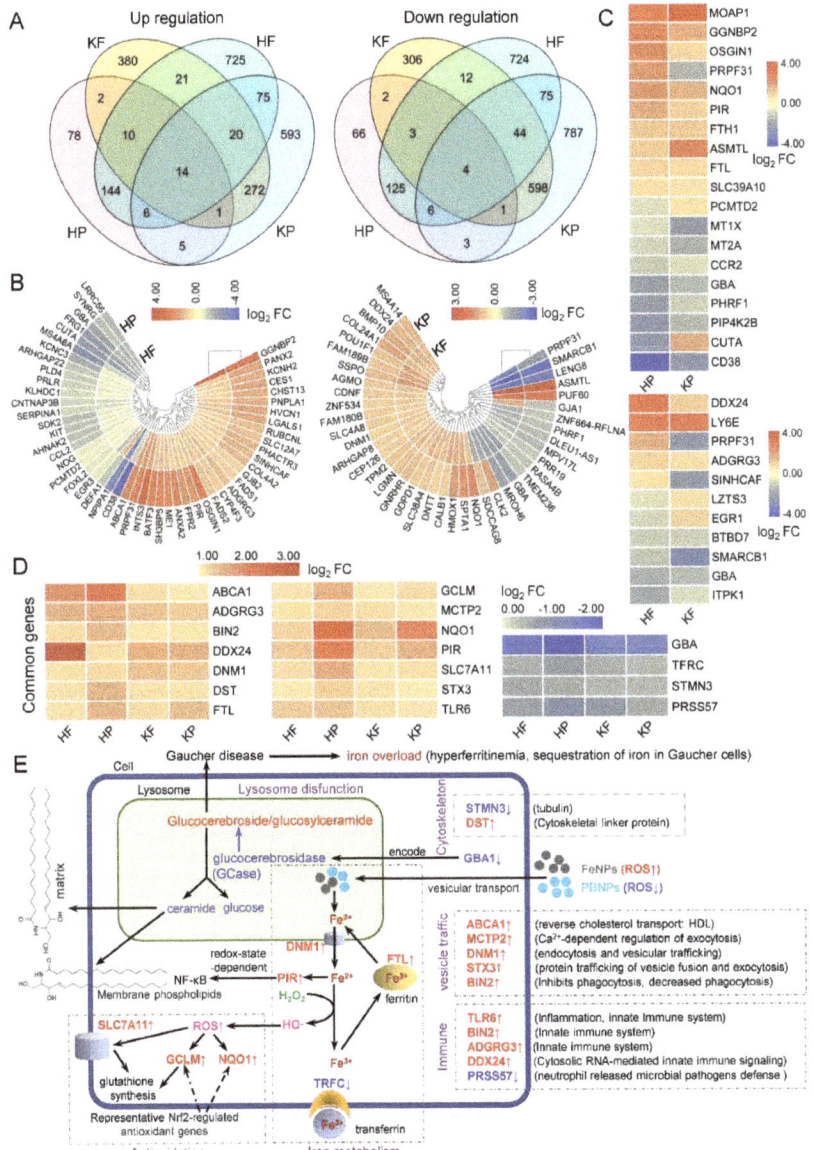

Figure 2. Comparisons of differentially expressed genes (DEGs) in two Leukemia cells treated with two kinds of iron nanoparticles: (**A**) number of upregulated and downregulated DEGs (fold change > 1.0) in the PBNP- and FeNP-treated HL60 and KG1a cells and their relationship, (**B**) common DEGs (fold change > 1.5) in a cell treated by two kinds of nanoparticles, (**C**) common DEGs (fold change > 1.5) in two cells treated by a nanoparticle, (**D**) common DEGs (fold change > 1.0) in two cells treated by two kinds of nanoparticles, and (**E**) schematic of cellular functions of common DEGs (fold change > 1.0) in two cells treated by two kinds of nanoparticles. The detailed information of all DEGs is shown in File S1 (Supplementary Materials). HF, FeNP-treated HL60 cells; HP, PBNP-treated HL60 cells; KF, FeNP-treated KG1a cells; and KP, PBNP-treated KG1a cells.

It was interesting that GBA was significantly downregulated in two cells by two kinds of nanoparticles (Figure 2D). GBA/GBA1 codes for glucerebrosidase (GCase), which plays a central role in the degradation of complex lipids and the turnover of cellular membranes [21]. Deficiency in GCase activity leads to accumulation of glucosylceramide/glucocerebroside in lysosome and compromised lysosomal activity, which would eventually affect lipid metabolism and trafficking [22]. GBA drives autophagy-dependent cell death [23], and the GBA mutation has a close relationship with Gaucher and Parkinson's diseases [24]. Besides GBA1, the expression of other important lysosomal function-related genes was also changed by iron nanoparticles, such as LYST, CLN3, LAMP1, LAMP5, LAPTM5, LAPTM4A, LAPTM4B, and HPS6 in HF, HP, and KP. The compromised lysosomal activity also affects the intracellular iron metabolism because the stored iron in ferritin has to be released as Fe^{2+} in lysosome. This is coincident with the iron overload (hyperferritinemia) that occurs in Gaucher cells [25]. The ceramide produced by GCase decomposing of glucocerebroside in lysosome plays a critical role in forming membrane phospholipids and the intracellular matrix. The significant iron nanoparticle-induced downregulation of GBA1 expression thus affects membrane maintenance and repair. This effect may contribute to iron nanoparticles-induced ferroptosis. However, the molecular mechanism of how iron nanoparticles inhibit GBA1 expression still remains unclear.

GCLM and NQO1 are representative Nrf2-regulated antioxidant genes [26]. The expression of these two genes was significantly upregulated by two kinds of iron nanoparticles in two cells, suggesting that cell internalization of iron nanoparticles resulted in oxidative stress by the increase of ROS via a Fenton reaction. The cells had to upregulate these antioxidation genes and SLC7A11 to neutralize the increased ROS for maintaining redox balance. In response to the cell internalization of iron nanoparticles, cells also changed the expressions of several key iron metabolism-related genes including FTH, PIR, DNM1, and TRFC. Because iron nanoparticles were internalized into cells by phagocytosis and finally trafficked to lysosome, together with glucocerebroside accumulation in cells resulting from the iron nanoparticle-induced downregulation of the GBA1 gene, cells upregulated several important genes involved in phagocytosis, exocytosis, endocytosis, and vesicular trafficking, such as ABCA1, MCTP2, DNM1, STX3, and BIN2. The interaction of iron nanoparticles with cells also induced upregulation of several genes related to the innate immune system, such as TLR6, BIN2, ADGRG3, and DDX24. This is in agreement with a previous report that iron nanoparticles could induce virus-like immune responses [27].

To further establish a high-confidence gene signature of the two Leukemia cells treated by two kinds of iron nanoparticles, the DEGs that were most significantly regulated by the nanoparticle treatments were screened (Figure 3A). These DEGs had fold changes over 2.0. The top ones of these genes were schematically shown in cells with different treatments (Figure 3B) to indicate their distributions and relationship. It was found that GBA was the only common signature gene highly downregulated in two cells under the treatment of two kinds of iron nanoparticles. CD38 was commonly downregulated and GGNBP2 was commonly upregulated in HF, HP, and KP, respectively. SMACB1 was commonly downregulated in HF, KF, and KP. SMACB1 is a core subunit of the SWI/SNF (BAF) chromatin-remodeling complex and is well-recognized as a tumor suppressor gene, which is inactivated in aggressive cancers such as nearly all pediatric rhabdoid tumors [28,29]. These highly regulated common genes represent the typical gene signatures of various cells and nanoparticles. Besides these common genes, each cell showed some unique highly regulated genes when treated by different iron nanoparticles.

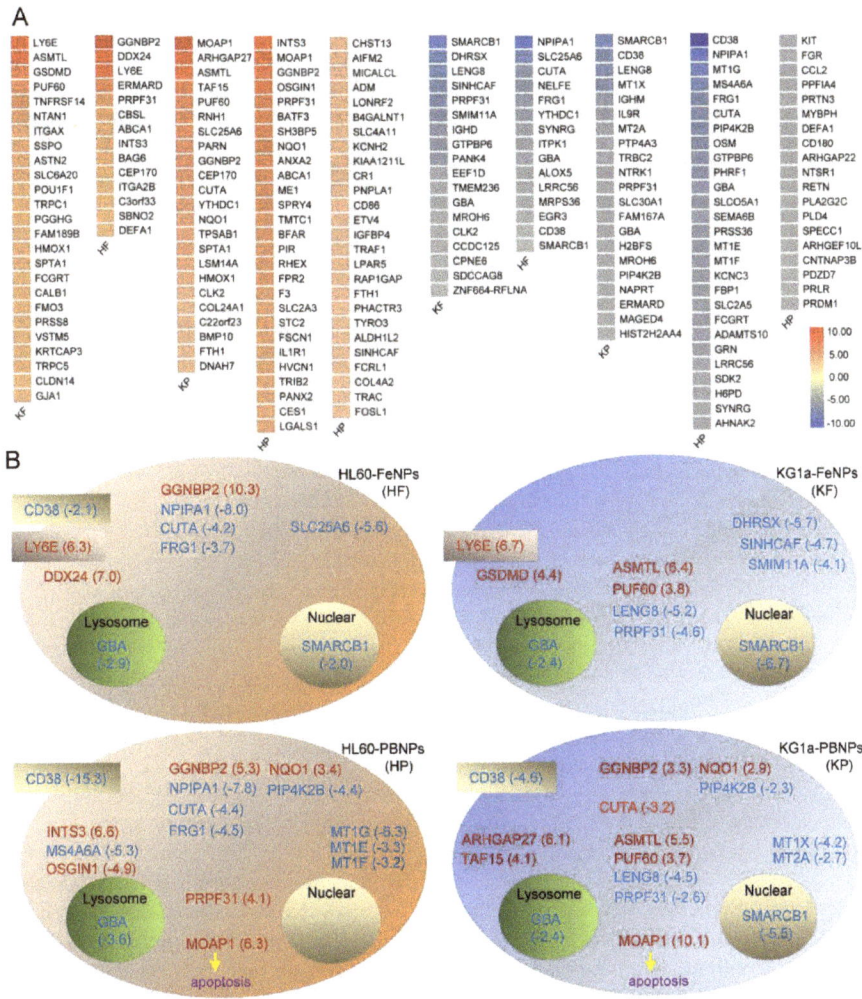

Figure 3. Gene signatures of two Leukemia cells treated by two kinds of iron nanoparticles: (**A**) most significantly regulated DEGs (fold change > 2.0) in two cell lines treated by two kinds of iron nanoparticles and (**B**) schematic of signature genes (fold change > 2.0) in two cell lines treated by two kinds of iron nanoparticles. The common genes were placed at the same positions in schematic cells for comparing.

In gene signatures, it is very interesting that CD38 was significantly downregulated in HF, HP, and KP and that LY6E was highly upregulated in HF and KF (Figure 3B). CD38 is an LSC marker gene, and LSC is marked by $CD34^+CD38^{low/-}$. The above qPCR detection indicated that KG1a expressed high-level CD34 and low-level CD38 whereas HL60 expressed no CD34 and relatively high-level CD38 (Figure 1C), showing that KG1a has much higher stemness than HL60. The treatment of two kinds of nanoparticles all significantly downregulated CD38 in two leukemia cells, especially, PBNPs most significantly downregulated CD38 in HL60 (Figure 3B). These data suggested that both iron nanoparticles preferentially killed non-stemness leukemia cells, which thus increased the relative proportion of stemness leukemia cells in live cells after iron nanoparticle treatment. On the contrary,

Ly6E was highly upregulated by FeNPs in two leukemia cells (Figure 3B). The human LY6 genes highly expressed in various cancers represent novel biomarkers for poor cancer prognosis, are required for cancer progression, and play an important role in immune escape [30–35]. More importantly, overexpression of certain Ly6 genes (Ly6D, Ly6E, Ly6K, and Ly6H) turned cancer cells into aggressive stem-like cells or allowed cancer cells to act like cancer stem cells [30]. In agreement with the downregulation of CD38, the significant upregulation of Ly6E in the two FeNP-treated leukemia cells also suggested that FeNPs preferentially killed non-stemness leukemia cells and thus allowed the proportion of stemness leukemia cells to increase in live cells. These data suggested the resistance of LSC to iron nanoparticle-induced cell death such as ferroptosis and nanoptosis [36].

3.4. GO Term Analysis of DEGs

To clarify the functions of the DEGs (|fold change| > 1.5, FDR < 0.05), GO function enrichment analysis was performed in Metascape (File S2 (Supplementary Materials)) [18]. The top 20 GO terms of four groups (HF: HL60-FeNPs, HP: HL60-PBNPs, KF: KG1a-FeNPs, and KP: KG1a-PBNPs) are displayed in Figures 4 and 5, respectively. Because PBNPs can effectively scavenge ROS via multienzyme-like activity including peroxidase (POD), catalase (CAT), and superoxide dismutase (SOD) activity while FeNPs produced hydroxyl radicals ($\cdot$OH) through the Fenton reaction and peroxidized lipids [15,37], the difference of GO terms between these two kinds of iron nanoparticles in one cell line (HL60 or KG1a) was firstly characterized. The most significant GO term in HF, HP, KF, and KP was the regulation of the lipid metabolic process, myeloid leukocyte activation, the HFE–transferrin receptor complex, and negative regulation of megakaryocyte, respectively. Interestingly, 25% of GO terms of HF was mainly enriched in "lipids", including regulation of lipid metabolic process, intracellular lipid transport, lipid biosynthetic process, cytoplasmic vesicle membrane, long-chain fatty acid metabolic process, and lipase activity (Figure 4A,B). In comparison, only 10% of GO terms of HP were related to "lipids", including regulation of lipid metabolic process and plasma membrane repair (Figure 4C,D). The results showed that the capability of FeNPs to produce ROS made it easier for FeNPs to regulate lipid metabolism than PBNPs. To further show the roles of genes in lipid metabolism, the DEGs in these GO terms are listed in Table 1. There were 28 (20 up- and 8 downregulated) genes in HF and 13 (9 up- and 4 downregulated) genes in HP involved in lipids regulation, of which 6 shared genes (ABCA1, FPR2, KIT, FADS1, ME1, and AHNAK2) were found. Particularly, the expression of ABCA1 was most significantly upregulated in lipid metabolism of HF and HP. ABCA1 was an important membrane-associated protein and actively participated to phosphatidylcholine, phosphatidylserine, and sphingomyelin transfer [38]. However, ABCA1 and 5 other shared genes were not found in the lipid-associated GO terms of KG1a. Besides these shared genes, ACACA was the unique gene that frequently appeared in lipid metabolism-related GO terms of HF. ACACA, acetyl-CoA carboxylase, was the first and rate-limiting step of de novo fatty acid biosynthesis [39]. This gene was also upregulated in HF and HP. This kind of significant effect of FeNPs on lipid metabolism was also found in the HepG2 cell treated by Fe_3O_4 nanoparticles in a previous study [36]. This previous study and this study all revealed that the treatment of Fe_3O_4 nanoparticles induced lipid accumulation in cells. In consistence with the previous study [36], this study also found that several lipid synthesis-related genes were upregulated in HF, including FDFT1, ACAT2, and HMGCS1. In contrast, the most significant biological process was myeloid leukocyte activation and cation homeostasis in the PBNP-treated HL60 cells (Figure 4C,D).

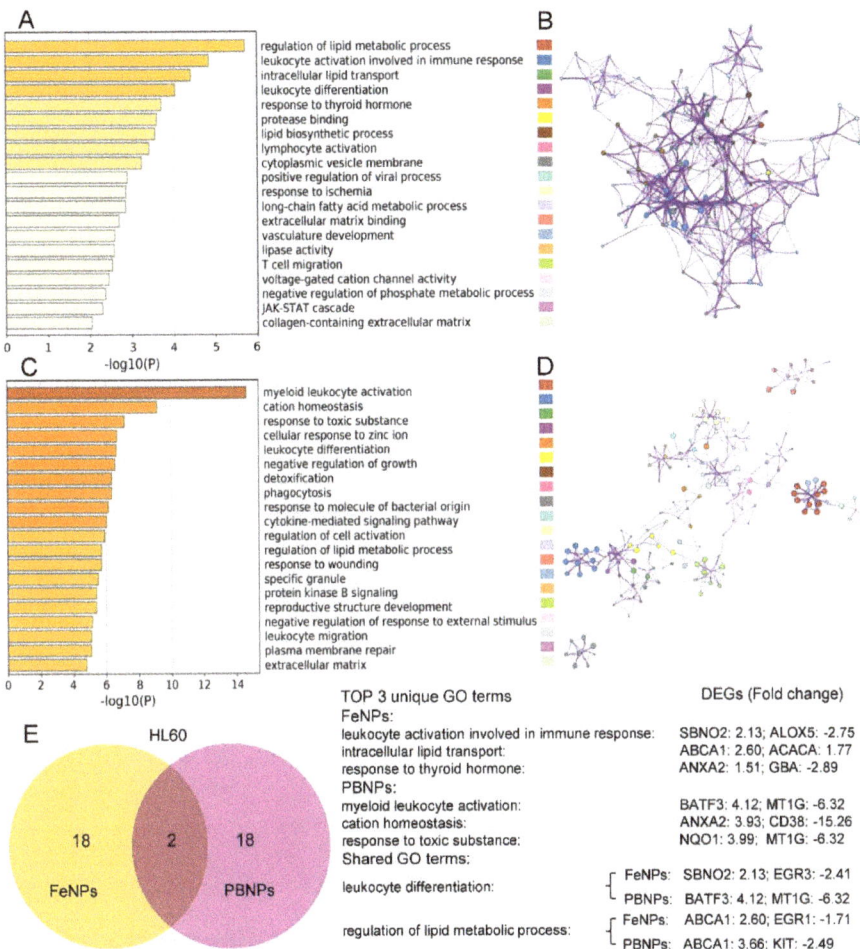

Figure 4. Top 20 Gene Ontology (GO) terms of the HL60 cells treated with two kinds of iron nanoparticles: (A,B) heatmap (A) and enrichment network (B) colored by the same cluster of GO terms in the FeNP-treated HL60 cells, and (C,D) heatmap (C) and enrichment network (D) colored by the same cluster of GO terms in the PBNP-treated HL60 cells. The colored labels followed the order of top 20 GO terms. (E) The Venn analysis of top 20 GO terms in the HL60 cells treated with PBNPs and FeNPs. The detailed information of all GO terms is shown in File S2 (Supplementary Materials).

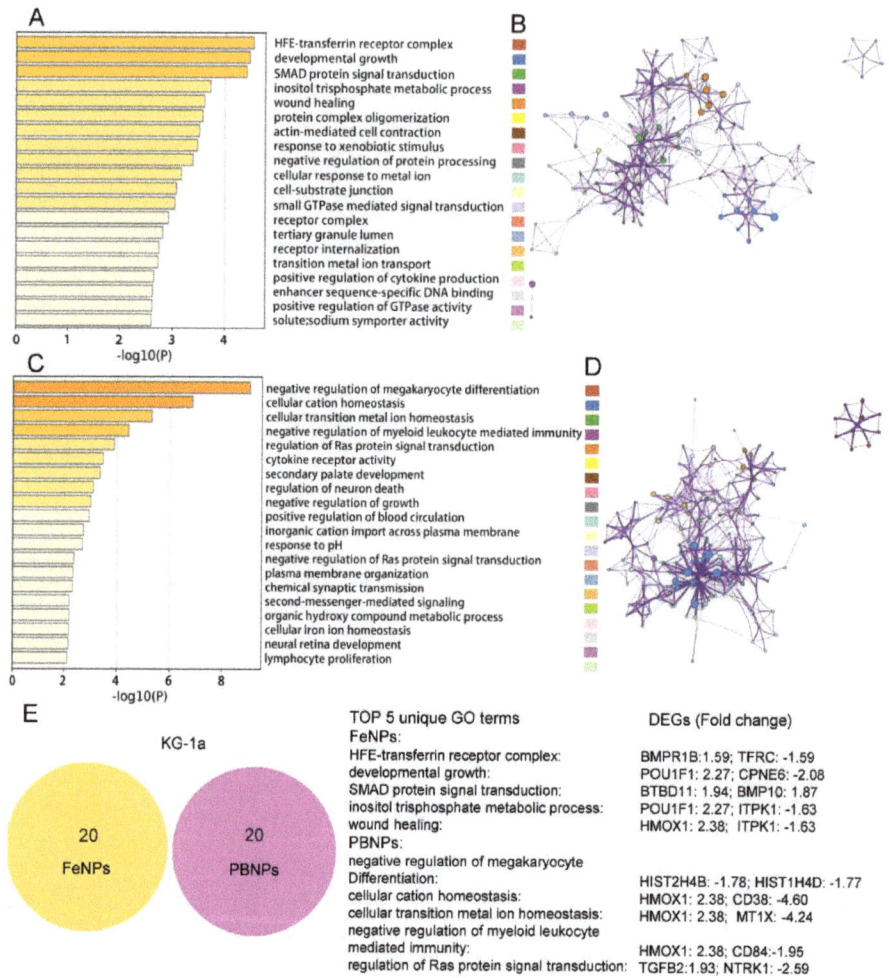

Figure 5. Top 20 GO terms of the KG1a cells treated with two kinds of iron nanoparticles: (**A**,**B**) heatmap (**A**) and enrichment network (**B**) colored by the same cluster of GO terms in the FeNP-treated KG1a cells, and (**C**,**D**) heatmap (**C**) and enrichment network (**D**) colored by the same cluster of GO terms in the PBNP-treated KG1a cells. The colored labels followed the order of top 20 GO terms. (**E**) Venn analysis of top 20 GO terms in the KG1a cells treated with PBNPs and FeNPs. The detailed information of all GO terms is shown in File S2 (Supplementary Materials).

For KG1a, there was few GO terms related to lipid metabolism. Only three genes (ITPK1, PLCG2, and POU1F1) were involved in inositol triphosphate metabolic process in KF, and four genes (SPTA1, TGFB2, CXCR4, and EHD2) mediated plasma membrane organization in KP. In contrast, GO terms that responded to metal ions were highly enriched in KG1a (Figure 5A–D). As listed in Table 2, 4 GO terms (containing 13 genes) were found in KF and just one term (containing 4 genes) was found in HF. It implied that KG1a was more sensitive to metal ions than HL60 under the FeNP treatment. For example, TFRC and TFR2 genes were over-suppressed in KF, which belong to the transferrin receptor-like family and are necessary for cellular iron uptake [40]. Another receptor, BMPR1B, overexpressed in KF, can specifically bind the bone morphogenetic protein (BMP) to regulate a wide range of biological processes including iron homeostasis, fat and bone development, and ovulation [41].

Table 1. GO terms of lipid metabolisms in KG1a and HL60 exposed to FeNPs or PBNPs (Top 20, $p < 0.01$).

Group	Category	GO Term	LogP	NO.	Gene Symbol
HF	BP	GO:0019216~regulation of lipid metabolic process	−5.71	11	ABCA1, ACACA, CHRM5, EGR1, FPR2, KIT, FADS1, ME1, SOCS7, LPCAT1, RUBCNL
	BP	GO:0032365~intracellular lipid transport	−4.42	4	ABCA1, ACACA, ANXA2, CES1
	BP	GO:0008610~lipid biosynthetic process	−3.55	10	ACACA, ALOX5, CES1, EGR1, FPR2, FADS1, PRLR, FADS2, LPCAT1, MBOAT2
	CC	GO:0030659~cytoplasmic vesicle membrane	−3.23	11	CD38, FPR2, IFNGR2, ITGA2B, TGFA, SH3BP5, SYNRG, LPCAT1, HVCN1, AHNAK2, ADGRG3
	MF	GO:0016298~lipase activity	−2.57	4	CES1, CHRM5, PLD4, PNPLA1
HP	BP	GO:0019216~regulation of lipid metabolic process	−5.52	9	ABCA1, ADM, FGR, FPR2, KIT, FADS1, ME1, PPARG, SMARCD3
	BP	GO:0001778~plasma membrane repair	−5.07	4	DYSF, SYT11, MYOF, AHNAK2
KF	BP	GO:0032957~inositol trisphosphate metabolic process	−2.92	3	ITPK1, PLCG2, POU1F1
KP	BP	GO:0007009~plasma membrane organization	−2.35	4	SPTA1, TGFB2, CXCR4, EHD2

Note: HF: HL60-FeNPs, HP: HL60-PBNPs, KF: KG1a-FeNPs, KP: KG1a-PBNPs.

Table 2. GO terms of metal ion metabolisms in KG1a and HL60 exposed to FeNPs or PBNPs (Top 20, $p < 0.01$).

Groups	Category	GO Terms	LogP	NO.	Gene Symbol
HF	MF	GO:0022843~voltage-gated cation channel activity	−2.45	4	ANXA2, KCNC3, KCNH2, HVCN1
HP	BP	GO:0055080~cation homeostasis	−9.14	31	ADM, ANXA2, ATP6V0A1, CD38, ELANE, FPR2, FTH1, FTL, FYN, GATA2, GRN, GSTM2, KCNH2, MT1E, MT1F, MT1G, MT1X, MT2A, NTSR1, PLCB2, TFRC, STC2, SLC12A7, NCS1, SLC7A8, MCUB, JPH1, SLC39A10, SLC4A11, SLC24A4, CCR2
	BP	GO:0071294~cellular response to zinc ion	−6.68	6	MT1E, MT1F, MT1G, MT1X, MT2A, HVCN1
KF	CC	GO:1990712~HFE-transferrin receptor complex	−4.54	3	BMPR1B, TFR2, TFRC
	BP	GO:0071248~cellular response to metal ion	−3.17	6	NQO1, HMOX1, LGMN, TFR2, CPNE6, RASA4B
	BP	GO:0000041~transition metal ion transport	−2.72	4	TFR2, TFRC, TRPC1, TRPC5
	MF	GO:0015370~solute sodium symporter activity	−2.60	3	SLC22A1, SLC4A8, SLC6A20
KP	BP	GO:0030003~cellular cation homeostasis	−6.87	18	CALB1, CD38, FTH1, FTL, GJA1, LPAR4, HMOX1, MT1X, MT2A, PTGER3, SLC8A1, SLC30A1, CXCR4, F2RL3, SLC4A8, SLC39A10, ROGDI, CCR2
	BP	GO:0046916~cellular transition metal ion homeostasis	−5.29	7	FTH1, FTL, HMOX1, MT1X, MT2A, SLC30A1, SLC39A10
	BP	GO:0098659~inorganic cation import across plasma membrane	−2.75	4	SLC8A1, SLC30A1, SLC39A10, SLC12A8
	BP	GO:0006879~cellular iron ion homeostasis	−2.19	3	FTH1, FTL, HMOX1

Note: HF: HL60-FeNPs, HP: HL60-PBNPs, KF: KG1a-FeNPs, KP: KG1a-PBNPs.

It was found that the antioxidation-related genes were highly regulated in two cells treated by two kinds of iron nanoparticles. NQO1 and GCLM were commonly upregulated in two cells treated by two kinds of nanoparticles (Figure 2D). Two genes (NQO1 and HMOX1) that was closely associated with antioxidant metabolism were in upregulated by two kinds of nanoparticles in KG1a (File S1 (Supplementary Materials)). NQO1 and HMOX1 are representative NRF2-regulated antioxidation genes [26]. NQO1 reduces quinone to hydroquinone, and HMOX1 catalyzes the degradation of heme to biliverdin, CO, and Fe^+. If either one of the two genes was knocked out, it would enhance erastin- and sorafenib-induced ferroptosis in hepatocellular carcinoma cells [7]. The two genes may help KG1a cells to scavenge ROS and thus resist iron nanoparticle-induced ferroptosis. Another antioxidation gene, GPX3, was only upregulated in HF. Together with the upregulated GCLM and GCLC in HF, these three typical NRF2-regulated antioxidation genes [26] revealed high oxidative stress in HF, which agrees with the decrease of cell viability of only HF in all treatments (Figure 1C). In addition, iron nanoparticles-induced oxidative stress was also demonstrated by the wide regulation of the expression of as many as 15 (HF), 42 (KF), 50 (HP), and 70 (KP) genes coding oxidase, reductase, peroxidase, dehydrogenase, epoxidase, and oxidoreductase (File S4 (Supplementary Materials)). It was interesting that a recently identified anti-ferroptosis gene, AIFM2 (renamed as ferroptosis suppressor protein 1, FSP1, a CoQ oxidoreductase) [42,43], was also upregulated in KF and HP. Many proteins sequester transition metals or transport them and thus indirectly act as antioxidants by suppressing formation of HO· from H_2O_2 by Fenton chemistry [44]. These proteins include ferritin (comprising light FTL1 and heavy FTH1 subunits), ferroportin (FPN1/SLC40A1), metallothionein, and ceruloplasmin. FTL was commonly upregulated by two kinds of nanoparticles in two cells (Figure 2D). FTH1 was upregulated in KF, HP, and KP (File S1 (Supplementary Materials)). Another an important antioxidation gene, SLC7A11, was commonly significantly upregulated in two cells treated by two kinds of nanoparticles (Figure 2D). SLC7A11 imported cysteine into cells for glutathione synthesis and thus plays key role in antioxidation of cells. Besides SLC7A11, as many as 13, 40, 48, and 56 soluble carrier (SLC) family genes were differentially regulated in HF, HP, KF, and KP, respectively (File S1 (Supplementary Materials)). These SLC family genes encoding passive transporters, ion coupled transporters, and exchangers were crucial for intracellular ion homeostasis [45,46]. It was worthy to note that metallothioneins (MTs) were generally downregulated in HL60 and KG1a exposed to PBNPs, including MT1E, MT1F, MT1G, MT1X, and MT2A in HL60, and MT1X and MT2A in KG1a. With a high content of cysteine residues, metallothioneins bound various heavy metals for detoxification in cells and acted as antioxidants to protect against hydroxyl free radicals [47]. The inhibited metallothioneins further supported the low metal toxicity and good antioxidant capacity of PBNPs in HL60 and KG1a. When exposed to PBNPs, this iron nanoparticle can effectively scavenge ROS via multienzyme-like activity to reduce the burden of cellular antioxidants.

3.5. Pathway Analysis of DEGs

To find the pathways regulated by iron nanoparticles, the DEGs with over 1.5-fold change were annotated by the KEGG database. As a result, 106 DEGs in HF, 283 DEGs in HP, 199 DEGs in KF, and 152 DEGs in KP were enriched in 10, 25, 18, and 12 KEGG pathways, respectively (File S3 (Supplementary Materials)). The comparison of the top 10 pathways revealed that there was great difference between HF and KF, but some similarity between HP and KP (Figure 6A,B). Only the pathways in cancer were enriched in four treatments (Figure 6C).

In HF, the fatty acid metabolism was the most significantly enriched pathway, in which the ACACA, FADS1, and FADS2 genes play important roles in cell membrane formation and repair. The metabolic pathways mainly involved in lipid metabolism and glycerophospholipid metabolism were also enriched in HF. In contrast, the HIF-1 signaling way was most prominently enriched in KF, which consisted of CDKN1A, FLT1, HMOX1, IGF1R, PLCG2, TFRC, STAT3, LDHA, ENO1, PGK1, and ELOB genes (Figure S4). This signaling way can mediate adaptive responses to reduced oxygen availability; it was crucial for angiogenesis, vascular reactivity and remodeling, glucose and energy metabolism, inflammation, tumor, and iron homeostasis [48]. The hypoxia and free radicals can activate the function of HIF-1 [49]. By producing ROS, the HIF-1 signaling way was activated by FeNPs in KG1a. PLCG2 was induced by ROS to affect the IP3/DAG pathways, the ubiquitination of HIF-1α was inhibited by the downregulated ELOB, and the activity of HIF-1α was enhanced by the upregulated receptor tyrosine kinase (RTK). The iron deprivation can stimulate TFRC transcription through HIF-1 [50]. LY6E, highly upregulated in HF and KF (Figure 3B), was identified as an activator of HIF-1 and functioned as a novel conductor of tumor growth through its modulation of the PTEN/PI3K/Akt/HIF-1 axis [35].

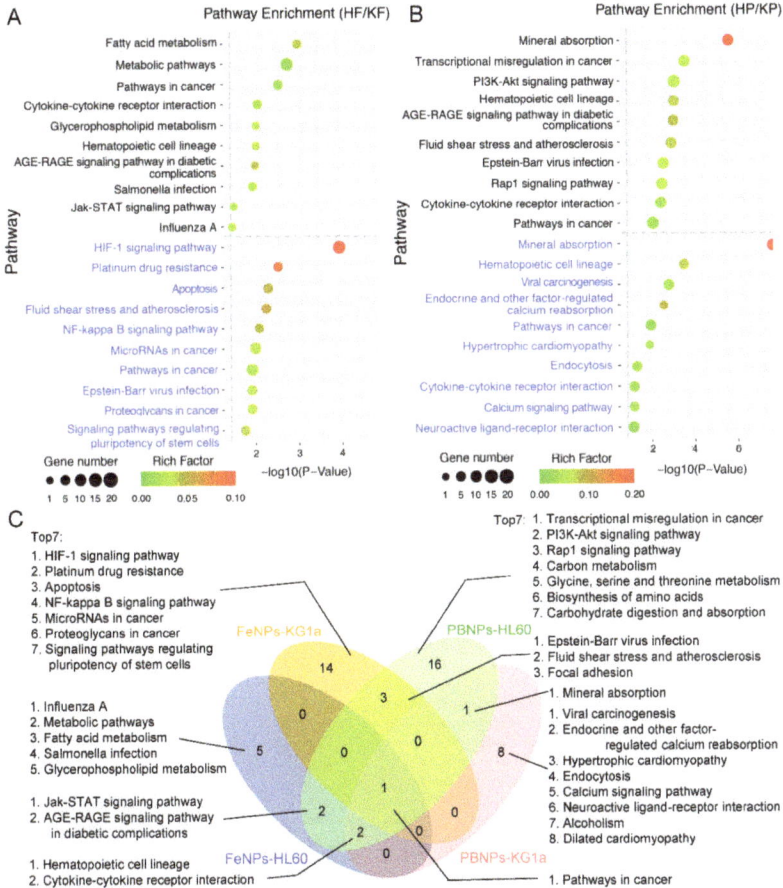

Figure 6. Comparative Kyoto Encyclopedia of Genes and Genomes (KEGG) pathway enrichment analysis of the DEGs ($p < 0.05$): (A) comparative top 10 enriched pathways of HL60 and KG1a treated with FeNPs and (B) comparative top 10 enriched pathways of HL60 and KG1a treated with PBNPs. The pathways in black and blue were HL60 and KG1a cells, respectively. (C) Four-way Venn analysis of all KEGG pathways in four groups. The detailed information of all KEGG pathways is shown in File S3 (Supplementary Materials). HF, FeNP-treated HL60 cells; HP, PBNP-treated HL60 cells; KF, FeNP-treated KG1a cells; and KP, PBNP-treated KG1a cells.

It is interesting that the Platinum drug resistance pathway was also highly enriched in KF, in which several genes involved in platinum drug resistance were upregulated, including BIRC3, CDKN1A, GSTM2, and BBC3 (File S1 (Supplementary Materials)). ROS increase plays a key role in both platinum and iron nanoparticle-induced cancer cell death. Therefore, the activation of the platinum drug resistance pathway in KF may underline the resistance of KG1a cell to FeNP treatment (Figure 1C). Interestingly, CDKN1A and GSTM2 were also upregulated in HP and BIRC3 and CDKN1A were also upregulated in KP (File S1 (Supplementary Materials)). However, none of these genes were regulated in HF. This contributed to the decrease of cell viability of HF and no significant decrease of cell viability of HP, KF, and KP (Figure 1C).

When exposed to PBNPs, 40% top 10 pathways were identical between KG1a and HL60, in which the mineral absorption was most significantly enriched in two cells (Figure 6B). In HP and KP, Ferritin (FTH1 and FTL) and MTs were changed to regulate cellular metal ions concentration due to increased iron ions (File S3 and Figure S5 (Supplementary Materials)). In contrast, the mineral absorption pathway in KG1a was more complex (File S3 and Figure S5 (Supplementary Materials)), including the multi-responses of HMOX1 to Fe^{2+}, SLC8A1(NCX1) to Na^+ and Ca^{2+}, and SLC30A1(ZNT1) to Zn^{2+} [7,51,52]. The activation of the mineral absorption pathway made the two cells survive under the treatment of PBNPs (Figure 1C); however, the significant change of lipid metabolism induced by FeNPs made HL60 easy to kill (Figure 1C) although FTL was upregulated and TFRC was downregulated (Figure 2).

3.6. Validation of RNA-Seq Gene Expression Levels Using RT-qPCR

To validate the accuracy of RNA-Seq results, ten genes in HL60 and KG1a were also detected by RT-qPCR. As a result, the RNA-Seq-detected expression regulation of 20 genes were verified by RT-qPCR detection (Figure 7A,B). Additionally, the qPCR-detected CD38 expression (Figure 1E) was also in agreement with that detected by RNA-Seq (Figure 3B). These data indicated that the RNA-Seq results were reliable.

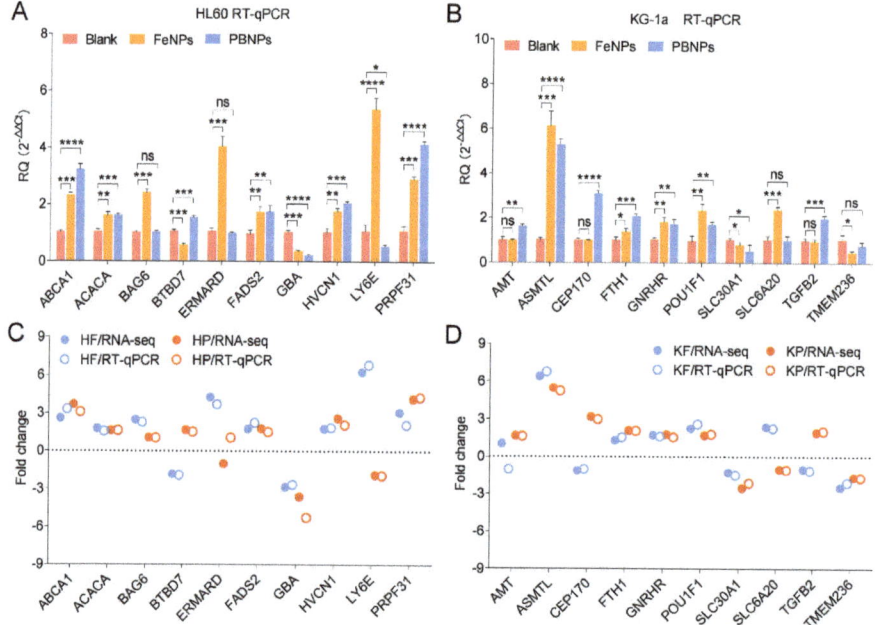

Figure 7. Validation of RNA-Seq DEGs using RT-qPCR: (**A**,**B**) the expression levels of 10 selected DEGs in the iron nanoparticle-treated HL60 (**A**) and KG1a (**B**) cells. All values are mean ± SD with $n = 3$. ns, no significance; *, $p < 0.05$; **, $p < 0.01$, ***, $p < 0.001$, ****, and $p < 0.0001$. (**C**,**D**) The comparison of fold change detected by RT-qPCR and RNA-Seq in the iron nanoparticle-treated HL60 and (**C**,**D**) KG1a cells.

4. Conclusions

This study provided the transcriptomic profiles of two leukemia cells (KG1a and HL60) that had different stemness treated by two kinds of iron nanoparticles (FeNPs and PBNPs) that had different ROS regulation capabilities. The results indicated that the expression of many genes was significantly regulated. More genes were regulated by PBNPs than FeNPs. The unique and common genes were determined. The gene signatures were established. The common genes in all treatments were closely related with iron metabolism, antioxidation, lipid metabolism, vesicle traffic, innate immune system, and cytoskeleton. The mineral absorption pathway was most significantly regulated by PBNPs in both cells, whereas the lipid metabolism pathway was most significantly regulated by FeNPs in HL60. This study shed new insights into the cytotoxicity at the gene transcription level of iron nanoparticles that differently regulate ROS in leukemia cells with different stemness. This study demonstrated why the leukemia cell with low stemness is sensitive and with high stemness is resistant to FeNPs as a ROS inducer. This study also suggested the potential resistance of stemness leukemia cells to iron nanoparticles as a ferroptosis inducer.

Supplementary Materials: The following are available online at http://www.mdpi.com/2079-4991/10/10/1951/s1, Table S1. The qPCR primers sequences used in this study; Table S2. Mapping statistics of RNA-Seq (each sample had two biological replicates); Table S3. The mRNA peak insert size in all samples; Figure S1. Statistics of the distribution of reads in different regions of the genome; Figure S2. Correlation analysis of gene expression in 12 samples; Figure S3. Density map of gene expression levels of all samples; Figure S4. KEGG analysis of the HIF-1 signaling pathway in Pathview; Figure S5. KEGG analysis of the mineral absorption pathway in Pathview; File S1. DEGs; File S2. GO terms; File S3. KEGG pathways; File S4. Redox-related DEGs.

Author Contributions: J.W. conceived the study and designed the experiments. T.L. performed data analysis, qPCR detection, and wrote the manuscript. J.G. performed wet experiments of RNA-Seq. N.L. provided support in data analysis. J.W. edited the manuscript with support from all authors. All authors have read and agreed to the published version of the manuscript.

Funding: This work was supported by the National Key Research and Development Program of China (2017YFA0205502) and the National Natural Science Foundation of China (61971122).

Conflicts of Interest: The authors declare no conflict of interest.

References

1. Xu, R.; Yu, S.; Zhu, D.; Huang, X.; Xu, Y.; Lao, Y.; Tian, Y.; Zhang, J.; Tang, Z.; Zhang, Z.; et al. hCINAP regulates the DNA-damage response and mediates the resistance of acute myelocytic leukemia cells to therapy. *Nat. Commun.* **2019**, *10*, 3812. [CrossRef] [PubMed]
2. Chen, B.; Lee, J.B.; Kang, H.; Minden, M.D.; Zhang, L. Targeting chemotherapy-resistant leukemia by combining DNT cellular therapy with conventional chemotherapy. *J. Exp. Clin. Cancer Res.* **2018**, *37*, 88. [CrossRef] [PubMed]
3. Strese, S.; Hassan, S.B.; Velander, E.; Haglund, C.; Hoglund, M.; Larsson, R.; Gullbo, J. In vitro and in vivo anti-leukemic activity of the peptidasepotentiated alkylator melflufen in acute myeloid leukemia. *Oncotarget* **2016**, *8*, 6341–6352. [CrossRef] [PubMed]
4. Sang, M.; Luo, R.; Bai, Y.; Dou, J.; Zhang, Z.; Liu, F.; Feng, F.; Xu, J.; Liu, W. Mitochondrial membrane anchored photosensitive nano-device for lipid hydroperoxides burst and inducing ferroptosis to surmount therapy-resistant cancer. *Theranostics* **2019**, *9*, 6209–6223. [CrossRef]
5. Yang, R.; Li, Y.; Wang, X.; Yan, J.; Pan, D.; Xu, Y.; Wang, L.; Yang, M. Doxorubicin loaded ferritin nanoparticles for ferroptosis enhanced targeted killing of cancer cells. *RSC Adv.* **2019**, *9*, 28548–28553. [CrossRef]
6. Song, J.; Lin, L.; Yang, Z.; Zhu, R.; Zhou, Z.; Li, Z.W.; Wang, F.; Chen, J.; Yang, H.; Chen, X. Self-Assembled Responsive Bilayered Vesicles with Adjustable Oxidative Stress for Enhanced Cancer Imaging and Therapy. *J. Am. Chem. Soc.* **2019**, *141*, 8158–8170. [CrossRef]
7. Hassannia, B.; Vandenabeele, P.; Vanden Berghe, T. Targeting Ferroptosis to Iron Out Cancer. *Cancer Cell* **2019**, *35*, 830–849. [CrossRef]
8. Dixon, S.J.; Lemberg, K.M.; Lamprecht, M.R.; Skouta, R.; Zaitsev, E.M.; Gleason, C.E.; Patel, D.N.; Bauer, A.J.; Cantley, A.M.; Yang, W.S.; et al. Ferroptosis: An iron-dependent form of nonapoptotic cell death. *Cell* **2012**, *149*, 1060–1072. [CrossRef]

9. Louandre, C.; Ezzoukhry, Z.; Godin, C.; Barbare, J.C.; Maziere, J.C.; Chauffert, B.; Galmiche, A. Iron-dependent cell death of hepatocellular carcinoma cells exposed to sorafenib. *Int. J. Cancer* **2013**, *133*, 1732–1742. [CrossRef]
10. Hangauer, M.J.; Viswanathan, V.S.; Ryan, M.J.; Bole, D.; Eaton, J.K.; Matov, A.; Galeas, J.; Dhruv, H.D.; Berens, M.E.; Schreiber, S.L.; et al. Drug-tolerant persister cancer cells are vulnerable to GPX4 inhibition. *Nature* **2017**, *551*, 247–250. [CrossRef]
11. Mai, T.T.; Hamai, A.; Hienzsch, A.; Caneque, T.; Muller, S.; Wicinski, J.; Cabaud, O.; Leroy, C.; David, A.; Acevedo, V.; et al. Salinomycin kills cancer stem cells by sequestering iron in lysosomes. *Nat. Chem.* **2017**, *9*, 1025–1033. [CrossRef]
12. Wang, W.; Green, M.; Choi, J.E.; Gijon, M.; Kennedy, P.D.; Johnson, J.K.; Liao, P.; Lang, X.; Kryczek, I.; Sell, A.; et al. CD8(+) T cells regulate tumour ferroptosis during cancer immunotherapy. *Nature* **2019**, *569*, 270–274. [CrossRef]
13. Shen, Z.; Liu, T.; Li, Y.; Lau, J.; Yang, Z.; Fan, W.; Zhou, Z.; Shi, C.; Ke, C.; Bregadze, V.I.; et al. Fenton-Reaction-Acceleratable Magnetic Nanoparticles for Ferroptosis Therapy of Orthotopic Brain Tumors. *ACS Nano* **2018**, *12*, 11355–11365. [CrossRef]
14. Trujillo-Alonso, V.; Pratt, E.C.; Zong, H.; Lara-Martinez, A.; Kaittanis, C.; Rabie, M.O.; Longo, V.; Becker, M.W.; Roboz, G.J.; Grimm, J.; et al. FDA-approved ferumoxytol displays anti-leukaemia efficacy against cells with low ferroportin levels. *Nat. Nanotechnol.* **2019**, *14*, 616–622. [CrossRef]
15. Zhang, W.; Hu, S.; Yin, J.J.; He, W.; Lu, W.; Ma, M.; Gu, N.; Zhang, Y. Prussian Blue Nanoparticles as Multienzyme Mimetics and Reactive Oxygen Species Scavengers. *J. Am. Chem. Soc.* **2016**, *138*, 5860–5865. [CrossRef]
16. Atashrazm, F.; Lowenthal, R.M.; Woods, G.M.; Holloway, A.F.; Karpiniec, S.S.; Dickinson, J.L. Fucoidan Suppresses the Growth of Human Acute Promyelocytic Leukemia Cells In Vitro and In Vivo. *J. Cell. Physiol.* **2016**, *231*, 688–697. [CrossRef]
17. Chen, Z.P.; Zhang, Y.; Zhang, S.; Xia, J.G.; Liu, J.W.; Xu, K.; Gu, N. Preparation and characterization of water-soluble monodisperse magnetic iron oxide nanoparticles via surface double-exchange with DMSA. *Colloids Surf. A* **2008**, *316*, 210–216. [CrossRef]
18. Zhou, Y.; Zhou, B.; Pache, L.; Chang, M.; Khodabakhshi, A.H.; Tanaseichuk, O.; Benner, C.; Chanda, S.K. Metascape provides a biologist-oriented resource for the analysis of systems-level datasets. *Nat. Commun.* **2019**, *10*, 1523. [CrossRef]
19. Luo, W.; Brouwer, C. Pathview: An R/Bioconductor package for pathway-based data integration and visualization. *Bioinformatics* **2013**, *29*, 1830–1831. [CrossRef]
20. Trapnell, C.; Williams, B.A.; Pertea, G.; Mortazavi, A.; Kwan, G.; van Baren, M.J.; Salzberg, S.L.; Wold, B.J.; Pachter, L. Transcript assembly and quantification by RNA-Seq reveals unannotated transcripts and isoform switching during cell differentiation. *Nat. Biotechnol.* **2010**, *28*, 511–515. [CrossRef]
21. Magalhaes, J.; Gegg, M.E.; Migdalska-Richards, A.; Doherty, M.K.; Whitfield, P.D.; Schapira, A.H. Autophagic lysosome reformation dysfunction in glucocerebrosidase deficient cells: Relevance to Parkinson disease. *Hum. Mol. Genet.* **2016**, *25*, 3432–3445. [CrossRef] [PubMed]
22. Westbroek, W.; Gustafson, A.M.; Sidransky, E. Exploring the link between glucocerebrosidase mutations and parkinsonism. *Trends Mol. Med.* **2011**, *17*, 485–493. [CrossRef] [PubMed]
23. Ma, Y.; Adjemian, S.; Mattarollo, S.R.; Yamazaki, T.; Aymeric, L.; Yang, H.; Portela Catani, J.P.; Hannani, D.; Duret, H.; Steegh, K.; et al. Anticancer chemotherapy-induced intratumoral recruitment and differentiation of antigen-presenting cells. *Immunity* **2013**, *38*, 729–741. [CrossRef] [PubMed]
24. Almeida Mdo, R. Glucocerebrosidase involvement in Parkinson disease and other synucleinopathies. *Front. Neurol.* **2012**, *3*, 65. [CrossRef]
25. Weisberger, J.; Emmons, F.; Gorczyca, W. Cytochemical diagnosis of Gaucher's disease by iron stain. *Br. J. Haematol.* **2004**, *124*, 696. [CrossRef] [PubMed]
26. Tonelli, C.; Chio, I.I.C.; Tuveson, D.A. Transcriptional Regulation by Nrf2. *Antioxid. Redox Signal.* **2018**, *29*, 1727–1745. [CrossRef] [PubMed]
27. Liu, Y.; Chen, Z.; Gu, N.; Wang, J. Effects of DMSA-coated Fe_3O_4 magnetic nanoparticles on global gene expression of mouse macrophage RAW264.7 cells. *Toxicol. Lett.* **2011**, *205*, 130–139. [CrossRef]
28. Kim, K.H.; Roberts, C.W.M. Mechanisms by which SMARCB1 loss drives rhabdoid tumor growth. *Cancer Genet.* **2014**, *207*, 365–372. [CrossRef]

29. Weissmiller, A.M.; Wang, J.; Lorey, S.L.; Howard, G.C.; Martinez, E.; Liu, Q.; Tansey, W.P. Inhibition of MYC by the SMARCB1 tumor suppressor. *Nat. Commun.* **2019**, *10*, 2014. [CrossRef]
30. Luo, L.; McGarvey, P.; Madhavan, S.; Kumar, R.; Gusev, Y.; Upadhyay, G. Distinct lymphocyte antigens 6 (Ly6) family members Ly6D, Ly6E, Ly6K and Ly6H drive tumorigenesis and clinical outcome. *Oncotarget* **2016**, *7*, 11165–11193. [CrossRef] [PubMed]
31. Upadhyay, G. Emerging Role of Lymphocyte Antigen-6 Family of Genes in Cancer and Immune Cells. *Front. Immunol.* **2019**, *10*, 819. [CrossRef] [PubMed]
32. Upadhyay, G. Emerging Role of Novel Biomarkers of Ly6 Gene Family in Pan Cancer. *Adv. Exp. Med. Biol.* **2019**, *1164*, 47–61.
33. Benti, S.; Tiwari, P.B.; Goodlett, D.W.; Daneshian, L.; Kern, G.B.; Smith, M.D.; Uren, A.; Chruszcz, M.; Shimizu, L.S.; Upadhyay, G. Small Molecule Binds with Lymphocyte Antigen 6K to Induce Cancer Cell Death. *Cancers* **2020**, *12*, 509. [CrossRef]
34. AlHossiny, M.; Luo, L.; Frazier, W.R.; Steiner, N.; Gusev, Y.; Kallakury, B.; Glasgow, E.; Creswell, K.; Madhavan, S.; Kumar, R.; et al. Ly6E/K Signaling to TGFbeta Promotes Breast Cancer Progression, Immune Escape, and Drug Resistance. *Cancer Res.* **2016**, *76*, 3376–3386. [CrossRef]
35. Yeom, C.J.; Zeng, L.H.; Goto, Y.; Morinibu, A.; Zhu, Y.X.; Shinomiya, K.; Kobayashi, M.; Itasaka, S.; Yoshimura, M.; Hur, C.G.; et al. LY6E: A conductor of malignant tumor growth through modulation of the PTEN/PI3K/Akt/HIF-1 axis. *Oncotarget* **2016**, *7*, 65837–65848. [CrossRef]
36. Wang, P.X.; Liu, S.L.; Hu, M.X.; Zhang, H.W.; Duan, D.M.; He, J.Y.; Hong, J.J.; Lv, R.T.; Choi, H.S.; Yan, X.Y.; et al. Peroxidase-Like Nanozymes Induce a Novel Form of Cell Death and Inhibit Tumor Growth In Vivo. *Adv. Funct. Mater.* **2020**, *30*, 2000647. [CrossRef]
37. Peng, Q.; Huo, D.; Li, H.; Zhang, B.; Li, Y.; Liang, A.; Wang, H.; Yu, Q.; Li, M. ROS-independent toxicity of Fe_3O_4 nanoparticles to yeast cells: Involvement of mitochondrial dysfunction. *Chem. Biol. Interact.* **2018**, *287*, 20–26. [CrossRef]
38. Quazi, F.; Molday, R.S. Differential phospholipid substrates and directional transport by ATP-binding cassette proteins ABCA1, ABCA7, and ABCA4 and disease-causing mutants. *J. Biol. Chem.* **2013**, *288*, 34414–34426. [CrossRef]
39. Colbert, C.L.; Kim, C.W.; Moon, Y.A.; Henry, L.; Palnitkar, M.; McKean, W.B.; Fitzgerald, K.; Deisenhofer, J.; Horton, J.D.; Kwon, H.J. Crystal structure of Spot 14, a modulator of fatty acid synthesis. *Proc. Natl. Acad. Sci. USA* **2010**, *107*, 18820–18825. [CrossRef]
40. Shen, Y.; Li, X.; Dong, D.; Zhang, B.; Xue, Y.; Shang, P. Transferrin receptor 1 in cancer: A new sight for cancer therapy. *Am. J. Cancer Res.* **2018**, *8*, 916–931.
41. Wang, C.Y.; Canali, S.; Bayer, A.; Dev, S.; Agarwal, A.; Babitt, J.L. Iron, erythropoietin, and inflammation regulate hepcidin in Bmp2-deficient mice, but serum iron fails to induce hepcidin in Bmp6-deficient mice. *Am. J. Hematol.* **2019**, *94*, 240–248. [CrossRef] [PubMed]
42. Doll, S.; Freitas, F.P.; Shah, R.; Aldrovandi, M.; da Silva, M.C.; Ingold, I.; Grocin, A.G.; da Silva, T.N.X.; Panzilius, E.; Scheel, C.H.; et al. FSP1 is a glutathione-independent ferroptosis suppressor. *Nature* **2019**, *575*, 693–698. [CrossRef] [PubMed]
43. Bersuker, K.; Hendricks, J.M.; Li, Z.P.; Magtanong, L.; Ford, B.; Tang, P.H.; Roberts, M.A.; Tong, B.Q.; Maimone, T.J.; Zoncu, R.; et al. The CoQ oxidoreductase FSP1 acts parallel to GPX4 to inhibit ferroptosis. *Nature* **2019**, *575*, 688–692. [CrossRef] [PubMed]
44. John, D.; Hayes, A.T.D.-K.; Kenneth, D.T. Oxidative Stress in Cancer. *Cancer Cell* **2020**, *38*, 167–197.
45. Hediger, M.A.; Romero, M.F.; Peng, J.B.; Rolfs, A.; Takanaga, H.; Bruford, E.A. The ABCs of solute carriers: Physiological, pathological and therapeutic implications of human membrane transport proteinsIntroduction. *Pflug. Arch.* **2004**, *447*, 465–468. [CrossRef] [PubMed]
46. Liu, Y.; Wang, J. Effects of DMSA-coated Fe_3O_4 nanoparticles on the transcription of genes related to iron and osmosis homeostasis. *Toxicol. Sci.* **2013**, *131*, 521–536. [CrossRef] [PubMed]
47. Raudenska, M.; Gumulec, J.; Podlaha, O.; Sztalmachova, M.; Babula, P.; Eckschlager, T.; Adam, V.; Kizek, R.; Masarik, M. Metallothionein polymorphisms in pathological processes. *Metallomics* **2014**, *6*, 55–68. [CrossRef]
48. Semenza, G.L. Hypoxia-inducible factor 1: Oxygen homeostasis and disease pathophysiology. *Trends Mol. Med.* **2001**, *7*, 345–350. [CrossRef]
49. Dewhirst, M.W.; Cao, Y.; Moeller, B. Cycling hypoxia and free radicals regulate angiogenesis and radiotherapy response. *Nat. Rev. Cancer* **2008**, *8*, 425–437. [CrossRef]

50. Bianchi, L.; Tacchini, L.; Cairo, G. HIF-1-mediated activation of transferrin receptor gene transcription by iron chelation. *Nucleic Acids Res.* **1999**, *27*, 4223–4227. [CrossRef]
51. Rose, C.R.; Ziemens, D.; Verkhratsky, A. On the special role of NCX in astrocytes: Translating Na^+-transients into intracellular Ca^{2+} signals. *Cell Calcium* **2020**, *86*, 102154. [CrossRef] [PubMed]
52. Malavolta, M.; Costarelli, L.; Giacconi, R.; Basso, A.; Piacenza, F.; Pierpaoli, E.; Provinciali, M.; Ogo, O.A.; Ford, D. Changes in Zn homeostasis during long term culture of primary endothelial cells and effects of Zn on endothelial cell senescence. *Exp. Gerontol.* **2017**, *99*, 35–45. [CrossRef] [PubMed]

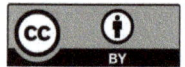

© 2020 by the authors. Licensee MDPI, Basel, Switzerland. This article is an open access article distributed under the terms and conditions of the Creative Commons Attribution (CC BY) license (http://creativecommons.org/licenses/by/4.0/).

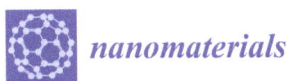

Review

Antioxidant Functionalized Nanoparticles: A Combat against Oxidative Stress

Harsh Kumar [1], Kanchan Bhardwaj [2], Eugenie Nepovimova [3], Kamil Kuča [3,*], Daljeet Singh Dhanjal [4], Sonali Bhardwaj [4], Shashi Kant Bhatia [5], Rachna Verma [2] and Dinesh Kumar [1,*]

1. School of Bioengineering & Food Technology, Shoolini University of Biotechnology and Management Sciences, Solan 173229, Himachal Pradesh, India; microharshs@gmail.com
2. School of Biological and Environmental Sciences, Shoolini University of Biotechnology and Management Sciences, Solan 173229, Himachal Pradesh, India; kanchankannu1992@gmail.com (K.B.); rachnaverma@shooliniuniversity.com (R.V.)
3. Department of Chemistry, Faculty of Science, University of Hradec Kralove, 50003 Hradec Kralove, Czech Republic; eugenie.nepovimova@uhk.cz
4. School of Biotechnology and Biosciences, Lovely Professional University, Phagwara 144411, Punjab, India; daljeetdhanjal92@gmail.com (D.S.D.); sonali.bhardwaj1414@gmail.com (S.B.)
5. Biotransformation and Biomaterials Laboratory, Department of Microbial Engineering, Konkuk University, Seoul 05029, Korea; shashikonkukuni@konkuk.ac.kr
* Correspondence: kamil.kuca@uhk.cz or kamil.kuca@fnhk.cz (K.K.); dineshkumar@shooliniuniversity.com (D.K.); Tel.: +420-603-289-166 (K.K.)

Received: 7 June 2020; Accepted: 6 July 2020; Published: 8 July 2020

Abstract: Numerous abiotic stresses trigger the overproduction of reactive oxygen species (ROS) that are highly toxic and reactive. These ROS are known to cause damage to carbohydrates, DNA, lipids and proteins, and build the oxidative stress and results in the induction of various diseases. To resolve this issue, antioxidants molecules have gained significant attention to scavenge these free radicals and ROS. However, poor absorption ability, difficulty in crossing the cell membranes and degradation of these antioxidants during delivery are the few challenges associated with both natural and synthetic antioxidants that limit their bioavailability. Moreover, the use of nanoparticles as an antioxidant is overlooked, and is limited to a few nanomaterials. To address these issues, antioxidant functionalized nanoparticles derived from various biological origin have emerged as an important alternative, because of properties like biocompatibility, high stability and targeted delivery. Algae, bacteria, fungi, lichens and plants are known as the producers of diverse secondary metabolites and phenolic compounds with extraordinary antioxidant properties. Hence, these compounds could be used in amalgamation with biogenic derived nanoparticles (NPs) for better antioxidant potential. This review intends to increase our knowledge about the antioxidant functionalized nanoparticles and the mechanism by which antioxidants empower nanoparticles to combat oxidative stress.

Keywords: oxidative stress; antioxidants; nanoparticles; biological nano-antioxidants

1. Introduction

In the twenty-first century, age-related diseases have become a major health concern worldwide. Ageing is a natural and progressive process which involves the degeneration of the functioning and structure of vital organs and is one of the risk factors responsible for numerous chronic diseases and accounts for the high mortality rate [1–4]. Among various theories thatunveil and elucidate the ageing process, the free radical theory holds an exceptional rank [5]. This theory states that the ageing occurs due to successive failure of the defense mechanism to resort the damage induced by the reactive oxygen species (ROS), especially in the mitochondria [6].

It is well comprehended that oxidative stress plays a significant role in degenerative senescence. ROS have been found to be involved in the pathogenesis of various cellular processes, and is also associated with numerous diseases like cardiovascular, cancer, neurodegenerative and respiratory diseases, as depicted in Figure 1 [7]. The rise in ROS concentration in cells have also been associated with ageing, however, it cannot be considered as the only determining factor responsible for ageing. Moreover, in age-related diseases, the elevated concentration of ROS has been involved in the impairment of mitochondria and cellular oxidative damage [2,8].

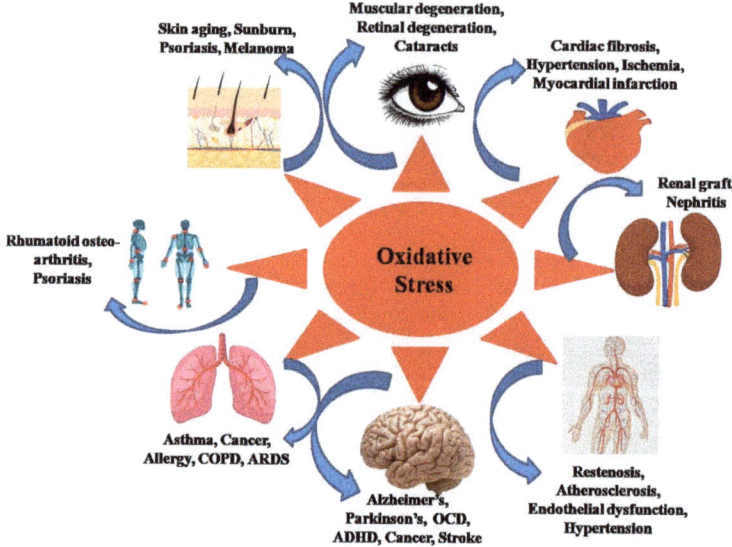

Figure 1. Side effects of oxidative stress on human body. COPD—Chronic obstructive pulmonary disease; ARDS—Acute respiratory distress syndrome; OCD—Obsessive-compulsive disorder; ADHD—Attention-deficit/hyperactivity disorder.

The production of ROS generally relies on both enzymatic as well as non-enzymatic reactions. The enzymatic reactions involved in various cellular processes, like phagocytosis, prostaglandin synthesis and respiratory chain system, are known to generate ROS [9–19]. The superoxide radical ($O2^{\bullet-}$) is synthesized during the activity of enzymes, like NADPH oxidase, peroxidase and xanthine oxidase, in various cellular processes. It has also been found that various other ROS, like hydrogen peroxide (H_2O_2), hydroxyl radical ($OH^{\bullet}$), hypochlorous acid (HOCl), peroxynitrite ($ONOO^-$), etc., are also formed during enzymatic reaction, and the action of enzymes like xanthine oxidase and amino acid oxidase leads to the formation of H_2O_2. Furthermore, $OH^{\bullet}$ is regarded as a highly reactive free radical species formed during the "Fenton reaction" between H_2O_2 and $O2^{\bullet-}$, in the presence Cu^+ or Fe^{2+}, which acts as the catalyst [11–18]. On the other hand, the non-enzymatic reactions between organic compounds and oxygen, or when cells are exposed to ionizing radiations and during mitochondrial respiration, have also been found to be involved in ROS formation [14,15,18]. At present, extensive research is being conducted to explore the natural compounds that can control oxidative stress and improve the immune system [20]. The search for novel molecules with antioxidant properties is an effective way to promote healthy ageing and counteract oxidative stress. Hence, this review focuses on highlighting the effectiveness of antioxidants functionalized nanoparticles. The first section of the review discusses synergism between ROS and age-related diseases, antioxidants and sources of antioxidants. The section following that discusses the role of nano-antioxidants; antioxidant functionalized nanoparticles and challenges associate with them.

2. Synergism between ROS and Age-Related Diseases

The overproductions of ROS have been found to be associated with numerous chronic diseases like cancer, cardiovascular, neurodegenerative and respiratory ailments. The synergism between ROS and chronic diseases is discussed in the following sections.

2.1. Cancer

Cancer, a fatal disease involves the malignant growth of tumors because of chromosomal alteration and lead to unregulated growth of the cells [21]. This deadly disease has a complex relationship with ROS and is involved at three different levels of cancer development, i.e., initiation, progression and promotion [22]. During the initiation stage, the ROS causes a mutation in DNA, which keeps on accumulating when the affected tissue does not get repaired [23]. The overproduction of ROS triggers the mutation in an oncogene, which potentially contributes to the initiation of cancer [24].

The cancer cells favor the excessive production of ROS in comparison to healthy cells, because of the alteration in the metabolic processes [25]. ROS-induced oxidative stresses in tumor triggers the cell signaling pathways and build resistance in tumor cells and elevate the supply of blood to tumor cells and promote their metastasis [26]. The elevated level of ROS plays a significant role in expanding tumor cells by altering the genes associated with apoptosis, cell proliferation and transcription factors [27]. Furthermore, ROS also downregulate the pro-apoptotic proteins by interfering with the Akt/PI3K and ERK cell signaling pathway, and upregulate the anti-apoptotic genes [28,29]. During the cancer progression stage, ROS interferes with cellular processes and upregulates the production of metalloproteinases by obstructing the angiogenesis process and, by anti-proteases, results in the metastasis of cancer cells [23,25,30].

2.2. Cardiovascular Disease

Cardiovascular disease, another fatal ailment, has a strong association with ROS during the development stage [31]. The overproduction of ROS in vascular cells during the reactions involving enzymes like NADPH oxidase, nitric oxide synthases causes the modification in low-density lipoproteins (LDL) [32]. Furthermore, ROS are also found to be involved in cardiac hypertrophy development, myocyte apoptosis and ischemia-reperfusion injury, which ultimately lead to cardiac arrest [33–35].

2.3. Neurodegenerative Diseases

Neurons are fundamental units of the brain and play a significant role in coordinating the actions and reactions of bodily functions. These neurons are highly vulnerable to ROS, as they weaken the antioxidants defense system, elevate the fatty acid (polyunsaturated) content in the cell membrane and increase the oxygen demand [36]. The significant research conducted in this direction revealed that ROS generation takes place through numerous mechanisms, and play a vital role in developing neurodegenerative diseases like Alzheimer's, Huntington's and Parkinson's disease. These ROS considerably affects the neuron and other cellular processes, the controlling of ROS level may serve as a potential treatment to restrain neurodegenerative disorder and provide relief from its associated symptoms [37].

2.4. Respiratory Disorders

Asthma and chronic obstructive pulmonary disease (COPD) are major respiratory disorders, accounting for high mortality worldwide [38]. Exposure to cigarette smoke and air pollutants significantly contributes to the overproduction of ROS in both asthma and COPD patients. The ROS primarily affects and damages the alveolar and connective tissues of the pulmonary system [39]. The overproduction of ROS also triggers the inflammatory cells, which, as a result, shows production of ROS in the pulmonary system. The ROS are predominantly observed during pathophysiology analysis for both asthma and COPD [40]. It is still unclear how increased ROS is a causative factor for these respiratory diseases [41]. Researchers are extensively working in this direction to decipher the role of these ROS in progression of these fatal diseases.

This synergism between ROS and these chronic diseases shows the major challenge associated with oxidative stress induced by ROS, and requires the effective solution to meet the challenges imposed by the overproduction of ROS.

3. Antioxidants

An antioxidant can be described as any substance or compound capable of inhibiting the oxidation of suitable substrate even when present in low concentrations [42]. During the late 19th and early 20th century, the exploration of antioxidants resulted in a boom, due to their involvement in various industrial processes like the prevention of corrosion, the polymerization of fuels, fouling in combustion engines and the vulcanization of rubber [43]. The application of antioxidants was limited for the prevention of the oxidation of unsaturated fats, as it resulted in the rancidity of fats [44]. The general procedure to determine the antioxidant potential of any compound involves the assessment of the rate of oxygen consumption when fat is kept in an enclosed container with oxygen. The identification of vitamins A, C and E, which act as antioxidant agents, has revolutionized the field and highlighted the significance of antioxidants in the biochemistry of living beings [45,46].

Another way to understand the antioxidant is that it is a stable molecule, which donates an electron to unwanted free radical species and neutralizes it, and curbs its ability to cause damage. In general, these antioxidants either inhibit or delay the cellular damage because of their scavenging properties [47]. The low molecular weight of these antioxidants allows them to interact with ROS (free radicals) easily and terminate their chain reaction before damaging vital molecules. Glutathione, uric acid and ubiquinol are few antioxidant molecules that are generated by our body during normal metabolic processes [48]. There are various enzymes are present in our body that can scavenge free radicals, and micronutrients like ascorbic acid (vitamin C), β-carotene and α-tocopherol (vitamin E) [49]. The body cannot produce these micronutrients on its own, therefore, these molecules are obtained from the consumed food.

4. Sources of Antioxidants

Dietary supplements are key source of antioxidants, which could aid in maintaining good health and prevent the onset of fatal diseases triggered by ROS. Even though some synthetic antioxidants have been developed, their carcinogenic and toxic nature has prompted the exploration for natural antioxidants like vitamins A, C and E [50]. Additionally, population studies have also revealed that the consumption of fruits, tea, vegetables and wine are a reliable source of natural antioxidants, and are effective in regulating the risk of cardiovascular diseases, which has intrigued researchers to exploring their potential as natural antioxidants [51]. Dietary supplements contain antioxidant compounds in the form of phytochemicals i.e., α-tocopherol, β-carotene, vitamin C, vitamin E and various phenolic compounds [52]. Numerous ethnomedicinal plants, fruits, vegetables, mushrooms and other spices have been well-documented as sources of natural antioxidants, which play a significant role in promoting healthy life and treating various fatal diseases [53].

Phenolic compounds obtained from natural sources are considered far better than synthesized chemicals. Microbes are also being explored for synthesizing organic compounds with antioxidant potential. Various fungal strains have been reported to produce compounds like ellagic acid, ferulic acid and gallic acid under solid-state fermentation and submerged fermentation conditions [54]. All these compounds are known to contain 2–4 reactive hydroxyl groups, which impart them the antioxidant potential. In addition, algae and lichens are active producers of different secondary metabolites, including antioxidants (Table 1).

Table 1. Antioxidants from different biological sources.

Source	Antioxidants	Ref.
Bacteria	Thiazostatins A, 5-(2,4-Dimethylbenzyl) Pyrrolidin-2-One, Phenazoviridin, Benthophoenin, Benthocyanins A, B and C, Benzastatins A, B and C, Benzastatins C, (Z)-1-((1-Hydroxypenta-2,4-Dien-1-Yl)Oxy)Anthracene-9,10-Dione	[53]
Plants	Gallic acid, Protocatechuic acid, p-Coumaric acid, Caffeic acid, Rosmarinic acid, Carnosol, Carnosic acid, Rosmanol, Rutin, Epicatechin gallate, Epigallocatechin gallate, Epicatechin, Quercetin (flavanol), Eugenol, Carvacrol, Safrole, Thymol, Myristicin, Menthol, 1,8-Cineol, α-Terpineol, p-Cymene, Cinnamaldehyde, Piperine, Flavone, Flavonol, Chalcone, Flavanone, Anthocyanin, Anthocyanidin-3,5-glucoside, Alpha tocopherol, Gamma tocopherol, Ascorbic acid, Ascorbyl palmitate, Propyl gallate, Resveratrol	[55]
Fungi	Isopestacin, Pestacin, Atrovenetin, 2-Acetonyl-2,4,9,-Trihydroxy-6-Methoxy-7-Methyl-1HPhenalene-1,3(2H)-Dione, Graphislactone, 4,6-dihydroxy-5-methoxy-7-methyl-1,3-dihydroisobenzofuran, 4,5,6-trihydroxy-7-methyl-1,3-dihydroisobenzofuran, 3″-Dihydroxyterphenyllin and 3-Hydroxyterphenyllin, p-Hydroxybenzoic acid, Protocatechuic acid, Gallic acid, Gentisic acid, Vanillic acid, 5-Sulfosalicylic acid, Syringic acid, Veratric acid, Vanillin, Cinnamic acid, p-Coumaric acid, o-Coumaric acid, Caffeic acid, Ferulic acid, 3-O-Caffeoylquinic acid, 4-O-Caffeoylquinic acid, 5-O-Caffeoylquinic acid, Quercetin, Rutin, Kaempferol, Myricetin, Chrysin, Catechin, Hesperetin, Naringenin, Naringin, Formometin, Biochanin, Pyrogallol, Resveratrol, Ellagic acid, Tannic acid, Sinapic acid, Flavonols, Flavones, Isoflavones, Flavanones, Anthocyanidins, Flavanols, Vitamin C, Vitamin E, Homogentisic acid	[53,56,57]
Algae	β-carotene, Lutein, Bromophenol, Carrageenan, Fucophlorethols, Fucoxanthin, Galactan sulphate, Phlorotannins, Phycoerythrin, Porphyran, Shinorine, Catechin, Epicatechin, Gallate, Alginic acid, Laminaran, Vitamin A, Phloroglucinol, Eckol, Fucodiphlorethol G, Phlorofucofuroeckol A, 7-phloroeckol, Dieckol, 6,6′-bieckol, Triphlorethol-A, 2,7′-phloroglucinol-6,6′-bieckol	[58,59]
Lichens	1-Chloropannarin, 2-O-Methylsekikaic acid, Atranol, Atranorin, Barbatic acid, Boninic acid, Chloroatranol, Chloroatranorin, Chlorohematommic acid, Cryptostictinolide, Divaricatic acid, Ergosterol peroxide, Ethyl chlorohematommate, Evernic acid, Fumarprotocetraric acid, Gyrophoric acid, Hematommic acid, Lecanoric acid, Lecanoric acid, Methyl orsellinate, Orcinol, Physodic acid, Protrocetraric acid, Sekikaic acid, Umbilicaric acid	[60]

185

5. Nano-Antioxidants

Antioxidants have been accorded as effective therapeutic and prophylactic agents for various diseases. However, these antioxidants have received very limited success until now, as most of the antioxidants show low permeability, and are poorly soluble in water, demonstrate instability during storage and gastrointestinal degradation, which are some of their limitations [61]. The amalgamation of material sciences with nanotechnology has substantially improved and reduced the free radical synthesis during nanoparticle production in different areas and the nanoparticles synthesized for this purpose are regarded as nano-antioxidants [62,63]. Carbon nanotubes, metal and metal oxide nanoparticles and various types of polymer-loaded antioxidant nanoparticles, have been reported to exhibit antioxidant properties [63]. In the past few decades, various preparation protocols, such as emulsion/solvent evaporation, supercritical fluid technology, solvent displacement method, templating method and nanoprecipitation techniques, have been used for synthesizing nano-oxidants [63]. Some oxide nanoparticles can scavenge the reactive nitrogen and reactive oxygen species (RNS/ROS) and mimic the antioxidant molecule, due to their intrinsic physicochemical properties [64]. In the biomedical field, cerium oxide nanoparticles (CONPs) have gathered special attention for their multi-enzymatic scavenging of ROS and their regenerative abilities [65]. These CONPs have unique properties, like the coexistence in both oxidation states i.e., Ce^{3+} and Ce^{4+}, the ability to reversibly switch between both oxidation states and the reduction potential of ~1.52 V [66]. Cerium dioxide as a bulk crystal primarily contains Ce^{4+}, but during its reduction to nano-size, substantially enhances the relative amount of Ce^{3+}, therefore, leading to higher catalytic activity, in contrast to various biological processes and biological antioxidants [67,68]. Hirst et al. (2013) conducted an in vivo test on mice to assess the antioxidant potential of nanoceria, which were injected intravenously in the subject, and the result of the study revealed that nanoceria significantly decreased the lipoperoxidation after the three weeks, which indicates that CONPs are effective in treating oxidative stress [69]. Caputo et al. (2015) conducted a comparative study to assess the antioxidant potential between CONPs and NAC (N-acetyl-cysteine) and Trolox (soluble analogues of vitamin E) [70]. The results of this study revealed that NAC and Trolox reduced the oxidative 2′-7′-Dichlorofluorescein (DCF) signal triggered by irradiated TiO_2 nanoparticles, but the antioxidant potential was significantly lower in comparison to CONPs. This result also highlights the stability of CONPs because of their auto-regenerative redox cycle, which allows them to surpass the challenges related to the stability of the antioxidants molecules.

On the other hand, synthetic polymeric NPs have emerged as the promising nano-drug delivery system, as they can encapsulate the therapeutic agent and progressively release the therapeutic compound at the target site. Poly-D, L-lactide (PLA) and poly (lactic-co-glycolic acid) (PLGA) are some examples of synthetic biodegradable polymers that have been approved safe by the European Medicine Agency (EMA) and U.S. Food and Drug Administration (FDA) for administration (Table 2).

Table 2. In vivo and in vitro delivery of antioxidants by different nanoparticles.

Nanoparticles	Delivered Antioxidant/Enzyme	Method of Preparation	Characterization	Size	Test System	Biological Effects	Ref.
Poly(lactide-co glycolide) (PLGA) and Polycaprolactone (PCL)	Ellagic acid	Emulsion-diffusion-evaporation	DLS, Zeta potential	ND	Overnight fasted male Sprague Dawley (SD) rats	Prevent cyclosporine A (CyA)-induced nephrotoxicity	[71]
Polybutylcyanoacrylate, Liposomes, Poly(Lactide-co-Glycolide)	Superoxide dismutase (SOD)	Emulsion solvent evaporation	DLS, Zeta potential	ND	C57BL/6 mice	Nanoparticles displayed protection against reperfusion injury and ischemia when applied after injury reduced in infarct volume with a 50% to 60%, lowered inflammatory markers, and improved in mice behavior	[72]
Iron oxide (magnetite)	Catalase and SOD	Nanoprecipitation	Zeta potential, TEM	303 ± 38 nm (Catalase loaded), 350 ± 10 nm (SOD loaded)	Bovine aortic endothelial cells (BAEC), Primary human umbilical vein endothelial cells (HUVEC)	Cultured endothelial cells rapidly take magnetically responsive nanoparticles (MNP) under magnetic guidance catalase-loaded providing increased resistance to oxidative stress (62 ± 12% cells rescued from hydrogen peroxide induced cell death vs. 10 ± 4% under non-magnetic conditions)	[73]
Poly(lactide-co glycolide) (PLGA)	SOD	Emulsion solvent evaporation	TEM, DLS, Zeta potential	81 ± 4 nm	Male Sprague-Dawley rats	NPs encapsulated by superoxide dismutase helps in reduction of cerebral injury and promote neurological recovery in a rat cerebral ischemia-reperfusion model	[74]
Bovine serum albumin (BSA)-dextran	Curcumin	Self-assembly	TEM, DLS, Zeta potential	115 nm	Caco-2 cells	At 5 µg/mL curcumin in BSA-dextran nanoparticle the CAA (cellular antioxidant activity) value was 65.35, significantly more that of free curcumin (48.61) at the same concentration, showing that nanoencapsulation increased the uptake of curcumin ($p < 0.05$). Curcumin-loaded BSA-dextran nanoparticle EC_{50} values was 3.27 µg/mL, indicating the CAA of curcumin was enhanced by nanoparticle-based delivery systems	[75]
Mesoporous silica	Caffeic acid, Rutin	ND	TEM, Zeta potential	200 nm	Caco-2 and the epidermal HaCaT cell lines	After 24 h incubation of cells with grafted nanoparticles the best results were given by Rutin in terms of antioxidant capacities preservation during coupling procedures, decrease of ROS level and cellular toxicity alleviation. Rutin protective effects were found more apparated in HaCaT than in Caco-2 cells, revealing much cellular specificity towards defense against oxidative stress; MSN-RUT has ability to stimulate a strong Nrf2 protective response in HaCaT cells, accompanied by a comparable induction of HO-1 mRNA. These responses level in Caco-2 cells was again less important.	[76]
Chitosan/alginate	Quercetin	Gelation	Zeta potential	ND	Human hepatocellular carcinoma HepG2 cells and Male Wistar rats (paracetamol-induced liver injury)	Pretreatment of HepG2 cells with (10 µg/mL) encapsulated quercetin significantly reduction in cell viability in H_2O_2-induced oxidative stress (0.1 mM H_2O_2), thus showing an efficacious in vitro protection; oral pretreatment with encapsulated quercetin (0.18 mg/kg b.w. 7 days) significantly reduced the increased serum transaminases ALT and AST levels, reduced the lipid peroxidation and restored the gluthation (a marker of cell antioxidant defence system) levels	[77]
Stearic acid- and stearyl ferulate-based solid lipid	Trans-ferulic acid	Microemulsion	DLS, TEM	505 ± 8.2 (SLN-FA), 600 ± 3.4 nm (SLN-SF-FA)	Male rats	Both SLN-SF-FA and SLN-FA dose-dependently reduced lipid peroxidation induced by the three oxidants (NADPH/ADP-Fe^{3+}, AAPH and SIN-1). SLN-SF-FA showed high efficiency (EC_{50}) and potency (maximal activity) against NADPH/ADPFe^{3+} and AAPH-induced lipid peroxidation	[78]

TEM—transmission electron microscopy; DLS—dynamic light scattering; ND—not defined.

Liposomes are also used for delivering the antioxidant agents to the target site. The amphiphilic and biocompatible nature of these liposomes allows them to load both hydrophilic and lipophilic compounds and favor the encapsulation of the water-soluble and water-insoluble antioxidant enzymes [79].

Furthermore, chitosan is the material predominantly used for synthesizing nanoparticles as a sole material or in amalgamation with another [80]. Chitosan shows mucoadhesive properties, which improves the targeted delivery in mucosal surfaces such as intestinal and nasal epithelium [81]. Curcumin encapsulated in nanocarrier and covered and stabilized with chitosan has also been developed and evaluated for free radical scavenging in comparison with free curcumin, and showed the protective effect of chitosan on the antioxidant activity of curcumin [82]. Pu et al. (2014) reported the encapsulation of curcumin antioxidant compounds within the nanocarrier and regulation of release of antioxidant compounds, by changing the pH and oxidative stress of inflamed tissues to increase the overproduction of RNS/ROS synthesized by lipopolysaccharide (LPS)-stimulated macrophage [83].

6. Antioxidant Functionalized Nanoparticles

Bacteria, algae, fungi, lichens and plants are known to contain diverse bioactive compounds like terpenoids, alkaloids, polyphenols, phenolic acids etc. These bioactive compounds show potential antioxidant activity, and are known to reduce and stabilize the metallic ions. The diverse types of antioxidant functionalized nanoparticles derived from various biological extracts (Table 3) are discussed in the following sections.

Table 3. Antioxidant potential of functionalized nanoparticles.

Antioxidant Source	Types of Nanoparticles	Biological Extract	Temperature	Reaction Time	Characterizations	Morphology	Size	Stability	Antioxidant Activity	Ref.
Plant	Silver	*Lantana camara* L. leaves extract (terpenes rich)	RT	24 h	UV-Vis, XRD, Zeta potential, SEM	Sphere	425 nm	Nd	A10 μL of AgNP (2 mg/mL), spot intensity was found good and comparable with ascorbic acid	[84]
	Silver	*Taraxacum officinale* leaf extract	RT	15 min	UV-Vis, XRD, FTIR, HRTEM	Sphere	15 nm	4 months	The efficiency of AgNPs were found against ABTS radicals, displayed an IC_{50} value of 45.6 μg/mL; scavenging potential of Nitric Oxide is 72.1% at 100 μg/mL concentration with IC_{50} value of 55.2 μg/mL	[85]
	Silver	*Bergenia ciliate* crude extract	RT	3 h	UV-Vis, SEM, FTIR	Sphere	35 nm	Nd	Results of DPPH activity showed the effective free radical % scavenging potential of *Bergenia ciliate* AgNPs is 59.31%	[86]
	Silver	*Clerodendrum phlomidis* L. leaves extract	RT	10 min	UV-Vis, SEM, TEM, EDAX, FT-IR	Sphere	23–42 nm	Nd	AgNPs exhibited remarkable antioxidant activity than the crude extract using phosphomolybdate assay, ferric reducing power, superoxide radical scavenging activity and DPPH assay	[87]
	Silver	*Hippophae rhamnoides* L. leaves extract	RT	24 h	UV-Vis, TEM, HRTEM, FTIR	Sphere	10–40 nm	1 year	The SBT@AgNPs showed excellent DPPH radical scavenging capacity. The results also revealed that the antioxidant properties of the samples depends on dose as their concentrations (5–25 μg mL^{-1}) increase their percentage DPPH radical scavenging abilities also increased	[88]
	Gold	*Hippophae rhamnoides* ssp. *Turkestanica* leaves and berries extract	RT	2 min (LE), 15 min (BE)	UV-Vis, HRTEM, FTIR, XRD	Triangles, hexagon and sphere (BE AuNPs), Sphere (LE AuNPs)	55 nm (BE AuNPs), 27 nm (LE AuNPs)	5 months	Colorimetric DPPH assay at (80 μg/mL) concentration showed, free radical scavenging activity was found maximum in LE AuNPs (81%) and BE (70%) AuNPs. LE AuNPs nanospheres (IC_{50} 49 μg) revealed a little better (14%) antioxidant capacity as compared to BE nanotriangles (IC_{50} 57 μg)	[89]
	Silver	*Morus alba* leaf extract	RT	10 min	UV-Vis, FTIR, SEM, FESEM, EDX, HRTEM, XRD, DLS	Sphere	12–39 nm	Nd	Dose dependent antioxidant activity against free radicals like DPPH, ABTS$^+$, superoxide and nitric oxide	[90]
	Gold	*Couroupita guianensis* Aubl. fruit extract	70 °C	60 min	UV-Vis, FTIR, TEM, XRD, DLS, Zeta potential	Cubic	26 nm	45 days	For DPPH assay, CGAuNPs IC_{50} was 37 μg/mL; CGAuNPs were potent in scavenging the hydroxyl radicals with IC_{50} values of 30 and 36 μg/mL respectively; CGAuNPs superoxide scavenging activity increased with increasing concentrations and was observed as 89.8% inhibition rate	[91]

Table 3. Cont.

Antioxidant Source	Types of Nanoparticles	Biological Extract	Temperature	Reaction Time	Characterizations	Morphology	Size	Stability	Antioxidant Activity	Ref.
	Silver	Citrullus lanatus rind extract	RT	24 h	UV-Vis, SEM, EDX, FTIR, XRD	Sphere	109.97 nm	Nd	AgNPs DPPH free radical scavenging activity at 20–100 µg/mL ranged from 21.65% to 60.97%; AgNPs ABTS radical scavenging activity was 11.25% to 55.26% at a concentration of 20–100 µg/mL; AgNPs Nitric oxide scavenging activity was 9.05% to 54.15% at a concentration of 20–100 µg/mL.	[92]
	Silver	Erythrina suberosa (Roxb.) leaf extract	RT	Over night	UV-Vis, ATR-FTIR, DLS, TEM,	Sphere	12–115 nm	Nd	AgNPs antioxidant potential was estimated by DPPH radical scavenging assay having IC_{50} 30.04 µg/mL	[93]
	Silver	Thymus kotschyanus extract	RT	30 min	UV-Vis, FTIR, XRD, EDS, SEM, AFM, HRTEM	Sphere	50–60 nm	Nd	AgNPs DPPH free radical scavenging activities demonstrate effective inhibition as compared to BHT as the standard antioxidant	[94]
	Zinc Oxide	Berberis aristata leaf extract	70 °C	ND	UV-Vis, XRD, FTIR, SEM, EDX, DLS	Needle	90–110 nm	Nd	B. aristata leaves extract ZnO nanoparticles showed percent inhibition of 32.06% at the concentration of 1 µg/mL and for 5 µg/mL it was to be 61.63%	[95]
	Gold	Vitex negundo leaf extract	RT	ND	UV-Vis, XRD, FTIR, TEM	Sphere	20–70 nm	Nd	Radical scavenging activity of DPPH shown that at a 120 µg/mL concentration, the scavenging activity NPs reached 84.64% and the IC_{50} of the NPs was found to be 62.18 µg; The nitric oxide assay results revealed that the antioxidant property of NPs at a concentration of 120 µg/mL, the NPs scavenging activity reached 69.79% with IC_{50} estimated at 70.45 µg	[96]
	Silver	Cestrum nocturnum leaf extract	RT	1 week	XRD, TEM, EDS, SEM, FTIR,	Sphere	20 nm	Nd	AgNPs antioxidant activity for DPPH method was 29.55%	[97]
	Copper Oxide	Hibiscus rosasinensis leaf extract	RT	48 h	UV-Vis, FTIR, TEM	ND	ND	Nd	Good antioxidant activity from FRAP assay	[98]
	Copper Oxide	Dioscorea bulbifera tuber extract	40 °C	5 h	UV-Vis, TEM, EDS, XRD, DLS	Sphere	86–126 nm	Nd	Showed 40.81 ± 1.44%, 79.06 ± 1.02% and 48.39 ± 1.46% scavenging activity against DPPH, nitric oxide and superoxide radicals respectively	[99]
	Copper Oxide	Adiantum lunulatum whole plant extract	RT	1 h	UV-Vis, DLS, TEM, EDX, XRD, FTIR	Sphere	6.5 nm	Nd	CAT, APX, and SOD activities have steadily increased according to the increasing concentration of copper nanoparticles treatment to Lens culinaris	[100]
	Copper Oxide	Galeopsitis herba. G. herba extract	25 °C	24 h	UV-Vis, SEM, FTIR, TEM	Sphere	10 nm	Nd	Showed good scavenging activity against DPPH	[101]

Table 3. Cont.

Antioxidant Source	Types of Nanoparticles	Biological Extract	Temperature	Reaction Time	Characterizations	Morphology	Size	Stability	Antioxidant Activity	Ref.
	Copper Oxide	*Cissus arnotiana* leaf extract	RT	4 h	UV-Vis, XRD, SEM, TEM	Sphere	80–90 nm	Nd	The antioxidant property observed was comparatively equal with the standard antioxidant agent ascorbic acid at a maximum concentration of 40 µg/mL DPPH assay	[102]
	Iron	*Amaranthus dubius* leaf extract	60 °C	90 min	UV-Vis, FTIR, XRD, SEM	Sphere	43–220 nm	Nd	Showed high antioxidant activity against DPPH	[103]
	Iron	*Amaranthus spinosus* leaf extract	RT	90 min	UV-Vis, FTIR, TEM, EDX, XRD	Sphere	ND	Nd	Antioxidant efficiency was observed to be 93% against DPPH	[104]
	Iron	*Asphodelus aestivus* Brot. extract	50–60 °C	20 min	UV-Vis, FTIR, TEM, EDX, SEM, XRD	NS	20–25 nm	Nd	Antioxidant activity against DPPH (IC$_{50}$: 3.48 µg/mL) and ABTS (60.52%)	[105]
	Nickel Oxide	*Stevia rebaudiana* Bertoni leaf extract	100 °C	2 h	UV-Vis, XRD, SEM, TEM, FTIR	Sphere	20–50 nm	Nd	Antioxidant efficiency was observed to be 70% against DPPH	[106]
	Gold	*Lactobacillus kimchicus* DCY51^T biomass	RT	12 h	UV-Vis, FE-TEM, XRD, DLS, FTIR	Sphere	13 nm	NS	Lowest concentration of the biosynthesized AuNps DPPH percentage scavenging ability was 15.85 ± 0.49 and when concentration was increased to 500 µg/mL this scavenging ability was increased to 60 ± 1.82	[107]
	Silver	*Streptomyces griseorubens* AU2 cell free supernatant	RT	48 h	UV-Vis, FTIR, TEM, SEM, XRD	Sphere	5–20 nm	Nd	DPPH free radical scavenging activity of AgNPs showed at various concentrations viz. 9.66, 14.27, 15.59, 23.46 and 54.99%	[108]
	Gold	*Enterococcus* species cell free extract	RT	30 min	UV-Vis, TEM, EDX, FTIR	Sphere	8–50 nm	Nd	AuNPs have ability to scavenge DPPH at all the investigated concentrations (1–40 µg/mL), yielding activities of 33.24–51.47%	[109]
Bacteria	Gold and Silver	*Escherichia coli* cell protein	RT	ND	UV-Vis, XRD, FTIR, TEM	Triangular, circular, hexagonal (AuNPs), Sphere (AgNPs)	10–100 nm (AuNPs), 10–50 nm (AgNPs)	3 months	EC$_{75}$ (for scavenging 75% effective concentration) of protein capped gold nanoparticles is 916 µg/mL	[110]
	Silver	*Streptomyces rugosisii* MA7 biomass	RT	72 h	UV-Vis, FTIR, XRD, EDX, AFM, SEM, TEM, HRTEM	Sphere	5–50 nm	Nd	At a concentration of 1000 µg/mL, AgNPs showed good reducing power comparatively than ascorbic acid (vitamin C)	[111]
	Selenium	*Streptomyces minutiscleroticus* M10A62 biomass	RT	72 h	UV-Vis, XRD, HRTEM, FTIR, EDX	Sphere	10–250 nm	Nd	SeNPs actinobacterially synthesized were found strong free radical scavenging activity compared with standard ascorbic acid was proved by positive DPPH activity. Free radical scavenging activity depends on concentration as increases with increased concentration of SeNPs	[112]
	Selenium	*Pantoea agglomerans* UC-32	RT	24 h	TEM, EDS, SEM	Sphere	100 nm	Nd	High antioxidant activity in human umbilical vein endothelial cells	[113]

Table 3. Cont.

Antioxidant Source	Types of Nanoparticles	Biological Extract	Temperature	Reaction Time	Characterizations	Morphology	Size	Stability	Antioxidant Activity	Ref.
	Gold and Silver	*Gordonia amicalis* HS-11 cell free supernatant	100 °C	10 min	UV-Vis, XRD, TEM, FTIR	Grain	5–25 nm	Nd	CPS synthesized AgNPs and AuNPs respectively, showed 88.5 and 87.75% inhibition towards hydroxyl radicals; CPS mediated AuNPs inhibited nitric oxide radicals by 67.5% and with AgNPs the inhibited by 61.5%	[114]
	Silver	*Streptomyces violaceus* MM72 exopolysaccharides	RT	1 h	TEM, EDX, XRD	ND	30 nm	Nd	The DPPH radical scavenging activity shown by SNPs of 89.5% at 50 µg/mL concentration; SNPs exhibited the more total antioxidant activity of 0.730 at 50 µg/mL concentration; H_2O_2 scavenging activity of SNPs was evaluated at different concentrations, 50 µg/mL exhibited a higher activity of 72.5% which was significantly higher than that of the standard L-ascorbic acid; SNPs (50 µg/mL) had a nitric oxide scavenging activity of 60.1%; Ferric reducing power of the SNPs was estimated by the reduction of Fe/ferricyanide and the inhibition was observed at 0.390 AU at 50 µg/mL	[115]
	Zinc Oxide	*Pichia kudriavzevii* cell free extract	RT	36 h	UV-Vis, XRD, TEM, Zeta potential	Hexagonal	10–61 nm	Nd	DPPH radical scavenging activities IC_{50} values were 10 ± 0.52, 5.26 ± 0.42 and 25.46 ± 0.35 µg/mL for ZnO/T1, ZnO/T2 and ZnO/T3 respectively	[116]
Fungi	Silver	*Pestalotiopsis microspora* filtrate	RT	24 h	UV-Vis, FTIR, XRD, TEM, DLS	Sphere	2–10 nm	Nd	IC_{50} concentrations (the concentration of the sample required to scavenge 50% radicals) of the biosynthesized AgNPs were found to be 76.95 ± 2.96 µg/mL; Biosynthesized AgNPs also exhibited effective scavenging activity against H_2O_2 radicals and the maximum scavenging activity of $51.14\% \pm 1.78\%$ was observed at the highest concentration of 100 µg/mL	[117]
	Gold	*Cladosporium cladosporioides* filtrate	RT	ND	UV-Vis, FESEM, EDX, XRD, FTIR, DLS, AFM	Cubic	100 nm	6 months	DPPH radical scavenging capacity of the AuNPs was found to be dose dependent; AuNPs was subjected to reducing power assay where it showed moderate activity of 1.51 ± 0.03 mg of AAE/g sample	[118]
	Silver	*Cladosporium cladosporioides* filtrate	RT	ND	UV-Vis, FESEM, XRD, FTIR, DLS, AFM	Sphere	100 nm	Nd	AgNPs showed potent antioxidant potential and their radical scavenging ability was increasing with increment in their concentration	[119]

Table 3. Cont.

Antioxidant Source	Types of Nanoparticles	Biological Extract	Temperature	Reaction Time	Characterizations	Morphology	Size	Stability	Antioxidant Activity	Ref.
	Silver	*Aspergillus versicolor* ENT7 filtrate	RT	24 h	UV-Vis, TEM, XRD, FTIR	Sphere	3–40 nm	Nd	The radical scavenging activity for the AgNPs at 100 µg/mL was determined as 60.04% which is close to 68.52% obtained for the standard ascorbic acid at the same concentration. IC_{50} value for the AgNPs is found to be 60.64 µg/mL	[120]
	Silver	*Trichoderma atroviride* cell free filtrate	40 °C	ND	UV-Vis, TEM, EDS, FTIR	Variables	15–25 nm	Nd	AgNPs exhibited quite higher DPPH scavenging activity at concentration dependent manner with IC_{50} of 45.6 µg/mL	[121]
	Zinc Oxide	*Aspergillus niger* cell free filtrate	RT	24 h	UV-Vis, FTIR, XRD, DLS, SEM	Rod and cluster	80–130 nm	Nd	Maximum DPPH scavenging of 57.74% was obtained at 100 µg/mL concentration of ZnONPs; ABTS assay scavenging of 73.58% was obtained at 100 µg/mL concentration of ZnONPs	[122]
	Silver	*Penicillium* species extract	RT	10 min	UV-Vis, SEM, XRD	Sphere	18 nm	Nd	FRAP reducing ability potentially reduced by PsAgNPs was 1109.41 where the standard ascorbic acid shows 1648.52 µm	[123]
	Silver	*Inonotus obliquus* extract	RT	80 min	UV-Vis, SEM, EDX, TEM, XRD, FTIR	Sphere	14.2–35.2 nm	8 months	Free radical scavenging activity of the AgNPs on ABTS radicals was found to increase with increase in the concentration, showing maximum inhibition (76.57%) at 1 mM and minimum inhibition (60.98%) at 0.125 mM solution	[124]
	Silver	*Cladosporium* species extract	RT	1 h	UV-Vis, SEM, XRD, FTIR	Sphere	24 nm	Nd	CsAgNPs exhibited potent antioxidant potential and as the concentration increases the radical scavenging ability also increases	[125]
	Silver	*Ganoderma lucidum* and *Agaricus Bisporus* extract	RT and 60 °C	12 h (RT), 5 h (60 °C)	UV-Vis, SEM, XRD, FTIR	Rod	10–80 nm	Nd	EHT synthesized AgNPs shows higher antioxidant activity (75% ± 0.24%) in comparison of standard (70.34% ± 0.03%)	[126]
	Gold	*Inonotus obliquus* extract	RT	30 min	UV-Vis, SEM, EDX, TEM, AFM, XRD, FTIR	Sphere, triangle, hexagonal and rod	23 nm	Nd	ABTS scavenging effect increased with increasing concentration of AuNPs. The ABTS radical scavenging activity showed a maximum and minimum at 1 mM and 0.125 mM, respectively	[127]
	Silver	*Ganoderma lucidum* extract	RT	ND	UV-Vis, TEM, XRD, FTIR, XPS	Sphere	15–22 nm	Nd	DPPH free radicals scavenging activity of AgNPs raised from 32.57% to 54.16% when concentration raised from 50 mg/L to 100 mg/L	[128]
	Silver	*Ganoderma lucidum* extract	60 °C	24 h	UV-Vis, XRD, SEM, FTIR	Sphere	10–30 nm	Nd	Percentage of inhibition by silver nanoparticles showing maximum with 73.49% and minimum with 55.34% at 100 and 10 µg/mL respectively	[129]

Table 3. Cont.

Antioxidant Source	Types of Nanoparticles	Biological Extract	Temperature	Reaction Time	Characterizations	Morphology	Size	Stability	Antioxidant Activity	Ref.
Algae	Gold	*Gracilaria corticata* extract	40 °C	4 h	UV-Vis, SEM	ND	45–57 nm	Nd	Synthesized AuNPs revealed a good capacity of DPPH free radical scavenging	[130]
	Gold	*Lemanea fluviatilis* (L.) C. Ag. extract	RT	12 h	UV-Vis, XRD, TEM, HRTEM, DLS, FTIR	Sphere	5–15 nm	Up to 3 months	DPPH scavenging (%) vs. different weights of the sample was found to be 18.10 mg	[131]
	Silver	*Ecklonia cava* extract	RT	72 h	UV-Vis, FTIR, XRD, TEM, DLS	Sphere	43 nm	Nd	250 μg/mL of *Ecklonia cava* extract or biosynthesized AgNPs was mixed with DPPH solution, ca. 50% of scavenging activity was achieved. DPPH radical scavenging activities of *Ecklonia cava* extract and biosynthesized AgNPs were similar at the same concentrations (e.g. 100, 250, and 500 μg/mL).	[59]
Lichens	Silver	*Parmeliopsis ambigua*, *Punctelia subrudecta*, *Evernia mesomorpha*, *Xanthoparmelia plittii* mycelia mats	RT	24 h	UV-Vis, SEM, FTIR	Variables	150–250 nm	Nd	SNPs samples total antioxidant capacity are 2.55 ± 0.05, 3.35 ± 0.04, 2.90 ± 0.01, 2.22 ± 0.01 μg AA/g respectively. *Punctelia subrudecta* displayed a higher activity (3.35 ± 0.04 μg AA/g) than the remaining samples; The hydroxyl radical scavenging activity showed that values were 7.75 ± 0.10, 34.48 ± 1.19, 31.97 ± 1.87 and 27.21 ± 1.39 μg/mL for all four samples respectively; Among the tested lichen SNPs, *Punctelia subrudecta* (*Punctelia subrudecta*) gave highest reducing power	[132]
	Gold	*Acroscyphus sphaerophoroides* Lev, *Sticta nylanderiana* extract	RT	12 h	UV-Vis, FTIR, XRD, TEM	Quasi-spherical and prismatic (*Acroscyphus* sp.), Twinned (*Sticta* sp.)	5–35 nm (*Acroscyphus* sp.), 20–50 nm (*Sticta* sp.)	Up to 3 months	1.66 and 4.48 mg sample concentration (SC$_{50}$) were found	[133]

RT—room temperature; Uiv-vis—ultraviolet-visible spectroscopy; TEM—transmission electron microscopy; SEM—scanning electron microscopy; FT-IR—Fourier-transform infrared spectroscopy; XRD—X-ray powder diffraction; EDX—energy dispersive X-ray spectroscopy; DLS—dynamic light scattering; HRTEM—high-resolution transmission electron microscopy; AFM—atomic force microscopy; ND—not defined; NS—not specified; Nd—not determ.

6.1. Silver Nanoparticles (AgNPs)

The silver nanoparticles (AgNPs), show a substantial biochemical and catalytic activity, which can be attributed to their significantly large surface area, as compared with other particles with similar chemical structures [134]. The AgNPs synthesis occurs via two steps, at first, Ag^+ ions are reduced to $Ag°$, followed by the agglomeration of colloidal silver nanoparticles, to form the oligomeric clusters which are finally stabilized [134]. Biological catalysts (enzymes) are required to reduce the Ag^+ ions, and the production of AgNPs with characteristic antioxidant properties can be achieved with a variety of plant extracts, as shown in Table 3. Patra et al. (2016) extracted the aqueous portion of watermelon rind (WRA), and used it to synthesize the AgNPs under light-exposed conditions at room temperature [92].

In recent studies, actinobacteria have been identified from various ecosystems that are potential natural producers of AgNPs and the whole-cell biomass and cell free extract of *Streptomyces naganishii* MA7 and *Streptomyces griseorubens* AU2, respectively, were used to synthesize silver nanoparticles with potential antioxidant properties [108,111]. On the other hand, fungal species like *Aspergillus versicolor* ENT7, *Cladosporium cladosporioides* and *Pestalotiopsis microspore* have also been used for the production of antioxidant functionalized AgNPs [117,119,120]. Various researchers have also reported *Ganoderma lucidium* as a potential source of antioxidant functionalized AgNPs [126,128,129]. Venkatesan et al. (2016) prepared the extracts of *Ecklonia cava*, a marine alga known to be a reservoir of phenolic compounds that can act as capping and reducing agents, and used it for the synthesis of silver nanoparticles [59]. Several lichens have also been identified with potential antioxidant properties, and extracts of *Parmeliopsis ambigua*, *Punctelia subrudecta*, *Evernia mesomorpha*, and *Xanthoparmelia plitti* were used to synthesize AgNPs [132].

The AgNPs synthesized using the leaves extract of *Clerodendrum phlomidis*, are found to have ferric reducing power of 1.63 AU, which is higher than the leaves extract used alone [87]. Whereas, on comparing the IC_{50} value of the extract (i.e., 1920 µg/mL), the AgNPs synthesized using the leaves extract of *Clerodendrum phlomidis* showed higher scavenging activity as confirmed by IC_{50} value (i.e., 55.86 µg/mL). Furthermore, the DPPH radical scavenging activity of AgNPs was found to be dose-dependent, showing the maximum inhibition (85.74%) greater than that of the extract alone. The AgNPs IC_{50} value (9.12 µg/mL) was found to be significantly lower, as compared to the extract (IC_{50} value 388.4 µg/mL) and standard ferulic acid (182.8 µg/mL), which confirmed the AgNPs with high antioxidant potential. In 2019, Das and his colleagues reported that AgNPs synthesized using *Morus alba* leaves extract increased the DPPH scavenging activity to 47.81% against the ~56% of the activity shown by standard ascorbic acid at the same concentration. However, plant extract mediated AgNPs showed 95.08% $ABTS^+$ scavenging activity, which is the equivalent to that which was shown by the BTH standard i.e., 95.51% at 100µg/mL, therefore indicating its strong scavenging potential. On the other hand, for nitric oxide scavenging activity, AgNPs displayed 64.04% scavenging, as compared to 45.72% and 88.62% in plant extract and gallic acid standard, respectively, at 100 µg/mL. Similarly, AgNPs at 100µg/mL concentration have shown a significant superoxide scavenging activity of 81.92%, as compared to the 85.35% present in the tocopherol standard [90].

6.2. Gold Nanoparticles (AuNPs)

Gold nanoparticles (AuNPs) have attained significant attention, owing to their physical characteristics (size and shape), optical properties and biocompatibility [134]. Gold nanoparticles of varied sizes and diverse morphologies have been employed in the medical sector for various purposes, such as the detection of tumors, and as a carrier for drugs etc. (e.g., Paclitaxel) [134]. Antioxidant AuNPs are mostly derived from extracts of plant parts like leaves and fruits, as shown in Table 3. Markus et al. (2016) reported the identification of *Lactobacillus kimchicus* DCY51^T, a novel probiotic from Korean kimchi, using an intracellular membrane-bound approach, and synthesized antioxidant functionalized AuNPs from these bacteria [107]. It was observed that the AuNPs formed a capping layer which comprised of several amino acids, while the presence of surface-bound proteins rendered them harmless to cancerous cell lines i.e., human colorectal adenocarcinoma (HT29) and murine macrophage (RAW264.7). As compared with gold salts, biological produced gold nanoparticles were found to be better scavengers of free radicals, especially DPPH. A food inhabiting *Enterococcus* species was identified and used for the production of gold nanoparticles, and was further confirmed through techniques like Fourier transform infrared spectroscopy (FT-IR), UV-vis absorption spectroscopy and transmission electron microscopy (TEM) [109].

Veeraapandian et al. (2012) utilized extracellular proteins of *Escherichia coli* to synthesize gold nanoparticles of anisotropic nature [110]. The size and shape of AuNPs are greatly influenced by the quantity of protein, as extracellular proteins significantly increases the shelf life of nanoparticles by acting as a capping agent, and thereby conferring them with stability. Manjunath et al. (2017) in their study, used a fungal endophyte, *Cladosporium cladosporioides*, obtained from *Sargassum wightii*, seaweed, to synthesize gold nanoparticles [118]. The process of reduction of gold metal salts into gold nanoparticles involved the use of phenolic compounds, and was found to be mediated through the activity of NADPH-dependent reductase enzyme. Lee et al. (2015) used the extracts of a mushroom species, *Inonotus obliquus*, to develop AuNPs without application of deleterious agents [127]. In another study, AuNPs were synthesized from the extracts of *Gracilaria corticate*, a red alga inhabiting in the marine environment and using it as a reducing agent [130]. Sharma et al. (2014) used the desiccated biomass of *Lemanea fluviatilis* to reduce and stabilize the AuNPs [131]. Debnath et al. (2016) developed the gold nanoparticles without the use of extraneous stabilizing and reducing agents by using desiccated biomass of lichens inhabiting in the alpine region of Eastern Himalayas (India) at high altitudes [133]. The gold nanoparticles obtained from lichen *Acroscyphus* sp. comprised of prismatic and multiply twinned quasi-spherical shapes, while those synthesized from *Sticta* sp. were simply multiply twinned and, both of these exhibited antioxidant activity.

6.3. Copper Oxide Nanoparticles (Cu_2ONPs)

In recent years, copper (Cu) has intrigued researchers for its application in nanoparticle synthesis, due to its readily available nature, and characteristics like catalytic, electrical, optical and mechanical properties [135–137]. Copper oxide, being a vital inorganic material, is predominantly used in modern technologies, especially in the field of catalysis, ceramics and superconductor applications. Moreover, it can also be used as electrode active materials for the degradation of nitrous oxide with ammonia, and oxidizing carbon monoxide, hydrocarbon and phenol in the formation of supercritical water [138]. The phytogenic synthesis of Cu_2ONPs possessing antioxidant ability is compiled in Table 3. In 2019, Rajeshkumar and his colleagues also reported a similar radical scavenging property of copper nanoparticles synthesized using leaf extract of *Cissus arnotiana*, when compared with the standard ascorbic acid [102].

6.4. Iron Nanoparticles (INPs)

Iron is another imperative material used for synthesizing nanoparticles, because of unique physiochemical properties like high catalytic activity, low toxicity, high magnetism and microwave absorption ability [139–141]. The iron nanoparticles (INPs) are categorized into three groups i.e., (a) iron oxide nanoparticles (IONs), (b) iron oxide hydroxide (FeOOH) nanoparticles, and (c) zero-valent iron (ZVI) nanoparticles [142–145]. These nanoparticles are used for varied applications like bio-separation, bioprocess intensification, drug delivery, environmental remediation, ferrofluids, food preservation, gene therapy, hyperthermia, magnetic targeting, negative MRI contrast enhancement, pigments, stem cell sorting and manipulation, thermal-ablation and lithium-ion batteries [146]. Table 3 shows the plant mediated INPs with antioxidant potential. In 2015, Muthukumar and Manickam observed the high antioxidant potential of *Amaranthus spinosus* leaf extract mediated INPs, because of the presence of amaranthine and phenolic compounds in it, which act as the capping agent [104].

6.5. Zinc Oxide (ZnONPs), Selenium (SeNPs) and Nickel Oxide Nanoparticles (NiONPs)

Zinc oxide is a metal oxide generally used in n-type of semiconductors. In recent decades, ZnONPs have drawn significant attention, owing to their widespread application in various fields like electronics, optical and the biomedical sector [147]. The process of production of zinc oxide nanoparticles is cost-effective, safe and easy, and ZnO has been given the status of generally recognized as safe (GRAS) by the US Food and Drug Administration [148,149]. ZnONPs are primarily known for their exceptional semiconducting properties, which can be attributed to the wide band gap of 3.37 eV, high catalytic activity, UV filtering properties and large exciton binding energy of 60 meV, and also have good optical, wound healing and anti-inflammatory properties [147]. ZnONPs have been comprehensively used in the cosmetic industry, in products like sunscreen lotions, for their intrinsic UV filtering properties [150]. They also have widespread applications in the biomedical sector, such as in drug delivery, and also exhibit antidiabetic, antibacterial anticancer and antifungal properties [147]. Chandra et al. (2019) used the leaf extract of *Berberis aristata*, a plant of medicinal importance, to synthesize zinc oxide nanoparticles [95]. Other studies have employed the yeast species, *Pichia kudriavzevii* for the extracellular biosynthesis of ZnONPs and the development of ZnONPs by using the fungal strain, *Aspergillus niger* [116,122].

In addition to these materials, selenium nanoparticles (SeNPs) are also attracting researchers, owing to their enhanced properties like semi-conduction, photoelectrical, photoconduction, catalytic etc., and their potential in optical and electronic instruments. They are known to have lesser toxic effects than selenium (Se) compounds, and are used in the medical field, as they show high therapeutic and anticancer properties [151]. Ramya et al. (2015) used an actinomycetes species, *Streptomyces minutiscleroticus* M10A62, obtained from magnesite mine, to develop SeNPs [98]. In 2012, Torres and his colleagues used *Pantoea agglomerans* isolated from the Camarones River to synthesize Se nanoparticles [113]. In 2013, Li and team members fabricated 6-hydroxy-2,5,7,8-tetramethylchroman-2-carboxylic acid (Trolox) coated surface-functionalized nanoparticles of Selenium (Se@Trolox) with antioxidant potential [152]. Moreover, Se@Trolox was found to block the activation of the AKT and MAPK signaling pathway, cisplatin-induced reactive oxygen species (ROS) accumulation, and DNA damage-mediated p53 phosphorylation in HK-2 cells [152].

Recently, nickel oxide has been found to perform different functions in various fields like biomedicine, electronics and magnetism, owing to its properties like anti-bacterial, anti-inflammatory, eco-friendliness, easy usage and high reactiveness [153]. Being highly reactive, it is readily used for catalyzing various organic reactions, like the α-alkylation of methyl ketone, the chemo-selective oxidative coupling of thiols, the hydrogenation of olefins, the synthesis of stilbenes from alcohol through Wittig-type olefination and the reduction of ketones and aldehydes [154–158]. Moreover, it is also found to catalyze inorganic reactions, such as the decomposition of ammonia [159]. Recently, it has been used for developing carbon nanotubes (CNTs) [160]. The plant derived nickel oxide nanoparticles showing antioxidant potential are shown in Table 3.

7. Challenges

Apart from the widespread applications of metallic nanoparticles, owing to their size, chemical composition, shape, stability, functionalization, surface coating and purity, they also possess potential toxic effects [161]. Nanoparticles show characteristically distinct cellular uptake mechanisms, and also exhibit the ability to catalyze the synthesis of ROS, thus, leading to ROS associated toxic effects [162]. The size of the NPs is also known to affect the uptake of NPs and their distribution within the cell significantly, and it has been found that in NPs with the same dosage but having distinct sizes; the small-sized NPs are readily internalized within the cell than the large-sized NPs [163]. Moreover, it has been observed that the small-sized NPs possess relatively high reactivity, as they have a large surface area [164]. The size, surface charge and the material type of NPs determine the aggregating efficiency of MNPs, which further influences the internalization of NPs in the cell, and ultimately affects the NPs associated toxicity [165]. A lot of research is being carried out at a global scale to evaluate the NP's associated toxic effects. Cho et al. (2009) found that polyethyleneglycol (PEG)-coated AuNPs triggers acute inflammation, as well as apoptosis, in the liver after intravenous injection, and also leads to the aggregation of the AuNPs in the cytoplasmic vesicles, liver and spleen [166]. There are numerous transition metals like copper (Cu), chromium (Cr), iron (Fe), silicon (Si) and vanadium (V), which are also involved in the generation of ROS via the Fenton reaction and the Haber-Weiss mechanism [167]. Apart from this, ZnONPs have also been reported to increase the cytotoxicity, due to the formation of ROS, which causes oxidative damage, and evoke the release of inflammatory mediators, thus, resulting in the senescence of phagocytic RAW264.7 cells and the transformation of BEAS-2B (human bronchial epithelial) cells [168]. These are some of the challenges associated with the use of metallic and metalloid NPs, and continuous efforts are being made to eliminate and overcome these challenges.

8. Conclusions

A sedentary lifestyle and the consumption of high carbohydrate, proteins and fat have drastically changed the lives of humans, resulting in the production of ROS, which subsequently leads to oxidative stress. Moreover, these oxidative stresses are known to be linked with various diseases, and many attempts have been made to subside these with different medications. Although conventional therapies using antioxidants have been used in the past, they were mostly found ineffective in treating various diseases because of their incompetence in passing through the blood–brain barrier. To overcome these challenges, several antioxidant functionalized nanoparticles have been derived from biological sources, and evaluated by using scavenging assays under invitro conditions. Antioxidant properties of these nanocarriers make it a suitable candidate for targeted delivery, and can open new opportunities for combating oxidative stress in in vivo conditions. Furthermore, researchers are making continuous effort to slow down the toxic effects associated with the metallic and metalloid nanoparticles.

Author Contributions: Conceptualization, E.N., K.K., and D.K.; Manuscript writing, H.K. and K.B.; Manuscript editing, D.S.D., S.B., and R.V.; Critical revising, E.N., K.K., S.K.B. and D.K. All authors have read and agreed to the published version of the manuscript.

Funding: This research was funded by the University of Hradec Kralove (Faculty of Science VT2019-2021).

Acknowledgments: We acknowledge university of Hradec Kralove (Faculty of Science, VT2019-2021) for financial support.

Conflicts of Interest: The authors declare no conflict of interest.

References

1. Dabhade, P.; Kotwal, S. Tackling the aging process with biomolecules: A possible role for caloric restriction, food-derived nutrients, vitamins, amino acids, peptides, and minerals. *J. Nutr. Gerontol. Geriatr.* **2013**, *32*, 24–40. [CrossRef]
2. López-Otín, C.; Blasco, M.A.; Partridge, L.; Serrano, M.; Kroemer, G. The hallmarks of aging. *Cell* **2013**, *153*, 1194–1217. [CrossRef] [PubMed]
3. Shokolenko, I.N.; Wilson, G.L.; Alexeyev, M.F. Aging: A mitochondrial DNA perspective, critical analysis and an update. *World J. Exp. Med.* **2014**, *4*, 46. [CrossRef] [PubMed]
4. Chang, C.H.; Lee, K.Y.; Shim, Y.H. Normal aging: Definition and physiologic changes. *J. Korean Med. Assoc.* **2017**, *60*, 358–363. [CrossRef]
5. Harman, D. Aging: A theory based on free radical and radiation chemistry. *J. Gerontol.* **1956**, *11*, 298–300. [CrossRef] [PubMed]
6. Islam, M.T. Oxidative stress and mitochondrial dysfunction-linked neurodegenerative disorders. *Neurol. Res.* **2017**, *39*, 73–82. [CrossRef]
7. Valentão, P.; Fernandes, E.; Carvalho, F.; Andrade, P.B.; Seabra, R.M.; De Lourdes Bastos, M. Antioxidant activity of *Hypericum androsaemum* infusion: Scavenging activity against superoxide radical, hydroxyl radical and hypochlorous acid. *Biol. Pharm. Bull.* **2002**, *25*, 1320–1323. [CrossRef] [PubMed]

8. Dias, V.; Junn, E.; Mouradian, M.M. The role of oxidative stress in Parkinson's disease. *J. Parkinson's Dis.* **2013**, *3*, 461–491. [CrossRef] [PubMed]
9. Halliwell, B.; Gutteridge, J.M.C. *Free Radicals in Biology and Medicine*, 4th ed.; Clarendon Press: Oxford, UK, 2007.
10. Bahorun, T.; Soobrattee, M.A.; Luximon-Ramma, V.; Aruoma, O.I. Free radicals and antioxidants in cardiovascular health and disease. *Internet J. Med. Update* **2006**, *1*, 25–41. [CrossRef]
11. Kumar, S.; Pandey, A.K. Free radicals: Health implications and their mitigation by herbals. *Br. J. Med. Med. Res.* **2015**, *7*, 438–457. [CrossRef]
12. Kumar, S.; Pandey, A.K. Chemistry and biological activities of flavonoids: An overview. *Sci. World J.* **2013**, *2013*, 162750. [CrossRef] [PubMed]
13. Valko, M.; Izakovic, M.; Mazur, M.; Rhodes, C.J.; Telser, J. Role of oxygen radicals in DNA damage and cancer incidence. *Mol. Cell. Biochem.* **2004**, *266*, 37–56. [CrossRef] [PubMed]
14. Valko, M.; Leibfritz, D.; Moncola, J.; Cronin, M.D.; Mazur, M.; Telser, J. Free radicals and antioxidants in normal physiological functions and human disease. *Int. J. Biochem. Cell Biol.* **2007**, *39*, 44–84. [CrossRef] [PubMed]
15. Dröge, W. Free radicals in the physiological control of cell function. *Physiol. Rev.* **2002**, *82*, 47–95. [CrossRef]
16. Willcox, J.K.; Ash, S.L.; Catignani, G.L. Antioxidants and prevention of chronic disease. *Crit. Rev. Food Sci. Nutr.* **2004**, *44*, 275–295. [CrossRef]
17. Pacher, P.; Beckman, J.S.; Liaudet, L. Nitric oxide and peroxynitrite in health and disease. *Physiol. Rev.* **2007**, *87*, 315–424. [CrossRef]
18. Genestra, M. Oxyl radicals, redox-sensitive signaling cascades and antioxidants. *Cell. Signal.* **2007**, *19*, 1807–1819. [CrossRef]
19. Halliwell, B. Biochemistry of oxidative stress. *Biochem. Soc. Trans.* **2007**, *35*, 1147–1150. [CrossRef]
20. Ricordi, C.; Garcia-Contreras, M.; Farnetti, S. Diet and inflammation: Possible effects on immunity, chronic diseases, and life span. *J. Am. Coll. Nutr.* **2015**, *34*, 10–13. [CrossRef]
21. Sharma, P.; Mehta, M.; Dhanjal, D.S.; Kaur, S.; Gupta, G.; Singh, H.; Thangavelu, L.; Rajeshkumar, S.; Tambuwala, M.; Bakshi, H.A.; et al. Emerging trends in the novel drug delivery approaches for the treatment of lung cancer. *Chem. Biol. Interact.* **2019**, *309*, 108720. [CrossRef]
22. Aggarwal, V.; Tuli, H.S.; Varol, A.; Thakral, F.; Yerer, M.B.; Sak, K.; Varol, M.; Jain, A.; Khan, M.; Sethi, G. Role of reactive oxygen species in cancer progression: Molecular mechanisms and recent Advancements. *Biomolecules* **2019**, *9*, 735. [CrossRef]
23. Liou, G.Y.; Storz, P. Reactive oxygen species in cancer. *Free Radic. Res.* **2010**, *44*, 479–496. [CrossRef] [PubMed]
24. Qian, Q.; Chen, W.; Cao, Y.; Cao, Q.; Cui, Y.; Li, Y.; Wu, J. Targeting reactive oxygen species in cancer via Chinese herbal medicine. *Oxid. Med. Cell. Longev.* **2019**, *2019*, 9240426. [CrossRef] [PubMed]
25. Kumari, S.; Badana, A.K.; Murali, M.G.; Shailender, G.; Malla, R. Reactive oxygen species: A key constituent in cancer survival. *Biomark. Insights* **2018**, *13*, 1177271918755391. [CrossRef]
26. Yang, H.; Villani, R.M.; Wang, H.; Simpson, M.J.; Roberts, M.S.; Tang, M.; Liang, X. The role of cellular reactive oxygen species in cancer chemotherapy. *J. Exp. Clin. Cancer Res.* **2018**, *37*, 266. [CrossRef] [PubMed]
27. Schieber, M.; Chandel, N.S. ROS function in redox signaling and oxidative stress. *Curr. Biol.* **2014**, *24*, R453–R462. [CrossRef]
28. Redza-Dutordoir, M.; Averill-Bates, D.A. Activation of apoptosis signalling pathways by reactive oxygen species. *Biochim. Biophys. Acta* **2016**, *1863*, 2977–2992. [CrossRef]
29. Mehta, M.; Dhanjal, D.S.; Paudel, K.R.; Singh, B.; Gupta, G.; Rajeshkumar, S.; Thangavelu, L.; Tambuwala, M.M.; Bakshi, H.A.; Chellappan, D.K.; et al. Cellular signalling pathways mediating the pathogenesis of chronic inflammatory respiratory diseases: An update. *Inflammopharmacology* **2020**, 1–23. [CrossRef]
30. Kessenbrock, K.; Plaks, V.; Werb, Z. Matrix metalloproteinases: Regulators of the tumor microenvironment. *Cell* **2010**, *141*, 52–67. [CrossRef]
31. He, F.; Zuo, L. Redox roles of reactive oxygen species in cardiovascular diseases. *Int. J. Mol. Sci.* **2015**, *16*, 27770–27780. [CrossRef]
32. Panth, N.; Paudel, K.R.; Parajuli, K. Reactive oxygen species: A key hallmark of cardiovascular disease. *Adv. Med.* **2016**, *2016*, 9152732. [CrossRef]
33. Sag, C.M.; Santos, C.X.; Shah, A.M. Redox regulation of cardiac hypertrophy. *J. Mol. Cell Cardiol.* **2014**, *73*, 103–111. [CrossRef] [PubMed]

34. Zhou, T.; Prather, E.R.; Garrison, D.E.; Zuo, L. Interplay between ROS and antioxidants during ischemia-reperfusion injuries in cardiac and skeletal muscle. *Int. J. Mol. Sci.* **2018**, *19*, 417. [CrossRef] [PubMed]
35. Van der Pol, A.; Van Gilst, W.H.; Voors, A.A.; Van der Meer, P. Treating oxidative stress in heart failure: Past, present and future. *Eur. J. Heart Fail.* **2019**, *21*, 425–435. [CrossRef] [PubMed]
36. Uttara, B.; Singh, A.V.; Zamboni, P.; Mahajan, R.T. Oxidative stress and neurodegenerative diseases: A review of upstream and downstream antioxidant therapeutic options. *Curr. Neuropharmacol.* **2009**, *7*, 65–74. [CrossRef] [PubMed]
37. Liu, Z.; Zhou, T.; Ziegler, A.C.; Dimitrion, P.; Zuo, L. Oxidative stress in neurodegenerative diseases: From molecular mechanisms to clinical applications. *Oxid. Med. Cell. Longev.* **2017**, *2017*, 2525967. [CrossRef]
38. Khaltaev, N.; Axelrod, S. Chronic respiratory diseases global mortality trends, treatment guidelines, life style modifications, and air pollution: Preliminary analysis. *J. Thorac. Dis.* **2019**, *11*, 2643–2655. [CrossRef]
39. Boukhenouna, S.; Wilson, M.A.; Bahmed, K.; Kosmider, B. Reactive oxygen species in chronic obstructive pulmonary disease. *Oxid. Med. Cell. Longev.* **2018**, *2018*, 5730395. [CrossRef]
40. Thimmulappa, R.K.; Chattopadhyay, I.; Rajasekaran, S. Oxidative stress mechanisms in the pathogenesis of environmental lung diseases. In *Oxidative Stress in Lung Diseases*; Chakraborti, S., Chakraborti, T., Ghosh, R., Ganguly, N.K., Parinandni, N.L., Eds.; Springer: Singapore, 2020; Volume 2, pp. 103–137.
41. Pizzino, G.; Irrera, N.; Cucinotta, M.; Pallio, G.; Mannino, F.; Arcoraci, V.; Squadrito, F.; Altavilla, D.; Bitto, A. Oxidative stress: Harms and benefits for human health. *Oxid. Med. Cell. Longev.* **2017**, *2017*, 8416763. [CrossRef]
42. Young, I.S.; Woodside, J.V. Antioxidants in health and disease. *J. Clin. Pathol.* **2001**, *54*, 176–186. [CrossRef]
43. Matill, H.A. Antioxidants. *Annu. Rev. Biochem.* **1947**, *16*, 177–192. [CrossRef] [PubMed]
44. German, J. Food processing and lipid oxidation. *Adv. Exp. Med. Biol.* **1999**, *459*, 23–50. [PubMed]
45. Jacob, R. Three eras of vitamin C discovery. *Subcell. Biochem.* **1996**, *25*, 1–16.
46. Knight, J. Free radicals: Their history and current status in aging and disease. *Ann. Clin. Lab. Sci.* **1998**, *28*, 331–346.
47. Halliwell, B. How to characterize an antioxidant- An update. *Biochem. Soc. Symp.* **1995**, *61*, 73–101.
48. Shi, H.L.; Noguchi, N.; Niki, N. Comparative study on dynamics of antioxidative action of α- tocopheryl hydroquinone, ubiquinoland α- tocopherol, against lipid peroxidation. *Free Radic. Biol. Med.* **1999**, *27*, 334–346. [CrossRef]
49. Levine, M.; Ramsey, S.C.; Daruwara, R. Criteria and recommendation for vitamin C intake. *JAMA* **1991**, *281*, 1415–1423. [CrossRef]
50. Yang, X.; Sun, Z.; Wang, W.; Zhou, Q.; Shi, G.; Wei, F.; Jiang, G. Developmental toxicity of synthetic phenolic antioxidants to the early life stage of zebrafish. *Sci. Total. Environ.* **2018**, *643*, 559–568. [CrossRef]
51. Aguilera, Y.; Martin-Cabrejas, M.A.; González de Mejia, E. Phenolic compounds in fruits and beverages consumed as part of the mediterranean diet: Their role in prevention of chronic diseases. *Phytochem. Rev.* **2016**, *15*, 405–423. [CrossRef]
52. Faustino, M.; Veiga, M.; Sousa, P.; Costa, E.M.; Silva, S.; Pintado, M. Agro-food byproducts as a new source of natural food additives. *Molecules* **2019**, *24*, 1056. [CrossRef]
53. Chandra, P.; Sharma, R.K.; Arora, D.S. Antioxidant compounds from microbial sources: A review. *Food Res. Int.* **2020**, *129*, 108849. [CrossRef]
54. Dey, T.B.; Chakraborty, S.; Jain, K.K.; Sharma, A.; Kuhad, R.C. Antioxidant phenolics and their microbial production by submerged and solid state fermentation process: A review. *Trends Food Sci. Technol.* **2016**, *53*, 60–74.
55. Brewer, M.S. Natural antioxidants: Sources, compounds, mechanisms of action, and potential applications. *Compr. Rev. Food Sci. Food Saf.* **2011**, *10*, 221–247. [CrossRef]
56. Kozarski, M.; Klaus, A.; Jakovljevic, D.; Todorovic, N.; Vunduk, J.; Petrović, P.; Niksic, M.; Niksic, M.M.; Griensven, L.V. Antioxidants of edible mushrooms. *Molecules* **2015**, *20*, 19489–19525. [CrossRef]
57. Ferreira, I.C.F.R.; Barros, L.; Abreu, R.M.V. Antioxidants in wild mushrooms. *Curr. Med. Chem.* **2009**, *16*, 1543–1560. [CrossRef]
58. Munir, N.; Sharif, N.; Naz, S.; Manzoor, F. Algae: A potent antioxidant source. *Sky J. Microbiol. Res.* **2013**, *1*, 22–31.

59. Venkatesan, J.; Kim, S.K.; Shim, S.K. Antimicrobial, antioxidant, and anticancer activities of biosynthesized silver nanoparticles using marine algae *Ecklonia cava*. *Nanomaterials* **2016**, *6*, 235. [CrossRef]
60. Fernández-Moriano, C.; Gómez-Serranillos, M.P.; Crespo, A. Antioxidant potential of lichen species and their secondary metabolites. A systematic review. *Pharm. Biol.* **2015**, *54*, 1–17. [CrossRef]
61. Hu, B.; Liu, X.; Zhang, C.; Zeng, X. Food macromolecule based nanodelivery systems for enhancing the bioavailability of polyphenols. *J. Food Drug. Anal* **2017**, *25*, 3–15. [CrossRef] [PubMed]
62. Eftekhari, A.; Ahmadian, E.; Panahi-Azar, V.; Hosseini, H.; Tabibiazar, M.; Dizaj, S.M. Hepatoprotective and free radical scavenging actions of quercetin nanoparticles on aflatoxin B1-induced liver damage: In vitro/in vivo studies. *Artif. Cells Nanomed. Biotechnol.* **2017**, *46*, 411–420. [CrossRef] [PubMed]
63. Eftekhari, A.; Dizaj, S.M.; Chodari, L.; Sunar, S.; Hasanzadeh, A.; Ahmadian, E.; Hasanzadeh, M. The promising future of nano-antioxidant therapy against environmental pollutants induced-toxicities. *Biomed. Pharmacother.* **2018**, *103*, 1018–1027. [CrossRef] [PubMed]
64. Nelson, B.C.; Johnson, M.E.; Walker, M.L.; Riley, K.R.; Sims, C.M. Antioxidant cerium oxide nanoparticles in biology and medicine. *Antioxidants* **2016**, *5*, 15. [CrossRef] [PubMed]
65. Eriksson, P.; Tal, A.A.; Skallberg, A.; Brommesson, C.; Hu, Z.; Boyd, R.D.; Olovsson, W.; Fairley, N.; Abrikosov, I.A.; Zhang, X.; et al. Cerium oxide nanoparticles with antioxidant capabilities and gadolinium integration for MRI contrast enhancement. *Sci. Rep.* **2018**, *8*, 6999. [CrossRef]
66. Das, S.; Dowding, J.M.; Klump, K.E.; McGinnis, J.F.; Self, W.; Seal, S. Cerium oxide nanoparticles: Applications and prospects in nanomedicine. *Nanomedicine* **2013**, *8*, 1483–1508. [CrossRef]
67. Deshpande, S.; Patil, S.; Kuchibhatla, S.V.N.T.; Seal, S. Size dependency variation in lattice parameter and valency states in nanocrystalline cerium oxide. *Appl. Phys. Lett.* **2005**, *87*, 133113. [CrossRef]
68. Kim, C.K.; Kim, T.; Choi, I.Y.; Soh, M.; Kim, D.; Kim, Y.J.; Jang, H.; Yang, H.S.; Kim, J.Y.; Park, H.K.; et al. Ceria nanoparticles that can protect against ischemic stroke. *Angew. Chem. Int. Ed. Engl.* **2012**, *51*, 11039–11043. [CrossRef] [PubMed]
69. Hirst, S.M.; Karakoti, A.; Singh, S.; Self, W.; Tyler, R.; Seal, S.; Reilly, C.M. Bio-distribution and in vivo antioxidant effects of cerium oxide nanoparticles in mice. *Envrion. Toxicol.* **2013**, *28*, 107–118. [CrossRef]
70. Caputo, F.; Nicola, M.D.; Sienkiewicz, A.; Giovanetti, A.; Bejarano, I.; Licoccia, S.; Traversa, E.; Ghibelli, L. Cerium oxide nanoparticles, combining antioxidant and UV shielding properties, prevent UV-induced cell damage and mutagenesis. *Nanoscale* **2015**, *7*, 15643–15656. [CrossRef]
71. Sonaje, K.; Italia, J.L.; Sharma, G.; Bhardwaj, V.; Tikoo, K.; Kumar, M.N.V.R. Development of biodegradable nanoparticles for oral delivery of ellagic acid and evaluation of their antioxidant efficacy against cyclosporine A-induced nephrotoxicity in rats. *Pharm. Res.* **2007**, *24*, 899–908. [CrossRef]
72. Yun, X.; Maximov, V.D.; Yu, J.; Zhu, H.; Vertegel, A.A.; Kindly, M.S. Nanoparticles for targeted delivery of antioxidant enzymes to the brain after cerebral ischemia and reperfusion injury. *J. Cereb. Blood Flow. Metab.* **2013**, *33*, 583–592. [CrossRef]
73. Chorny, M.; Hood, E.; Levy, R.J.; Muzykantov, V.R. Endothelial delivery of antioxidant enzymes loaded into non-polymeric magnetic nanoparticles. *J. Control. Release* **2010**, *146*, 144–151. [CrossRef]
74. Reddy, M.K.; Labhasetwar, V. Nanoparticle-mediated delivery of superoxide dismutase to the brain: An effective strategy to reduce ischemia-reperfusion injury. *FASEB J.* **2009**, *23*, 1384–1395. [CrossRef]
75. Fan, Y.; Yi, J.; Zhang, Y.; Yokoyama, W. Fabrication of curcumin-loaded bovine serum albumin (BSA)-dextran nanoparticles and the cellular antioxidant activity. *Food Chem.* **2018**, *239*, 1210–1218. [CrossRef] [PubMed]
76. Elle, R.E.; Rahmani, S.; Lauret, C.; Morena, M.; Bidel, L.P.R.; Boulahtouf, A.; Balaguer, P.; Cristol, J.P.; Durand, J.O.; Charnay, C.; et al. Functionalized mesoporous silica nanoparticle with antioxidants as a new carrier that generates lower oxidative stress impact on cells. *Mol. Pharm.* **2016**, *13*, 2647–2660. [CrossRef] [PubMed]
77. Tzankova, V.; Aluani, D.; Kondeva-Burdina, M.; Yordanov, Y.; Odzhakov, F.; Apostolov, A.; Yoncheva, K. Hepatoprotective and antioxidant activity of quercetin loaded chitosan/alginate particles in vitro and in vivo in a model of paracetamol-induced toxicity. *Biomed. Pharmacother.* **2017**, *92*, 569–579. [CrossRef]
78. Trombino, S.; Cassano, R.; Ferrarelli, T.; Barone, E.; Picci, N.; Mancuso, C. *Trans*-ferulic acid-based solid lipid nanoparticles and their antioxidant effect in rat brain microsomes. *Colloids Surf. B Biointerfaces* **2013**, *109*, 273–279. [CrossRef]
79. Du, L.; Li, J.; Chen, C.; Liu, Y. Nanocarrier: A potential tool for future antioxidant therapy. *Free Radic. Res.* **2014**, *48*, 1061–1069. [CrossRef] [PubMed]

80. Hans, M.; Lowman, A. Biodegradable nanoparticles for drug delivery and targeting. *Curr. Opin. Solid State Mater. Sci.* **2002**, *6*, 319–327. [CrossRef]
81. Vila, A.; Sanchez, A.; Tobıo, M.; Calvo, P.; Alonso, M. Design of biodegradable particles for protein delivery. *J. Control. Release* **2002**, *78*, 15–24. [CrossRef]
82. Shah, B.R.; Zhang, C.; Li, Y.; Li, B. Bioaccessibility and antioxidant activity of curcumin after encapsulated by nano and pickering emulsion based on chitosan-tripolyphosphate nanoparticles. *Food Res. Int.* **2016**, *89*, 399–407. [CrossRef]
83. Pu, H.L.; Chiang, W.L.; Maiti, B.; Liao, Z.X.; Ho, Y.C.; Shim, M.S.; Chuang, E.Y.; Xia, Y.; Sung, H.W. Nanoparticles with dual responses to oxidative stress and reduced pH for drug release and anti-inflammatory applications. *ACS Nano* **2014**, *8*, 1213–1221. [CrossRef] [PubMed]
84. Patil, S.P.; Kumbhar, S.T. Antioxidant, antibacterial and cytotoxic potential of silver nanoparticles synthesized using terpenes rich extract of *Lantana camara* L. leaves. *Biochem. Biophys. Rep.* **2017**, *10*, 76–81.
85. Saratale, R.G.; Benelli, G.; Kumar, G.; Kim, D.S.; Saratale, G.D. Bio-fabrication of silver nanoparticles using the leaf extract of an ancient herbal medicine, dandelion (*Taraxacum officinale*), evaluation of their antioxidant, anticancer potential, and antimicrobial activity against phytopathogens. *Environ. Sci. Pollut. Res.* **2018**, *25*, 10392–10406. [CrossRef] [PubMed]
86. Phull, A.R.; Abbas, Q.; Ali, A.; Raza, H.; Kim, S.J.; Zia, M.; Haq, I.U. Antioxidant, cytotoxic and antimicrobial activities of green synthesized silver nanoparticles from crude extract of *Bergenia ciliata*. *Future J. Pharm. Sci.* **2016**, *2*, 31–36. [CrossRef]
87. Sriranjani, R.; Srinithya, B.; Vellingiri, V.; Brindha, P.; Anthony, S.P.; Sivasubramanian, A.; Muthuraman, M.S. Silver nanoparticle synthesis using *Clerodendrum phlomidis* leaf extract and preliminary investigation of its antioxidant and anticancer activities. *J. Mol. Liq.* **2016**, *220*, 926–930. [CrossRef]
88. Kalaiyarasan, T.; Bharti, V.K.; Chaurasia, O.P. One pot green preparation of Seabuckthorn silver nanoparticles (SBT@AgNPs) featuring high stability and longevity, antibacterial, antioxidant potential: A nano disinfectant future perspective. *RSC Adv.* **2017**, *7*, 51130–51141. [CrossRef]
89. Sharma, B.; Deswal, R. Single pot synthesized gold nanoparticles using *Hippophae rhamnoides* leaf and berry extract showed shape-dependent differential nanobiotechnological applications. *Artif. Cells Nanomed. Biotechnol.* **2018**, *46*, 408–418. [CrossRef]
90. Das, D.; Ghosh, R.; Mandal, P. Biogenic synthesis of silver nanoparticles using S1 genotype of *Morus alba* leaf extract: Characterization, antimicrobial and antioxidant potential assessment. *SN Appl. Sci.* **2019**, *1*, 498. [CrossRef]
91. Sathishkumar, G.; Jha, P.K.; Vignesh, V.; Rajkuberan, C.; Jeyaraj, M.; Selvakumar, M.; Jha, R.; Sivaramakrishnan, S. Cannonball fruit (*Couroupita guianensis*, Aubl.) extract mediated synthesis of gold nanoparticles and evaluation of its antioxidant activity. *J. Mol. Liq.* **2016**, *215*, 229–236.
92. Patra, J.K.; Das, G.; Baek, K.H. Phyto-mediated biosynthesis of silver nanoparticles using the rind extract of watermelon (*Citrullus lanatus*) under photo-catalyzed condition and investigation of its antibacterial, anticandidal and antioxidant efficacy. *J. Photochem. Photobiol. B* **2016**, *161*, 200–210. [CrossRef]
93. Mohanta, Y.K.; Panda, S.K.; Jayabalan, R.; Sharma, N.; Bastia, A.K.; Mohanta, T.K. Antimicrobial, antioxidant and cytotoxic activity of silver nanoparticles synthesized by leaf extract of *Erythrina suberosa* (Roxb.). *Front. Mol. Biosci.* **2017**, *4*, 14. [CrossRef]
94. Hamelian, M.; Zangeneh, M.M.; Amisama, A.; Varmira, K.; Veisi, H. Green synthesis of silver nanoparticles using *Thymus kotschyanus* extract and evaluation of their antioxidant, antibacterial and cytotoxic effects. *Appl. Organomet. Chem.* **2018**, *32*, e4458. [CrossRef]
95. Chandra, H.; Patel, D.; Kumari, P.; Jangwan, J.S.; Yadav, S. Phyto-mediated synthesis of zinc oxide nanoparticles of *Berberis aristata*: Characterization, antioxidant activity and antibacterial activity with special reference to urinary tract pathogens. *Mater. Sci. Eng. C Mater. Biol. Appl.* **2019**, *102*, 212–220. [CrossRef]
96. Veena, S.; Devasena, T.; Sathak, S.S.M.; Yasasve, M.; Vishal, L.A. Green synthesis of gold nanoparticles from *Vitex negundo* leaf extract: Characterization and in vitro evaluation of antioxidant-antibacterial activity. *J. Clust. Sci.* **2019**, *30*, 1591–1597. [CrossRef]
97. Keshari, A.K.; Srivastava, R.; Singh, P.; Yadav, V.B.; Nath, G. Antioxidant and antibacterial activity of silver nanoparticles synthesized by *Cestrum nocturnum*. *J. Ayurveda Integr. Med.* **2020**, *11*, 37–44. [CrossRef] [PubMed]

98. Subbaiy, R.; Selvam, M.M. Green synthesis of copper nanoparticles from *Hibicus rosasinensis* and their antimicrobial, antioxidant activities. *Res. J. Pharm. Biol. Chem. Sci.* **2015**, *6*, 1183–1190.
99. Ghosh, S.; More, P.; Nitnavare, R.; Jagtap, S.; Chippalkatti, R.; Derle, A.; Kitture, R.; Asok, A.; Kale, S.; Singh, S.; et al. Antidiabetic and antioxidant properties of copper nanoparticles synthesized by medicinal plant *Dioscorea bulbifera*. *J. Nanomed. Nanotechnol.* **2015**, *S6*, 007.
100. Sarkar, J.; Chakraborty, N.; Chatterjee, A.; Bhattacharjee, R.; Dasgupta, D.; Acharya, K. Green synthesized copper oxide nanoparticles ameliorate defence and antioxidant enzymes in *Lens culinaris*. *Nanomaterials* **2020**, *10*, 312. [CrossRef]
101. Dobrucka, R. Antioxidant and catalytic activity of biosynthesized CuO nanoparticles using extract of *Galeopsidis herba*. *J. Inorg. Organomet. Polym. Mater.* **2018**, *28*, 812–819. [CrossRef]
102. Rajeshkumar, S.; Menon, S.; Kumar, S.V.; Tambuwala, M.M.; Bakshi, H.A.; Mehta, M.; Satija, S.; Gupta, G.; Chellappan, D.K.; Thangavelu, L.; et al. Antibacterial and antioxidant potential of biosynthesized copper nanoparticles mediated through *Cissus arnotiana* plant extract. *J. Photochem. Photobiol.* **2019**, *197*, 111531. [CrossRef]
103. Harshiny, M.; Iswarya, C.N.; Matheswaran, M. Biogenic synthesis of iron nanoparticles using *Amaranthus dubius* leaves extract as reducing agents. *Powder Technol.* **2015**, *286*, 744–749. [CrossRef]
104. Muthukumar, H.; Manickam, M. Amaranthus spinosus leaf extract mediated FeO nanoparticles: Physicochemical traits, photocatalytic and antioxidant activity. *ACS Sustain. Chem. Eng.* **2015**, *3*, 3149–3156. [CrossRef]
105. Tuzun, B.S.; Fafal, T.; Tastan, P.; Kivcak, B.; Yelken, B.O.; Kayabasi, C.; Susluer, S.Y.; Gunduz, C. Structural characterization, antioxidant and cytotoxic effects of iron nanoparticles synthesized using *Asphodelus aestivus* Brot. aqueous extract. *Green Process. Synth.* **2020**, *9*, 153–163. [CrossRef]
106. Srihasam, S.; Thyagarajan, K.; Korivi, M.; Lebaka, V.R.; Mallem, S.P.R. Phytogenic generation of NiO nanoparticles using *Stevia* leaf extract and evaluation of their in-vitro antioxidant and antimicrobial properties. *Biomolecules* **2020**, *10*, 89. [CrossRef] [PubMed]
107. Markus, J.; Mathiyalagan, R.; Kim, Y.J.; Abbai, R.; Singh, P.; Ahn, S.; Perez, Z.E.J.; Hurh, J.; Yang, D.C. Intracellularsynthesis of goldnanoparticles with antioxidantactivity by probiotic *Lactobacillus kimchicus* DCY51^T isolated from Koreankimchi. *Enzym. Microb. Technol.* **2016**, *95*, 85–93. [CrossRef] [PubMed]
108. Baygar, T.; Ugur, A. Biosynthesis of silver nanoparticles by *Streptomyces griseorubens* isolated from soil and their antioxidant activity. *IET Nanobiotechnol.* **2017**, *11*, 286–291. [CrossRef]
109. Oladipo, I.C.; Lateef, A.; Elegbede, J.A.; Azeez, M.A.; Asafa, T.M.; Yekeen, T.A.; Akinboro, A.; Gueguim-Kana, E.B.; Beukes, L.S.; Oluyide, T.O.; et al. Enterococcus species for the one-pot biofabrication of gold nanoparticles: Characterization and nanobiotechnological applications. *J. Photochem. Photobiol. B* **2017**, *173*, 250–257. [CrossRef]
110. Veeraapandian, S.; Sawant, S.N.; Doble, M. Antibacterial and antioxidant activity of protein capped silver and gold nanoparticles synthesized with *Escherichia coli*. *J. Bimed. Nanotechnol.* **2012**, *8*, 140–148. [CrossRef]
111. Shanmugasundaram, T.; Radhakrishnan, M.; Gopikrishnan, V.; Pazhanimurugan, R.; Balagurunathan, R. A study of the bactericidal, anti-biofouling, cytotoxic and antioxidant properties of actinobacterially synthesised silver nanoparticles. *Colloids Surf. B Biointerfaces* **2013**, *111*, 680–687. [CrossRef]
112. Ramya, S.; Shanmugasundaram, T.; Balagurunathan, R. Biomedical potential of actinobacterially synthesised selenium nanoparticles with special reference to anti-biofilm, anti-oxidant, wound healing, cytotoxic and anti-viral activities. *J. Trace Elem. Med. Biol.* **2015**, *32*, 30–39. [CrossRef]
113. Torres, S.K.; Campos, V.L.; León, C.G.; Rodríguez-Llamazares, S.M.; Rajos, S.M.; González, M.; Smith, C.; Mondaca, M.A. Biosynthesis of selenium nanoparticles by *Pantoea agglomerans* and their antioxidant activity. *J. Nanopart Res.* **2012**, *14*, 1236. [CrossRef]
114. Sowani, H.; Mohite, P.; Munot, H.; Shouche, Y.; Bapat, T.; Kumar, A.R.; Kulkarni, M.; Zinjarde, S. Green synthesis of gold and silver nanoparticles by an Actinomycete *Gordonia amicalis* HS-11: Mechanistic aspects and biological application. *Process Biochem.* **2016**, *51*, 374–383. [CrossRef]
115. Sivasankar, P.; Seedevi, P.; Poongodi, S.; Sivakumar, M.; Murugan, T.; Sivakumar, L.; Sivakumar, K. Characterization, antimicrobial and antioxidant property of exopolysaccharide mediated silver nanoparticles synthesized by *Streptomyces violaceus* MM72. *Carbohydr. Polym.* **2018**, *181*, 752–759. [CrossRef] [PubMed]

116. Moghaddam, A.B.; Moniri, M.; Azizi, S.; Rahim, R.A.; Ariff, A.B.; Saad, W.Z.; Namvar, F.; Navaderi, M.; Mohamad, R. Biosynthesis of ZnO nanoparticles by a new *Pichia kudriavzevii* yeast strain and evaluation of their antimicrobial and antioxidant activities. *Molecules* **2017**, *22*, 872. [CrossRef] [PubMed]
117. Netala, V.R.; Bethu, M.S.; Pushpalatha, B.; Baki, V.B.; Aishwarya, S.; Rao, J.V.; Tartte, V. Biogenesis of silver nanoparticles using endophytic fungus *Pestalotiopsis microspora* and evaluation of their antioxidant and anticancer activities. *Int. J. Nanomed.* **2016**, *11*, 5683–5696. [CrossRef] [PubMed]
118. Manjunath, H.M.; Joshi, C.G.; Danagoudar, A.; Poyya, J.; Kudva, A.K.; Dhananjaya, B.L. Biogenic synthesis of gold nanoparticles by marine endophytic fungus-*Cladosporium cladosporioides* isolated from seaweed and evaluation of their antioxidant and antimicrobial properties. *Process Biochem.* **2017**, *63*, 137–144.
119. Manjunath, H.M.; Joshi, C.G. Characterization, antioxidant and antimicrobial activity of silver nanoparticles synthesized using marine endophytic fungus- *Cladosporium cladosporioides*. *Process Biochem.* **2019**, *82*, 199–204. [CrossRef]
120. Netala, V.R.; Kotakadi, V.S.; Bobbu, P.; Gaddam, S.A.; Tartte, V. Endophytic fungal isolate mediated biosynthesis of silver nanoparticles and their free radical scavenging activity and anti microbial studies. *3Biotech* **2016**, *6*, 132. [CrossRef]
121. Saravanakumar, K.; Wang, M.H. *Trichoderma* based synthesis of anti-pathogenic silver nanoparticles and their characterization, antioxidant and cytotoxicity properties. *Microb. Pathog.* **2018**, *114*, 269–273. [CrossRef]
122. Gao, Y.; Anand, M.A.V.; Ramachandran, V.; Karthikkumar, V.; Shalini, V.; Vijayalakshmi, S.; Ernest, D. Biofabrication of zinc oxide nanoparticles from *Aspergillus niger*, their antioxidant, antimicrobial and anticancer activity. *J. Clust. Sci.* **2019**, *30*, 937–946. [CrossRef]
123. Govindappa, M.; Farheen, H.; Chandrappa, C.P.; Rai, R.V.; Raghavendra, V.B. Mycosynthesis of silver nanoparticles using extract of endophytic fungi, *Penicillium* species of *Glycosmis mauritiana*, and its antioxidant, antimicrobial, anti-inflammatory and tyrokinase inhibitory activity. *Adv. Nat. Sci. Nanosci. Nanotechnol.* **2016**, *7*, 035014. [CrossRef]
124. Nagajyothi, P.C.; Sreekanth, T.V.M.; Lee, J.I.; Lee, K.D. Mycosynthesis: Antibacterial, antioxidant and antiproliferative activities of silver nanoparticles synthesized from *Inonotus obliquus* (Chaga mushroom) extract. *J. Photochem. Photobiol. B* **2014**, *130*, 299–304. [CrossRef]
125. Popli, D.; Anil, V.; Subramanyam, A.B.; Namratha, M.N.; Ranjitha, V.R.; Rao, S.N.; Rai, R.V.; Govindappa, M. Endophyte fungi, *Cladosporium* species-mediated synthesis of silver nanoparticles possessing in vitro antioxidant, anti-diabetic and anti-Alzheimer activity. *Artif. Cells Nanomed. Biotechnol.* **2018**, *46*, 676–683. [CrossRef] [PubMed]
126. Sriramulu, M.; Sumathi, S. Photocatalytic, antioxidant, antibacterial and anti-inflammatory activity of silver nanoparticles synthesised using forest and edible mushroom. *Adv. Nat. Sci. Nanosci. Nanotechnol.* **2017**, *8*, 045012. [CrossRef]
127. Lee, K.D.; Nagajyothi, P.C.; Sreekanth, T.V.M.; Park, S. Eco-friendly synthesis of gold nanoparticles (AuNPs) using *Inonotus obliquus* and their antibacterial, antioxidant and cytotoxic activities. *J. Ind. Eng. Chem.* **2015**, *26*, 67–72. [CrossRef]
128. Aygün, A.; Özdemir, S.; Gülcan, M.; Cellat, K.; Şen, F. Synthesis and characterization of Reishi mushroom-mediated green synthesis of silver nanoparticles for the biochemical applications. *J. Pharm. Bimed. Anal.* **2020**, *178*, 112970. [CrossRef]
129. Poudel, M.; Pokharel, R.; Sudip, K.C.; Awal, S.C.; Pradhananga, R. Biosynthesis of silver nanoparticles using *Ganoderma Lucidum* and assessment of antioxidant and antibacterial activity. *Int. J. Appl. Sci. Biotechnol.* **2017**, *5*, 523–531. [CrossRef]
130. Naveena, B.E.; Prakash, S. Biological synthesis of gold nanoparticles using marine algae *Gracilaria corticata* and its application as a potent antimicrobial and antioxidant agent. *Asian J. Pharm. Clin. Res.* **2013**, *6*, 179–182.
131. Sharma, B.; Purkayastha, D.D.; Hazra, S.; Thajamanbi, M.; Bhattacharjee, C.R.; Ghosh, N.N.; Rout, J. Biosynthesis of fluorescent gold nanoparticles using an edible freshwater red alga, Lemanea fluviatilis (L.) C.Ag. and antioxidant activity of biomatrix loaded nanoparticles. *Bioprocess Biosyst. Eng.* **2014**, *37*, 2559–2565. [CrossRef]
132. Dasari, S.; Suresh, K.A.; Rajesh, M.; Reddy, C.S.S.; Hemalatha, C.S.; Wudayagiri, R.; Valluru, L. Biosynthesis, characterization, antibacterial and antioxidant activity of silver nanoparticles produced by lichens. *J. Bionanosci.* **2013**, *7*, 237–244. [CrossRef]

133. Debnath, R.; Purkayastha, D.D.; Hazra, S.; Ghosh, N.N.; Bhattacharjee, C.R.; Rout, J. Biogenic synthesis of antioxidant, shape selective gold nanomaterials mediated by high altitude lichens. *Mater. Lett.* **2016**, *169*, 58–61. [CrossRef]
134. Kumar, H.; Bhardwaj, K.; Kuča, K.; Kalia, A.; Nepovimova, E.; Verma, R.; Kumar, D. Flower-basedgreensynthesis of metallicnanoparticles: Applicationsbeyondfragrance. *Nanomaterials* **2020**, *10*, 766. [CrossRef] [PubMed]
135. Guajardo-Pachecoa, M.J.; Morales-Sanchz, J.E.; González-Hernándezc, J.; Ruiz, F. Synthesis of copper nanoparticles using soybeans as a chelant agent. *Mater. Lett.* **2010**, *64*, 1361–1364. [CrossRef]
136. Xi, Y.; Hu, C.; Gao, P.; Yang, R.; He, X.; Wang, X.; Wan, B. Morphology and phase selective synthesis of Cu_xO (x = 1, 2) nanostructures and their catalytic degradation activity. *Mater. Sci. Eng. B* **2010**, *166*, 113–117. [CrossRef]
137. He, Y. A novel solid-stabilized emulsion approach to CuO nanostructures microspheres. *Mater. Res. Bull.* **2007**, *42*, 190–195. [CrossRef]
138. Motogoshi, R.; Oku, T.; Suzuki, A.; Kikuchi, K.; Kikuchi, S.; Jeyadevan, B.; Cuya, J. Fabrication and characterization of cupprious oxide: Fullerene solar cells. *Synth. Met.* **2010**, *160*, 1219–1222. [CrossRef]
139. Herlekar, M.; Barve, S.; Kumar, R. Plant-mediated green synthesis of iron nanoparticles. *J. Nanopart. Res.* **2014**, *2014*, 140614. [CrossRef]
140. Huber, D.L. Synthesis, properties, and applications of iron nanoparticles. *Small* **2005**, *1*, 482–501. [CrossRef]
141. Guo, J.; Wang, R.; Tjiu, W.W.; Pan, J.; Liu, T. Synthesis of Fe nanoparticles@ graphene composites for environmental applications. *J. Hazard. Mater.* **2012**, *225*, 63–73. [CrossRef]
142. Babay, S.; Mhiri, T.; Toumi, M. Synthesis, structural and spectroscopic characterizations of maghemite γ-Fe_2O_3 prepared by one-step coprecipitation route. *J. Mol. Struct.* **2015**, *1085*, 286–293. [CrossRef]
143. Saleh, N.; Kim, H.J.; Phenrat, T.; Matyjaszewski, K.; Tilton, R.D.; Lowry, G.V. Ionic strength and composition affect the mobility of surface-modified Fe^0 nanoparticles in water-saturated sand columns. *Environ. Sci. Technol.* **2008**, *42*, 3349–3355. [CrossRef] [PubMed]
144. Kim, H.J.; Kim, D.G.; Yoon, H.; Choi, Y.S.; Yoon, J.; Lee, J.C. Polyphenol/Fe^{III} complex coated membranes having multifunctional properties prepared by a one-step fast assembly. *Adv. Mater. Interfaces* **2015**, *2*, 1500298. [CrossRef]
145. Yang, L.; Cao, Z.; Sajja, H.K.; Mao, H.; Wang, L.; Geng, H.; Xu, H.; Jiang, T.; Wood, W.C.; Nie, S.; et al. Development of receptor targeted magnetic iron oxide nanoparticles for efficient drug delivery and tumor imaging. *J. Biomed. Nanotechnol.* **2008**, *4*, 439–449. [CrossRef] [PubMed]
146. Ebrahiminezhad, A.; Zare-Hoseinabadi, A.; Sarmah, A.K.; Taghizadeh, S.; Ghasemi, Y.; Berenjian, A. Plant-mediated synthesis and applications of iron nanoparticles. *Mol. Biotechnol.* **2018**, *60*, 154–168. [CrossRef]
147. Agarwal, H.; Kumar, S.V.; Rajeshkumar, S. A review on green synthesis of zinc oxide nanoparticles -An eco-friendly approach. *Res. Effic. Technol.* **2017**, *3*, 406–413. [CrossRef]
148. Jayaseelan, C.; Rahuman, A.A.; Kirthi, A.V.; Marimuthu, S.; Santhoshkumar, T.; Bagavan, A.; Guarav, K.; Karthik, L.; Rao, K.V. Novel microbial route to synthesize ZnO nanoparticles using *Aeromonas hydrophila* and their activity against pathogenic bacteria and fungi. *Spectrochim. Acta A Mol. Biomol. Spectrosc.* **2012**, *90*, 78–84. [CrossRef]
149. Pulit-prociak, J.; Chwastowski, J.; Kucharski, A.; Banach, M. Applied surface science functionalization of textiles with silver and zinc oxide nanoparticles. *Appl. Surf. Sci.* **2016**, *385*, 543–553. [CrossRef]
150. Wodka, D.; Bielaníska, E.; Socha, R.P.; Elzbieciak-Wodka, M.; Gurgul, J.; Nowak, P.; Warszyński, P.; Kumakiri, I. Photocatalytic activity of titanium dioxide modified by silver nanoparticles. *ACS Appl. Mater. Interfaces* **2010**, *2*, 1945–1953. [CrossRef]
151. Wadhwani, S.A.; Shedbalkar, U.U.; Singh, R.; Chopade, B.A. Biogenic selenium nanoparticles: Current status and future prospects. *Appl. Microbiol. Biotechnol.* **2016**, *100*, 2555–2566. [CrossRef]
152. Li, Y.; Li, X.; Zheng, W.; Fan, C.; Zhang, Y.; Chen, T. Functionalized selenium nanoparticles with nephroprotective activity, the important roles of ROS mediated signaling pathways. *J. Mater. Chem.* **2013**, *1*, 6365–6372. [CrossRef]
153. Din, M.I.; Rani, A. Recent advances in the synthesis and stabilization of nickel and nickel oxide nanoparticles: A green adeptness. *Int. J. Anal. Chem.* **2016**, *2016*, 3512145.
154. Saxena, A.; Kumar, K.; Mozumdar, S. Ni-nanoparticles: An efficient green catalyst for chemo-selective oxidative couplingof thiols. *J. Mol. Catal. A Chem.* **2007**, *269*, 35–40. [CrossRef]

155. Alonso, F.; Riente, P.; Yus, M. Hydrogen-transfer reduction of carbonyl compounds promoted by nickel nanoparticles. *Tetrahedron* **2008**, *64*, 1847–1852. [CrossRef]
156. Dhakshinamoorthy, A.; Pitchumani, K. Clay entrapped nickel nanoparticles as efficient and recyclable catalysts forhydrogenation of olefins. *Tetrahedron Lett.* **2008**, *49*, 1818–1823. [CrossRef]
157. Alonso, F.; Riente, P.; Yus, M. Wittig-type olefination of alcohols promoted by nickel nanoparticles: Synthesis ofpolymethoxylated and polyhydroxylated stilbenes. *Eur. J. Org. Chem.* **2009**, *2009*, 6034–6042. [CrossRef]
158. Alonso, F.; Riente, P.; Yus, M. Alcohols for the α-alkylationof methyl ketones and indirect aza-wittig reaction promoted bynickel nanoparticles. *Eur. J. Org. Chem.* **2008**, *2008*, 4908–4914. [CrossRef]
159. Li, X.K.; Ji, W.J.; Zhao, J.; Wang, S.J.; Au, C.T. Ammonia decomposition over Ru and Ni catalysts supported on fumed SiO_2, MCM-41, and SBA-15. *J. Catal.* **2005**, *236*, 181–189. [CrossRef]
160. Li, Y.; Zhang, B.; Xie, X.; Liu, J.; Xu, Y.; Shen, W. Novel Nicatalysts for methane decomposition to hydrogen and carbonnanofibers. *J. Catal.* **2006**, *238*, 412–424. [CrossRef]
161. Al-Rawi, M.; Diabaté, S.; Weiss, C. Uptake and intracellular localization of submicron and nano-sized SiO_2 particles in HeLa cells. *Arch Toxicol.* **2011**, *85*, 813–826. [CrossRef]
162. Hussain, S.M.; Hess, K.L.; Gearhart, J.M.; Geiss, K.T.; Schlager, J.J. In vitro toxicity of nanoparticles in BRL 3A rat liver cells. *Toxicol. Vitr.* **2005**, *19*, 975–983. [CrossRef]
163. Clift, M.J.D.; Rothen-Rutishauser, B.; Brown, D.M.; Duffin, R.; Ronaldson, K.; Proudfoot, L.; Guy, K.; Stone, V. The impact of different nanoparticle surface chemistry and size on uptake and toxicity in a murine macrophage cell line. *Toxicol. Appl. Pharmacol.* **2008**, *232*, 418–427. [CrossRef] [PubMed]
164. Rabolli, V.; Thomassen, L.C.; Uwambayinema, F.; Martens, J.A.; Lison, D. The cytotoxic activity of amorphous silica nanoparticles is mainly influenced by surface area and not by aggregation. *Toxicol. Lett.* **2011**, *206*, 197–203. [CrossRef] [PubMed]
165. Morais, T.; Soares, M.E.; Duarte, J.A.; Soares, L.; Maia, S.; Gomes, P.; Pereira, E.; Fraga, S.; Carmo, H.; De Lourdes Bastos, M. Effect of surface coating on the biodistribution profile of gold nanoparticles in the rat. *Eur. J. Pharm. Biopharm.* **2012**, *80*, 185–193. [CrossRef]
166. Cho, W.S.; Cho, M.; Jeong, J.; Choi, M.; Cho, H.Y.; Han, B.S.; Kim, S.H.; Kim, H.O.; Lim, Y.T.; Chung, B.H.; et al. Acute toxicity and pharmacokinetics of 13 nm-sized PEG-coated gold nanoparticles. *Toxicol. Appl. Pharmacol.* **2009**, *236*, 16–24. [CrossRef]
167. Knaapen, A.M.; Borm, P.J.; Albrecht, C.; Schins, R.P. Inhaled particles and lung cancer. Part A: Mechanisms. *Int. J. Cancer* **2004**, *109*, 799–809. [CrossRef] [PubMed]
168. Xia, T.; Kovochich, M.; Liong, M.; Mädler, L.; Gilbert, B.; Shi, H.; Yeh, J.I.; Zink, J.I.; Nel, A.E. Comparison of the mechanism of toxicity of zinc oxide and cerium oxide nanoparticles based on dissolution and oxidative stress properties. *ACS Nano* **2008**, *2*, 2121–2134. [CrossRef] [PubMed]

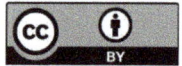

© 2020 by the authors. Licensee MDPI, Basel, Switzerland. This article is an open access article distributed under the terms and conditions of the Creative Commons Attribution (CC BY) license (http://creativecommons.org/licenses/by/4.0/).

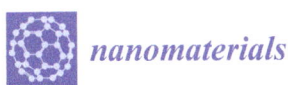

Review

Recent Advances in Nanomedicine for the Diagnosis and Therapy of Liver Fibrosis

Xue Bai [1,2], Gaoxing Su [3,*] and Shumei Zhai [1,*]

1. School of Chemistry and Chemical Engineering, Shandong University, Jinan 250100, China; baixue1013@163.com
2. School of Public Health, Cheeloo College of Medicine, Shandong University, Jinan 250012, China
3. School of Pharmacy, Nantong University, Nantong 226001, China
* Correspondence: sugaoxing@ntu.edu.cn (G.S.); smzhai@sdu.edu.cn (S.Z.); Tel.: +86-513-8505-1749 (G.S.); +86-531-8836-4464 (S.Z.)

Received: 31 August 2020; Accepted: 27 September 2020; Published: 29 September 2020

Abstract: Liver fibrosis, a reversible pathological process of inflammation and fiber deposition caused by chronic liver injury and can cause severe health complications, including liver failure, liver cirrhosis, and liver cancer. Traditional diagnostic methods and drug-based therapy have several limitations, such as lack of precision and inadequate therapeutic efficiency. As a medical application of nanotechnology, nanomedicine exhibits great potential for liver fibrosis diagnosis and therapy. Nanomedicine enhances imaging contrast and improves tissue penetration and cellular internalization; it simultaneously achieves targeted drug delivery, combined therapy, as well as diagnosis and therapy (i.e., theranostics). In this review, recent designs and development efforts of nanomedicine systems for the diagnosis, therapy, and theranostics of liver fibrosis are introduced. Relative to traditional methods, these nanomedicine systems generally demonstrate significant improvement in liver fibrosis treatment. Perspectives and challenges related to these nanomedicine systems translated from laboratory to clinical use are also discussed.

Keywords: nanomedicine; liver fibrosis; diagnosis; therapy; theranostics; targeted drug delivery

---

1. Introduction

Liver fibrosis is an important pathological and repair process in chronic liver disease, which is caused by chronic viral hepatitis, alcohol, and non-alcoholic steatohepatitis (NASH), and autoimmune liver disease [1–3]. It has been reported that liver diseases caused 4.6% of all deaths in the Asia-Pacific region, 2.7% in the USA, and 2.1% in Europe in 2015. The Asia-Pacific region holds more than half of the global population and accounted for 62.6% of all deaths due to liver diseases globally in 2015. Chronic hepatitis B virus (HBV) infection caused more than half of the deaths due to cirrhosis and other chronic liver diseases, followed by alcohol consumption, non-alcoholic fatty liver disease, and chronic infection with hepatitis C virus [4]. With persistent damage, live fibrosis develops into cirrhosis and, even to hepatocellular carcinoma, together with a series of complications, including hepatic encephalopathy, hepatic failure, and portal hypertension [5,6].

Liver fibrosis is currently diagnosed based on ultrasound imaging and blood testing, both of which lack precision [7]. Chemical drugs [8], Chinese herbal medicines [9], and monoclonal antibodies [10] are also being developed for the treatment of liver fibrosis. These approaches aim to remove injurious stimuli, suppress hepatic inflammation, down regulate hepatic stellate cell (HSC) activation, and promote matrix degradation [11]. However, these approaches exhibit limited therapeutic efficiency and have side effects. Therapeutic methods with enhanced therapeutic efficiency and targeted capabilities need to be developed. Precise diagnostic methods are also needed to monitor the progression of the disease.

Nanomedicine involves the design and application of nanoparticles (NPs) in the diagnosis and treatment of diseases [12–14]. As an important area of nanotechnology research, nanomedicine has greatly contributed to biomedicine in recent decades. Finely designed nanostructures have been fabricated as effective therapeutic agents for liver fibrosis with specific site-targeting abilities [15–17]. Nanostructures have also been developed as nanoagents for contrast enhancement or nanoprobes for the diagnosis of liver fibrosis [18]. Numerous inorganic or organic NPs have thus far been extensively investigated for the diagnosis and treatment of liver fibrosis, including metal oxide NPs [18], metal NPs [19], lipid NPs [20], polymer NPs [21], and protein NPs [22]. The various composition, controllable shape, size, and modifiable surface properties of NPs provide to them superior advantages, including controlled drug release, cell-tissue gap penetration, high contrast, prolonged duration in the bloodstream, improvement of the pharmacokinetics of drugs, and reduction of toxic side effects [23]. A greater significance of such systems is that they allow the integration of diagnosis and therapy in one nanoplatform [24].

The current review summarizes potential targets and the application of emerging nanomedicine systems for liver fibrosis diagnosis and therapy, including liposomes, polymer NPs, protein NPs, inorganic NPs, and hybrid NPs. Major research gaps, challenges, and coping strategies for the treatment of liver fibrosis by using nanomedicine are also discussed.

2. Potential Targets of Liver Fibrosis

Activated HSCs are involved in the inflammatory response, fibrogenesis, and angiogenesis in liver fibrosis (Figure 1). They are at the center of liver fibrosis. Therefore, HSC-targeted strategies can be developed for the treatment of liver fibrosis. Alternative strategies include anti-inflammatory agents and inhibition of collagen deposition.

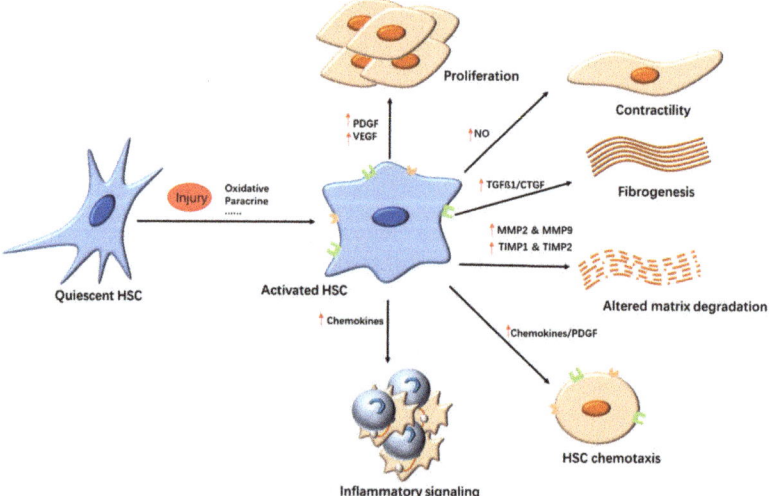

Figure 1. Hepatic stellate cell (HSC) activation. The pathways of HSC activation include initiation and perpetuation stages. Initiation is stimulated by reactive oxygen species (ROS), paracrine stimuli, and so on. The continuous stimulation could induce HSCs into myofibroblast cells, and the perpetuation phase occurs, which is involved in the change of HSC behavior, including proliferation, contractility, fibrogenesis, altered matrix degradation, chemotaxis, and inflammatory signaling. Abbreviations: CTGF, connective tissue growth factor; HSC, hepatic stellate cell; MMP, matrix metalloproteinase; NO, nitric oxide; PDGF, platelet-derived growth factor; TGF-β1, transforming growth factor β1; TIMP, tissue inhibitor of metalloproteinase; VEGF, vascular endothelial growth factor.

2.1. Targeting HSCs

Comprising about 13% of total liver cells, HSCs exist in the sinus space and come in direct contact with hepatic epithelial cells and endothelial cells [25]. In their normal state, HSCs are quiescent and mainly participate in vitamin A (VA) metabolism and fat storage. If the liver suffers from injuries, HSCs are activated and transformed into myofibroblasts. Activation of HSCs is a hallmark of liver fibrosis. Activated HSCs typically express smooth muscle actin (α-SMA); in addition, they synthesize and secrete the extracellular matrix (ECM). ECM deposition changes the structure and function of liver tissue, which is the root cause of liver fibrosis [26,27]. Therefore, activated HSCs are among the important targets for liver fibrosis therapy. Numerous signaling molecules are involved in the activation of HSCs, with TGF-β and PDGF being the important ones [27–29]. Therefore, blocking the TGF-β or PDGF signaling pathways is an effective strategy for the treatment of liver fibrosis. Protease inhibitors, such as camostat mesilate (FOY305), can neutralize TGF-β [30]. As a multi-target receptor tyrosine kinase inhibitor, sorafenib, targets the Raf/ERK signaling pathways and PDGF receptor and can effectively attenuate experimental liver fibrosis, inflammation, and angiogenesis [31]. Moreover, many anti-fibrosis drugs, such as the semisynthetic analog of fumagillin-TNP-470 [32] and the fungal metabolite-OPC-15161 [33], suppress the activation and proliferation of HSCs. Moreover, ROS contributes to liver fibrosis by promoting the activation and proliferation of fibroblasts and myofibroblasts, as well as the activating the TGF-β pathway in an autocrine manner [34]. Antioxidants, such as vitamin E [35], silymarin [36], N-acetylcysteine [8], resveratrol [37], quercetin [9], phosphatidylcholine [38], and glutathione [39], can inhibit the activation of HSCs and reduce liver fibrosis. These drugs benefit patients with alcoholic liver disease and NASH.

HSCs are also involved in hepatic angiogenesis and hepatic sinus vascular remodeling. When stimulated by inflammatory factors or hypoxia, HSCs can directly express VEGF and angiopoietin-1, influencing angiogenesis in the liver [40,41]. Pathological angiogenesis is related to the process of liver fibrosis and cirrhosis [42]. During liver fibrosis, fibrous scar tissue presses against the portal vein and central vein, leading to increased intrahepatic resistance. Simultaneously, liver sinus capillarization and fibrous scar obstruction also increase the resistance of blood flow and oxygen diffusion. These processes result in low oxygen conditions in the liver and gene expression, which are sensitive to oxygen concentration such as hypoxia-inducible factors (HIFs). Pathological angiogenesis cannot improve the oxygen level in the liver because of the high permeability of new blood vessels induced by VEGF. Therefore, pathologic angiogenesis and hypoxemia interfere with normal tissue repair and promote the development of liver fibrosis [43]. Pathological angiogenesis plays an important role in liver fibrosis and thus has been considered as an important therapeutic target for the reversal of liver fibrosis. One study found that the knockout of HIF-1α in rats significantly ameliorated liver fibrosis, indicating that improving intrahepatic hypoxia could effectively treat such a disease [44].

2.2. Anti-Inflammatory Response

An inflammatory response to autocrine or paracrine stimulation prompts HSC activation and proliferation. HSC activation consists of two stages: initiation and perpetuation [25,27]. Early changes in gene expression and phenotype represent the initiation stage. Initiation is mainly induced by cytokines, or other stimuli from cells around HSCs and act as paracrine pathways [27]. Reactive oxygen species (ROS) released from Kupffer cells can directly stimulate and activate HSCs [45]. By cascade amplification of inflammatory response, a large number of inflammatory cells infiltrate the damaged sites, and secrete inflammatory cytokines, leading to HSC activation and proliferation [46]. Continuous stimulation can induce HSCs into myofibroblast cells, inducing the perpetuation stage. The activated HSCs subsequently release chemokines, further aggravating the inflammatory response. In this stage, HSC promotes inflammation, fibrosis, and cell proliferation in the autocrine and/or paracrine pathway. Therefore, the inflammation response plays an important role in liver fibrosis. Anti-inflammatory drugs such as corticosteroids [47], colchicine [48], and ursodeoxycholic acid [49] have been used to treat liver fibrosis. Another anti-inflammatory strategy involves the application of specific receptor antagonists to neutralize inflammatory cytokines. In one study, the antifibrotic and anti-inflammatory effects of IL-10 were observed in patients infected with hepatitis C [50]. Moreover, hepatic macrophages participate in the pathogenesis of liver fibrosis by the secretion of inflammatory factors. Targeting hepatic macrophages is also an effective anti-inflammatory technique for the treatment of liver fibrosis [51].

2.3. Inhibition of Collagen Deposition

The main clinical feature of liver fibrosis is the excessive deposition of ECM, particularly collagen. Collagen I is the main component in ECM, and the cross-linking of collagen I is significantly increased in liver fibrosis. Therefore, collagen I reduction has been adopted to treat liver fibrosis. In one study, the monoclonal antibody AB0023, which is an inhibitor of the matrix remodeling enzyme LOXL2, inhibited liver fibrosis by regulating the cross-linking of collagen I [52]. In another study, the human monoclonal antibody GS-6624 was used for the treatment of NASH-induced liver fibrosis [11].

3. Nanomedicine in Liver Fibrosis Diagnosis

For liver diseases, early detection of liver fibrosis would be helpful for treatment. Unfortunately, most cases of liver disease are diagnosed late because of no symptoms. Current strategies for the diagnosis of liver fibrosis rely on an invasive biopsy which would cause damage for the patients [53]. Recently, magnetic resonance imaging (MRI) has been developed as a method with high diagnostic accuracy for the detection of fibrosis [54]. Magnetic NPs play an important role in the diagnosis and imaging of liver fibrosis [55]. For example, dextran stabilized superparamagnetic iron oxide NPs (D-SPIONs) with high blood compatibility and low cytotoxicity was used as an MRI contrast agent for liver fibrosis detection [56]. D-SPIONs enhanced image contrast of tissue and led to a 55% decrease in the pixel intensity, and therefore improved the contrast difference between the fibrotic tissue and the rest of the extracellular matrix rich hepatic parenchyma at the fibrosis stage significantly. Citrate-coated ultrasmall iron oxide NPs were also shown to provide a good MRI of liver fibrosis [57]. In one study, Fe_3O_4 NPs coated with SiO_2 and then coupled with indocyanine green (ICG) and arginine–glycine–aspartic acid (SPIO@SiO$_2$–ICG–RGD) were constructed for HSC targeting and early detection of liver fibrosis (Figure 2) [18]. Fe_3O_4 NPs and ICG as the photographic developers for T_2 MRI and near-infrared (NIR) imaging, respectively. NIR fluorescence (NIR) and MRI revealed that SPIO@SiO$_2$–ICG–RGD could elicit accurate identification of fibrotic regions in the liver. These NIR hybrid NPs combined imaging and MRI and provided higher sensitivity and spatial resolution for liver fibrosis detection, compared with MRI alone.

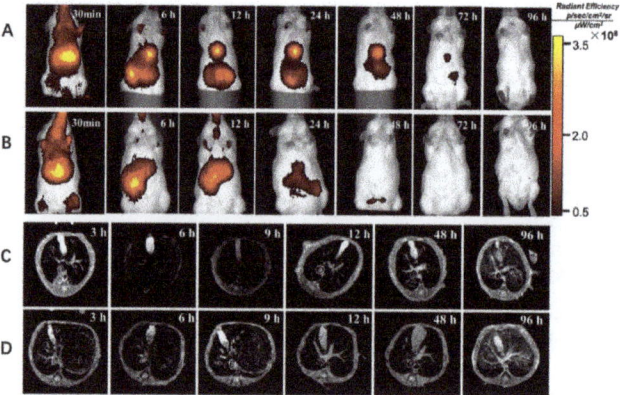

Figure 2. In vivo optical imaging and MRI of liver fibrosis using SPIO@SiO$_2$–ICG–RGD. (**A,C**) A model of hepatic fibrosis in mice. (**B,D**) Healthy mouse model (control). Adapted with permission from [18]. Copyright RSC publishing, 2018.

Furthermore, zero-valent iron (ZVI)-based NPs were also fabricated as novel contrast agents for MRI. After functionalized with liver specific polysaccharide pullulan and fluorescent carbon dots, a dual imaging contrast agent (P@ZVI-Cdts) was obtained. The efficiency of the developed systems for targeted liver imaging and optical imaging has been successfully demonstrated in vivo. The high r1 relaxivity enables ZVI NPs to be a competent T_1 MRI contrast agent for various clinical applications including diagnosis of liver fibrosis [58].

In addition to MRI, the combination of an ultrasound agent with a targeting peptide has been reported for the early and non-invasive diagnosis of liver fibrosis. One study found that core–shell perfluorooctyl bromide (PFOB) coated with poly(lactic-co-glycolic acid) (PLGA) polymers and modified with a cyclic RGD (cRGD–PLGA–PFOB NPs) exhibited powerful ultrasound molecular imaging features, including high-contrast imaging among liver fibrotic stages and adjacent tissues [59].

4. Nanomedicine for Liver Fibrosis Therapy

4.1. NPs as Therapeutic Agents

Owing to their distinctive bioactive properties, inorganic NPs alone can be used as therapeutic agents for liver fibrosis therapy [60–62]. Both titanium dioxide NPs (TiO_2 NPs) and silicon dioxide NPs (SiO_2 NPs) can inhibit the expression of collagen I and α-SMA. They also facilitate collagen I degradation by upregulating matrix metalloproteinases (MMPs) and downregulating tissue inhibitors of metalloproteinases (TIMPs), indicating the potential antifibrotic activities of TiO_2 NPs and SiO_2 NPs in vitro [63]. These NPs further exhibit anti-adhesive and anti-migratory effects by regulating epithelial–mesenchymal transition (EMT) gene expression and revert TGF-β-activated HSCs to a quiescent state (Figure 3). Owing to their anti-inflammatory properties, cerium oxide NPs reduce liver steatosis, portal hypertension, and liver fibrosis in rats [64]. Oral exposure of citrate-functionalized Mn_3O_4 NPs can protect the liver from carbon tetrachloride (CCl_4)-induced cirrhosis, fibrosis, and oxidative stress because of the increased antioxidant properties of Mn_3O_4 NPs upon acid treatment in the stomach [65]. ZnO NPs also ameliorate liver fibrosis by reducing lipid peroxidation, oxidative stress, and inflammation in dimethylnitrosamine-induced liver damage [66].

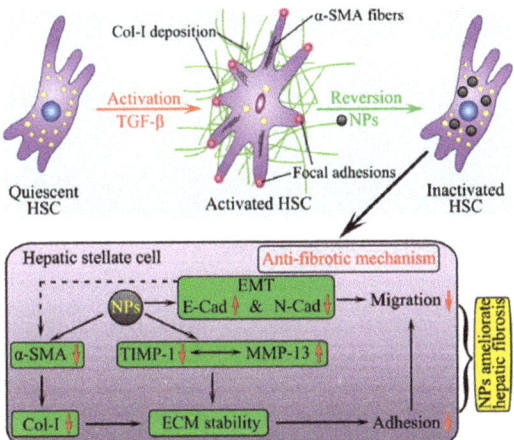

Figure 3. Model for TiO_2 NPs and SiO_2 NPs ameliorated fibrosis, adhesion and migration of HSCs. TiO_2 NPs and SiO_2 NPs can suppress the expression of α-SMA and deposition of Col-I induced by TGF-β. ECM was degraded by upregulating MMP-13 and downregulating TIMP-1. Therefore, adhesion of LX-2 cells was reduced. Furthermore, NPs stimulated the expression of E-Cad and reduced the expression of N-Cad, and, therefore, aggravated the migratory phenotype. Reproduced with permission from [63]. Copyright American Chemical Society, 2018.

In addition to metal oxide NPs, other types of inorganic NPs are also used to treat liver fibrosis. A study found that gold NPs reduced liver fibrosis in a rat model of ethanol- and methamphetamine-induced liver injury by inhibiting the activity of Kupffer cells and HSCs [67]. The mechanism involves the regulation of AKT/PI3K and MAPK signaling pathways by gold NPs, thereby reducing pro-inflammatory cytokine secretion and oxidative stress. Another study reported that vitamin E-modified selenium NPs can attenuate liver fibrosis by reducing oxidative stress [68].

4.2. NPs as Drug Carriers without Targeting Ligand for the Treatment of Liver Fibrosis

The liver is the main metabolic and excretory organ in the body in which NPs can accumulate and accomplish passive targeting because of their size. Thus, NPs have been widely used as drug carriers for the treatment of liver fibrosis. Lipid-based NPs have been recognized as the most powerful vehicles because of their good biocompatibility and low toxicity (Table 1) [69]. CCAAT/enhancer-binding protein alpha (CEBPA), a master transcriptional factor in the liver, resets the natural gene regulatory mechanism of hepatocytes to reduce fibrosis and reverse liver dysfunction. Small activating RNA oligonucleotide therapy (CEBPA-51) formulated in liposome NPs can upregulate CEBPA, thereby reducing fibrosis [70]. After Cur-mNLCs treatment, pro-inflammatory cytokines, collagen fibers and α-SMA were reduced, while hepatocyte growth factors (HGF) and MMP2 were increased. Cationic lipid NPs loaded with small interfering RNA to the procollagen $\alpha 1(I)$ gene (LNP-siCol1α1) can be retained in the liver of fibrotic mice and accumulate in nonparenchymal liver cells, specifically blocking procollagen $\alpha 1(I)$ expression and inhibiting liver fibrosis progression without noticeable side effects [20].

Table 1. NPs as drug carriers without targeting ligands in liver fibrosis treatment.

Nanoparticle Systems	NPs Formulation	Delivered Drug	Reference
Lipid-based NPs	RNA oligonucleotide-liposomal	MTL-CEBPA	[70]
	Cationic lipid NPs	small interfering RNA to the procollagen 1(I) gene	[20]
	Dexamethasone-liposomes	dexamethasone	[71]
Polymer-based NPs	Cationic nanohydrogel particles	anti-Col1α1 siRNA	[72]
	Ketal cross-linked cationic nanohydrogel	Cy5-labeled anti-col1α1 siRNA	[73]
	PLGA	phyllanthin	[74]
	PEG-PLGA or PEG-PLGA/PLGA NPs	sorafenib	[75]
	Eudragit(R) RS100 NPs (SMnps)	silymarin	[76]
Inorganic NPs	Rhodamine B (RhB)-mesoporous silica NPs (MSNs-RhB)	salvianolic acid B	[77]
	Mesoporous silica NPs	siTnC	[78]
	PEG-AuNPs	hesperetin	[79]
	AuNPs and SiNPs	NO donors	[80]
	PtNPs	Curcumin	[81]
	Calcium phosphate NPs (CaP@BSA NPs)	TSG-6	[82]
	Graphene nanostars linked to PAMAM-GS dendrimer	Plasmid	[83]
Protein NPs	Zein nanospheres	Curcumin	[84]
	Glucose modify albumin NPs	Berberine	[85]
	Albumin NPs	Bexamethasone	[22]
	Polyavidin-based NPs	Dexamethasone	[86]

Polymer-based NPs have been fabricated as drug carriers for the treatment of liver fibrosis (Table 1). In one study, ketal cross-linked cationic nanohydrogel particles were synthesized to deliver Cy5-labeled anti-col1α1 siRNA, which enhanced carrier and payload accumulation in the fibrotic tissue and prevented fibrosis progression [73]. PLGA and eudragit have also been employed as drug carriers. In one study, phyllanthin was carried by PLGA to reduce liver marker enzymes, namely alanine aminotransferase and aspartate aminotransferase, as well as collagen [74]. In another study, silymarin was delivered by eudragit NPs for the treatment of liver fibrosis by decreasing the expression of TNF-α, TGF-β1, TIMP-1, and CK-19. Moreover, nanoformulations were also found to increase HGF and MMP-2 expression and the MMP-2/TIMP-1 ratio [76].

In addition, inorganic NPs such as silica-based NPs were prepared as drug carriers because of their porous structures (Table 1). Salvianolic acid B (SAB) loaded rhodamine B covalently grafted mesoporous silica NPs (SAB@MSNs-RhB) were prepared for liver fibrosis therapy through the [77]. The SAB@MSNs-RhB formulation exhibited improved cellular uptake, sustained drug release, and enhanced efficacy in anti-ROS/hepatic fibrosis. Small interfering tenascin-C was delivered by mesoporous silica NPs to reduce the expression of TnC, an ECM glycoprotein, consequently reducing the secretion of inflammatory cytokines and hepatocyte migration [78]. Compared with hesperetin alone, hesperetin loaded on PEGylated gold NPs showed higher antioxidative, anti-inflammatory, anti-proliferative, and anti-fibrotic activities in diethylnitrosamine-induced hepatocarcinogenesis in rats [79]. Graphene nanostars conjugated with a PAMAM-G5 dendrimer were prepared for the selective targeting and delivery of a plasmid expressing collagenase metalloproteinase 9 under the CD11b promoter into inflammatory macrophages in cirrhotic livers. The nanoformulations promoted the macrophage switch from inflammatory M1 to proregenerative M2 and reduced selectively and locally the presence of collagen fibers in fibrotic tracts [83].

Protein-based NPs currently show great potential as drug carriers for the treatment of liver fibrosis because of their biocompatibility and low immunogenicity (Table 1) [87]. Algandaby et al. reported that curcumin-loaded zein nanospheres showed high efficiency in attenuating the hepatic gene expression of collagen I, the tissue inhibitor of MMP2, and TGF-β, as well as downregulating MMP2 expression [84]. Moreover, compared with free berberine, berberine entrapped in glucose-modified albumin NPs more efficiently inhibited the growth of the human hepatic stellate cell line LX-2 and reduced liver fibrosis in vivo [85]. Human serum albumin-dexamethasone NPs were also fabricated to deliver dexamethasone to non-parenchymal hepatic cells, which play an important role in the pathogenesis of liver fibrosis. This treatment efficiently inhibited TNF-α production, hence the significant decrease in fibrosis relative to that in rats treated with free dexamethasone treatment [22]. Another study reported on the preparation of avidin-nucleic-acid-nano-assemblies (ANANAS), which are NPs based on polyavidin. These NPs were generated from a nucleic acid filament and avidin, a protein in egg whites. These NPs were designed to selectively deliver dexamethasone to the liver, particularly to the liver immunocompetent cells, and thereby improve the therapeutic efficacy by reducing interlobular collagen I deposition and MMP13 [86].

4.3. NPs as Drug Carriers with Targeting Ligands for the Treatment of Liver Fibrosis

Non-specific drug disposition limits the effective clinical use of traditional anti-fibrotic drugs. Targeting drug delivery to the fibrotic region can thus far be achieved using nanoformulations. As the sole hepatic VA storage cells with a crucial role in liver fibrosis, HSCs have been actively targeted by conjugating NPs with VA.

Liposomes loaded with drugs and HSC targeting components have been developed to target HSCs for the treatment of liver fibrosis (Table 2). In one study, VA-coupled liposomes were prepared to deliver imatinib. The hepatic accumulation of imatinib increased by about 13.5-fold, compared with imatinib treatment alone [88]. The nanoformulations not only inhibited the expression of phosphorylated PDGFR-β but also reduced the expression of profibrotic mediators such as hydroxyproline, TGF-β, and MMP2 with fewer adverse effects. In another study, VA-coupled liposomes were used to deliver valsartan, an angiotensin II receptor antagonist [89]. The nanoformulations increased the expression of hepatic Mas-receptor and PPAR-γ and potently normalized the level of fibrogenic mediators by improving the permeability and efficacy of valsartan.

Table 2. NPs used in active targeting therapy of liver fibrosis.

Nanoparticle Systems	NPs Formulation	Delivered Drugs	Targeted Ligand	Targeted Structures	Reference
Lipid-based NPs	VA-liposomes	Imatinib	VA	HSC	[88]
	VA-liposomes	Valsartan	VA	HSC	[89]
	pPB-modified liposomes	Recombinant human TRAIL	pPB	HSC	[90]
	AMD3100-liposomes	Antiangiogenic siRNA	VEGF siRNAs	HSC	[91]
	M6P-bovine serum albumin (BSA)-conjugated-liposomes	Hesperidin	M6P	HSC	[92]
	VA-coupled liposomes	BMP4-siRNA	VA	HSC	[93]
	Cationic liposomes	Artificial microRNA	microRNA	CTGF	[94]
	Chol-PEG-VA-amphiphilic cationic hyperbranched lipoid (C15-PA)	SiCol I α1 and siTIMP-1	VA	HSC	[95]
	pPB-modified stable nucleic acid lipid	siRNAs against heat shock protein 47	pPB	HSC	[96]
	Galactosamine-phospholipid NPs	siRNA targets CTGF	galactosamine	hepatocytes and renal tubular epithelial cells	[97]
	SP94-LCPP (lipid/calcium/phosphate/protamine) nanoparticle	TRAIL plasmid DNA	hepato-cellular carcinoma (HCC)-targeting peptide (SP94)	hepatocellular carcinoma (HCC) cells	[98]
	Phosphatidylserine-modified nanostructured lipid NPs	Curcumin	phosphatidylserine	macrophage	[99]
Polymer-based NPs	VA-collagenase I-poly-(lactic-co-glycolic)-b-poly (ethylene glycol)-maleimide (PLGA-PEG-Mal) (named CRM) micelle	Nilotinib	VA	HSC	[100]
	Poly (lactide-co-glycolide)-polyspermine-poly (ethylene glycol)-vitamin A (PLGA-PSPE-PEG-VA) self-assembled into core-shell polymeric micelles (PVMs)	Silibinin genetic (siCol1 alpha 1) drugs	VA	HSC	[101]
	Retinoic acid-chondroitin sulfate micells	Doxorubicin	VA	HSC	[102]
	POEGMA-b-PVDM -VA micelle	NO	VA	HSC	[19]
	Retinol-conjugated polyetherimine (RcP) nanoparticle	Antisense oligonucleotide (ASO)	RcP	HSC	[103]
	PLGA NPs	R406	R406	Macrophages	[104]
	retinol-chitosan NPs	JQ1 and atorvastatin	VA	HSC	[105]
Inorganic NPs	pPB-MSNP	Erlotinib	pPB	PDGFRB	[106]

Abbreviations: VA, vitamin A; TRAIL, TNF-related apoptosis-inducing ligand; HSC, hepatic stellate cell; CTGF, connective tissue growth factor; MMP, matrix metalloproteinase; NO, nitric oxide; VEGF, vascular endothelial growth factor.

Polymer-based NPs have also been fabricated to target HSCs by coupling with VA for liver fibrosis therapy (Table 2). An article reported on the preparation of retinol and collagenase I co-decorated polymeric micelles (CRM) based on PLGA-b-poly(ethylene glycol)-maleimide (PLGA-PEG-Mal) to be used as HSC-targeting nanodrug delivery systems for liver fibrosis therapy [100]. In the current study, the decoration of collagenase I could facilitate the nanocarrier penetration of the fibrotic liver. Consistent with this finding, CRMs were found to efficiently degrade pericellular collagen I and exhibit excellent accumulation in the fibrotic liver and accurate targeting of activated HSCs in a mouse hepatic fibrosis model. CRM/NIL loaded with nilotinib (NIL), a second-generation tyrosine kinase inhibitor used for the treatment of liver fibrosis, showed excellent antifibrotic efficiency (Figure 4). In addition, polymeric micelles (PVMs) formed with PLGA-polyspermine-PEG-VA were used to target HSCs and deliver the chemical drug silibinin and genetic drug siCol1α1 to the liver fibrosis site [101]. The double-loaded polymer micelle more efficiently reduced collagen I and ameliorated liver fibrosis, compared with the PVMS loaded with either the chemical drug only or genetic drug only. Chondroitin sulfate micelles coupled with retinoic acid and doxorubicin (DOX) (DOX + RA–CS micelles) were selectively taken up in activated HSCs and hepatoma cells, but not in normal hepatocytes (LO2) [102]. DOX + RA–CS micelles preferentially accumulated in the Golgi apparatus, destroyed the Golgi structure, and ultimately downregulated collagen I production in vitro and exerted synergistic antifibrotic effects on CCl4-induced fibrotic rat models.

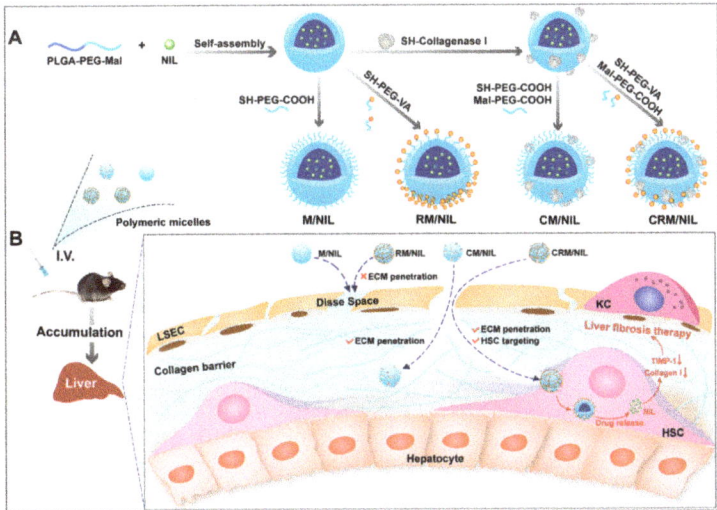

Figure 4. Extracellular matrix-penetrating polymeric micelles for liver fibrosis therapy. (**A**) Schematic illustration of the preparation of four different polymeric micelles. (**B**) Schematic illustration of the proposed destiny of the four different polymeric micelles in vivo. The CRM/NIL is able to penetrate the collagen barrier and target activated HSCs. Internalization of CRM/NIL allows the release of NIL, which reduces expression of the metallopeptidase inhibitor, TIMP-1, which in turn enhances collagen I degradation, thereby exerting therapeutic action against liver fibrosis. Reproduced with permission from [100]. Copyright Elsevier, 2020.

Apart from polymeric micelles, other polymer nanoformulations have also been constructed for the delivery of drugs, nucleic acid and other therapeutic moieties for the treatment of liver fibrosis (Table 2). In one study, retinol-conjugated polyetherimine NPs adsorbed plasma proteins, particularly retinol-binding protein 4 (RBP), forming a protein-coated complex [103]. The adsorbed RBP could direct the NPs into HSCs. After being loaded with antisense oligonucleotides, NPs effectively suppressed the expression of collagen I, consequently ameliorating hepatic fibrosis. Hassan et al. reported that chitosan NPs loaded with JQ1 (a small molecule that could abrogate the cytokine-induced activation of HSCs and reverse fibrotic response in animal models) and atorvastatin and further conjugated with retinol could target and prevent HSC activation [105].

In addition to VA, cyclic peptide pPB can particularly recognize PDGFRβ on the surface of HSCs (Table 2). A study used pPB-modified liposomes to deliver recombinant human tumor necrosis factor-related apoptosis-inducing ligand (rhTRAIL) to the HSC membrane, prolonging rhTRAIL circulation in vivo and alleviating fibrosis both in vitro and in vivo [90]. Similarly, the CXCR4 antagonist AMD3100 could target HSCs [91]. AMD3100-conjugated liposomes efficiently delivered therapeutic VEGF siRNAs to activate CXCR4-overexpressed HSCs both in vitro and in vivo. The nanoformulations downregulated the expression of VEGF, reduced the mean vessel density, and normalized the hepatic vascular structure in the livers of mice with CCl_4-induced liver fibrosis. Moreover, AMD3100 encapsulated in liposomes also exhibited antifibrotic effects by suppressing the proliferation and activation of HSCs. Mannose 6-phosphate (M6P)/insulin-like growth factor-II receptor, overexpressed in HSCs, was also used as the targeting site. Conjugation of M6P-modified albumin to hesperidin-loaded liposomes improved the efficacy of chemical drugs and attenuated liver fibrosis [92].

Hepatic macrophages play important roles in the pathogenesis of liver fibrosis and act as target sites for the treatment of liver fibrosis (Table 2). Scavenger receptors expressed on liver endothelial cells and Kupffer cells have also been targeted using nanoformulations. For instance, phosphatidylserine (PS), which acts as a specific recognition signal for the phagocytosis of apoptotic cells, can target macrophages. Wang et al. showed that PS-modified lipid carriers containing curcumin (Cur–mNLCs) exhibited enhanced retention time, bioavailability, and delivery efficiency of payload, as well as reduced liver damage and fibrosis in vivo [99].

5. Nanomedicine in Liver Fibrosis Theranostics

"Theranostics", a portmanteau word of "therapeutics" and "diagnostics", is achieved by incorporating diagnostic and therapeutic functions into a single nanoplatform. Theranostics has been proposed as a new and revolutionary therapeutic concept in several types of disease therapy, including that for liver fibrosis [107]. This strategy allows simultaneous diagnosis and treatment response by using personalized medicine with high accuracy and specificity. In one study, Hepatitis B core protein nanocages coated with RGD-targeting ligands (RGD–HBc/QR) exhibited selectivity to activated HSCs by targeting integrin $α_vβ_3$ and efficiently inhibited the proliferation and activation of HSCs both in vitro and in vivo [108]. By encapsulating a quercetin–gadolinium complex and/or labeling it with NIR fluorescent probes (Cy5.5), the resulted nanoformulations (RGD–HBc/QGd) showed great potential as MRI contrast agents and NIR fluorescent agents for liver fibrosis diagnosis in vivo. Another study reported that relaxin-conjugated PEGylated superparamagnetic iron oxide NPs (RLX-SPIONs) showed specific binding and uptake in TGFβ-activated HSCs, as well as strongly attenuated cirrhosis and showed enhanced contrast in MRI [20]. Micelles coupled with inorganic materials were also developed for theranostics to treat liver fibrosis. A pH-sensitive and VA-conjugated copolymer cationic micelle that was coupled with a superparamagnetic iron oxide nanoparticle could transport miRNA-29b and miRNA-112 to HSCs in an MRI-visible manner. Synergistic antifibrotic therapeutic efficacy was achieved by downregulating the expression of fibrosis-related genes, including collagen Iα1, α-SMA, and a tissue inhibitor of MMP1 (Figure 5) [109].

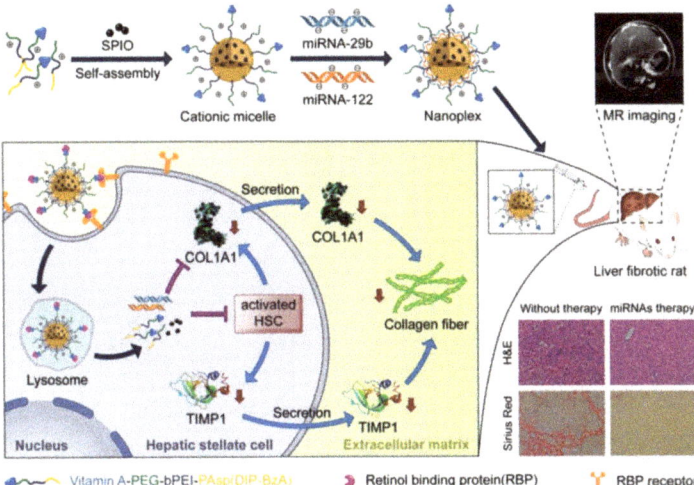

Figure 5. Vitamin A–decorated pH-sensitive and SPIO-loaded nanocomplex T-PBP@miRNA/SPIO (T-miRNA/S) for miRNA targeting delivery in the therapy of liver fibrosis. Expression of liver fibrosis-related genes for alleviating liver fibrosis were synergistically downregulated. The red arrows indicate the reduction of COL1A1, TIMP1, and collagen fiber. Abbreviations: COL1A1, collagen type I alpha 1 protein; TIMP1, tissue inhibitor of metalloproteinase 1; SPIO, superparamagnetic iron oxide. Reproduced with permission from [109]. Copyright John Wiley and Sons, 2019.

6. Conclusions and Future Perspectives

This review summarizes the strategies being used to develop novel methods for the treatment of liver fibrosis on the basis of multifunctional NPs. The application of nanomedicine systems in the diagnosis and treatment of liver fibrosis is widely reported in the literature and continues to be a rapidly growing research field, with emphasis on active targeted drug delivery and theranostics. Numerous types of inorganic and organic NPs have been extensively investigated, including metal oxide NPs, metal NPs, liposomes, polymer NPs, dendrimers, protein NPs, and organic–inorganic hybrid NPs. Each type has its advantages disadvantages. Inorganic NPs are intrinsically robust with relatively low manufacturing costs, but their design flexibility and functionality are limited. Organic NPs possess broad design flexibility for integrating multiple functions into one platform but show structural instability and involve high manufacturing cost and fabrication complexity. Organic–inorganic hybrid NPs combine the advantages of organic NPs and inorganic NPs and thus are preferred in the development of theranostic platforms.

Although NPs have shown great potential for liver fibrosis therapy, they also exhibit hepatotoxicity [110–114]. The long-term hepatotoxicity of NPs should be carefully and systemically evaluated, particularly when they are used in patients with liver disease. Patients are more sensitive to NPs because of reduced self-protective mechanisms, decreased immune function, and lack of ability for self-repair. Studies have shown that exposure to NPs increases pathological damage [115–117]. Therefore, the health risks involved in the use of NPs for liver fibrosis therapy should be given significant attention.

Until now, lipid-based NPs were the only nanomedicine system that in the clinical stages of studies for the treatment of liver fibrosis. Lipid NPs delivering siRNA against heat shock protein 47 were developed to target HSCs and treat advanced liver fibrosis caused by NASH or hepatitis C virus infection. This nanomedicine system was in clinical phase 1b/2 and study results were safe and effective [118,119]. To improve the clinical applicability of nanomedicine systems in the future, the following directions should be considered: (1) Developing stimuli-responsive nanomedicine systems with high sensitivity, which can intelligently respond to endogenous or exogenous stimuli and release payload at targeting sites. (2) Employing an "all-in-one" strategy to develop smart nanomedicine systems that combine multiple functionalities, including targeted delivery, prolonged blood retention, enhanced tissue penetration and cellular internalization, responsiveness to stimuli, and disease progressive monitoring. (3) Systematic evaluation of long-term toxicity, immunogenicity, and pharmacokinetics of medicine systems. Notably, from the clinical use of the reported nanomedicine systems, only one example was performed. All obstacles should be overcome by designing and fabricating nanomedicine systems with appropriate components, surface chemistry, sizes, payloads, and specific target ligands before clinical translation.

Author Contributions: X.B., G.S. and S.Z. designed this work of review. X.B. and G.S. performed the literature search of the databases. X.B. and G.S. wrote the manuscript. G.S. and S.Z. revised the manuscript. All authors have read and agreed to the published version of the manuscript.

Funding: This research received no external funding.

Acknowledgments: This research was funded by the National Natural Science Foundation of China (21677090, 22076085).

Conflicts of Interest: The authors declare no conflict of interest.

References

1. Lee, Y.A.; Wallace, M.C.; Friedman, S.L. Pathobiology of liver fibrosis: A translational success story. *Gut* **2015**, *64*, 830–841. [CrossRef] [PubMed]
2. Baffy, G.; Brunt, E.M.; Caldwell, S.H. Hepatocellular carcinoma in non-alcoholic fatty liver disease: An emerging menace. *J. Hepatol.* **2012**, *56*, 1384–1391. [CrossRef] [PubMed]
3. Mieli-Vergani, G.; Vergani, D.; Czaja, A.J.; Manns, M.P.; Krawitt, E.L.; Vierling, J.M.; Lohse, A.W.; Montano-Loza, A.J. Autoimmune hepatitis. *Nat. Rev. Dis. Primers* **2018**, *4*, 18017. [CrossRef] [PubMed]
4. Sarin, S.K.; Kumar, M.; Eslam, M.; George, J.; Al Mahtab, M.; Akbar, S.M.F.; Jia, J.; Tian, Q.; Aggarwal, R.; Muljono, D.H.; et al. Liver diseases in the Asia-Pacific region: A Lancet Gastroenterology & Hepatology Commission. *Lancet Gastroenterol. Hepatol.* **2020**, *5*, 167–228.
5. Trautwein, C.; Friedman, S.L.; Schuppan, D.; Pinzani, M. Hepatic fibrosis: Concept to treatment. *J. Hepatol.* **2015**, *62*, S15–S24. [CrossRef]
6. Zhang, D.Y.; Friedman, S.L. Fibrosis-dependent mechanisms of hepatocarcinogenesis. *Hepatology* **2012**, *56*, 769–775. [CrossRef]
7. Manning, D.S.; Afdhal, N.H. Diagnosis and Quantitation of Fibrosis. *Gastroenterology* **2008**, *134*, 1670–1681. [CrossRef]
8. De Oliveira, C.P.M.S.; Stefano, J.T.; De Siqueira, E.R.F.; Silva, L.S.; De Campos Mazo, D.F.; Lima, V.M.R.; Furuya, C.K.; Mello, E.S.; Souza, F.G.; Rabello, F.; et al. Combination of N-acetylcysteine and metformin improves histological steatosis and fibrosis in patients with non-alcoholic steatohepatitis. *Hepatol. Res.* **2008**, *38*, 159–165. [CrossRef]
9. Peres, W.; Tuñón, M.J.; Collado, P.S.; Herrmann, S.; Marroni, N.; González-Gallego, J. The flavonoid quercetin ameliorates liver damage in rats with biliary obstruction. *J. Hepatol.* **2000**, *33*, 742–750. [CrossRef]
10. Ogawa, S.; Ochi, T.; Shimada, H.; Inagaki, K.; Fujita, I.; Nii, A.; Moffat, M.A.; Katragadda, M.; Violand, B.N.; Arch, R.H.; et al. Anti-PDGF-B monoclonal antibody reduces liver fibrosis development. *Hepatol. Res.* **2010**, *40*, 1128–1141. [CrossRef]
11. Schuppan, D.; Kim, Y.O. Evolving therapies for liver fibrosis. *J. Clin. Investig.* **2013**, *123*, 1887–1901. [CrossRef]
12. Silva, C.; Pinho, J.; Lopes, J.M.; Almeida, A.J.; Reis, C.P. Current Trends in Cancer Nanotheranostics: Metallic, Polymeric, and Lipid-Based Systems. *Pharmaceutics* **2019**, *11*, 22. [CrossRef] [PubMed]
13. Pucek, A.; Tokarek, B.; Waglewska, E.; Bazylińska, U. Recent Advances in the Structural Design of Photosensitive Agent Formulations Using "Soft" Colloidal Nanocarriers. *Pharmaceutics* **2020**, *12*, 587. [CrossRef] [PubMed]
14. Wawrzyńczyk, D.; Cichy, B.; Zaręba, J.K.; Bazylińska, U. On the interaction between up-converting NaYF4:Er3+,Yb3+ nanoparticles and Rose Bengal molecules constrained within the double core of multifunctional nanocarriers. *J. Mater. Chem. C* **2019**, *7*, 15021–15034. [CrossRef]

15. Doane, T.L.; Burda, C. The unique role of nanoparticles in nanomedicine: Imaging, drug delivery and therapy. *Chem. Soc. Rev.* **2012**, *41*, 2885–2911. [CrossRef] [PubMed]
16. Surendran, S.P.; Thomas, R.G.; Moon, M.J.; Jeong, Y.Y. Nanoparticles for the treatment of liver fibrosis. *Int. J. Nanomed.* **2017**, *12*, 6997–7006. [CrossRef] [PubMed]
17. Reddy, L.H.; Couvreur, P. Nanotechnology for therapy and imaging of liver diseases. *J. Hepatol.* **2011**, *55*, 1461–1466. [CrossRef]
18. Li, Y.; Shang, W.; Liang, X.; Zeng, C.; Liu, M.; Wang, S.; Li, H.; Tian, J. The diagnosis of hepatic fibrosis by magnetic resonance and near-infrared imaging using dual-modality nanoparticles. *RSC Adv.* **2018**, *8*, 6699–6708. [CrossRef]
19. Duong, H.T.; Dong, Z.; Su, L.; Boyer, C.; George, J.; Davis, T.P.; Wang, J. The use of nanoparticles to deliver nitric oxide to hepatic stellate cells for treating liver fibrosis and portal hypertension. *Small Weinh. Der Bergstr. Ger.* **2015**, *11*, 2291–2304. [CrossRef]
20. Calvente, C.J.; Sehgal, A.; Popov, Y.; Kim, Y.O.; Zevallos, V.; Sahin, U.; Diken, M.; Schuppan, D. Specific hepatic delivery of procollagen α1(I) small interfering RNA in lipid-like nanoparticles resolves liver fibrosis. *Hepatology* **2015**, *62*, 1285–1297. [CrossRef]
21. Li, L.; Wang, H.; Ong, Z.Y.; Xu, K.; Ee, P.L.R.; Zheng, S.; Hedrick, J.L.; Yang, Y.-Y. Polymer- and lipid-based nanoparticle therapeutics for the treatment of liver diseases. *Nano Today* **2010**, *5*, 296–312. [CrossRef]
22. Melgert, B.N.; Olinga, P.; Jack, V.K.; Molema, G.; Meijer, D.K.F.; Poelstra, K. Dexamethasone coupled to albumin is selectively taken up by rat nonparenchymal liver cells and attenuates LPS-induced activation of hepatic cells. *J. Hepatol.* **2000**, *32*, 603–611. [CrossRef]
23. Petros, R.A.; DeSimone, J.M. Strategies in the design of nanoparticles for therapeutic applications. *Nat. Rev. Drug Discov.* **2010**, *9*, 615–627. [CrossRef]
24. Nagórniewicz, B.; Mardhian, D.F.; Booijink, R.; Storm, G.; Prakash, J.; Bansal, R. Engineered Relaxin as Theranostic nanomedicine to diagnose and ameliorate liver cirrhosis. *Nanomed. Nanotechnol. Biol. Med.* **2019**, *17*, 106–118. [CrossRef] [PubMed]
25. Yin, C.; Evason, K.J.; Asahina, K.; Stainier, D.Y.R. Hepatic stellate cells in liver development, regeneration, and cancer. *J. Clin. Investig.* **2013**, *123*, 1902–1910. [CrossRef]
26. Hernandez-Gea, V.; Friedman, S.L. Pathogenesis of Liver Fibrosis. *Annu. Rev. Pathol. Mech. Dis.* **2011**, *6*, 425–456. [CrossRef]
27. Tsuchida, T.; Friedman, S.L. Mechanisms of hepatic stellate cell activation. *Nat. Rev. Gastroenterol. Hepatol.* **2017**, *14*, 397–411. [CrossRef]
28. Meng, X.-M.; Nikolic-Paterson, D.J.; Lan, H.Y. TGF-β: The master regulator of fibrosis. *Nat. Rev. Nephrol.* **2016**, *12*, 325–338. [CrossRef]
29. Kocabayoglu, P.; Lade, A.; Lee, Y.A.; Dragomir, A.-C.; Sun, X.; Fiel, M.I.; Thung, S.; Aloman, C.; Soriano, P.; Hoshida, Y.; et al. β-PDGF receptor expressed by hepatic stellate cells regulates fibrosis in murine liver injury, but not carcinogenesis. *J. Hepatol.* **2015**, *63*, 141–147. [CrossRef]
30. Okuno, M.; Moriwaki, H.; Muto, Y.; Kojima, S. Protease inhibitors suppress TGF-β generation by hepatic stellate cells. *J. Hepatol.* **1998**, *29*, 1031–1032. [CrossRef]
31. Wang, Y.; Gao, J.; Zhang, D.; Zhang, J.; Ma, J.; Jiang, H. New insights into the antifibrotic effects of sorafenib on hepatic stellate cells and liver fibrosis. *J. Hepatol.* **2010**, *53*, 132–144. [CrossRef]
32. Wang, Y.Q.; Ikeda, K.; Ikebe, T.; Hirakawa, K.; Sowa, M.; Nakatani, K.; Kawada, N.; Kaneda, K. Inhibition of hepatic stellate cell proliferation and activation by the semisynthetic analogue of fumagillin TNP-470 in rats. *Hepatology* **2000**, *32*, 980–989. [CrossRef] [PubMed]
33. Sugawara, H.; Ueno, T.; Torimura, T.; Inuzuka, S.; Tanikawa, K. Inhibitory effect of OPC-15161, a component of fungus Thielavia minor, on proliferation and extracellular matrix production of rat cultured hepatic stellate cells. *J. Cell. Physiol.* **1998**, *174*, 398–406. [CrossRef]
34. Morry, J.; Ngamcherdtrakul, W.; Yantasee, W. Oxidative stress in cancer and fibrosis: Opportunity for therapeutic intervention with antioxidant compounds, enzymes, and nanoparticles. *Redox Biol.* **2017**, *11*, 240–253. [CrossRef] [PubMed]
35. Hickman, I.; Macdonald, G. Is vitamin E beneficial in chronic liver disease? *Hepatology* **2007**, *46*, 288–290. [CrossRef] [PubMed]

36. Sukalingam, K.; Ganesan, K.; Xu, B. Protective Effect of Aqueous Extract from the Leaves of Justicia tranquebariesis against Thioacetamide-Induced Oxidative Stress and Hepatic Fibrosis in Rats. *Antioxidants* **2018**, *7*, 78. [CrossRef]
37. Di Pascoli, M.; Diví, M.; Rodríguez-Vilarrupla, A.; Rosado, E.; Gracia-Sancho, J.; Vilaseca, M.; Bosch, J.; García-Pagán, J.C. Resveratrol improves intrahepatic endothelial dysfunction and reduces hepatic fibrosis and portal pressure in cirrhotic rats. *J. Hepatol.* **2013**, *58*, 904–910. [CrossRef]
38. Mezey, E. Prevention of alcohol-induced hepatic fibrosis by phosphatidylcholine. *Gastroenterology* **1994**, *106*, 257–259. [CrossRef]
39. Hirano, A.; Kaplowitz, N.; Tsukamoto, H.; Kamimura, S.; Fernandez-Checa, J.C. Hepatic mitochondrial glutathione depletion and progression of experimental alcoholic liver disease in rats. *Hepatology* **1992**, *16*, 1423–1427. [CrossRef]
40. Ankoma-Sey, V.; Wang, Y.; Dai, Z. Hypoxic stimulation of vascular endothelial growth factor expression in activated rat hepatic stellate cells. *Hepatology* **2000**, *31*, 141–148. [CrossRef]
41. Aleffi, S.; Petrai, I.; Bertolani, C.; Parola, M.; Colombatto, S.; Novo, E.; Vizzutti, F.; Anania, F.A.; Milani, S.; Rombouts, K.; et al. Upregulation of proinflammatory and proangiogenic cytokines by leptin in human hepatic stellate cells. *Hepatology* **2005**, *42*, 1339–1348. [CrossRef] [PubMed]
42. Fernández, M.; Semela, D.; Bruix, J.; Colle, I.; Pinzani, M.; Bosch, J. Angiogenesis in liver disease. *J. Hepatol.* **2009**, *50*, 604–620. [CrossRef] [PubMed]
43. Taura, K.; De Minicis, S.; Seki, E.; Hatano, E.; Iwaisako, K.; Osterreicher, C.H.; Kodama, Y.; Miura, K.; Ikai, I.; Uemoto, S.; et al. Hepatic Stellate Cells Secrete Angiopoietin 1 That Induces Angiogenesis in Liver Fibrosis. *Gastroenterology* **2008**, *135*, 1729–1738. [CrossRef] [PubMed]
44. Moon, J.-O.; Welch, T.P.; Gonzalez, F.J.; Copple, B.L. Reduced liver fibrosis in hypoxia-inducible factor-1α-deficient mice. *Am. J. Physiol. Gastrointest. Liver Physiol.* **2009**, *296*, G582–G592. [CrossRef] [PubMed]
45. Sánchez-Valle, V.; Chávez-Tapia, N.C.; Uribe, M.; Méndez-Sánchez, N. Role of oxidative stress and molecular changes in liver fibrosis: A review. *Curr. Med. Chem.* **2012**, *19*, 4850–4860. [CrossRef]
46. Seki, E.; Schwabe, R.F. Hepatic inflammation and fibrosis: Functional links and key pathways. *Hepatology* **2015**, *61*, 1066–1079. [CrossRef] [PubMed]
47. Anand, L.; Choudhury, A.; Bihari, C.; Sharma, B.C.; Kumar, M.; Maiwall, R.; Tan, S.S.; Shah, S.R.; Hamid, S.; Butt, A.S.; et al. Flare of Autoimmune Hepatitis Causing Acute on Chronic Liver Failure: Diagnosis and Response to Corticosteroid Therapy. *Hepatology* **2019**, *70*, 587–596. [CrossRef]
48. Morgan, T.R.; Weiss, D.G.; Nemchausky, B.; Schiff, E.R.; Anand, B.; Simon, F.; Kidao, J.; Cecil, B.; Mendenhall, C.L.; Nelson, D.; et al. Colchicine treatment of alcoholic cirrhosis: A randomized, placebo-controlled clinical trial of patient survival. *Gastroenterology* **2005**, *128*, 882–890. [CrossRef]
49. Cheng, K.; Ashby, D.; Smyth, R.L. Ursodeoxycholic acid for cystic fibrosis-related liver disease. *Cochrane Database Syst. Rev.* **2017**, *2017*, CD000222. [CrossRef] [PubMed]
50. Nelson, D.R.; Lauwers, G.Y.; Lau, J.Y.N.; Davis, G.L. Interleukin 10 treatment reduces fibrosis in patients with chronic hepatitis C: A pilot trial of interferon nonresponders. *Gastroenterology* **2000**, *118*, 655–660. [CrossRef]
51. Heide, D.v.d.; Weiskirchen, R.; Bansal, R. Therapeutic Targeting of Hepatic Macrophages for the Treatment of Liver Diseases. *Front. Immunol.* **2019**, *10*, 2852. [CrossRef]
52. Van Bergen, T.; Spangler, R.; Marshall, D.; Hollanders, K.; Van de Veire, S.; Vandewalle, E.; Moons, L.; Herman, J.; Smith, V.; Stalmans, I. The Role of LOX and LOXL2 in the Pathogenesis of an Experimental Model of Choroidal Neovascularization. *Investig. Ophthalmol. Vis. Sci.* **2015**, *56*, 5280–5289. [CrossRef]
53. Yoshio, S.; Atsushi, N.; Yoshito, I. Limitations of liver biopsy and non-invasive diagnostic tests for the diagnosis of nonalcoholic fatty liver disease/nonalcoholic steatohepatitis. *World J. Gastroenterol* **2014**, *20*, 475–485.
54. Dulai, P.S.; Sirlin, C.B.; Loomba, R. MRI and MRE for non-invasive quantitative assessment of hepatic steatosis and fibrosis in NAFLD and NASH: Clinical trials to clinical practice. *J. Hepatol.* **2016**, *65*, 1006–1016. [CrossRef] [PubMed]
55. Sun, C.; Lee, J.S.H.; Zhang, M. Magnetic nanoparticles in MR imaging and drug delivery. *Adv. Drug Deliv. Rev.* **2008**, *60*, 1252–1265. [CrossRef] [PubMed]
56. Saraswathy, A.; Nazeer, S.S.; Nimi, N.; Arumugam, S.; Shenoy, S.J.; Jayasree, R.S. Synthesis and characterization of dextran stabilized superparamagnetic iron oxide nanoparticles for in vivo MR imaging of liver fibrosis. *Carbohydr. Polym.* **2014**, *101*, 760–768. [CrossRef]

57. Saraswathy, A.; Nazeer, S.S.; Jeevan, M.; Nimi, N.; Arumugam, S.; Harikrishnan, V.S.; Varma, P.R.; Jayasree, R.S. Citrate coated iron oxide nanoparticles with enhanced relaxivity for in vivo magnetic resonance imaging of liver fibrosis. *Colloids Surf. B Biointerfaces* **2014**, *117*, 216–224. [CrossRef]
58. Nimi, N.; Saraswathy, A.; Nazeer, S.S.; Francis, N.; Shenoy, S.J.; Jayasree, R.S. Multifunctional hybrid nanoconstruct of zerovalent iron and carbon dots for Magnetic Resonance Angiography and Optical Imaging: An In vivo study. *Biomaterials* **2018**, *171*, 46–56. [CrossRef]
59. Xuan, J.; Chen, Y.; Zhu, L.; Guo, Y.; Ao, M. Ultrasound molecular imaging with cRGD-PLGA-PFOB nanoparticles for liver fibrosis staging in a rat model. *Oncotarget* **2017**, *8*, 108676–108691. [CrossRef]
60. Anselmo, A.C.; Mitragotri, S. A Review of Clinical Translation of Inorganic Nanoparticles. *AAPS J.* **2015**, *17*, 1041–1054. [CrossRef]
61. Xu, Z.P.; Zeng, Q.H.; Lu, G.Q.; Yu, A.B. Inorganic nanoparticles as carriers for efficient cellular delivery. *Chem. Eng. Sci.* **2006**, *61*, 1027–1040. [CrossRef]
62. Tee, J.K.; Peng, F.; Ho, H.K. Effects of inorganic nanoparticles on liver fibrosis: Optimizing a double-edged sword for therapeutics. *Biochem. Pharmacol.* **2019**, *160*, 24–33. [CrossRef] [PubMed]
63. Peng, F.; Tee, J.K.; Setyawati, M.I.; Ding, X.; Yeo, H.L.A.; Tan, Y.L.; Leong, D.T.; Ho, H.K. Inorganic Nanomaterials as Highly Efficient Inhibitors of Cellular Hepatic Fibrosis. *ACS Appl. Mater. Interfaces* **2018**, *10*, 31938–31946. [CrossRef] [PubMed]
64. Oró, D.; Yudina, T.; Fernández-Varo, G.; Casals, E.; Reichenbach, V.; Casals, G.; González de la Presa, B.; Sandalinas, S.; Carvajal, S.; Puntes, V.; et al. Cerium oxide nanoparticles reduce steatosis, portal hypertension and display anti-inflammatory properties in rats with liver fibrosis. *J. Hepatol.* **2016**, *64*, 691–698. [CrossRef] [PubMed]
65. Adhikari, A.; Polley, N.; Darbar, S.; Bagchi, D.; Pal, S.K. Citrate functionalized Mn3O4 in nanotherapy of hepatic fibrosis by oral administration. *Future Sci. OA* **2016**, *2*, 2056–5623. [CrossRef] [PubMed]
66. Rani, V.; Verma, Y.; Rana, K.; Rana, S.V.S. Zinc oxide nanoparticles inhibit dimethylnitrosamine induced liver injury in rat. *Chem. Biol. Interact.* **2018**, *295*, 84–92. [CrossRef] [PubMed]
67. De Carvalho, T.G.; Garcia, V.B.; de Araújo, A.A.; da Silva Gasparotto, L.H.; Silva, H.; Guerra, G.C.B.; de Castro Miguel, E.; de Carvalho Leitão, R.F.; da Silva Costa, D.V.; Cruz, L.J.; et al. Spherical neutral gold nanoparticles improve anti-inflammatory response, oxidative stress and fibrosis in alcohol-methamphetamine-induced liver injury in rats. *Int. J. Pharm.* **2018**, *548*, 1–14. [CrossRef] [PubMed]
68. Hamza, R.Z.; EL-Megharbel, S.M.; Altalhi, T.; Gobouri, A.A.; Alrogi, A.A. Hypolipidemic and hepatoprotective synergistic effects of selenium nanoparticles and vitamin. E against acrylamide-induced hepatic alterations in male albino mice. *Appl. Organomet. Chem.* **2020**, *34*, e5458. [CrossRef]
69. Böttger, R.; Pauli, G.; Chao, P.-H.; Al Fayez, N.; Hohenwarter, L.; Li, S.-D. Lipid-based nanoparticle technologies for liver targeting. *Adv. Drug Deliv. Rev.* **2020**, in press.
70. Reebye, V.; Huang, K.-W.; Lin, V.; Jarvis, S.; Cutilas, P.; Dorman, S.; Ciriello, S.; Andrikakou, P.; Voutila, J.; Saetrom, P.; et al. Gene activation of CEBPA using saRNA: Preclinical studies of the first in human saRNA drug candidate for liver cancer. *Oncogene* **2018**, *37*, 3216–3228. [CrossRef]
71. Bartneck, M.; Scheyda, K.M.; Warzecha, K.T.; Rizzo, L.Y.; Hittatiya, K.; Luedde, T.; Storm, G.; Trautwein, C.; Lammers, T.; Tacke, F. Fluorescent cell-traceable dexamethasone-loaded liposomes for the treatment of inflammatory liver diseases. *Biomaterials* **2015**, *37*, 367–382. [CrossRef] [PubMed]
72. Kaps, L.; Nuhn, L.; Aslam, M.; Brose, A.; Foerster, F.; Rosigkeit, S.; Renz, P.; Heck, R.; Kim, Y.O.; Lieberwirth, I.; et al. In Vivo Gene-Silencing in Fibrotic Liver by siRNA-Loaded Cationic Nanohydrogel Particles. *Adv. Healthc. Mater.* **2015**, *4*, 2809–2815. [CrossRef]
73. Leber, N.; Kaps, L.; Aslam, M.; Schupp, J.; Brose, A.; Schäffel, D.; Fischer, K.; Diken, M.; Strand, D.; Koynov, K.; et al. SiRNA-mediated in vivo gene knockdown by acid-degradable cationic nanohydrogel particles. *J. Control. Release* **2017**, *248*, 10–23. [CrossRef] [PubMed]
74. Krithika, R.; Vhora, I.; Verma, R.J. Preparation, toxicity analysis and in vivo protective effect of phyllanthin-loaded PLGA nanoparticles against CCl4-induced hepatic fibrosis. *J. Drug Deliv. Sci. Technol.* **2019**, *51*, 364–371. [CrossRef]
75. Lin, T.-T.; Gao, D.-Y.; Liu, Y.-C.; Sung, Y.-C.; Wan, D.; Liu, J.-Y.; Chiang, T.; Wang, L.; Chen, Y. Development and characterization of sorafenib-loaded PLGA nanoparticles for the systemic treatment of liver fibrosis. *J. Control. Release* **2016**, *221*, 62–70. [CrossRef]

76. Younis, N.; Shaheen, M.A.; Abdallah, M.H. Silymarin-loaded Eudragit® RS100 nanoparticles improved the ability of silymarin to resolve hepatic fibrosis in bile duct ligated rats. *Biomed. Pharmacother.* **2016**, *81*, 93–103. [CrossRef]
77. He, Q.; Zhang, J.; Chen, F.; Guo, L.; Zhu, Z.; Shi, J. An anti-ROS/hepatic fibrosis drug delivery system based on salvianolic acid B loaded mesoporous silica nanoparticles. *Biomaterials* **2010**, *31*, 7785–7796. [CrossRef]
78. Vivero-Escoto, J.L.; Vadarevu, H.; Juneja, R.; Schrum, L.W.; Benbow, J.H. Nanoparticle mediated silencing of tenascin C in hepatic stellate cells: Effect on inflammatory gene expression and cell migration. *J. Mater. Chem. B* **2019**, *7*, 7396–7405. [CrossRef]
79. Krishnan, G.; Subramaniyan, J.; Chengalvarayan Subramani, P.; Muralidharan, B.; Thiruvengadam, D. Hesperetin conjugated PEGylated gold nanoparticles exploring the potential role in anti-inflammation and anti-proliferation during diethylnitrosamine-induced hepatocarcinogenesis in rats. *Asian J. Pharm. Sci.* **2017**, *12*, 442–455. [CrossRef]
80. Das, A.; Mukherjee, P.; Singla, S.K.; Guturu, P.; Frost, M.C.; Mukhopadhyay, D.; Shah, V.H.; Patra, C.R. Fabrication and characterization of an inorganic gold and silica nanoparticle mediated drug delivery system for nitric oxide. *Nanotechnology* **2010**, *21*, 305102. [CrossRef]
81. Yu, X.; Yuan, L.; Zhu, N.; Wang, K.; Xia, Y. Fabrication of antimicrobial curcumin stabilized platinum nanoparticles and their anti-liver fibrosis activity for potential use in nursing care. *J. Photochem. Photobiol. B Biol.* **2019**, *195*, 27–32. [CrossRef] [PubMed]
82. Wang, M.; Zhang, M.; Fu, L.; Lin, J.; Zhou, X.; Zhou, P.; Huang, P.; Hu, H.; Han, Y. Liver-targeted delivery of TSG-6 by calcium phosphate nanoparticles for the management of liver fibrosis. *Theranostics* **2020**, *10*, 36–49. [CrossRef] [PubMed]
83. Melgar-Lesmes, P.; Luquero, A.; Parra-Robert, M.; Mora, A.; Ribera, J.; Edelman, E.R.; Jiménez, W. Graphene–Dendrimer Nanostars for Targeted Macrophage Overexpression of Metalloproteinase 9 and Hepatic Fibrosis Precision Therapy. *Nano Lett.* **2018**, *18*, 5839–5845. [CrossRef] [PubMed]
84. Algandaby, M.M.; Al-Sawahli, M.M.; Oaa, A.; Fahmy, U.A.; Abdallah, H.M.; Hattori, M.; Ashour, O.M.; Abdel-Naim, A.B. Curcumin-Zein Nanospheres Improve Liver Targeting and Antifibrotic Activity of Curcumin in Carbon Tetrachloride-Induced Mice Liver Fibrosis. *J. Biomed. Nanotechnol.* **2016**, *12*, 1746–1757. [CrossRef] [PubMed]
85. Lam, P.L.; Kok, S.H.L.; Gambari, R.; Kok, T.W.; Leung, H.Y.; Choi, K.L.; Wong, C.S.; Hau, D.K.P.; Wong, W.Y.; Lam, K.H.; et al. Evaluation of berberine/bovine serum albumin nanoparticles for liver fibrosis therapy. *Green Chem.* **2015**, *17*, 1640–1646. [CrossRef]
86. Violatto, M.B.; Casarin, E.; Talamini, L.; Russo, L.; Baldan, S.; Tondello, C.; Messmer, M.; Hintermann, E.; Rossi, A.; Passoni, A.; et al. Dexamethasone Conjugation to Biodegradable Avidin-Nucleic-Acid-Nano-Assemblies Promotes Selective Liver Targeting and Improves Therapeutic Efficacy in an Autoimmune Hepatitis Murine Model. *ACS Nano* **2019**, *13*, 4410–4423. [CrossRef]
87. Hawkins, M.J.; Soon-Shiong, P.; Desai, N. Protein nanoparticles as drug carriers in clinical medicine. *Adv. Drug Deliv. Rev.* **2008**, *60*, 876–885. [CrossRef]
88. El-Mezayen, N.S.; El-Hadidy, W.F.; El-Refaie, W.M.; Shalaby, T.I.; Khattab, M.M.; El-Khatib, A.S. Hepatic stellate cell-targeted imatinib nanomedicine versus conventional imatinib: A novel strategy with potent efficacy in experimental liver fibrosis. *J. Control. Release* **2017**, *266*, 226–237. [CrossRef]
89. El-Mezayen, N.S.; El-Hadidy, W.F.; El-Refaie, W.M.; Shalaby, T.I.; Khattab, M.M.; El-Khatib, A.S. Oral vitamin-A-coupled valsartan nanomedicine: High hepatic stellate cell receptors accessibility and prolonged enterohepatic residence. *J. Control. Release* **2018**, *283*, 32–44. [CrossRef]
90. Li, Q.; Ding, Y.; Guo, X.; Luo, S.; Zhuang, H.; Zhou, J.; Xu, N.; Yan, Z. Chemically modified liposomes carrying TRAIL target activated hepatic stellate cells and ameliorate hepatic fibrosis in vitro and in vivo. *J. Cell. Mol. Med.* **2019**, *23*, 1951–1962. [CrossRef]
91. Liu, C.-H.; Chan, K.-M.; Chiang, T.; Liu, J.-Y.; Chern, G.-G.; Hsu, F.-F.; Wu, Y.-H.; Liu, Y.-C.; Chen, Y. Dual-Functional Nanoparticles Targeting CXCR4 and Delivering Antiangiogenic siRNA Ameliorate Liver Fibrosis. *Mol. Pharm.* **2016**, *13*, 2253–2262. [CrossRef] [PubMed]
92. Morsy, M.A.; Nair, A.B. Prevention of rat liver fibrosis by selective targeting of hepatic stellate cells using hesperidin carriers. *Int. J. Pharm.* **2018**, *552*, 241–250. [CrossRef]

93. Omar, R.; Yang, J.; Alrushaid, S.; Burczynski, F.J.; Minuk, G.Y.; Gong, Y. Inhibition of BMP4 and Alpha Smooth Muscle Actin Expression in LX-2 Hepatic Stellate Cells by BMP4-siRNA Lipid Based Nanoparticle. *J. Pharm. Pharm. Sci.* **2018**, *21*, 119–134. [CrossRef] [PubMed]
94. Yang, D.; Gao, Y.H.; Tan, K.B.; Zuo, Z.X.; Yang, W.X.; Hua, X.; Li, P.J.; Zhang, Y.; Wang, G. Inhibition of hepatic fibrosis with artificial microRNA using ultrasound and cationic liposome-bearing microbubbles. *Gene Ther.* **2013**, *20*, 1140–1148. [CrossRef]
95. Qiao, J.-B.; Fan, Q.-Q.; Zhang, C.-L.; Lee, J.; Byun, J.; Xing, L.; Gao, X.-D.; Oh, Y.-K.; Jiang, H.-L. Hyperbranched lipoid-based lipid nanoparticles for bidirectional regulation of collagen accumulation in liver fibrosis. *J. Control. Release* **2020**, *321*, 629–640. [CrossRef]
96. Jia, Z.; Gong, Y.; Pi, Y.; Liu, X.; Gao, L.; Kang, L.; Wang, J.; Yang, F.; Tang, J.; Lu, W.; et al. pPB Peptide-Mediated siRNA-Loaded Stable Nucleic Acid Lipid Nanoparticles on Targeting Therapy of Hepatic Fibrosis. *Mol. Pharm.* **2018**, *15*, 53–62. [CrossRef] [PubMed]
97. Khaja, F.; Jayawardena, D.; Kuzmis, A.; Önyüksel, H. Targeted Sterically Stabilized Phospholipid siRNA Nanomedicine for Hepatic and Renal Fibrosis. *Nanomaterials* **2016**, *6*, 8. [CrossRef]
98. Liu, C.-H.; Chern, G.-J.; Hsu, F.-F.; Huang, K.-W.; Sung, Y.-C.; Huang, H.-C.; Qiu, J.T.; Wang, S.-K.; Lin, C.-C.; Wu, C.-H.; et al. A multifunctional nanocarrier for efficient TRAIL-based gene therapy against hepatocellular carcinoma with desmoplasia in mice. *Hepatology* **2018**, *67*, 899–913. [CrossRef]
99. Wang, J.; Pan, W.; Wang, Y.; Lei, W.; Feng, B.; Du, C.; Wang, X.J. Enhanced efficacy of curcumin with phosphatidylserine-decorated nanoparticles in the treatment of hepatic fibrosis. *Drug Deliv.* **2018**, *25*, 1–11. [CrossRef]
100. Fan, Q.-Q.; Zhang, C.-L.; Qiao, J.-B.; Cui, P.-F.; Xing, L.; Oh, Y.-K.; Jiang, H.-L. Extracellular matrix-penetrating nanodrill micelles for liver fibrosis therapy. *Biomaterials* **2020**, *230*, 119616. [CrossRef]
101. Qiao, J.-B.; Fan, Q.-Q.; Xing, L.; Cui, P.-F.; He, Y.-J.; Zhu, J.-C.; Wang, L.; Pang, T.; Oh, Y.-K.; Zhang, C.; et al. Vitamin A-decorated biocompatible micelles for chemogene therapy of liver fibrosis. *J. Control. Release* **2018**, *283*, 113–125. [CrossRef] [PubMed]
102. Luo, J.; Zhang, P.; Zhao, T.; Jia, M.; Yin, P.; Li, W.; Zhang, Z.-R.; Fu, Y.; Gong, T. Golgi Apparatus-Targeted Chondroitin-Modified Nanomicelles Suppress Hepatic Stellate Cell Activation for the Management of Liver Fibrosis. *ACS Nano* **2019**, *13*, 3910–3923. [CrossRef]
103. Zhang, Z.; Wang, C.; Zha, Y.; Hu, W.; Gao, Z.; Zang, Y.; Chen, J.; Zhang, J.; Dong, L. Corona-Directed Nucleic Acid Delivery into Hepatic Stellate Cells for Liver Fibrosis Therapy. *ACS Nano* **2015**, *9*, 2405–2419. [CrossRef] [PubMed]
104. Kurniawan, D.W.; Jajoriya, A.K.; Dhawan, G.; Mishra, D.; Argemi, J.; Bataller, R.; Storm, G.; Mishra, D.P.; Prakash, J.; Bansal, R. Therapeutic inhibition of spleen tyrosine kinase in inflammatory macrophages using PLGA nanoparticles for the treatment of non-alcoholic steatohepatitis. *J. Control. Release* **2018**, *288*, 227–238. [CrossRef] [PubMed]
105. Hassan, R.; Tammam, S.N.; Safy, S.E.; Abdel-Halim, M.; Asimakopoulou, A.; Weiskirchen, R.; Mansour, S. Prevention of hepatic stellate cell activation using JQ1- and atorvastatin-loaded chitosan nanoparticles as a promising approach in therapy of liver fibrosis. *Eur. J. Pharm. Biopharm.* **2019**, *134*, 96–106. [CrossRef]
106. Deshmukh, M.; Nakagawa, S.; Higashi, T.; Vincek, A.; Venkatesh, A.; Ruiz de Galarreta, M.; Koh, A.P.; Goossens, N.; Hirschfield, H.; Bian, C.B.; et al. Cell type-specific pharmacological kinase inhibition for cancer chemoprevention. *Nanomedicine* **2018**, *14*, 317–325. [CrossRef]
107. Gou, Y.; Miao, D.D.; Zhou, M.; Wang, L.J.; Zhou, H.Y.; Su, G.X. Bio-Inspired Protein-Based Nanoformulations for Cancer Theranostics. *Front. Pharmacol.* **2018**, *9*, 421. [CrossRef]
108. Zhang, Q.; Xu, D.; Guo, Q.; Shan, W.; Yang, J.; Lin, T.; Ye, S.; Zhou, X.; Ge, Y.; Bi, S.; et al. Theranostic Quercetin Nanoparticle for Treatment of Hepatic Fibrosis. *Bioconjugate Chem.* **2019**, *30*, 2939–2946. [CrossRef]
109. Wu, J.; Huang, J.; Kuang, S.; Chen, J.; Li, X.; Chen, B.; Wang, J.; Cheng, D.; Shuai, X. Synergistic MicroRNA Therapy in Liver Fibrotic Rat Using MRI-Visible Nanocarrier Targeting Hepatic Stellate Cells. *Adv. Sci.* **2019**, *6*, 1801809. [CrossRef]
110. Yu, Y.; Duan, J.; Li, Y.; Li, Y.; Sun, Z. Silica nanoparticles induce liver fibrosis via TGF-β1/Smad3 pathway in ICR mice. *Int. J. Nanomed.* **2017**, *12*, 6045–6057. [CrossRef]
111. Zhang, Q.; Chang, X.; Wang, H.; Liu, Y.; Wang, X.; Wu, M.; Zhan, H.; Li, S.; Sun, Y. TGF-β1 mediated Smad signaling pathway and EMT in hepatic fibrosis induced by Nano NiO in vivo and in vitro. *Environ. Toxicol.* **2020**, *35*, 419–429. [CrossRef] [PubMed]

112. Bo, L.; Zhang, X.; Yang, J.; Zhang, Y.; Li, W.; Fan, C.; Huang, Q. Influence of polyethylene glycol coating on biodistribution and toxicity of nanoscale graphene oxide in mice after intravenous injection. *Int. J. Nanomed.* **2014**, *9*, 4697–4707.
113. Lee, I.-C.; Ko, J.-W.; Park, S.-H.; Shin, N.-R.; Shin, I.-S.; Moon, C.; Kim, S.-H.; Yun, W.-K.; Kim, H.-C.; Kim, J.-C. Copper nanoparticles induce early fibrotic changes in the liver via TGF-β/Smad signaling and cause immunosuppressive effects in rats. *Nanotoxicology* **2018**, *12*, 637–651. [CrossRef] [PubMed]
114. Wen, T.; Du, L.; Chen, B.; Yan, D.; Yang, A.; Liu, J.; Gu, N.; Meng, J.; Xu, H. Iron oxide nanoparticles induce reversible endothelial-to-mesenchymal transition in vascular endothelial cells at acutely non-cytotoxic concentrations. *Part. Fibre Toxicol.* **2019**, *16*, 30. [CrossRef]
115. Bartneck, M.; Ritz, T.; Keul, H.A.; Wambach, M.; Bornemann, J.; Gbureck, U.; Ehling, J.; Lammers, T.; Heymann, F.; Gassler, N.; et al. Peptide-Functionalized Gold Nanorods Increase Liver Injury in Hepatitis. *ACS Nano* **2012**, *6*, 8767–8777. [CrossRef] [PubMed]
116. Jia, J.; Li, F.; Zhou, H.; Bai, Y.; Liu, S.; Jiang, Y.; Jiang, G.; Yan, B. Oral Exposure to Silver Nanoparticles or Silver Ions May Aggravate Fatty Liver Disease in Overweight Mice. *Environ. Sci. Technol.* **2017**, *51*, 9334–9343. [CrossRef] [PubMed]
117. Li, J.; He, X.; Yang, Y.; Li, M.; Xu, C.; Yu, R. Risk assessment of silica nanoparticles on liver injury in metabolic syndrome mice induced by fructose. *Sci. Total Environ.* **2018**, *628*, 366–374. [CrossRef]
118. Soule, B.; Tirucherai, G.; Kavita, U.; Kundu, S.; Christian, R. Safety, tolerability, and pharmacokinetics of BMS-986263/ND-L02-s0201, a novel targeted lipid nanoparticle delivering HSP47 siRNA, in healthy participants: A randomised, placebo-controlled, double-blind, phase 1 study. *J. Hepatol.* **2018**, *68*, S112. [CrossRef]
119. Sakamoto, N.; Ogawa, K.; Suda, G.; Morikawa, K.; Sho, T.; Nakai, M.; Suzuki, H.; Yamagata, N.; Tanaka, Y.; Ying, W. Clinical phase 1b study results for safety, pharmacokinetics and efficacy of ND-L02-s0201, a novel targeted lipid nanoparticle delivering HSP47 SIRNA for the treatment of Japanese patients with advanced liver fibrosis. *J. Hepatol.* **2018**, *68*, S242. [CrossRef]

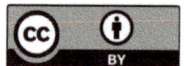

© 2020 by the authors. Licensee MDPI, Basel, Switzerland. This article is an open access article distributed under the terms and conditions of the Creative Commons Attribution (CC BY) license (http://creativecommons.org/licenses/by/4.0/).

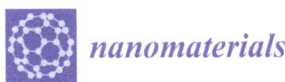

Review

Molecular Ultrasound Imaging

Gurbet Köse [1,†], **Milita Darguzyte** [1,†] **and Fabian Kiessling** [1,2,*]

[1] Institute for Experimental Molecular Imaging, University Hospital Aachen, Forckenbeckstrasse 55, 52074 Aachen, Germany; gkoese@ukaachen.de (G.K.); mdarguzyte@ukaachen.de (M.D.)
[2] Fraunhofer MEVIS, Institute for Medical Image Computing, Forckenbeckstrasse 55, 52074 Aachen, Germany
* Correspondence: fkiessling@ukaachen.de
† These authors contributed equally to this work.

Received: 28 August 2020; Accepted: 22 September 2020; Published: 28 September 2020

Abstract: In the last decade, molecular ultrasound imaging has been rapidly progressing. It has proven promising to diagnose angiogenesis, inflammation, and thrombosis, and many intravascular targets, such as VEGFR2, integrins, and selectins, have been successfully visualized in vivo. Furthermore, pre-clinical studies demonstrated that molecular ultrasound increased sensitivity and specificity in disease detection, classification, and therapy response monitoring compared to current clinically applied ultrasound technologies. Several techniques were developed to detect target-bound microbubbles comprising sensitive particle acoustic quantification (SPAQ), destruction-replenishment analysis, and dwelling time assessment. Moreover, some groups tried to assess microbubble binding by a change in their echogenicity after target binding. These techniques can be complemented by radiation force ultrasound improving target binding by pushing microbubbles to vessel walls. Two targeted microbubble formulations are already in clinical trials for tumor detection and liver lesion characterization, and further clinical scale targeted microbubbles are prepared for clinical translation. The recent enormous progress in the field of molecular ultrasound imaging is summarized in this review article by introducing the most relevant detection technologies, concepts for targeted nano- and micro-bubbles, as well as their applications to characterize various diseases. Finally, progress in clinical translation is highlighted, and roadblocks are discussed that currently slow the clinical translation.

Keywords: molecular ultrasound; nanobubbles; active targeting; targeted microbubbles; angiogenesis; inflammation; thrombosis; clinical translation; molecular imaging

1. Introduction

Ultrasound (US) imaging, also known as sonography, is used routinely in clinics for examining various organs of the body to diagnose, localize, and characterize diseases. Its advantages are low costs, real-time imaging capability, and the lack of exposure of the patient to radioactive rays. During US imaging the body is exposed to high-frequency sound waves, which are reflected by the tissues. The US probe is detecting the echoes and by calculating the amplitude and time of the reflected waves, an image is generated. Since tissue penetration decreases with increasing frequency of the sound waves but resolution increases, harmonic imaging was developed, which considers not only the center frequency of the echoes, but also their higher harmonics [1].

US contrast agents (UCA) can be used to visualize the vasculature of the tissue. The standard UCA are small gas-filled spheres, mainly referred to as microbubbles (MB), which are stabilized by a shell layer formed of lipids, proteins or polymers [2]. MB typically have a size between 1 and 10 µm. Therefore, they do not leave the vasculature. Due to the acoustic impedance difference between gas and blood, UCA can be easily distinguished from the tissue. Hereby, an increase in the signal to noise ratio is achieved.

Furthermore, decorating UCA with targeting moieties, specific disease markers can be detected and quantified. Various intravascular targets have been proposed for MB targeting such as integrins, selectins, and cell adhesion molecules. The preclinical results indicate that actively targeted MB can detect angiogenesis, inflammation, and thrombus formation [3]. In this context, even small changes in marker expression can be quantified by molecular US. Undoubtfully, molecular US imaging has high potential for clinical translation, and two targeted MB formulations are already in clinical trials. Complementary to MB, there is increasing research activity on molecular US imaging using nanobubbles (NB) and their targeting to extravascular markers [4]. UCA are also employed for US mediated drug and gene delivery. Drug or gene uptake is facilitiated by increasing the permeability of cell membranes and biological barriers with oscillating or bursting MB. However, this topic is already addressed in recent review articles [5–7].

Therefore, this review article focus on the evolution of molecular US, highlighting the newest molecular US imaging technologies, providing an overview of targeted contrast agent formulations, and summarizing their applications in preclinical and clinical studies. In the context of the latter, this paper also discusses challenges that have to be overcome to accelerate clinical translation.

2. Detection Technologies

UCA can be injected into the blood pool to increase the contrast during imaging. The detection of UCA relies on their non-linear response to US. When the sound waves are emitted from the transducer and hit the UCA they are backscattered with a different frequency (non-linearity), while for tissues the emitted and returning signals are more linear. By this, the signal from the UCA can be distinguished from the tissue signal (Figure 1).

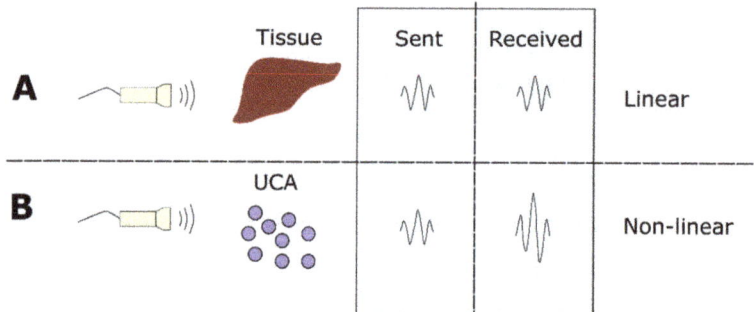

Figure 1. Non-linear response from UCA to US. The US transducer is transmitting ultrasound waves to tissue and UCA. For tissue (**A**) the sent and received signals are similar (linear response), while for UCA (**B**) the received signal has a different frequency than the initial frequency (non-linear response).

This nonlinearity originates from the nature of the response of the UCA to the US wave, which consists of high- and low-pressure phases. When the UCA is exposed to high pressure, it is compressed, and when it is exposed to low pressure it expands. With high wave amplitudes, the compression during the rise in pressure is bigger than the expansion during the pressure drop, which creates the non-linear response.

There are several techniques using non-linearity to detect UCA such as pulse/phase inversion, power modulation, or contrast pulse sequencing (Figure 2).

During pulse/phase inversion two pulses are transmitted. The second pulse is shifted by 180 degrees. Afterward, the responses to these pulses are summed up. For mostly linear responses as it is the case for tissue, the total is close to zero. For UCA the response does not cancel out due to irregularity in the backscattered US wave (non-linearity).

During power modulation, two identical pulses are sent out with a two-fold difference in amplitude. The response pulses are then summed up, while the second pulse is multiplied by two. With a linear response from tissue the total is again close to zero. With UCA, the total is not zero due to a difference in shape and amplitude (non-linearity) [8].

Contrast pulse sequencing is a combination of both above mentioned methods. Practically, during contrast pulse sequencing two pulses are used, where the second one is shifted 180 degrees and has an amplitude twice the magnitude as the first one. The advantage of this technique is that it can be used at low pressure [9,10].

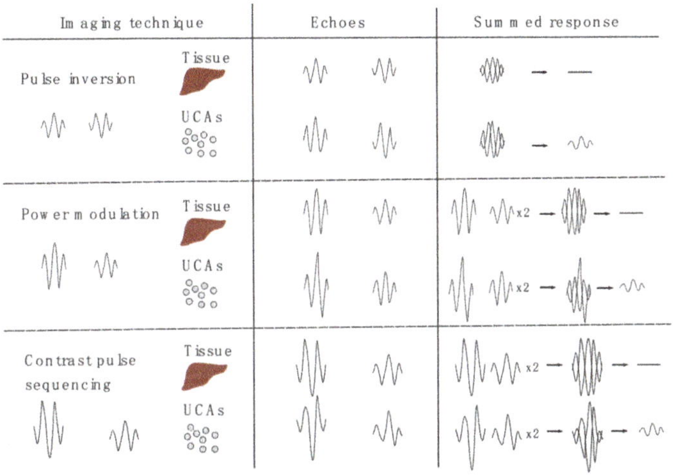

Figure 2. Theoretical background of imaging techniques based on the non-linear response of UCA. During pulse inversion two pulses are transmitted. The second pulse is shifted by 180 degrees. After receiving the echoes, the responses are summed up. In tissue the transmitted and received signals are the same and thus cancel out. For UCA the summed signal does not cancel out due to the non-linear response. During power modulation two pulses are transmitted. The second pulse has a two-fold difference in amplitude. For the summation of the responses the second pulse is multiplied by two. For tissue the response is near zero, for UCA the summed response is not zero due to the irregularity in UCA echoes. Contrast pulse sequencing is a combination of both mentioned methods. Two pulses are used where the second one is shifted by 180 degrees and has an amplitude twice the magnitude as the first one. Reproduced with permission from [11]. Copyright Elsevier, 2011.

While the imaging techniques mentioned above do not destroy the UCA, there are methods, which destroy the MB by US. In the field of molecular US imaging, a prominent example is the 3D SPAQ method.

SPAQ can be applied in cases where high local densities of bound MB are present in the tissue but the blood pool is already cleared from free circulating MB. After injection, the targeted MB are allowed to bind to their target and unbound MB are allowed to wash out (approximately after 10 min). Then, a destructive US pulse is applied in the tissue of interest. When MB are destroyed the resulting non-linear signal is construed as a strong movement and detected by Doppler imaging. Subsequently, the transducer is moved forward in the micrometer steps and Doppler imaging is applied to destroy the MB. From the second destructive pulse, MB are only present in the non-overlapping part of the sound field, which should be much smaller than the voxel size. Thus, signals of multiple MB within one voxel can be assessed separately. At the end, a 3D data set is generated that displays MB destruction events with higher resolution than is possible with a single image assessment [12].

Alternatively, to detect targeted MB the destruction - replenishment technique can be used. Targeted MB are injected and images are recorded. After the targeted MB are expected to have bound to their target, a high mechanical index pulse is applied that destroys the MB in the examined area. Images are recorded promptly after the destructive pulse. By subtracting the mean signal intensity of images after the destructive pulse from that directly before, the signals originating from target-bound MB can be assessed [6,13].

Another approach was suggested by Pysz and colleagues where targeted MB are identified by their dwelling time in one spot. To do so, the pixel intensities representing the MB in each frame during B-mode imaging are monitored over a specific time frame. First, it is evaluated whether there is an increase in pixel intensity indicating the presence of a MB. Then, it is evaluated if the pixel intensity stays constant and a time threshold is defined for which a MB is considered as target bound. This technique can be applied in real-time with minimum post-processing and without using a destructive pulse exposing the tissue to a high acoustic pressure [14].

3. Targeted Contrast Agents

The main UCA are MB, NB, and nanodroplets (Figure 3). To enhance their specificity, various ligands were coupled, including antibodies, peptides, and carbohydrates. Depending on their size, UCA have been targeted to intravascular or extravascular markers.

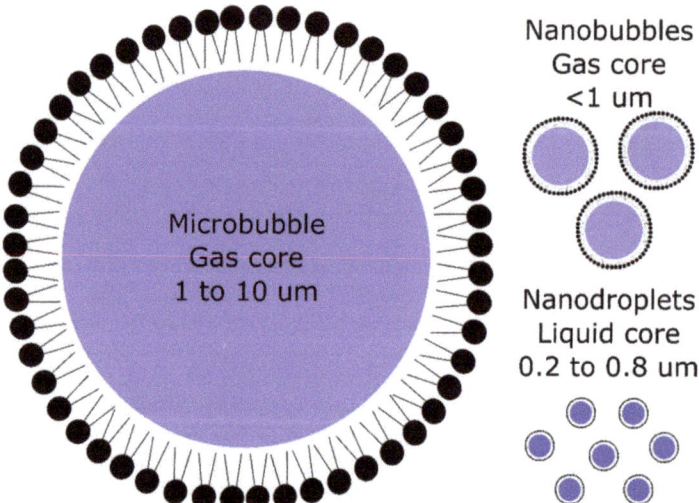

Figure 3. Schematic representation of microbubbles, nanobubbles, and nanodroplets.

3.1. Functionalization of Contrast Agents

The easiest way to functionalize UCA is to have the targeting ligand incorporated in the shell layer of the bubble (Figure 4). This method favorably works for lipid-bound ligands such as phosphatidylserine [15] and phospholipid-heteropeptides binding to the vascular endothelial growth factor receptors 2 (VEGFR2) [16], because they can withstand harsh MB synthesis conditions.

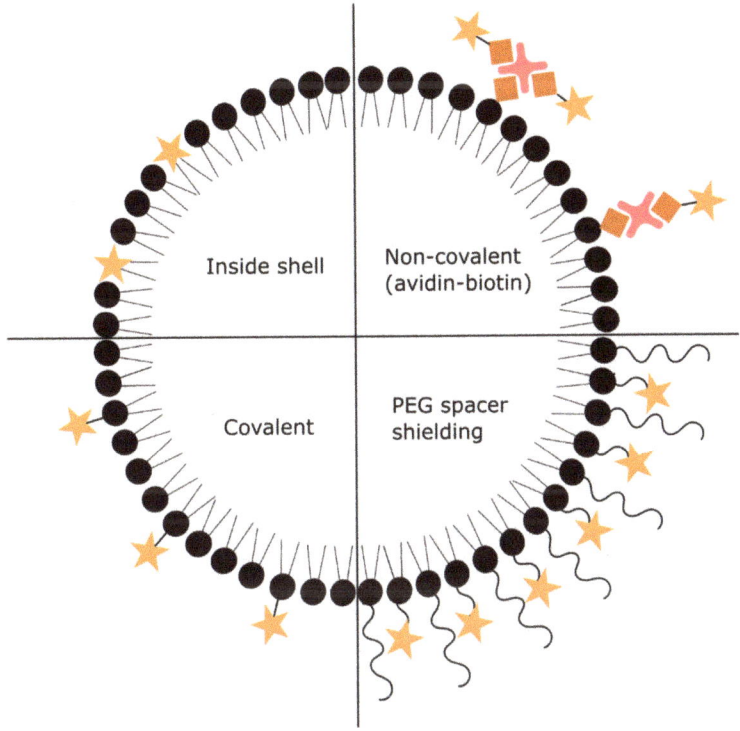

Figure 4. Schematic representation of different functionalization methods of UCA.

Another way of functionalizing UCA is to incorporate a reactive moiety into the shell that can be coupled via a non-covalent or covalent bond to the targeting ligand. For non-covalent coupling, an avidin-biotin bond has been extensively used. In this case, biotin is incorporated into the shell layer and with the use of avidin as a "bridging" moiety biotinylated ligands are coupled. Since avidin has four possible binding sites multiple ligands can be attached. Additionally, it was shown that avidin itself can be incorporated into the bubble shell layer. The major drawback of using a biotin-avidin bond for UCA functionalization is the immunogenicity of avidin. Thus, avidin-biotin bubbles can only be used in preclinical research and not in the clinics.

Furthermore, two covalent binding methods (Figure 4) for UCA functionalization have been used. The first one is the carbodiimide coupling. In this case, the carboxyl group located on the shell coat reacts with an amine group present in the targeting ligand forming an amide bond. Due to the low yield of the reaction, an excess of ligand has to be used, which can become expensive [17]. Additionally, if the ligand contains multiple amine groups (as it is the case for most proteins) the coupling can occur at several sites leading to uncontrolled conjugation and a possible reduction in targeting affinity. Hence, the second method using maleimide-thiol coupling is preferred. Maleimide can be easily conjugated to polyethylene glycol (PEG)-lipids that can be used for the bubble synthesis, while the thiol group has to be attached to the ligand. In single-step "click" reaction maleimide and thiol groups form a thioether bond. This method has higher yield compared to carbodiimide coupling, thus fewer ligands are needed. Moreover, due to the single thiol group introduction to the targeting ligand the coupling to the UCA is better controlled. Though covalent bond avoids immunogenic materials like avidin, the unreacted chemical groups on the shell layer might as well trigger an immune response. Thus, it is important to have all chemical groups bonded.

In some cases, PEG was used as a spacer between the bubble and the targeting ligand (Figure 4). A long chain of PEG gives the targeting ligand more flexibility and mobility to interact with its receptors. It has been shown that ligand interaction to its receptor was increased with the increasing length of the spacer [18,19]. Moreover, the ligand could be shielded by introducing additional longer PEG chains without targeting moieties [20,21]. This prevented specific interactions with the target. Only when US irradiation was applied the longer PEG chains unfolded and exposed the ligand to its receptor. Then MB were able to bind to the target. Thus, the bimodal structure produces stimulus-responsive, targeted UCA. The advantage is reduced immunogenicity and low binding at not insonated sites.

3.2. Intravascular Targeting (MB)

Due to their size, MB do not leave the vasculature, so targets should be located within the vessels. This is the case for many angiogenesis, inflammation, and thrombosis markers, for which several ligands have been investigated (Table 1).

Table 1. Summary of intravascular targets investigated for molecular US imaging.

Target	Binding Ligand	Model
$\alpha_v\beta_3$ integrin	Echistatin peptide	Malignant glioma in rats [22] Cremaster muscle in mice [23] Ischemic muscle in rats [24]
	Knottin peptide	Ovarian cancer in mice [25]
	Cyclic RGD peptide	Breast cancer in mice [26] Spontaneous model of ovarian cancer in hens [27]
	RGD peptide	Prostate cancer in rats [28] Squamous cell carcinoma in mice [29]
	Anti-$\alpha_v\beta_3$ integrin antibody	Breast, ovarian and pancreatic cancers in mice [30] Skin cancer in mice [31] Cremaster muscle in mice [23]
	Cyclic RRL peptide	Prostate cancer in mice [32]
VEGFR2	Anti-VEGFR2 antibody	Squamous cell carcinoma in mice [29] Ovarian cancers in mice [30] Skin cancer in mice [31,33] Colon cancer in mice [34] Pancreatic cancer in mice [30,35] Malignant glioma in mice [36] Angiosarcoma in mice [36,37] Breast cancers in mice [30,38,39]
	10th type III domain of human fibronectin	Transgenic breast cancer in mice [40]
	Single-chain VEGF construct	Colon cancer in mice [41]
	VEGFR2-binding phospholipid-heteropeptides	Prostate cancer in rats [42] Breast cancer in rats [16] and mice [43–45] Transgenic breast cancer in mice [46] Transgenic pancreatic ductal cancer in mice [47] Colon cancer in mice [48] Squamous cell carcinoma in mice [49] Colon cancer in mice [50,51]
Neuropilin-1	CRPPR and ATWLPPR peptides	Pancreatic cancer in mice [35]
Endoglin	Anti-endoglin antibody	Breast cancer in mice [30,52] Ovarian cancers in mice [30] Pancreatic cancer in mice [30,35] Skin cancer in mice [31]
SFRP2	Anti-SFRP2 antibody	Angiosarcoma in mice [53]
B7-H3	Anti-B7-H3 antibody	Breast cancer in mice [54]
Nucleolin	F3 peptide	Breast cancer in mice [55]

Table 1. Cont.

Target	Binding Ligand	Model
Thy1	Anti-Thy1 antibody	Transgenic and implanted pancreatic cancer in mice [56]
Leukocytes	Phosphatidylserine	Inflammation in mice [57] and dogs [58]
	Anti-ICAM-1 antibody	Activated endothelial cells [59]
MAdCAM-1	Anti-MAdCAM-1 antibody	Inflammatory bowel disease in mice [60]
JAM-A	Anti-JAM-A antibody	Atherosclerosis in mice [61] and rabbits [62]
VCAM-1	Anti-VCAM-1 antibody	Atherosclerosis in mice [63–70] and swine [71]
	Nanobody targeting VCAM-1	Epidermoid carcinoma in mice [72]
		Atherosclerosis in mice [73]
	HGRANLRILARY peptide	Atherosclerosis in mice [74]
ICAM-1	Anti-ICAM-1 antibody	Endothelial cells [17]
		Inflammation in rats [75]
P-selectin	Anti-P-selectin antibody	Atherosclerosis in mice [63,65,69,70]
		Inflammation in mice [76,77] and flow chamber [78]
		Muscle inflammation in mice [79,80]
		Inflammatory bowel disease in mice [81,82]
		Myocardial ischemia in mice [83,84] and rats [85]
	LVSVLDLEPLDAAWL peptide	Atherosclerosis in mice [74]
	Sialyl Lewis X	Inflammation in mice [77]
E-selectin	IELLQAR peptide	Ovarian carcinoma in mice [86,87]
		Epidermoid carcinoma in mice [72,87]
	Anti-E-selectin antibody	Muscle inflammation in mice [80]
		Myocardial ischemia in rats [85]
	E-selectin affibody	Myocardial ischemia in rats [88]
GP Ibα	Anti-GP Ibα antibody	Atherosclerosis in mice [63,64]
	Dimeric murine recombinant A1 domain of VWF A1	Atherosclerosis in mice [69]
GP IIb/IIIa	Linear KQAGDV peptide	Thrombosis in flow chamber [89] and mongrels [90]
	Cyclic RGD	Thrombosis in mice [91,92]
	Anti-GP IIb/IIIa antibody	Thrombosis in mice artery [93]
GP VI	Anti-GP VI antibody	Atherosclerosis in mice [94]
VWF	Cell-derived peptide	Atherosclerosis in mice [69]
	RVVCEYVFGRGAVCS peptide	Atherosclerosis in mice [74]
LOX-1	LSIPPKA peptide	Atherosclerosis in mice [74]
Thrombin	Thrombin aptamer	Thrombosis in rabbit blood [95,96]
	Thrombin-sensitive ACPP	Thrombosis in rabbit blood [97]

Due to the fast flow of MB in larger vessels, it is important that the ligands bind quickly to the target. For this purpose, a high kinetic association for binding is needed. Alternatively, an increase in binding can be achieved by using multiple ligands on one bubble (more about it in Section 3.2.4) or by applying acoustic radiation force pulses.

Acoustic radiation forces (primary and secondary) are the forces affecting MB localization and distribution. They cause movement of MB (primary radiation force) and interaction of the MB with each other (secondary radiation force) [98,99]. The primary radiation force is experienced by single particles resulting from the acoustic pressure field. It leads to the movement of the MB in the acoustic field and also allows to push a MB streamline towards the vessel wall bringing the bubbles closer to the target, which might increment targeting efficiency [99–101]. In this regard, Dayton et al. showed that during this process the flow of the MB concentrating close to the vessel wall was reduced compared to the MB floating in the streamline [100]. Secondary or Bjerknes force affects neighboring bubbles. It is produced by the scattered field of a resonating bubble. This leads to a reversible attraction and clustering of MB [99,100]. Moreover, the clustering of MB is affected by the distance between two bubbles [98]. It is hypothesized that bound bubbles can attract other bubbles thus increasing targeting efficacy and the concentration of bound MB [100,101]. Following up, Zhao and colleagues showed in vitro that enhanced binding of targeted MB was observed when radiation force was applied [101]. In line with this, the in vivo study from Gessner et al. using a cyclic arginine–glycine–aspartic (RGD) peptide targeted to $\alpha_v\beta_3$ demonstrated a significant increase in targeting efficacy and US signal intensity, when acoustic radiation force was applied [102]. In addition, Wang et al. programmed a conventional US imaging device with an acoustic radiation force inducing sequence for pushing the MB to the vessel wall by using low pressure and long duty cycles. The experiments successfully demonstrated higher MB binding to P-selectin in large blood vessels in vitro and in vivo, where good binding efficiency is usually difficult to achieve due to low contact between MB and the vessel wall at the high physiological flow rates [103]. Furthermore, with the introduced sequence the signal between molecularly adherent, non-specific adherent and free floating MB can be distinguished [104]. This method could be very helpful since all molecular US imaging methods reported above cannot distinguish between unspecific adherent stationary MB and target-bound ones, which increases the unspecific background signal.

3.2.1. Angiogenesis

Angiogenesis describes the process of vessel formation and is crucial for tumor growth and metastasis. Among angiogenesis markers, VEGFR2 and $\alpha_v\beta_3$ integrin are the most addressed targets. VEGFR2 also known as KDR is an endothelium-specific receptor, that is highly expressed on tumor-associated endothelial cells [105]. Activation of the VEGFR2 pathway triggers multiple signaling cascades that result in endothelial cell survival, mitogenesis, migration, differentiation, and alterations in vascular permeability [103]. Moreover, overexpression of VEGFR2 has been linked to tumor progression and poor prognosis in several tumors [106]. Integrins are transmembrane receptors that are expressed on endothelial and tumor cells. They activate signaling cascades that regulate gene expression, cytoskeletal organization, cell adhesion and cell survival. This facilitates tumor growth, invasion and metastasis [107]. In particular, $\alpha_v\beta_3$ integrin expression is low on endothelial cells under normal conditions, but is elevated during tumor angiogenesis [108–110]. Another angiogenesis related marker is Endoglin, a transmembrane glycoprotein expressed in proliferating endothelial cells such as tumor endothelial cells [111]. It is a component of the transforming growth factor beta receptor complex involved in cell proliferation, differentiation and migration [111].

MB functionalized with ligands against VEGFR2, integrin and other angiogenesis markers have been successfully tested for molecular US imaging (Table 1). Moreover, the CEUS signal of the targeted MB could be correlated to the level of angiogenesis marker expression in the tissue. For example, CEUS signal using VEGFR2-targeted MB increased from hyperplasia to ductal carcinoma in situ and invasive breast cancer compared to normal tissue [46]. This was additionally confirmed by histological analysis.

During tumor angiogenesis, multiple endothelial markers are overexpressed [112]. These markers could be good targets for cancer detection. In this respect, E-selectin [86,87], secreted frizzled related protein 2 (SFRP2) [113], B7-H3 [54], nucleolin [55] and thymocyte differentiation antigen 1 (Thy1) [56] were tested for cancerous tissue detection and showed promising results. Since angiogenesis is an early event in tumor development [114], angiogenesis targeted MB should be able to detect tumors at early stages. Indeed, ovarian cancer at an early stage was sensitively detected using $\alpha_v\beta_3$ integrin-targeted MB [27]. Also, VEGFR2-targeted UCA were able to visualize breast cancer tumors as small as 2 mm in diameter [44,46] and pancreatic ductal adenocarcinoma lesions smaller than 3 mm in diameter [47]. Interestingly, a study showed that smaller breast cancer xenografts express the highest amount of VEGFR2, while with increasing tumor size the expression decreases [44]. Thus, current results suggest that VEGFR2 targeted MB are promising UCA for early tumor detection, though more research should be done.

Since angiogenesis plays an important role in tumor growth, it is not surprising that multiple anti-cancer drugs target angiogenesis. The idea is to stop tumors from developing new blood vessels and hopefully shrink them by cutting the nutrient and oxygen supply. CEUS imaging using targeted MB can provide information on the angiogenesis profile of the tumor and assess antiangiogenic therapy effects. Several groups showed successful monitoring of antiangiogenic therapy using VEGFR2-targeted MB [29,31,35,45,49,50]. In all cases, a clear decrease of VEGFR2-targeted MB accumulation was observed after treatment compared to untreated controls. These findings were further confirmed with immunohistochemistry analysis. Moreover, other therapies such as gemcitabine [35], nilotinib [45], and carbon ion treatment [28] were monitored using CEUS with angiogenesis targeted MB. Similarly, as for antiangiogenic therapy monitoring, CEUS was correlated to the target marker expression according to immunohistochemistry analysis. Hence, CEUS using angiogenesis targeted MB seems to be a promising tool for non-invasive antitumor therapy monitoring.

Furthermore, by combining functional and molecular US imaging, vascular responses in tumors can be comprehensively characterized. This is important since the percentage of angiogenic vessels—indicating angiogenic activity – cannot be assessed solely from the information on VEGFR2 bound MB. For, example, Palmowski and co-workers showed that VEGFR2 and $\alpha_v\beta_3$ integrin-targeted MB bound less after administration of a matrix metalloproteinase (MMP) inhibitor, which was in line with immunohistochemical analysis. However, when normalizing the molecular marker expression to vascular density no change in the percentage of angiogenic vessels was visible indicating that the MMP inhibitor did not decrease angiogenesis but induced a general decrease in vascularization [29]. To unravel these effects by US, Bzyl et al. injected long-circulating UCA (BR38) to derive functional information on vascularization and relative blood volume and VEGFR2-targeted MB (BR55) to assess angiogenesis [39]. Two breast cancer models with different aggressiveness and angiogenic activity were evaluated. The results showed that the more aggressive tumor model (MDA-MB-231) had the higher total expression of VEGFR2 compared to MCF-7 according to VEGFR2-targeted US measurements and immunohistochemistry. Also, the normalization of the molecular imaging data to the relative blood volume confirmed the higher angiogenic activity of the MDA-MB-231 model. A few years later Baetke et al. showed that functional and molecular US imaging can even be performed in one examination using only the targeted MB [49]. Here, antiangiogenic therapy effects were monitored in squamous cell carcinomas using BR55. It was shown, that the first-pass analysis of VEGFR2-targeted MB was not strongly affected by the targeting, and vascularization results were comparable to those obtained with non-targeted MB. Hence, in the early binding phase, functional information could be obtained and at the late phase, the molecular angiogenesis profile of the tumors could be assessed (Figure 5). Combining functional and molecular US in one examination would reduce measurement time and the need for multiple injections and multiple formulations of MB.

In summary, all these pre-clinical studies using angiogenesis-targeted MB showed promising results confirming that the targeted UCA can be used for angiogenesis profiling in various tumors. Most research has been done using VEGFR2-targeted MB, especially using the clinical-grade contrast agent BR55. These MB can detect tumors at early stages and can be used for antiangiogenic therapy monitoring combining functional and molecular US. BR55 is now evaluated in clinical trials and the initial results are summarized in Section 3.2.5.

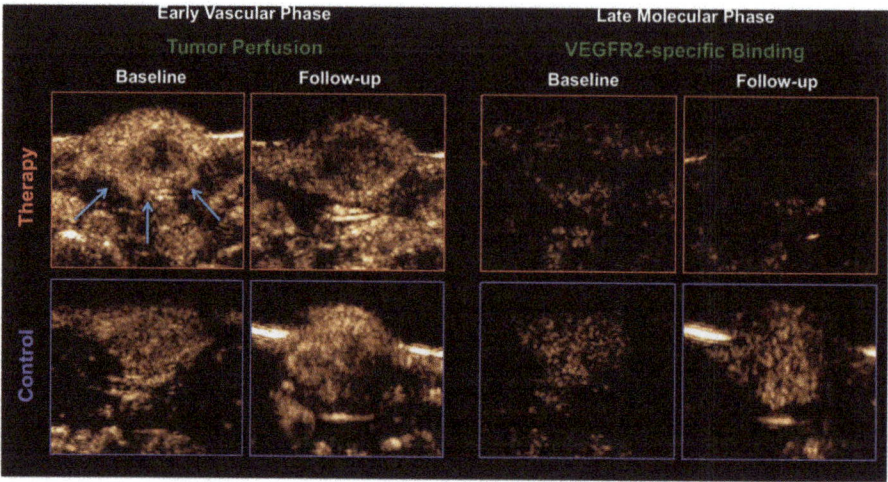

Figure 5. CEUS images of treated (top) and untreated tumors (bottom). Left side: early vascular phase with VEGFR2-targeted MB as a functional imaging biomarker; Right side: late phase of VEGFR2-specific binding with the targeted MB as a molecular imaging biomarker 8 min after contrast injection. Reproduced with permission from [51]. Copyright Eschbach et al., 2017.

3.2.2. Inflammation and Atherosclerosis

Atherosclerosis is an inflammatory disease that is driven by endothelial dysfunction. Many patients do not have symptoms for a long time until a plaque ruptures or severe narrowing or total blocking of the blood vessel occurs. Although there are biomarkers to identify atherosclerosis [115,116], tools that can predict the growth dynamics of a plaque or its risk to rupture are hardly available. CEUS with targeted MB could suit this purpose considering its high sensitivity and capability to quantify even low amounts of the inflammation-related markers. Vascular cell adhesion molecule 1 (VCAM-1) is known to be overexpressed and translocated to the luminal surface of endothelial cells at the early stages of atherosclerosis [117,118]. Thus, VCAM-1-targeted MB have been proposed for atherosclerosis imaging [63–71,73,74]. These UCA have successfully identified atherosclerosis and the CEUS signals could be correlated to the progression of the disease [65,67]. Moreover, molecular changes during apocynin [63,64,69] and statin [66] therapy were successfully monitored. Further, VCAM-1, platelet glycoprotein (GP) Ibα [63,64,69], junctional adhesion molecule A (JAM-A) [62], GP VI [94], lectin-type oxidized low-density lipoprotein receptor 1 (LOX-1) [74], and von Willebrand factor (VWF) [69,74] have been used for atherosclerosis imaging. Of these markers, JAM-A expression might be particularly associated with early plaque formation and vulnerability [119]. Indeed, in mice with partial ligation and atherogenic diet molecular US of JAM-A indicated atherosclerosis at a very early stage and was even capable of assessing vascular sites that underwent an immediate change in shear stress [61]. Moreover, another group demonstrated that plaque vulnerability can be assessed in rabbits [62]. Another interesting target is GP VI since it can be used for atherosclerosis therapy. It has been shown that administering soluble anti-GP VI antibody inhibits thrombus formation and progression of atherosclerosis [120–122]. Using high-frequency US, it is possible to disrupt MB and release the ligand coupled to the shell. Thus, GP VI-targeted MB could work as theranostic agents. A study showed that these MB help to diagnose atherosclerosis, and in combination with the high-frequency US work as a therapy [94].

Another pathology that would benefit from a broadly available reliable non-invasive detection technique is acute cardiac ischemia. Electrocardiogram and serological markers often have limited expressiveness or lead to misjudgment [123–126]. The gold standard in the clinics is cardiac magnetic resonance imaging (MRI) though it is time-consuming, requires multiple breath holds, and due to usage of gadolinium cannot be used in patients with renal dysfunction. Other diagnosis methods include scintigraphy and coronary CT. However, both techniques raise safety concerns due to usage of radioisotopes and/or radiation. Myocardial ischemia is associated with endothelial upregulation of adhesion molecules which persist after ischemia has resolved. Thus, it could be possible to identify post-ischemic myocardium using the molecular US. P-selectin seems to be a good target since it is expressed within minutes after ischemia or injury [127]. As expected, P-selectin-targeted MB strongly bound in post-ischemic myocardium in mice [74,83]. Similar results were also seen for E-selectin-targeted UCA in rats (Figure 6) [88]. Moreover, the researchers decided to target both, P- and E-selectins [84,85,128,129]. This proved to be particularly useful since P-selectin was present immediately after ischemia but only E-selectin was still overexpressed after 24 h [84]. Thus, the dual-targeted MB could detect myocardial ischemia for a longer time. Further in vivo experiments were performed in primates demonstrating that molecular US using selectin-targeted MB is a safe and effective method to detect myocardial ischemia [129]. However, despite these promising results, molecular US imaging of the heart is difficult to perform, user-dependent, and requires an experienced physician. Thus, it must be carefully evaluated whether a high diagnostic accuracy and reproducibility can also be achieved outside specialized centers and whether it can compete with the clinically established imaging methods.

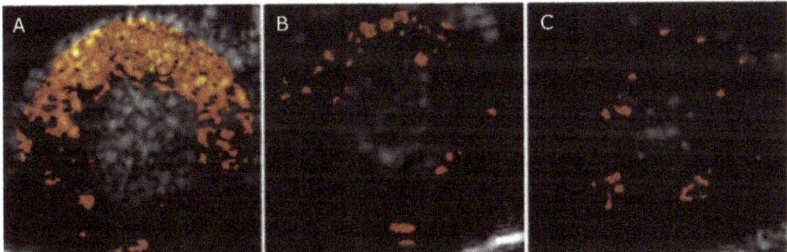

Figure 6. B-mode US images of the left ventricle 4 h after conorary occlusion overlayed with the signal of E-selectin targeted MB (**A**), non-targeted MB (**B**) and non-specific IgG targeted MB (**C**). Enhanced contrast signal is seen using E-selectin targeted MB. Reproduced with permission from [88]. Copyright SAGE Publications, 2014.

Inflammatory bowel disease (IBD) is currently assessed by endoscopic monitoring, US, and clinical chemistry. Endoscopy is invasive and cannot access major parts of the small intestine. US is applied to capture the enhanced thickness of the inflamed bowel wall and the enhanced perfusion by Doppler. However, this approach has limited sensitivity and only becomes prominent at advanced disease stages. Here, molecular US could be introduced as a complementary sensitive tool. Inflammation in patients with IBD is associated with increased expression of cell adhesion molecules. Initially, mucosal addressin cell adhesion molecule 1 (MAdCAM-1) targeted MB were proposed for IBD detection [60]. The CEUS signal using these MB positively correlated with the severity of ileal inflammation assessed by immunohistochemical analysis. However, no further research was published using these MB. Instead, molecular US of IBD was mostly approached using different selectin-targeted MB. For example, P-selectin-targeted MB were successfully applied for IBD detection and monitoring of anti-TNFα antibody therapy [81]. CEUS signal changes were observed already after 3 days of therapy, while there was no decrease in bowel wall thickness or perfusion yet. In another study, these MB were able to depict radiation-induced P-selectin expression in the colon [82]. Furthermore, clinical-scale P- and E-selectin-targeted UCA were tested for IBD detection. The experiments in colitis induced mice showed that molecular US assessment of IBD excellently correlated with ^{18}FDG-PET (positron emission tomography) and histological examination [130]. Further studies in swine demonstrated that dual-targeted UCA have the potential for clinical translation [131,132]. Wang and co-workers showed that, one hour after inflammation induction by exposing ileum to 2, 4, 6-trinitrobenzene sulfonic acid (TNBS) and ethanol, a significant increase in CEUS signal occurred [131]. The US signal changed in line with the increased selectin expression and further increased with the progression of the inflammation. Moreover, P- and E-selectin-targeted MB also proved promising for long-term monitoring of anti-inflammatory IBD treatment in swine [132]. The combination treatment of prednisone and meloxicam reduced inflammation and downregulated selectin expression in the inflamed vasculature in the bowel. This molecular change was clearly depicted by molecular US imaging. Interestingly, there was no difference in the inflammation score obtained from the histological analysis between treated and control groups. This underlines the high sensitivity of selectin-targeted US imaging for IBD assessment and highlights its potential for clinical translation.

3.2.3. Thrombosis

Thrombosis describes the formation of a blood clot in a vessel. In the clinics, Doppler US is a standard method for detecting deep venous thrombosis (DVT). However, the blood clot has to be big enough to produce visible circulation defects and the thrombus activity cannot be assessed. Moreover, the examination is user-dependent and hence the accuracy in detecting DVT varies [133]. MB targeting activated platelets have been proposed for thrombus detection and characterization. Acute thrombus should have a higher number of activated platelets than the chronic state. Hence, ligands, which only bind to activated platelets, have been proposed for targeting: lysine-glutamine-alanine-glycine-aspartate-valine (KQAGDV) [89,90], glycoprotein (GP) IIa/IIIb [93] and cyclic arginine-glycine-aspartate (RGD) [91,92]. All targeted MB formulations showed thrombus-specific US contrast in vitro and in vivo. Nonetheless, the exact concentration of activated platelets required to successfully identify a thrombus by targeted MB still needs to be elucidated, which is crucial for evaluating the potential of the method for early thrombus detection.

Furthermore, stimulus-responsive MB have been suggested for thrombus detection. The first group proposed MB decorated with aptamers [95,96]. When exposed to thrombin, the aptamers were detached and the bubble stiffness was reduced. The change in shell stiffness alters the harmonic signals generated by the bubble. For thrombus formation a critical concentration of 25 nmol is required [134,135]. At this concentration it was seen that all aptamers detach from the MB making the shell soft, while at lower concentrations (10 to 25 nmol) only a partial softness change was observed. Hence, these MB become active and give US contrast only when thrombin levels exceed the critical threshold. In vitro and in vivo experiments proved the concept. The stimulus-responsive MB increased the CEUS signal five-fold in presence of clots and even small lesions that were not visible by non-specific UCA were detected. Another group proposed MB with thrombin-sensitive activatable cell-penetrating peptides (ACPP) [97]. In this case, thrombin cleaved ACPP making the UCA positively charged. Due to Coulomb interaction, activated MB adhere to negatively charged surfaces like red blood cells, fibrin, and platelets. The concept of these UCA was confirmed in vitro using rabbit blood and an increase in the US signal was only seen if thrombin was present (Figure 7). Therefore, ACPP MB detect only acute blood clots. Both stimulus-responsive MB formulations can distinguish between acute and chronic thrombosis according to thrombin levels in the blood.

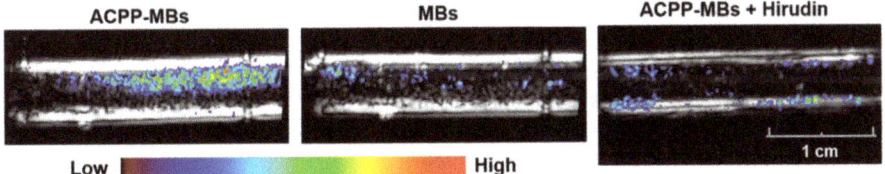

Figure 7. Molecular US imaging of thrombosis. Spatial maps of the molecular US signal color-coded and overlaid on B-mode images acquired at baseline after infusion of MB and washing with saline using targeted MB (left), non-targeted MB (middle), and targeted MB co-injected with hirudin (right). Targeted MB give specific signal only in the presence of thrombin. Reproduced with permission from [97]. Copyright American Chemical Society, 2017.

3.2.4. Multiple Targets

Besides single targeted UCA, few groups have synthesized and tested multi-targeted ones (Table 2). The idea is that addressing multiple targets at the same time improves MB binding affinity and avidity. This would reduce the amount of unbound bubbles, meaning a lower concentration would be needed to achieve similar results as with single-targeted MB, and the bubbles would persist for a longer time. Furthermore, in the case of a disease with heterogeneous expression of the individual markers, multi-targeted UCA could improve the accuracy of diagnosis.

Table 2. Summary of multi-targeted MB investigated for molecular US imaging.

Targets	Binding Ligands	Model
ICAM-1 and selectins	Anti-ICAM-1 antibody and sialyl Lewis X	Flow chamber [136]
VCAM-1 and P-selectin	Anti-VCAM-1 and anti-P-selectin antibodies	Flow chamber [137]
VEGFR2 and $\alpha_v\beta_3$ integrin	Anti-VEGFR2 and anti- $\alpha_v\beta_3$ integrin antibodies	Ovarian cancer in mice [138]
Selectins	Sialyl Lewis X	Muscle inflammation in mice [80]
Selectins	Sialyl Lewis X	Myocardial ischemia in rats [128]
Selectins	PSGL-Ig	Muscle inflammation in mice [80]
Selectins	PSGL-Ig	Inflammatory bowel disease in mice [130] and swine [131,132]
Selectins	PSGL-Ig	Myocardial ischemia in mice [84], rats [85] and macaques [129]
VEGFR2, $\alpha_v\beta_3$ integrin and P-selectin	Anti-VEGFR2, anti- $\alpha_v\beta_3$ integrin and anti-P-selectin antibodies	Breast cancer in mice [139,140]

First multi-targeted MB were functionalized using anti-ICAM-1 antibodies and sialyl Lewis X [133]. These dual-targeted MB had greater adhesion to inflammatory endothelial cells compared to their single targeted counterparts under shear flow. Similar results were reported for MB modified with anti-VCAM-1 and anti-P-selectin antibodies in flow chamber experiments [137]. Moreover, VEGFR2 and $\alpha_v\beta_3$ integrin-targeted MB for angiogenesis imaging showed the benefits of dual-targeting in vivo [138]. Since dual-targeted MB comprise of two ligands it was expected that its binding affinity and avidity would be an average of the single-targeted MB counterparts. Interestingly, in all three studies, dual-targeted MB showed significantly higher binding affinity than their single targeted counterparts. Hence, the ligands on MB seem to synergistically increase the binding affinity.

The main drawback of dual-targeted UCA is the synthesis route. In the case of attaching two ligands to the MB, a ratio between the ligands has to be chosen. Controlling this ratio during synthesis can be difficult. This challenge can be overcome by using a single ligand that targets multiple markers, such as sialyl Lewis X that binds to P- and E-selectin. MB decorated with this natural ligand identified postischemic myocardium better than UCA targeted to just P- or E-selectin [128]. Moreover, even better results were achieved using P-selectin glycoprotein ligand-1 analog (PSGL-Ig) instead of sialyl Lewis X [80]. PSGL-Ig-targeted MB enabled the detection and quantification of inflammation in colitis induced mice [130] and swine [131,132]. Moreover, post-ischemic myocardium was detected in mice [84], rats [85], and even macaques [129]. Hence, inflammation detection using P- and E-selectin-targeted MB is possible and preferential over single-targeted UCA.

Furthermore, MB modified with VEGFR2, $\alpha_v\beta_3$ integrin and P-selectin have been synthesized [139,140]. These triple-targeted UCA possess better binding to target cells than single- or even double-targeted MB (Figure 8). The in vivo experiments further confirmed these results. Interestingly, in vivo US intensity using triple-targeted UCA was higher than the cumulative intensity of all single-targeted MB [139]. Similar to dual-targeted MB, the ligands synergistically increased the efficiency of the binding. Moreover, these MB were used for monitoring antiangiogenic therapy in breast cancer-bearing mice [140]. Due to the high US signal produced by multi-targeted UCA, even small changes in angiogenesis could be detected. Therefore, an early response to the therapy can be assessed. However, no further studies using this triple-targeted MB have been reported so far.

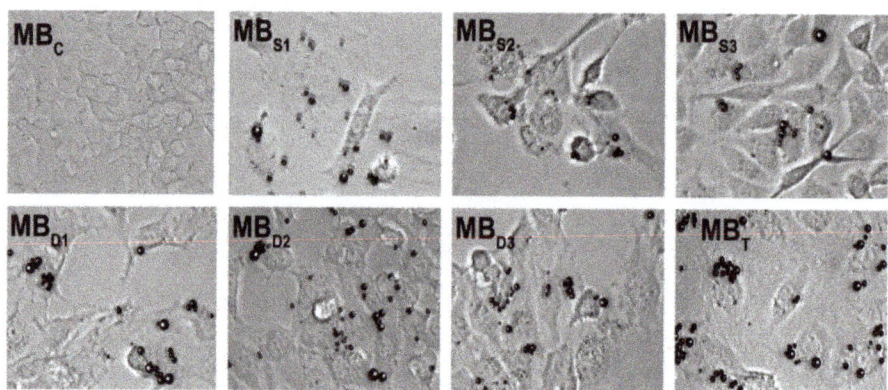

Figure 8. In vitro microscopy images of control (MB$_C$), single (MB$_S$), double (MB$_D$), and triple (MB$_T$) targeted MB adhered on cells. Triple targeted MB adhere more on the cells than single or double targeted ones. Reproduced with permission from [139]. Copyright John Wiley and Sons, 2011.

3.2.5. Targeted MB in The Clinics

Although there are many successful pre-clinical studies using targeted MB, the translation to the clinics is slow. Most of the targeted MB used in research have been functionalized using biotin-avidin or covalent coupling. As discussed before, avidin can cause severe allergic reactions in patients and thus its use should be avoided [141–145]. However, free chemical groups sticking out of the MB shell can as well cause an immune response. Thus, it is not surprising that the only two targeted MB (Sonazoid™ and BR55) currently in clinical trials have the ligand incorporated in the shell layer.

Sonazoid™ (Daiichi Sankyo Company Ltd.) is not specifically advertised as a targeted MB. However, due to phosphatidylserine in the shell layer, these MB circulate for a longer time in the blood and accumulate in Kupffer cells and macrophages of the liver. These MB are clinically approved in Japan for CEUS imaging of hepatic tumors. They are also in phase I clinical trial in the United States (ClinicalTrials.gov identifier: NCT02968680) for detecting sentinel lymph nodes in patients with melanoma and in phase III clinical trial in China (NCT03335566) for liver lesion detection.

The second targeted MB in the clinical translation is BR55 (Bracco Suisse SA, Geneva, Switzerland). These MB contain VEGFR2-binding phospholipid-heteropeptides. The first clinical trials in women with ovarian or breast cancer showed that BR55 is safe to use in patients, and the CEUS signal correlated with the VEGFR2 amount in tumor lesions [146]. Further clinical trials are ongoing to evaluate its specificity and sensitivity in the prostate (NCT02142608 and NCT01253213), ovarian cancer (NCT03493464 and NCT04248153) and pancreatic lesions (NCT03486327).

3.3. Extravascular Targeting (NB)

Since MB are trapped in the bloodstream due to their size, extravascular imaging is not possible. This is not necessarily a drawback, since many promising targets are still accessible. Furthermore, the intravascular distribution minimizes the unspecific MB accumulation in tissues leading to a low background. However, if extravascular targeting is desired one can adapt the UCA size to the size of the vascular fenestrations. In leaky tumor vessels fenestrations are known to be around 400–800 nm large [147]. Therefore, bubbles in the nanoscale were introduced, which can leak from the vasculature into the tumor tissue [148–150]. Due to their accumulation via the enhanced permeability and retention effect (EPR), they show prolonged persistence at tumor site compared to MB. By targeting over-expressed tumor markers, the retention of the NB in the tumor tissue can be enhanced [7,151]. An overview of targeted NB is provided in Table 3.

Table 3. Summary of extravascular targets investigated for molecular US imaging.

Targets	Binding Ligands	Model
HER2	HER2-affibody	Breast cancer in mice [152,153]
	Anti-HER2 antibody	Breast cancer in mice [154]
CAIX	Aptamer	Adenocarcinoma in mice [7]
PSMA	PSMA-1 ligand	Prostate cancer in mice [151]
CD3	Anti-CD3 antibody	T-lymphocyte in rats [155]
CA-125	Anti-CA-125 antibody	Epithelial ovarian cancer in mice [156]
proGRP	Anti- proGRP antibody	Small cell lung cancer in mice [149]
Phosphatidylserine	Annexin V	Apoptosis in mice [157]
VEGFR2 and HER2	Anti-HER2 and anti-VEGFR2 antibodies	Breast cancer in mice [158]

Due to their small size, NB are expected to backscatter less and, thus, show less signal during US imaging [159]. Furthermore, for smaller bubbles higher frequencies are needed, which can hamper imaging, since high frequencies do not reach deep into tissue [160]. Moreover, US devices used in the clinics usually do not have the transducers for high frequencies.

Surprisingly, some studies report that NB show similar echogenicity as MB (Figure 9) [148,161]. There are no clear explanations for this observation. However, one group discusses that there might be an underestimation of NB concentrations in the phantoms because NB are difficult to count [161].

Furthermore, highly flexible shells of some NB may increase the echogenicity significantly, even at lower frequencies than their resonance frequency [159–162]. For instance, Perera and colleagues designed a new shell, which was inspired by nature, where shells with several layers exist. The layers differ in their elastic properties such as in bacterial cell envelopes [163]. Perera adapted this concept and designed a shell consisting of two layers differing in elasticity, one compliant layer, another stiff adlayer with PEG on top. This composition provides high shell stability, which reduces air loss during oscillation and improves better persistence in the blood circulation. Together, these properties promise an extended effective visualization of the tumor.

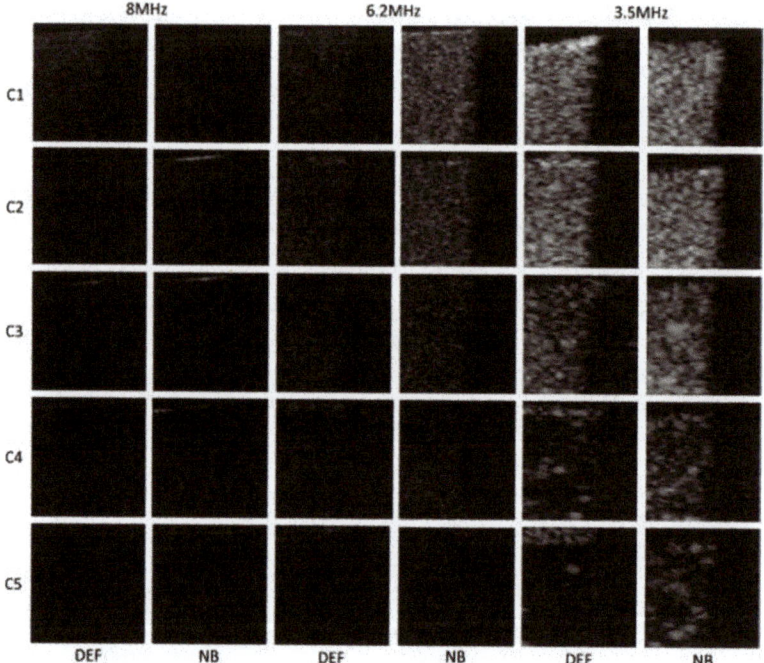

Figure 9. Contrast harmonic images of NB and commercially available Definity® MB (DEF) at different concentrations and frequencies. Reproduced with permission from [161]. Copyright Elsevier, 2013.

By targeting NB a longer tumor persistence but not necessarily a big difference in US signals was observed [152,157]. This is in line with results on other nanoparticles, were targeting only improved retention but not accumulation, the latter being mostly mediated via the EPR effect [164]. Thus, obtaining exact information about extravascular molecular marker expression with particles of this size will remain difficult. However, the exploration of the diagnostic benefits resulting from NB accumulation is just beginning and needs further research and reasonable conceptual considerations.

3.4. Phase Shift Nanodroplets

Nanodroplets were introduced as UCA to prolong circulation time and enhance extravasation to tissue. Since their application mainly focuses on drug delivery rather than imaging, only a brief overview of their functional principle is given in this review.

Nanodroplets have a perfluorocarbon liquid core stabilized by lipids, polymers, or proteins [165]. The emulsion is injected in liquid form, not showing much contrast during US imaging compared to MB. However, when US is applied as an external trigger, the core solution shifts from liquid to gas phase forming MB and achieving high echogenicity [166,167]. This process is called acoustic droplet vaporization (ADV). This comes with several advantages. The solution in its liquid phase has a higher circulation time and can leave the vasculature. Additionally, the phase shift can be activated at the target site. Two elements are important for ADV, namely the temperature to reach the boiling point of the liquid and the pressure. The boiling point is usually already reached at body temperature. For instance, the boiling point for perfluorocarbon gas starts from 29 °C. Hence, small bubbles might already be forming when the emulsion is injected in the body. By additionally applying the US, the surrounding pressure is lowered and less than the vapor pressure, this enhances the phase shift and formation of MB [165,168].

A chemotherapeutic drug can be added to the emulsion and thus, encapsulated in the MB after ADV. By using US, the MB collapse and the drug will be released at the target site. Since the nanodroplets are capable of extravasating into tumor tissue, they can be used for contrast-enhanced tumor imaging combined with drug delivery all in once [169–171]. Furthermore, there have been targeted nanodroplets approaches [172–174]. As targeting ligands, folate [172,173] and anti-Her2/*neu* peptide [174] were used. By adding these targeting ligands, the formed bubbles stayed attached at the vaporized area visualizing the subject area aimed for therapy. However, more research is needed to evaluate the added value of targeted nanodroplets over NB or MB regarding their imaging abilities.

4. Conclusions

Molecular US has broadened the application spectrum of standard US. Multiple effective endovascular targeting strategies have been explored using MB, and are now complemented by NB that open access to extravascular targets. Unfortunately, of the many pre-clinically explored actively targeted MB, only few meet the criteria for clinical translation. Furthermore, important questions about MB pharmacokinetics and the fate of shell components, but also about upscaling of MB production, batch reproducibility, storage stability, and sterilization, often remain open. Without these questions being answered by our scientific community, it will be difficult to convince investors or pharmaceutical industry to consider these agents as potential clinical products. In addition, the clinical indications must be very carefully chosen. High comfort to the patient, lack of radiation, excellent availability of US devices, and low costs are arguments speaking for the clinical implementation of molecular US imaging. However, to have a chance for broad acceptance, the molecular US methods need to be at least equivalent to or able to provide a clear added value over the clinical diagnostic standard methods. This can be reflected in higher sensitivity and specificity in disease detection, classification, and therapy response monitoring. Taking these arguments into consideration, indications in the fields of angiogenesis in cancer, inflammatory diseases, and arteriosclerosis/thrombosis appear highly meaningful. Ideally, the chosen applications should already use US in the clinical diagnostic routine. The molecular US examination then increases the power and expressiveness of the routine examination, enables faster therapeutic decision making, and reduces the need for further diagnostic analyses. Unfortunately, often, the most promising indications do not address huge markets, and thus are financially not interesting for big pharmaceutical companies. In addition, academia faces the dilemma that third-party funding is often only available for basic research and clinical phase II/III studies, but hard to get for closing the critical translational gap in between. Nonetheless, to move this exciting technology into clinical application, in our opinion, the translational process must be actively promoted by academia together with spin offs and small and medium enterprises, for which smaller markets are still attractive. Then, molecular US imaging could evolve to its full potential as a highly sensitive, specific, and real-time molecular imaging tool to the benefit of patients suffering from various diseases.

Author Contributions: G.K. and M.D. researched the data for the article and wrote the manuscript. F.K. reviewed and edited the manuscript. All authors have read and agreed to the published version of the manuscript.

Funding: This research was supported by the Deutsche Forschungsgemeinschaft (DFG) in the framework of the Research Training Group 2375 "Tumor-targeted Drug Delivery" grant 331065168, DFG FOR 2591 to F.K. grant No. 321137804 and grant No. KI 1072/11-3.

Conflicts of Interest: The authors declare no conflict of interest.

Abbreviations

The following abbreviations are used in this manuscript:

^{18}FDG	Fluorodeoxyglucose
ACPP	Activatable cell-penetrating peptides
ATWLPPR	Alanine-threonine-tryptophan-leucine-proline-proline-arginine
CAIX	Carbonic anhydrase IX
CEUS	Contrast-enhanced ultrasound
CRPPR	Cysteine-arginine-proline-proline-arginine
CT	Computed tomography
DVT	Deep venous thrombosis
EPR	Enhanced permeability and retention
GP	Glycoprotein
HER2	Human epidermal growth factor receptor 2
IBD	Inflammatory bowel disease
ICAM-1	Intercellular adhesion molecule - 1
IgG	Immunoglobulin G
JAM-A	Junctional adhesion molecule - A
KDR	Kinase insert domain receptor
KQAGDV	Lysine-glutamine-alanine-glycine-aspartate-valine
LOX-1	Lectin-like oxidized low-density lipoprotein receptor-1
MAdCAM-1	Mucosal addressin cellular adhesion molecule - 1
MB	Microbubbles
MMP	Matrix metalloproteinase
MRI	Magnetic resonance imaging
NB	Nanobubbles
PEG	Polyethylene glycol
PET	Positron emission tomography
proGRP	Pro-gastrin releasing peptide
PSGL-Ig	P-selectin glycoprotein ligand-1 analog
PSMA	Prostate specific membrane antigen
RGD	Arginine-glycine-aspartate
RRL	Arginine-arginine-leucine
SFRP2	Secreted frizzled related protein 2
SPAQ	Sensitive particle acoustic quantification
Thy 1	Thymocyte differentiation antigen 1
TNBS	2, 4, 6-trinitrobenzene sulfonic acid
UCA	Ultrasound contrast agents
US	Ultrasound
VCAM-1	Vascular cell adhesion molecule - 1
VEGF	Vascular endothelial growth factor
VEGFR2	Vascular endothelial growth factor receptor 2
VWF	Von Willebrand factor

References

1. Uppal, T. Tissue harmonic imaging. *Australas. J. Ultrasound Med.* **2010**, *13*, 29–31. [CrossRef] [PubMed]
2. Frinking, P.; Segers, T.; Luan, Y.; Tranquart, F. Three Decades of Ultrasound Contrast Agents: A Review of the Past, Present and Future Improvements. *Ultrasound Med. Biol.* **2020**, *46*, 892–908. [CrossRef] [PubMed]
3. Guevener, N.; Appold, L.; de Lorenzi, F.; Golombek, S.K.; Rizzo, L.Y.; Lammers, T.; Kiessling, F. Recent advances in ultrasound-based diagnosis and therapy with micro-and nanometer-sized formulations. *Methods* **2017**, *130*, 4–13. [CrossRef] [PubMed]
4. Zhu, L.; Wang, L.; Liu, Y.; Xu, D.; Fang, K.; Guo, Y. CAIX aptamer-functionalized targeted nanobubbles for ultrasound molecular imaging of various tumors. *IJN* **2018**, *13*, 6481–6495. [CrossRef]

5. Roovers, S.; Segers, T.; Lajoinie, G.; Deprez, J.; Versluis, M.; De Smedt, S.C.; Lentacker, I. The Role of Ultrasound-Driven Microbubble Dynamics in Drug Delivery: From Microbubble Fundamentals to Clinical Translation. *Langmuir* **2019**, *35*, 10173–10191. [CrossRef]
6. Yu, J.; Chen, Z.; Yan, F. Advances in mechanism studies on ultrasonic gene delivery at cellular level. *Prog. Biophys. Mol. Biol.* **2019**, *142*, 1–9. [CrossRef]
7. Omata, D.; Unga, J.; Suzuki, R.; Maruyama, K. Lipid-based microbubbles and ultrasound for therapeutic application. *Adv. Drug Deliv. Rev.* **2020**. [CrossRef]
8. Mor-Avi, V.; Caiani, E.G.; Collins, K.A.; Korcarz, C.E.; Bednarz, J.E.; Lang, R.M. Combined assessment of myocardial perfusion and regional left ventricular function by analysis of contrast-enhanced power modulation images. *Circulation* **2001**, *104*, 352–357. [CrossRef]
9. Whittingham, T.A. Contrast-Specific Imaging Techniques: Technical Perspective. In *Contrast Media in Ultrasonography: Basic Principles and Clinical Applications*; Quaia, E., Ed.; Springer: Berlin/Heidelberg, Germany, 2005; pp. 43–70. ISBN 978-3-540-27214-4.
10. Phillips, P.J. Contrast Pulse Sequences (CPS): Imaging Nonlinear Microbubbles. In Proceedings of the 2001 IEEE Ultrasonics Symposium, Atlanta, GA, USA, 7–10 October 2001; pp. 1739–1745.
11. Caskey, C.F.; Hu, X.; Ferrara, K.W. Leveraging the power of ultrasound for therapeutic design and optimization. *J. Control. Release* **2011**, *156*, 297–306. [CrossRef]
12. Reinhardt, M.; Hauff, P.; Briel, A.; Uhlendorf, V.; Linker, R.A.; Mäurer, M.; Schirner, M. Sensitive particle acoustic quantification (SPAQ): A new ultrasound-based approach for the quantification of ultrasound contrast media in high concentrations. *Invest. Radiol.* **2005**, *40*, 2–7.
13. Wei, K.; Jayaweera, A.R.; Firoozan, S.; Linka, A.; Skyba, D.M.; Kaul, S. Quantification of Myocardial Blood Flow With Ultrasound-Induced Destruction of Microbubbles Administered as a Constant Venous Infusion. *Circulation* **1998**, *97*, 473–483. [CrossRef]
14. Pysz, M.A.; Guracar, I.; Tian, L.; Willmann, J.K. Fast microbubble dwell-time based ultrasonic molecular imaging approach for quantification and monitoring of angiogenesis in cancer. *Quant. Imaging Med. Surg.* **2012**, *2*, 16.
15. Zhao, R.; Jiang, J.; Li, H.; Chen, M.; Liu, R.; Sun, S.; Ma, D.; Liang, X.; Wang, S. Phosphatidylserine-microbubble targeting-activated microglia/macrophage in inflammation combined with ultrasound for breaking through the blood–brain barrier. *J. Neuroinflamm.* **2018**, *15*, s12974–s018. [CrossRef] [PubMed]
16. Pochon, S.; Tardy, I.; Bussat, P.; Bettinger, T.; Brochot, J.; von Wronski, M.; Passantino, L.; Schneider, M. BR55: A Lipopeptide-Based VEGFR2-Targeted Ultrasound Contrast Agent for Molecular Imaging of Angiogenesis. *Investig. Radiol.* **2010**, *45*, 89–95. [CrossRef] [PubMed]
17. Villanueva, F.S.; Jankowski, R.J.; Klibanov, S.; Pina, M.L.; Alber, S.M.; Watkins, S.C.; Brandenburger, G.H.; Wagner, W.R. Microbubbles Targeted to Intercellular Adhesion Molecule-1 Bind to Activated Coronary Artery Endothelial Cells. *Circulation* **1998**, *98*, 1–5. [CrossRef] [PubMed]
18. Ham, A.S.; Klibanov, A.L.; Lawrence, M.B. Action at a distance: Lengthening adhesion bonds with poly(ethylene glycol) spacers enhances mechanically stressed affinity for improved vascular targeting of microparticles. *Langmuir* **2009**, *25*, 10038–10044. [CrossRef]
19. Kim, D.H.; Klibanov, A.L.; Needham, D. The Influence of Tiered Layers of Surface-Grafted Poly(ethylene glycol) on Receptor–Ligand-Mediated Adhesion between Phospholipid Monolayer-Stabilized Microbubbles and Coated Glass Beads. *Langmuir* **2000**, *16*, 2808–2817. [CrossRef]
20. Borden, M.A.; Sarantos, M.R.; Stieger, S.M.; Simon, S.I.; Ferrara, K.W.; Dayton, P.A. Ultrasound radiation force modulates ligand availability on targeted contrast agents. *Mol. Imaging* **2006**, *5*, 139–147. [CrossRef]
21. Borden, M.A.; Zhang, H.; Gillies, R.J.; Dayton, P.A.; Ferrara, K.W. A stimulus-responsive contrast agent for ultrasound molecular imaging. *Biomaterials* **2008**, *29*, 597–606. [CrossRef]
22. Ellegala, D.B.; Leong-Poi, H.; Carpenter, J.E.; Klibanov, A.L.; Kaul, S.; Shaffrey, M.E.; Sklenar, J.; Lindner, J.R. Imaging Tumor Angiogenesis With Contrast Ultrasound and Microbubbles Targeted to $\alpha v \beta 3$. *Circulation* **2003**, *108*, 336–341. [CrossRef]
23. Leong-Poi, H.; Christiansen, J.; Klibanov, A.L.; Kaul, S.; Lindner, J.R. Noninvasive Assessment of Angiogenesis by Ultrasound and Microbubbles Targeted to αv-Integrins. *Circulation* **2003**, *107*, 455–460. [CrossRef] [PubMed]

24. Leong-Poi, H.; Christiansen, J.; Heppner, P.; Lewis, C.W.; Klibanov, A.L.; Kaul, S.; Lindner, J.R. Assessment of Endogenous and Therapeutic Arteriogenesis by Contrast Ultrasound Molecular Imaging of Integrin Expression. *Circulation* **2005**, *111*, 3248–3254. [CrossRef] [PubMed]
25. Willmann, J.K.; Kimura, R.H.; Deshpande, N.; Lutz, A.M.; Cochran, J.R.; Gambhir, S.S. Targeted Contrast-Enhanced Ultrasound Imaging of Tumor Angiogenesis with Contrast Microbubbles Conjugated to Integrin-Binding Knottin Peptides. *J. Nucl. Med.* **2010**, *51*, 433–440. [CrossRef] [PubMed]
26. Anderson, C.R.; Hu, X.; Zhang, H.; Tlaxca, J.; Declèves, A.-E.; Houghtaling, R.; Sharma, K.; Lawrence, M.; Ferrara, K.W.; Rychak, J.J. Ultrasound Molecular Imaging of Tumor Angiogenesis With an Integrin Targeted Microbubble Contrast Agent. *Investig. Radiol.* **2011**, *46*, 215–224. [CrossRef]
27. Barua, A.; Yellapa, A.; Bahr, J.M.; Machado, S.A.; Bitterman, P.; Basu, S.; Sharma, S.; Abramowicz, J.S. ATL: A Preclinical Model of Spontaneous Ovarian Cancer. *Int. J. Gynecol. Cancer* **2014**, *24*, 19–28. [CrossRef]
28. Palmowski, M.; Peschke, P.; Huppert, J.; Hauff, P.; Reinhardt, M.; Maurer, M.; Karger, C.P.; Scholz, M.; Semmler, W.; Huber, P.E.; et al. Molecular Ultrasound Imaging of Early Vascular Response in Prostate Tumors Irradiated with Carbon Ions. *Neoplasia* **2009**, *11*, 856–863. [CrossRef] [PubMed]
29. Palmowski, M.; Huppert, J.; Ladewig, G.; Hauff, P.; Reinhardt, M.; Mueller, M.M.; Woenne, E.C.; Jenne, J.W.; Maurer, M.; Kauffmann, G.W.; et al. Molecular profiling of angiogenesis with targeted ultrasound imaging: Early assessment of antiangiogenic therapy effects. *Mol. Cancer Ther.* **2008**, *7*, 101–109. [CrossRef]
30. Deshpande, N.; Ren, Y.; Foygel, K.; Rosenberg, J.; Willmann, J.K. Tumor Angiogenic Marker Expression Levels during Tumor Growth: Longitudinal Assessment with Molecularly Targeted Microbubbles and US Imaging. *Radiology* **2011**, *258*, 804–811. [CrossRef]
31. Leguerney, I.; Scoazec, J.-Y.; Gadot, N.; Robin, N.; Pénault-Llorca, F.; Victorin, S.; Lassau, N. Molecular Ultrasound Imaging Using Contrast Agents Targeting Endoglin, Vascular Endothelial Growth Factor Receptor 2 and Integrin. *Ultrasound Med. Biol.* **2015**, *41*, 197–207. [CrossRef]
32. Weller, G.E.R.; Wong, M.K.K.; Modzelewski, R.A.; Lu, E.; Klibanov, A.L.; Wagner, W.R.; Villanueva, F.S. Ultrasonic Imaging of Tumor Angiogenesis Using Contrast Microbubbles Targeted via the Tumor-Binding Peptide Arginine-Arginine-Leucine. *Cancer Res.* **2005**, *65*, 533–539.
33. Rychak, J.J.; Graba, J.; Cheung, A.M.Y.; Mystry, B.S.; Lindner, J.R.; Kerbel, R.S.; Foster, F.S. Microultrasound Molecular Imaging of Vascular Endothelial Growth Factor Receptor 2 in a Mouse Model of Tumor Angiogenesis. *Mol. Imaging* **2007**, *6*. [CrossRef]
34. Wang, S.; Herbst, E.B.; Mauldin, F.W.; Diakova, G.B.; Klibanov, A.L.; Hossack, J.A. Ultra–Low-Dose Ultrasound Molecular Imaging for the Detection of Angiogenesis in a Mouse Murine Tumor Model: How Little Can We See? *Investig. Radiol.* **2016**, *51*, 758–766. [CrossRef] [PubMed]
35. Korpanty, G.; Carbon, J.G.; Grayburn, P.A.; Fleming, J.B.; Brekken, R.A. Monitoring Response to Anticancer Therapy by Targeting Microbubbles to Tumor Vasculature. *Clin. Cancer Res.* **2007**, *13*, 323–330. [CrossRef] [PubMed]
36. Willmann, J.K.; Paulmurugan, R.; Chen, K.; Gheysens, O.; Rodriguez-Porcel, M.; Lutz, A.M.; Chen, I.Y.; Chen, X.; Gambhir, S.S. US Imaging of Tumor Angiogenesis with Microbubbles Targeted to Vascular Endothelial Growth Factor Receptor Type 2 in Mice. *Radiology* **2008**, *246*, 508–518. [CrossRef]
37. Willmann, J.K.; Cheng, Z.; Davis, C.; Lutz, A.M.; Schipper, M.L.; Nielsen, C.H.; Gambhir, S.S. Targeted Microbubbles for Imaging Tumor Angiogenesis: Assessment of Whole-Body Biodistribution with Dynamic Micro-PET in Mice. *Radiology* **2008**, *249*, 212–219. [CrossRef]
38. Lyshchik, A.; Fleischer, A.C.; Huamani, J.; Hallahan, D.E.; Brissova, M.; Gore, J.C. Molecular Imaging of Vascular Endothelial Growth Factor Receptor 2 Expression Using Targeted Contrast-Enhanced High-Frequency Ultrasonography. *J. Ultrasound Med.* **2007**, *26*, 1575–1586. [CrossRef]
39. Bzyl, J.; Lederle, W.; Rix, A.; Grouls, C.; Tardy, I.; Pochon, S.; Siepmann, M.; Penzkofer, T.; Schneider, M.; Kiessling, F.; et al. Molecular and functional ultrasound imaging in differently aggressive breast cancer xenografts using two novel ultrasound contrast agents (BR55 and BR38). *Eur. Radiol.* **2011**, *21*, 1988–1995. [CrossRef]
40. Abou-Elkacem, L.; Wilson, K.E.; Johnson, S.M.; Chowdhury, S.M.; Bachawal, S.; Hackel, B.J.; Tian, L.; Willmann, J.K. Ultrasound Molecular Imaging of the Breast Cancer Neovasculature using Engineered Fibronectin Scaffold Ligands: A Novel Class of Targeted Contrast Ultrasound Agent. *Theranostics* **2016**, *6*, 1740–1752. [CrossRef]

41. Anderson, C.R.; Rychak, J.J.; Backer, M.; Backer, J.; Ley, K.; Klibanov, A.L. scVEGF Microbubble Ultrasound Contrast Agents: A Novel Probe for Ultrasound Molecular Imaging of Tumor Angiogenesis. *Investig. Radiol.* **2010**, *45*, 579–585. [CrossRef]
42. Tardy, I.; Pochon, S.; Theraulaz, M.; Emmel, P.; Passantino, L.; Tranquart, F.; Schneider, M. Ultrasound molecular imaging of VEGFR2 in a rat prostate tumor model using BR55. *Investig. Radiol.* **2010**, *45*, 573–578. [CrossRef]
43. Patel, M.; Vadlapatla, R.K.; Pal, D.; Mitra, A.K. Molecular and functional characterization of riboflavin specific transport system in rat brain capillary endothelial cells. *Brain Res.* **2012**, *1468*, 1–10. [CrossRef] [PubMed]
44. Bzyl, J.; Palmowski, M.; Rix, A.; Arns, S.; Hyvelin, J.-M.; Pochon, S.; Ehling, J.; Schrading, S.; Kiessling, F.; Lederle, W. The high angiogenic activity in very early breast cancer enables reliable imaging with VEGFR2-targeted microbubbles (BR55). *Eur. Radiol.* **2013**, *23*, 468–475. [CrossRef] [PubMed]
45. Zafarnia, S.; Bzyl-Ibach, J.; Spivak, I.; Li, Y.; Koletnik, S.; Doleschel, D.; Rix, A.; Pochon, S.; Tardy, I.; Koyadan, S.; et al. Nilotinib Enhances Tumor Angiogenesis and Counteracts VEGFR2 Blockade in an Orthotopic Breast Cancer Xenograft Model with Desmoplastic Response. *Neoplasia* **2017**, *19*, 896–907. [CrossRef] [PubMed]
46. Bachawal, S.V.; Jensen, K.C.; Lutz, A.M.; Gambhir, S.S.; Tranquart, F.; Tian, L.; Willmann, J.K. Earlier detection of breast cancer with ultrasound molecular imaging in a transgenic mouse model. *Cancer Res.* **2013**, *73*, 1689–1698. [CrossRef] [PubMed]
47. Pysz, M.A.; Machtaler, S.B.; Seeley, E.S.; Lee, J.J.; Brentnall, T.A.; Rosenberg, J.; Tranquart, F.; Willmann, J.K. Vascular Endothelial Growth Factor Receptor Type 2–targeted Contrast-enhanced US of Pancreatic Cancer Neovasculature in a Genetically Engineered Mouse Model: Potential for Earlier Detection. *Radiology* **2015**, *274*, 790–799. [CrossRef]
48. Wang, H.; Kaneko, O.F.; Tian, L.; Hristov, D.; Willmann, J.K. Three-Dimensional Ultrasound Molecular Imaging of Angiogenesis in Colon Cancer Using a Clinical Matrix Array Ultrasound Transducer. *Investig. Radiol.* **2015**, *50*, 322–329. [CrossRef]
49. Baetke, S.C.; Rix, A.; Tranquart, F.; Schneider, R.; Lammers, T.; Kiessling, F.; Lederle, W. Squamous Cell Carcinoma Xenografts: Use of VEGFR2-targeted Microbubbles for Combined Functional and Molecular US to Monitor Antiangiogenic Therapy Effects. *Radiology* **2016**, *278*, 430–440. [CrossRef]
50. Zhou, J.; Wang, H.; Zhang, H.; Lutz, A.M.; Tian, L.; Hristov, D.; Willmann, J.K. VEGFR2-Targeted Three-Dimensional Ultrasound Imaging Can Predict Responses to Antiangiogenic Therapy in Preclinical Models of Colon Cancer. *Cancer Res.* **2016**, *76*, 4081–4089. [CrossRef]
51. Eschbach, R.S.; Clevert, D.-A.; Hirner-Eppeneder, H.; Ingrisch, M.; Moser, M.; Schuster, J.; Tadros, D.; Schneider, M.; Kazmierczak, P.M.; Reiser, M.; et al. Contrast-Enhanced Ultrasound with VEGFR2-Targeted Microbubbles for Monitoring Regorafenib Therapy Effects in Experimental Colorectal Adenocarcinomas in Rats with DCE-MRI and Immunohistochemical Validation. *PLoS ONE* **2017**, *12*, e0169323. [CrossRef]
52. Zhang, H.; Tam, S.; Ingham, E.S.; Mahakian, L.M.; Lai, C.-Y.; Tumbale, S.K.; Teesalu, T.; Hubbard, N.E.; Borowsky, A.D.; Ferrara, K.W. Ultrasound molecular imaging of tumor angiogenesis with a neuropilin-1-targeted microbubble. *Biomaterials* **2015**, *56*, 104–113. [CrossRef]
53. Tsuruta, J.K.; Klauber-DeMore, N.; Streeter, J.; Samples, J.; Patterson, C.; Mumper, R.J.; Ketelsen, D.; Dayton, P. Ultrasound Molecular Imaging of Secreted Frizzled Related Protein-2 Expression in Murine Angiosarcoma. *PLoS ONE* **2014**, *9*, e86642. [CrossRef] [PubMed]
54. Bachawal, S.V.; Jensen, K.C.; Wilson, K.E.; Tian, L.; Lutz, A.M.; Willmann, J.K. Breast Cancer Detection by B7-H3-Targeted Ultrasound Molecular Imaging. *Cancer Res.* **2015**, *75*, 2501–2509. [CrossRef] [PubMed]
55. Zhang, H.; Ingham, E.S.; Gagnon, M.K.J.; Mahakian, L.M.; Liu, J.; Foiret, J.L.; Willmann, J.K.; Ferrara, K.W. In Vitro Characterization and In Vivo Ultrasound Molecular Imaging of Nucleolin-Targeted Microbubbles. *Biomaterials* **2017**, *118*, 63–73. [CrossRef] [PubMed]
56. Abou-Elkacem, L.; Wang, H.; Chowdhury, S.M.; Kimura, R.H.; Bachawal, S.V.; Gambhir, S.S.; Tian, L.; Willmann, J.K. Thy1-Targeted Microbubbles for Ultrasound Molecular Imaging of Pancreatic Ductal Adenocarcinoma. *Clin Cancer Res.* **2018**, *24*, 1574–1585. [CrossRef] [PubMed]
57. Lindner, J.R.; Song, J.; Xu, F.; Klibanov, A.L.; Singbartl, K.; Ley, K.; Kaul, S. Noninvasive Ultrasound Imaging of Inflammation Using Microbubbles Targeted to Activated Leukocytes. *Circulation* **2000**, *102*, 2745–2750. [CrossRef]

58. Christiansen, J.P.; Leong-Poi, H.; Klibanov, A.L.; Kaul, S.; Lindner, J.R. Noninvasive Imaging of Myocardial Reperfusion Injury Using Leukocyte-Targeted Contrast Echocardiography. *Circulation* **2002**, *105*, 1764–1767. [CrossRef]
59. Weller, G.E.R.; Villanueva, F.S.; Klibanov, A.L.; Wagner, W.R. Modulating Targeted Adhesion of an Ultrasound Contrast Agent to Dysfunctional Endothelium. *Ann. Biomed. Eng.* **2002**, *30*, 1012–1019. [CrossRef]
60. Bachmann, C.; Klibanov, A.L.; Olson, T.S.; Sonnenschein, J.R.; Rivera-Nieves, J.; Cominelli, F.; Ley, K.F.; Lindner, J.R.; Pizarro, T.T. Targeting mucosal addressin cellular adhesion molecule (MAdCAM)-1 to noninvasively image experimental Crohn's disease. *Gastroenterology* **2006**, *130*, 8–16. [CrossRef]
61. Curaj, A.; Wu, Z.; Rix, A.; Gresch, O.; Sternkopf, M.; Alampour-Rajabi, S.; Lammers, T.; van Zandvoort, M.; Weber, C.; Koenen, R.R.; et al. Molecular Ultrasound Imaging of Junctional Adhesion Molecule A Depicts Acute Alterations in Blood Flow and Early Endothelial Dysregulation. *Arterioscler. Thromb. Vasc. Biol.* **2018**, *38*, 40–48. [CrossRef]
62. Zhang, Y.-J.; Bai, D.-N.; Du, J.-X.; Jin, L.; Ma, J.; Yang, J.-L.; Cai, W.-B.; Feng, Y.; Xing, C.-Y.; Yuan, L.-J.; et al. Ultrasound-guided imaging of junctional adhesion molecule-A-targeted microbubbles identifies vulnerable plaque in rabbits. *Biomaterials* **2016**, *94*, 20–30. [CrossRef]
63. Liu, Y.; Davidson, B.P.; Yue, Q.; Belcik, T.; Xie, A.; Inaba, Y.; McCarty Owen, J.T.; Tormoen Garth, W.; Zhao, Y.; Ruggeri, Z.M.; et al. Molecular Imaging of Inflammation and Platelet Adhesion in Advanced Atherosclerosis Effects of Antioxidant Therapy With NADPH Oxidase Inhibition. *Circ. Cardiovasc. Imaging* **2013**, *6*, 74–82. [CrossRef] [PubMed]
64. Khanicheh, E.; Qi, Y.; Xie, A.; Mitterhuber, M.; Xu, L.; Mochizuki, M.; Daali, Y.; Jaquet, V.; Krause, K.-H.; Ruggeri, Z.M.; et al. Molecular imaging reveals rapid reduction of endothelial activation in early atherosclerosis with apocynin independent of antioxidative properties. *Arterioscler. Thromb. Vasc. Biol.* **2013**, *33*, 2187–2192. [CrossRef] [PubMed]
65. Kaufmann, B.A.; Carr, C.L.; Belcik, J.T.; Xie, A.; Yue, Q.; Chadderdon, S.; Caplan, E.S.; Khangura, J.; Bullens, S.; Bunting, S.; et al. Molecular imaging of the initial inflammatory response in atherosclerosis: Implications for early detection of disease. *Arterioscler. Thromb. Vasc. Biol.* **2010**, *30*, 54–59. [CrossRef] [PubMed]
66. Khanicheh, E.; Mitterhuber, M.; Xu, L.; Haeuselmann, S.P.; Kuster, G.M.; Kaufmann, B.A. Noninvasive Ultrasound Molecular Imaging of the Effect of Statins on Endothelial Inflammatory Phenotype in Early Atherosclerosis. *PLoS ONE* **2013**, *8*, e58761. [CrossRef]
67. Kaufmann, B.A.; Sanders, J.M.; Davis, C.; Xie, A.; Aldred, P.; Sarembock, I.J.; Lindner, J.R. Molecular imaging of inflammation in atherosclerosis with targeted ultrasound detection of vascular cell adhesion molecule-1. *Circulation* **2007**, *116*, 276–284. [CrossRef]
68. Curaj, A.; Wu, Z.; Fokong, S.; Liehn, E.A.; Weber, C.; Burlacu, A.; Lammers, T.; van Zandvoort, M.; Kiessling, F. Noninvasive Molecular Ultrasound Monitoring of Vessel Healing After Intravascular Surgical Procedures in a Preclinical Setup. *Arterioscler. Thromb. Vasc. Biol.* **2015**, *35*, 1366–1373. [CrossRef]
69. Moccetti, F.; Brown, E.; Xie, A.; Packwood, W.; Qi, Y.; Ruggeri, Z.; Shentu, W.; Chen, J.; López, J.A.; Lindner, J.R. Myocardial Infarction Produces Sustained Proinflammatory Endothelial Activation in Remote Arteries. *J. Am. Coll. Cardiol.* **2018**, *72*, 1015–1026. [CrossRef]
70. Wang, S.; Unnikrishnan, S.; Herbst, E.B.; Klibanov, A.L.; Mauldin, F.W.; Hossack, J.A. Ultrasound Molecular Imaging of Inflammation in Mouse Abdominal Aorta. *Investig. Radiol* **2017**, *52*, 499–506. [CrossRef]
71. Masseau, I.; Davis, M.J.; Bowles, D.K. Carotid inflammation is unaltered by exercise in hypercholesterolemic swine. *Med. Sci. Sports Exerc.* **2012**, *44*, 2277–2289. [CrossRef]
72. Koczera, P.; Appold, L.; Shi, Y.; Liu, M.; Dasgupta, A.; Pathak, V.; Ojha, T.; Fokong, S.; Wu, Z.; van Zandvoort, M.; et al. PBCA-based Polymeric Microbubbles for Molecular Imaging and Drug Delivery. *J. Control. Release* **2017**, *259*, 128–135. [CrossRef]
73. Punjabi, M.; Xu, L.; Ochoa-Espinosa, A.; Kosareva, A.; Wolff, T.; Murtaja, A.; Broisat, A.; Devoogdt, N.; Kaufmann, B.A. Ultrasound Molecular Imaging of Atherosclerosis With Nanobodies: Translatable Microbubble Targeting Murine and Human VCAM (Vascular Cell Adhesion Molecule) 1. *Arterioscler. Thromb. Vasc. Biol.* **2019**, *39*, 2520–2530. [CrossRef] [PubMed]
74. Moccetti, F.; Weinkauf, C.C.; Davidson, B.P.; Belcik, J.T.; Marinelli, E.R.; Unger, E.; Lindner, J.R. Ultrasound Molecular Imaging of Atherosclerosis Using Small-Peptide Targeting Ligands Against Endothelial Markers of Inflammation and Oxidative Stress. *Ultrasound Med. Biol.* **2018**, *44*, 1155–1163. [CrossRef] [PubMed]

75. Weller, G.E.; Wong, M.K.; Modzelewski, R.A.; Lu, E.; Klibanov, A.L.; Wagner, W.R.; Villanueva, F.S. Ultrasound Imaging of Acute Cardiac Transplant Rejection With Microbubbles Targeted to Intercellular Adhesion Molecule-1. *Circulation* **2003**, *108*, 218–224. [CrossRef] [PubMed]
76. Lindner, J.R.; Song, J.; Christiansen, J.; Klibanov, A.L.; Xu, F.; Ley, K. Ultrasound Assessment of Inflammation and Renal Tissue Injury With Microbubbles Targeted to P-Selectin. *Circulation* **2001**, *104*, 2107–2112. [CrossRef]
77. Klibanov, A.L.; Rychak, J.J.; Yang, W.C.; Alikhani, S.; Li, B.; Acton, S.; Lindner, J.R.; Ley, K.; Kaul, S. Targeted ultrasound contrast agent for molecular imaging of inflammation in high-shear flow. *Contrast Media Mol. Imaging* **2006**, *1*, 259–266. [CrossRef]
78. Takalkar, A.M.; Klibanov, A.L.; Rychak, J.J.; Lindner, J.R.; Ley, K. Binding and detachment dynamics of microbubbles targeted to P-selectin under controlled shear flow. *J. Control. Release* **2004**, *96*, 473–482. [CrossRef]
79. Rychak, J.J.; Lindner, J.R.; Ley, K.; Klibanov, A.L. Deformable gas-filled microbubbles targeted to P-selectin. *J. Control. Release* **2006**, *114*, 288–299. [CrossRef]
80. Bettinger, T.; Bussat, P.; Tardy, I.; Pochon, S.; Hyvelin, J.-M.; Emmel, P.; Henrioud, S.; Biolluz, N.; Willmann, J.K.; Schneider, M.; et al. Ultrasound Molecular Imaging Contrast Agent Binding to Both E- and P-Selectin in Different Species. *Investig. Radiol.* **2012**, *47*, 516–523. [CrossRef]
81. Deshpande, N.; Lutz, A.M.; Ren, Y.; Foygel, K.; Tian, L.; Schneider, M.; Pai, R.; Pasricha, P.J.; Willmann, J.K. Quantification and Monitoring of Inflammation in Murine Inflammatory Bowel Disease with Targeted Contrast-enhanced US. *Radiology* **2012**, *262*, 172–180. [CrossRef]
82. El Kaffas, A.; Smith, K.; Pradhan, P.; Machtaler, S.; Wang, H.; von Eyben, R.; Willmann, J.K.; Hristov, D. Molecular Contrast-Enhanced Ultrasound Imaging of Radiation-Induced P-Selectin Expression in Healthy Mice Colon. *Int. J. Radiat. Oncol. Biol. Phys.* **2017**, *97*, 581–585. [CrossRef]
83. Kaufmann, B.A.; Lewis, C.; Xie, A.; Mirza-Mohd, A.; Lindner, J.R. Detection of recent myocardial ischaemia by molecular imaging of P-selectin with targeted contrast echocardiography. *Eur. Heart J.* **2007**, *28*, 2011–2017. [CrossRef] [PubMed]
84. Davidson, B.P.; Kaufmann, B.A.; Belcik, J.T.; Xie, A.; Qi, Y.; Lindner, J.R. Detection of Antecedent Myocardial Ischemia With Multiselectin Molecular Imaging. *J. Am. Coll. Cardiol.* **2012**, *60*, 1690–1697. [CrossRef] [PubMed]
85. Hyvelin, J.-M.; Tardy, I.; Bettinger, T.; von Wronski, M.; Costa, M.; Emmel, P.; Colevret, D.; Bussat, P.; Lassus, A.; Botteron, C.; et al. Ultrasound Molecular Imaging of Transient Acute Myocardial Ischemia With a Clinically Translatable P- and E-Selectin Targeted Contrast Agent: Correlation With the Expression of Selectins. *Investig. Radiol.* **2014**, *49*, 224–235. [CrossRef] [PubMed]
86. Fokong, S.; Fragoso, A.; Rix, A.; Curaj, A.; Wu, Z.; Lederle, W.; Iranzo, O.; Gätjens, J.; Kiessling, F.; Palmowski, M. Ultrasound Molecular Imaging of E-Selectin in Tumor Vessels Using Poly n-Butyl Cyanoacrylate Microbubbles Covalently Coupled to a Short Targeting Peptide. *Investig. Radiol.* **2013**, *48*, 843–850. [CrossRef] [PubMed]
87. Spivak, I.; Rix, A.; Schmitz, G.; Fokong, S.; Iranzo, O.; Lederle, W.; Kiessling, F. Low-Dose Molecular Ultrasound Imaging with E-Selectin-Targeted PBCA Microbubbles. *Mol. Imaging Biol.* **2016**, *18*, 180–190. [CrossRef]
88. Leng, X.; Wang, J.; Carson, A.; Chen, X.; Fu, H.; Ottoboni, S.; Wagner, W.R.; Villanueva, F.S. Ultrasound Detection of Myocardial Ischemic Memory Using an E-Selectin Targeting Peptide Amenable to Human Application. *Mol. Imaging* **2014**, *13*. [CrossRef]
89. Unger, E.C.; McCreery, T.P.; Sweitzer, R.H.; Shen, D.; Wu, G. In vitro studies of a new thrombus-specific ultrasound contrast agent. *Am. J. Cardiol.* **1998**, *81*, 58G–61G. [CrossRef]
90. Unger, E.; Metzger, P.; Krupinski, E.; Baker, M.; Hulett, R.; Gabaeff, D.; Mills, J.; Ihnat, D.; McCreery, T. The use of a thrombus-specific ultrasound contrast agent to detect thrombus in arteriovenous fistulae. *Investig. Radiol.* **2000**, *35*, 86–89. [CrossRef]
91. Wu, W.; Wang, Y.; Shen, S.; Wu, J.; Guo, S.; Su, L.; Hou, F.; Wang, Z.; Liao, Y.; Bin, J. In Vivo Ultrasound Molecular Imaging of Inflammatory Thrombosis in Arteries With Cyclic Arg-Gly-Asp–Modified Microbubbles Targeted to Glycoprotein IIb/IIIa. *Investig. Radiol.* **2013**, *48*, 803–812. [CrossRef]
92. Hu, G.; Liu, C.; Liao, Y.; Yang, L.; Huang, R.; Wu, J.; Xie, J.; Bundhoo, K.; Liu, Y.; Bin, J. Ultrasound molecular imaging of arterial thrombi with novel microbubbles modified by cyclic RGD in vitro and in vivo. *Thromb. Haemost.* **2012**, *107*, 172–183. [CrossRef]

93. Wang, X.; Hagemeyer, C.E.; Hohmann, J.D.; Leitner, E.; Armstrong, P.C.; Jia, F.; Olschewski, M.; Needles, A.; Peter, K.; Ahrens, I. Novel single-chain antibody-targeted microbubbles for molecular ultrasound imaging of thrombosis: Validation of a unique noninvasive method for rapid and sensitive detection of thrombi and monitoring of success or failure of thrombolysis in mice. *Circulation* **2012**, *125*, 3117–3126. [CrossRef] [PubMed]
94. Metzger, K.; Vogel, S.; Chatterjee, M.; Borst, O.; Seizer, P.; Schönberger, T.; Geisler, T.; Lang, F.; Langer, H.; Rheinlaender, J.; et al. High-frequency ultrasound-guided disruption of glycoprotein VI-targeted microbubbles targets atheroprogressison in mice. *Biomaterials* **2015**, *36*, 80–89. [CrossRef] [PubMed]
95. Nakatsuka, M.A.; Mattrey, R.F.; Esener, S.C.; Cha, J.N.; Goodwin, A.P. Aptamer-Crosslinked Microbubbles: Smart Contrast Agents for Thrombin-Activated Ultrasound Imaging. *Adv. Mater.* **2012**, *24*, 6010–6016. [CrossRef] [PubMed]
96. Nakatsuka, M.A.; Barback, C.V.; Fitch, K.R.; Farwell, A.R.; Esener, S.C.; Mattrey, R.F.; Cha, J.N.; Goodwin, A.P. In Vivo Ultrasound Visualization of Non-Occlusive Blood Clots with Thrombin-Sensitive Contrast Agents. *Biomaterials* **2013**, *34*, 9559–9565. [CrossRef] [PubMed]
97. Lux, J.; Vezeridis, A.M.; Hoyt, K.; Adams, S.R.; Armstrong, A.M.; Sirsi, S.R.; Mattrey, R.F. Thrombin-Activatable Microbubbles as Potential Ultrasound Contrast Agents for the Detection of Acute Thrombosis. *ACS Appl. Mater. Interfaces* **2017**, *9*, 37587–37596. [CrossRef] [PubMed]
98. Dayton, P.A.; Morgan, K.E.; Klibanov, A.L.; Brandenburger, G.; Nightingale, K.R.; Ferrara, K.W. A preliminary evaluation of the effects of primary and secondary radiation forces on acoustic contrast agents. *IEEE Trans. Ultrason. Ferroelectr. Freq. Control* **1997**, *44*, 1264–1277. [CrossRef]
99. Doinikov, A.A. Acoustic radiation forces: Classical theory and recent advances. *Recent Res. Dev. Acoust.* **2003**, *37661*, 39–61.
100. Dayton, P.; Klibanov, A.; Brandenburger, G.; Ferrara, K. Acoustic radiation force in vivo: A mechanism to assist targeting of microbubbles. *Ultrasound Med. Biol.* **1999**, *25*, 1195–1201. [CrossRef]
101. Zhao, S.; Borden, M.; Bloch, S.H.; Kruse, D.; Ferrara, K.W.; Dayton, P.A. Radiation-Force Assisted Targeting Facilitates Ultrasonic Molecular Imaging. *Mol. Imaging* **2004**, *3*, 14. [CrossRef]
102. Gessner, R.C.; Streeter, J.E.; Kothadia, R.; Feingold, S.; Dayton, P.A. An In Vivo Validation of the Application of Acoustic Radiation Force to Enhance the Diagnostic Utility of Molecular Imaging Using 3-D Ultrasound. *Ultrasound Med. Biol.* **2012**, *38*, 651–660. [CrossRef]
103. Wang, S.; Wang, C.Y.; Unnikrishnan, S.; Klibanov, A.L.; Hossack, J.A.; Mauldin, F.W. Optical Verification of Microbubble Response to Acoustic Radiation Force in Large Vessels With In Vivo Results. *Investig. Radiol.* **2015**, *50*, 772–784. [CrossRef] [PubMed]
104. Wang, S.; Mauldin, F.W.; Unnikrishnan, S.; Klibanov, A.L.; Hossack, J.A. Ultrasound quantification of molecular marker concentration in large blood vessels. In Proceedings of the 2014 IEEE International Ultrasonics Symposium, Chicago, IL, USA, 3–6 September 2014; pp. 831–834.
105. Ferrara, N. Vascular Endothelial Growth Factor: Basic Science and Clinical Progress. *Endocr. Rev.* **2004**, *25*, 581–611. [CrossRef] [PubMed]
106. Hicklin, D.J.; Ellis, L.M. Role of the Vascular Endothelial Growth Factor Pathway in Tumor Growth and Angiogenesis. *J. Clin. Oncol.* **2005**, *23*, 1011–1027. [CrossRef] [PubMed]
107. Hood, J.D.; Cheresh, D.A. Role of integrins in cell invasion and migration. *Nat. Rev. Cancer* **2002**, *2*, 91–100. [CrossRef] [PubMed]
108. Brooks, P.C.; Montgomery, A.M.; Rosenfeld, M.; Reisfeld, R.A.; Hu, T.; Klier, G.; Cheresh, D.A. Integrin alpha v beta 3 antagonists promote tumor regression by inducing apoptosis of angiogenic blood vessels. *Cell* **1994**, *79*, 1157–1164. [CrossRef]
109. Brooks, P.C.; Clark, R.A.; Cheresh, D.A. Requirement of vascular integrin alpha v beta 3 for angiogenesis. *Science* **1994**, *264*, 569–571. [CrossRef]
110. Van Waes, C. Cell adhesion and regulatory molecules involved in tumor formation, hemostasis, and wound healing. *Head Neck* **1995**, *17*, 140–147. [CrossRef]
111. Fonsatti, E.; Altomonte, M.; Arslan, P.; Maio, M. Endoglin (CD105): A target for anti-angiogenetic cancer therapy. *Curr. Drug Targets* **2003**, *4*, 291–296. [CrossRef]
112. Pircher, A.; Hilbe, W.; Heidegger, I.; Drevs, J.; Tichelli, A.; Medinger, M. Biomarkers in Tumor Angiogenesis and Anti-Angiogenic Therapy. *Int. J. Mol. Sci.* **2011**, *12*, 7077–7099. [CrossRef]

113. Bhati, R.; Patterson, C.; Livasy, C.A.; Fan, C.; Ketelsen, D.; Hu, Z.; Reynolds, E.; Tanner, C.; Moore, D.T.; Gabrielli, F.; et al. Molecular characterization of human breast tumor vascular cells. *Am. J. Pathol.* **2008**, *172*, 1381–1390. [CrossRef]
114. Bergers, G.; Benjamin, L.E. Tumorigenesis and the angiogenic switch. *Nat. Rev. Cancer* **2003**, *3*, 401–410. [CrossRef] [PubMed]
115. Fernández-Ortiz, A.; Jiménez-Borreguero, L.J.; Peñalvo, J.L.; Ordovás, J.M.; Mocoroa, A.; Fernández-Friera, L.; Laclaustra, M.; García, L.; Molina, J.; Mendiguren, J.M.; et al. The Progression and Early detection of Subclinical Atherosclerosis (PESA) study: Rationale and design. *Am. Heart J.* **2013**, *166*, 990–998. [CrossRef] [PubMed]
116. Blankenberg, S.; Zeller, T.; Saarela, O.; Havulinna, A.S.; Kee, F.; Tunstall-Pedoe, H.; Kuulasmaa, K.; Yarnell, J.; Schnabel, R.B.; Wild, P.S.; et al. Contribution of 30 Biomarkers to 10-Year Cardiovascular Risk Estimation in 2 Population Cohorts. *Circulation* **2010**, *121*, 2388–2397. [CrossRef]
117. Nakashima, Y.; Raines, E.W.; Plump, A.S.; Breslow, J.L.; Ross, R. Upregulation of VCAM-1 and ICAM-1 at Atherosclerosis-Prone Sites on the Endothelium in the ApoE-Deficient Mouse. *Arterioscler. Thromb. Vasc. Biol.* **1998**, *18*, 842–851. [CrossRef] [PubMed]
118. Iiyama, K.; Hajra, L.; Iiyama, M.; Li, H.; DiChiara, M.; Medoff, B.D.; Cybulsky, M.I. Patterns of vascular cell adhesion molecule-1 and intercellular adhesion molecule-1 expression in rabbit and mouse atherosclerotic lesions and at sites predisposed to lesion formation. *Circ. Res.* **1999**, *85*, 199–207. [CrossRef] [PubMed]
119. Babinska, A.; Azari, B.; Salifu, M.; Liu, R.; Jiang, X.-C.; Sobocka, M.; Boo, D.; Khoury, G.; Deitch, J.; Marmur, J.; et al. The F11 receptor (F11R/JAM-A) in atherothrombosis: Overexpression of F11R in atherosclerotic plaques. *Thromb. Haemost.* **2007**, *97*, 272–281. [CrossRef]
120. Schönberger, T.; Siegel-Axel, D.; Bußl, R.; Richter, S.; Judenhofer, M.S.; Haubner, R.; Reischl, G.; Klingel, K.; Münch, G.; Seizer, P.; et al. The immunoadhesin glycoprotein VI-Fc regulates arterial remodelling after mechanical injury in ApoE−/− mice. *Cardiovasc. Res.* **2008**, *80*, 131–137. [CrossRef]
121. Bültmann, A.; Li, Z.; Wagner, S.; Peluso, M.; Schönberger, T.; Weis, C.; Konrad, I.; Stellos, K.; Massberg, S.; Nieswandt, B.; et al. Impact of glycoprotein VI and platelet adhesion on atherosclerosis—A possible role of fibronectin. *J. Mol. Cell. Cardiol.* **2010**, *49*, 532–542. [CrossRef]
122. Ungerer, M.; Li, Z.; Baumgartner, C.; Goebel, S.; Vogelmann, J.; Holthoff, H.-P.; Gawaz, M.; Münch, G. The GPVI—Fc Fusion Protein Revacept Reduces Thrombus Formation and Improves Vascular Dysfunction in Atherosclerosis without Any Impact on Bleeding Times. *PLoS ONE* **2013**, *8*, e71193. [CrossRef]
123. Hamm, C.W.; Goldmann, B.U.; Heeschen, C.; Kreymann, G.; Berger, J.; Meinertz, T. Emergency room triage of patients with acute chest pain by means of rapid testing for cardiac troponin T or troponin I. *N. Engl. J. Med.* **1997**, *337*, 1648–1653. [CrossRef]
124. Pope, J.H.; Aufderheide, T.P.; Ruthazer, R.; Woolard, R.H.; Feldman, J.A.; Beshansky, J.R.; Griffith, J.L.; Selker, H.P. Missed diagnoses of acute cardiac ischemia in the emergency department. *N. Engl. J. Med.* **2000**, *342*, 1163–1170. [CrossRef] [PubMed]
125. Mehta, R.H.; Eagle, K.A. Missed diagnoses of acute coronary syndromes in the emergency room–continuing challenges. *N. Engl. J. Med.* **2000**, *342*, 1207–1210. [CrossRef] [PubMed]
126. Lev, E.I.; Battler, A.; Behar, S.; Porter, A.; Haim, M.; Boyko, V.; Hasdai, D. Frequency, characteristics, and outcome of patients hospitalized with acute coronary syndromes with undetermined electrocardiographic patterns. *Am. J. Cardiol.* **2003**, *91*, 224–227. [CrossRef]
127. Chukwuemeka, A.O.; Brown, K.A.; Venn, G.E.; Chambers, D.J. Changes in P-selectin expression on cardiac microvessels in blood-perfused rat hearts subjected to ischemia-reperfusion. *Ann. Thorac. Surg.* **2005**, *79*, 204–211. [CrossRef]
128. Villanueva, F.S.; Lu, E.; Bowry, S.; Kilic, S.; Tom, E.; Wang, J.; Gretton, J.; Pacella, J.J.; Wagner, W.R. Myocardial Ischemic Memory Imaging With Molecular Echocardiography. *Circulation* **2007**, *115*, 345–352. [CrossRef]
129. Davidson, B.P.; Chadderdon, S.M.; Belcik, J.T.; Gupta, S.; Lindner, J.R. Ischemic Memory Imaging in Nonhuman Primates with Echocardiographic Molecular Imaging of Selectin Expression. *J. Am. Soc. Echocardiogr.* **2014**, *27*, 786–793. [CrossRef]
130. Wang, H.; Machtaler, S.; Bettinger, T.; Lutz, A.M.; Luong, R.; Bussat, P.; Gambhir, S.S.; Tranquart, F.; Tian, L.; Willmann, J.K. Molecular Imaging of Inflammation in Inflammatory Bowel Disease with a Clinically Translatable Dual-Selectin–targeted US Contrast Agent: Comparison with FDG PET/CT in a Mouse Model. *Radiology* **2013**, *267*, 818–829. [CrossRef]

131. Wang, H.; Felt, S.A.; Machtaler, S.; Guracar, I.; Luong, R.; Bettinger, T.; Tian, L.; Lutz, A.M.; Willmann, J.K. Quantitative Assessment of Inflammation in a Porcine Acute Terminal Ileitis Model: US with a Molecularly Targeted Contrast Agent. *Radiology* **2015**, *276*, 809–817. [CrossRef]
132. Wang, H.; Hyvelin, J.-M.; Felt, S.A.; Guracar, I.; Vilches-Moure, J.G.; Cherkaoui, S.; Bettinger, T.; Tian, L.; Lutz, A.M.; Willmann, J.K. US Molecular Imaging of Acute Ileitis: Anti-Inflammatory Treatment Response Monitored with Targeted Microbubbles in a Preclinical Model. *Radiology* **2018**, *289*, 90–100. [CrossRef]
133. Goodacre, S.; Sampson, F.; Thomas, S.; van Beek, E.; Sutton, A. Systematic review and meta-analysis of the diagnostic accuracy of ultrasonography for deep vein thrombosis. *BMC Med. Imaging* **2005**, *5*, 6. [CrossRef]
134. Nesheim, M. Thrombin and Fibrinolysis. *Chest* **2003**, *124*, 33S–39S. [CrossRef] [PubMed]
135. Kessels, H.; Béguin, S.; Andree, H.; Hemker, H.C. Measurement of thrombin generation in whole blood—The effect of heparin and aspirin. *Thromb. Haemost.* **1994**, *72*, 78–83. [CrossRef] [PubMed]
136. Weller, G.E.R.; Villanueva, F.S.; Tom, E.M.; Wagner, W.R. Targeted ultrasound contrast agents: In vitro assessment of endothelial dysfunction and multi-targeting to ICAM-1 and sialyl Lewisx. *Biotechnol. Bioeng.* **2005**, *92*, 780–788. [CrossRef] [PubMed]
137. Ferrante, E.A.; Pickard, J.E.; Rychak, J.; Klibanov, A.; Ley, K. Dual targeting improves microbubble contrast agent adhesion to VCAM-1 and P-selectin under flow. *J. Control. Release* **2009**, *140*, 100–107. [CrossRef] [PubMed]
138. Willmann, J.K.; Lutz, A.M.; Paulmurugan, R.; Patel, M.R.; Chu, P.; Rosenberg, J.; Gambhir, S.S. Dual-targeted Contrast Agent for US Assessment of Tumor Angiogenesis in Vivo1. *Radiology* **2008**, *248*, 936–944. [CrossRef] [PubMed]
139. Warram, J.M.; Sorace, A.G.; Saini, R.; Umphrey, H.R.; Zinn, K.R.; Hoyt, K. A Triple-Targeted Ultrasound Contrast Agent Provides Improved Localization to Tumor Vasculature. *J. Ultrasound Med.* **2011**, *30*, 921–931. [CrossRef]
140. Sorace, A.G.; Saini, R.; Mahoney, M.; Hoyt, K. Molecular Ultrasound Imaging Using a Targeted Contrast Agent for Assessing Early Tumor Response to Antiangiogenic Therapy. *J. Ultrasound Med.* **2012**, *31*, 1543–1550. [CrossRef]
141. Ferrara, K.; Pollard, R.; Borden, M. Ultrasound microbubble contrast agents: Fundamentals and application to gene and drug delivery. *Annu Rev. Biomed. Eng* **2007**, *9*, 415–447. [CrossRef]
142. Meyer, D.L.; Schultz, J.; Lin, Y.; Henry, A.; Sanderson, J.; Jackson, J.M.; Goshorn, S.; Rees, A.R.; Graves, S.S. Reduced antibody response to streptavidin through site-directed mutagenesis. *Protein Sci.* **2001**, *10*, 491–503. [CrossRef]
143. Paganelli, G.; Chinol, M.; Maggiolo, M.; Sidoli, A.; Corti, A.; Baroni, S.; Siccardi, A.G. The three-step pretargeting approach reduces the human anti-mouse antibody response in patients submitted to radioimmunoscintigraphy and radioimmunotherapy. *Eur. J. Nucl. Med.* **1997**, *24*, 350–351. [CrossRef]
144. Breitz, H.B.; Weiden, P.L.; Beaumier, P.L.; Axworthy, D.B.; Seiler, C.; Su, F.-M.; Graves, S.; Bryan, K.; Reno, J.M. Clinical Optimization of Pretargeted Radioimmunotherapy with Antibody-Streptavidin Conjugate and 90Y-DOTA-Biotin. *J. Nucl. Med.* **2000**, *11*, 131–140.
145. Stieger, S.M.; Dayton, P.A.; Borden, M.A.; Caskey, C.F.; Griffey, S.M.; Wisner, E.R.; Ferrara, K.W. Imaging of angiogenesis using Cadence contrast pulse sequencing and targeted contrast agents. *Contrast Media Mol. Imaging* **2008**, *3*, 9–18. [CrossRef] [PubMed]
146. Willmann, J.K.; Bonomo, L.; Testa, A.C.; Rinaldi, P.; Rindi, G.; Valluru, K.S.; Petrone, G.; Martini, M.; Lutz, A.M.; Gambhir, S.S. Ultrasound Molecular Imaging With BR55 in Patients With Breast and Ovarian Lesions: First-in-Human Results. *J. Clin. Oncol.* **2017**, *35*, 2133–2140. [CrossRef] [PubMed]
147. Hobbs, S.K.; Monsky, W.L.; Yuan, F.; Roberts, W.G.; Griffith, L.; Torchilin, V.P.; Jain, R.K. Regulation of transport pathways in tumor vessels: Role of tumor type and microenvironment. *Proc. Natl. Acad. Sci. USA* **1998**, *95*, 4607. [CrossRef]
148. Yin, T.; Wang, P.; Zheng, R.; Zheng, B.; Cheng, D.; Zhang, X.; Shuai, X. Nanobubbles for enhanced ultrasound imaging of tumors. *Int. J. Nanomed.* **2012**, *7*, 895–904. [CrossRef]
149. Wang, J.-P.; Zhou, X.-L.; Yan, J.-P.; Zheng, R.-Q.; Wang, W. Nanobubbles as ultrasound contrast agent for facilitating small cell lung cancer imaging. *Oncotarget* **2017**, *8*, 78153–78162. [CrossRef] [PubMed]
150. Cai, W.B.; Yang, H.L.; Zhang, J.; Yin, J.K.; Yang, Y.L.; Yuan, L.J.; Zhang, L.; Duan, Y.Y. The Optimized Fabrication of Nanobubbles as Ultrasound Contrast Agents for Tumor Imaging. *Sci. Rep.* **2015**, *5*, 13725. [CrossRef]

151. Perera, R.; de Leon, A.; Wang, X.; Wang, Y.; Ramamurthy, G.; Peiris, P.; Abenojar, E.; Basilion, J.P.; Exner, A.A. Real Time Ultrasound Molecular Imaging of Prostate Cancer with PSMA-targeted Nanobubbles. *Nanomed. Nanotechnol. Biol. Med.* **2020**, *28*, 102213. [CrossRef]
152. Yang, H.; Cai, W.; Xu, L.; Lv, X.; Qiao, Y.; Li, P.; Wu, H.; Yang, Y.; Zhang, L.; Duan, Y. Nanobubble–Affibody: Novel ultrasound contrast agents for targeted molecular ultrasound imaging of tumor. *Biomaterials* **2015**, *37*, 279–288. [CrossRef]
153. Lv, W.; Shen, Y.; Yang, H.; Yang, R.; Cai, W.; Zhang, J.; Yuan, L.; Duan, Y.; Zhang, L. A Novel Bimodal Imaging Agent Targeting HER2 Molecule of Breast Cancer. *J. Immunol. Res.* **2018**, *2018*, 1–10. [CrossRef]
154. Jiang, Q.; Hao, S.; Xiao, X.; Yao, J.; Ou, B.; Zhao, Z.; Liu, F.; Pan, X.; Luo, B.; Zhi, H. Production and characterization of a novel long-acting Herceptin-targeted nanobubble contrast agent specific for Her-2-positive breast cancers. *Breast Cancer* **2016**, *23*, 445–455. [CrossRef]
155. Liu, J.; Chen, Y.; Wang, G.; Lv, Q.; Yang, Y.; Wang, J.; Zhang, P.; Liu, J.; Xie, Y.; Zhang, L.; et al. Ultrasound molecular imaging of acute cardiac transplantation rejection using nanobubbles targeted to T lymphocytes. *Biomaterials* **2018**, *162*, 200–207. [CrossRef] [PubMed]
156. Gao, Y.; Hernandez, C.; Yuan, H.-X.; Lilly, J.; Kota, P.; Zhou, H.; Wu, H.; Exner, A.A. Ultrasound molecular imaging of ovarian cancer with CA-125 targeted nanobubble contrast agents. *Nanomed. Nanotechnol. Biol. Med.* **2017**, *13*, 2159–2168. [CrossRef] [PubMed]
157. Zhou, T.; Cai, W.; Yang, H.; Zhang, H.; Hao, M.; Yuan, L.; Liu, J.; Zhang, L.; Yang, Y.; Liu, X.; et al. Annexin V conjugated nanobubbles: A novel ultrasound contrast agent for in vivo assessment of the apoptotic response in cancer therapy. *J. Control. Release* **2018**, *276*, 113–124. [CrossRef] [PubMed]
158. Du, J.; Li, X.-Y.; Hu, H.; Xu, L.; Yang, S.-P.; Li, F.-H. Preparation and Imaging Investigation of Dual-targeted C3F8-filled PLGA Nanobubbles as a Novel Ultrasound Contrast Agent for Breast Cancer. *Sci. Rep.* **2018**, *8*, 3887. [CrossRef]
159. Gorce, J.-M.; Arditi, M.; Schneider, M. Influence of Bubble Size Distribution on the Echogenicity of Ultrasound Contrast Agents: A Study of SonoVue™. *Investig. Radiol.* **2000**, *35*, 661–671. [CrossRef]
160. JafariSojahrood, A.; Nieves, L.; Hernandez, C.; Exner, A.; Kolios, M.C. Theoretical and experimental investigation of the nonlinear dynamics of nanobubbles excited at clinically relevant ultrasound frequencies and pressures: The role of lipid shell buckling. In Proceedings of the 2017 IEEE International Ultrasonics Symposium (IUS), Washington, DC, USA, 6–9 September 2017.
161. Wu, H.; Rognin, N.G.; Krupka, T.M.; Solorio, L.; Yoshiara, H.; Guenette, G.; Sanders, C.; Kamiyama, N.; Exner, A.A. Acoustic Characterization and Pharmacokinetic Analyses of New Nanobubble Ultrasound Contrast Agents. *Ultrasound Med. Biol.* **2013**, *39*, 2137–2146. [CrossRef]
162. Wang, C.-W.; Yang, S.-P.; Hu, H.; Du, J.; Li, F.-H. Synthesis, characterization and in vitro and in vivo investigation of C3F8-filled poly(lactic-co-glycolic acid) nanoparticles as an ultrasound contrast agent. *Mol. Med. Rep.* **2015**, *11*, 1885–1890. [CrossRef]
163. De Leon, A.; Perera, R.; Hernandez, C.; Cooley, M.; Jung, O.; Jeganathan, S.; Abenojar, E.; Fishbein, G.; Sojahrood, A.J.; Emerson, C.C.; et al. Contrast enhanced ultrasound imaging by nature-inspired ultrastable echogenic nanobubbles. *Nanoscale* **2019**, *11*, 15647–15658. [CrossRef]
164. Kiessling, F.; Mertens, M.E.; Grimm, J.; Lammers, T. Nanoparticles for Imaging: Top or Flop? *Radiology* **2014**, *273*, 10–28. [CrossRef]
165. Kee, A.L.Y.; Teo, B.M. Biomedical applications of acoustically responsive phase shift nanodroplets: Current status and future directions. *Ultrason. Sonochem.* **2019**, *56*, 37–45. [CrossRef]
166. Rapoport, N. Phase-shift, stimuli-responsive perfluorocarbon nanodroplets for drug delivery to cancer. *Wires Nanomed. Nanobiotechnol.* **2012**, *4*, 492–510. [CrossRef] [PubMed]
167. O'Neill, B.E.; Rapoport, N. Phase-shift, stimuli-responsive drug carriers for targeted delivery. *Ther. Deliv.* **2011**, *2*, 1165–1187. [CrossRef] [PubMed]
168. Lin, C.-Y.; Pitt, W.G. Acoustic Droplet Vaporization in Biology and Medicine. *Biomed Res. Int.* **2013**, *2013*, 404361. [CrossRef]
169. Rapoport, N.Y.; Kennedy, A.M.; Shea, J.E.; Scaife, C.L.; Nam, K.-H. Controlled and targeted tumor chemotherapy by ultrasound-activated nanoemulsions/microbubbles. *J. Control. Release* **2009**, *138*, 268–276. [CrossRef] [PubMed]
170. Rapoport, N.; Kennedy, A.M.; Shea, J.E.; Scaife, C.L.; Nam, K.-H. Ultrasonic Nanotherapy of Pancreatic Cancer: Lessons from Ultrasound Imaging. *Mol. Pharm.* **2010**, *7*, 22–31. [CrossRef]

171. Gao, Z.; Kennedy, A.M.; Christensen, D.A.; Rapoport, N.Y. Drug-loaded nano/microbubbles for combining ultrasonography and targeted chemotherapy. *Ultrasonics* **2008**, *48*, 260–270. [CrossRef]
172. Chen, W.-T.; Kang, S.-T.; Lin, J.-L.; Wang, C.-H.; Chen, R.-C.; Yeh, C.-K. Targeted tumor theranostics using folate-conjugated and camptothecin-loaded acoustic nanodroplets in a mouse xenograft model. *Biomaterials* **2015**, *53*, 699–708. [CrossRef]
173. Zhang, G.; Lin, S.; Leow, C.H.; Pang, K.; Hernandez-Gil, J.; Chee, M.; Long, N.J.; Matsunaga, T.O.; Tang, M.-X. Acoustic response of targeted nanodroplets post-activation using high frame rate imaging. In Proceedings of the 2017 IEEE International Ultrasonics Symposium (IUS), Washington, DC, USA, 6–9 September 2017.
174. Gao, D.; Gao, J.; Xu, M.; Cao, Z.; Zhou, L.; Li, Y.; Xie, X.; Jiang, Q.; Wang, W.; Liu, J. Targeted Ultrasound-Triggered Phase Transition Nanodroplets for Her2-Overexpressing Breast Cancer Diagnosis and Gene Transfection. *Mol. Pharm.* **2017**, *14*, 984–998. [CrossRef]

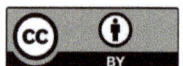

© 2020 by the authors. Licensee MDPI, Basel, Switzerland. This article is an open access article distributed under the terms and conditions of the Creative Commons Attribution (CC BY) license (http://creativecommons.org/licenses/by/4.0/).

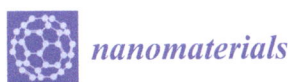

Article

In-Situ Biofabrication of Silver Nanoparticles in *Ceiba pentandra* Natural Fiber Using *Entada spiralis* Extract with Their Antibacterial and Catalytic Dye Reduction Properties

Wan Khaima Azira Wan Mat Khalir [1], Kamyar Shameli [1,*], Seyed Davoud Jazayeri [2,*], Nor Azizi Othman [1], Nurfatehah Wahyuny Che Jusoh [1] and Norazian Mohd Hassan [3]

[1] Malaysia-Japan International Institute of Technology, Universiti Teknologi Malaysia, Jalan Sultan Yahya Petra, Kuala Lumpur 54100, Malaysia; wkawmk_2505@yahoo.com (W.K.A.W.M.K.); norazizio.kl@utm.my (N.A.O.); nurfatehah@utm.my (N.W.C.J.)
[2] Centre for Virus and Vaccine Research, Sunway University, Bandar Sunway 47500, Malaysia
[3] Department of Pharmaceutical Chemistry, Kulliyyah of Pharmacy, International Islamic University Malaysia, Kuantan 25200, Malaysia; norazianmh@iium.edu.my
* Correspondence: kamyarshameli@gmail.com (K.S.); sjazayeri@sunway.edu.my (S.D.J.); Tel.: +60-173-443-492 (K.S.); Fax: +60-322-031-266 (K.S.)

Received: 5 March 2020; Accepted: 7 April 2020; Published: 3 June 2020

Abstract: It is believed of great interest to incorporate silver nanoparticles (Ag-NPs) into stable supported materials using biological methods to control the adverse properties of nanoscale particles. In this study, in-situ biofabrication of Ag-NPs using *Entada spiralis (E. spiralis)* aqueous extract in *Ceiba pentandra* (*C. pentandra*) fiber as supporting material was used in which, the *E. spiralis* extract acted as both reducing and stabilizing agents to incorporate Ag-NPs in the *C. pentandra* fiber. The properties of Ag-NPs incorporated in the *C. pentandra* fiber (*C. pentandra*/Ag-NPs) were characterized using UV-visible spectroscopy (UV-vis), X-ray Diffraction (XRD), Field Emission Transmission Electron Microscope (FETEM), Scanning Electron Microscope (Scanning Electron Microscope (SEM), Energy Dispersive X-ray (EDX), Brunauer-Emmett-Teller (BET), Thermogravimetric (TGA) and Fourier Transform Infrared (FTIR) analyses. The average size of Ag-NPs measured using FETEM image was 4.74 nm spherical in shape. The *C. pentandra*/Ag-NPs was easily separated after application, and could control the release of Ag-NPs to the environment due to its strong attachment in *C. pentandra* fiber. The *C. pentandra*/Ag-NPs exposed good qualitative and quantitative antibacterial activities against *Staphylococcus aureus* (ATCC 25923), *Enterococcus faecalis* (ATCC 29212), *Escherichia coli* (ATCC 25922) and *Proteus vulgaris* (ATCC 33420). The dye catalytic properties of *C. pentandra*/Ag-NPs revealed the dye reduction time in which it was completed within 4 min for 20 mg/L rhodamine B and 20 min for 20 mg/L methylene blue dye, respectively. Based on the results, it is evident that *C. pentandra*/Ag-NPs are potentially promising to be applied in wound healing, textile, wastewater treatment, food packaging, labeling and biomedical fields.

Keywords: silver nanoparticles; *Entada spiralis*; *Ceiba pentandra*; antibacterial assay; catalytic dye reduction

---

1. Introduction

With the strong potential of nanotechnology, various types of nanomaterials as an antibacterial agent with strong antibacterial activity have been widely used in many applications to prevent or control the health hazard of microorganisms. The examples of metal and metal oxide nanoparticles with antibacterial properties are zinc oxide (ZnO-NPs), Copper oxide (CuO-NPs) and Ag-NPs [1]. Among these nanoparticles, Ag-NPs have been greatly used in many applications due to their special properties such as the broad spectrum of antibacterial activity, powerful and safe antibacterial nanoparticles, as well as stable nanoparticle dispersion [2]. Moreover, Ag-NPs exhibit special catalytic, chemical, structural, electronic and optical properties different from bulk materials due to the high surface to volume ratio [3]. Such properties of Ag-NPs allow it to be widely used in medical applications (reduce severe burn and human skin treatment), wound dressing, catheter, scaffold, industrial products (shampoo, toothpaste, soaps, detergent, cosmetic products and shoes), pharmaceutical, textile, catalysis, photography, optoelectronics, biological labeling and also photocatalytic applications [4–6]. With the increasing production of Ag-NPs in various applications, there are concerns about their release into the environment. High concentrations of Ag-NPs in the environment and small size of the particle can cause potential adverse effects especially on aquatic organisms and human health. In addition, Ag-NPs easily transform into aggregates and settle due to particle-particle interactions. The aggregation of Ag-NPs affects the bioavailability concentration of Ag-NPs, loss of its properties as well as causing ineffective release of more Ag^+ ions. Therefore, to achieve better stability, control the size of Ag-NPs, high recovery and minimize the release of Ag-NPs into the environment, Ag-NPs should be loaded on supporting materials.

Currently, the loading of the metal nanoparticles on the supporting materials such as natural fiber has become an intended subject in the field of nanomaterials. One reason is due to these material properties which are renewable, biodegradable and environmentally friendly. The natural fiber loaded with metal nanoparticles can combine the desirable properties of both nanoscale materials and metal nanoparticles. The examples of natural fiber are flax, hemp, jute, kenaf and sisal [7,8]. The loading of metal nanoparticles on the surface of natural fiber can be based on the electrostatic interactions between the negatively charged of the functional group on the fiber surface and positively charged metal nanoparticles [9]. On the other hand, the natural fiber loaded with Ag-NPs can improve its properties which are mechanical, biocompatibility, optical, electronic and magnetic [10]. However, the ability of the natural fiber to absorb a large amount of moisture makes it more prone to microbial attack under certain conditions of humidity and temperature [11]. Therefore, natural fiber facilitating with the antimicrobial agents can be solved the problem. In this study, *C. pentandra* natural fiber was chosen as supporting material for loading of Ag-NPs and is the first time reported in the literature. Comparing with other supporting materials, *C. pentandra* has advantages such as high cellulose content, biodegradability, non-toxicity, abundant availability, low cost and resistance to the microbial attack due to the hydrophobic properties of fiber. The *C. pentandra* fiber is a local plant and can be found abundantly in Malaysia. This plant belongs to the Bombacaceae family which is a white fine silky, lightweight and strong fiber that surrounds the seeds in the pods of the *C. pentandra* tree. The common use of this fiber is in pillow or mattress products, textile industries, water safety equipment, insulation material and upholstery due to their softness and buoyancy [8]. *C. pentandra* fiber consists of single cell fiber with high cellulose compositions [12].

Nowadays, due to the environmental damage and pollution resulting from the various industrial processes, many researchers are interested in developing an environmentally friendly method that minimizes and reduces the use of the toxic chemicals. This is because; the toxic chemicals present in the environment can threaten human health and the ecosystem. The conventional method used to synthesize Ag-NPs has some drawbacks in term of toxicity and stability. Therefore, it is worth considering the high potential of plant extracts as a source of reduction Ag^+ ions to Ag-NPs with their environmentally friendly nature, simplicity and cost-effectiveness. The ability of the *E. spiralis* stem extract to biosynthesis Ag-NPs in *C. pentandra* fiber should be investigated. The in-situ biofabrication of Ag-NPs in *C. pentandra* fiber using natural reducing and stabilizing agent from *E. spiralis* extract was never done or reported in the existing literature. The purpose of this study is to prepare *C. pentandra* fiber as supporting materials for Ag-NPs via in-situ biofabrication process using *E. spiralis* extract and silver nitrate as a silver precursor and to evaluate their antibacterial and catalytic dye reduction properties. The properties of plant-mediated of Ag-NPs deposited in the *C. pentandra* fiber were characterized using UV-vis, XRD, FETEM, SEM, EDX, BET, TGA and FTIR analyses. Their antibacterial and catalytic dye reduction properties of C. pentandra/Ag-NPs also were investigated for the potential application like wound healing, textile, wastewater treatment, food packaging and labeling and biomedical fields.

2. Materials and Methods

2.1. Plant Materials and Chemicals

The E. spiralis stem was collected from the forest in Tasik Chini, Pahang, Malaysia, while the C. pentandra fiber was collected during their season from February to April every year from their trees in Besut, Terengganu, Malaysia. The plant of E. spiralis and C. pentandra are shown in Figure 1. The collected C. pentandra fiber was separated from their seed and cleaned with distilled water in order to remove any adhering materials. After being cleaned, the C. pentandra fiber was then dried at 60 °C in the oven (Memmert, Germany) overnight. The dried C. pentandra fiber was stored in a plastic container for further experiments. Four species of bacteria including two Gram-positive species (*Staphylococcus aureus* (S. aureus) (ATCC 25923) and *Enterococcus faecalis* (E. faecalis) (ATCC 29212)), as well as two Gram-negative species (*Proteus Vulgaris* (P. vulgaris) (ATCC 33420) and *Escherichia coli* (E. coli) (ATCC 25922)), were bought from Choice Care Sdn. Bhd, Kuala Lumpur, Malaysia. The silver nitrate (99.85%) was purchased from Acros organic, Geel, Belgium. The sodium hydroxide pellet, nitric acid (69%) and sodium borohydride powder were bought from R&M, Birmingham, UK. The methylene blue dye was bought from (System, Malaysia) and Rhodamine B dye was bought from (R&M, Birmingham, UK). The Mueller Hinton agar (MHA), Mueller Hinton broth (MHB) and gentamicin antibiotic standard (disk) (10 µg) was bought from Difco, Detroit, Michigan, MI, USA. All the chemicals were used without any purification. The deionized water from ELGA Lab-Water/VWS (Buckinghamshire, UK) purification system was used throughout the experiment.

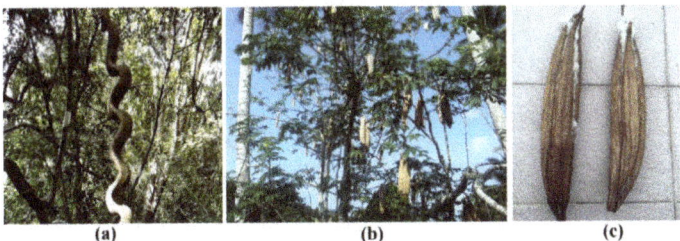

Figure 1. (a) E. spiralis plant, (b) C. pentandra plant and (c) C. pentandra fiber in the seed pod.

2.2. Alkaline Treatment of C. pentandra Fiber

This treatment process was performed using an alkaline solution of sodium hydroxide (NaOH). The mass of 2.0 g of untreated C. pentandra fiber and 200 mL of 1.0 M NaOH (1:100) was mixed in the 500 mL beaker as shown in Figure 2a. The mixture was soaked for 5 h at a temperature of ~90 °C. After the soaking process, the NaOH treated C. pentandra fiber was washed extensively with distilled water until the pH becomes neutral (pH 7) using pH meter. The washed NaOH treated C. pentandra fiber was then dried in an oven at 60 °C overnight. The NaOH treated C. pentandra fiber was stored in a plastic container at room temperature until further usage. The NaOH treated C. pentandra fiber was referred to as "treated C. pentandra fiber" hereafter.

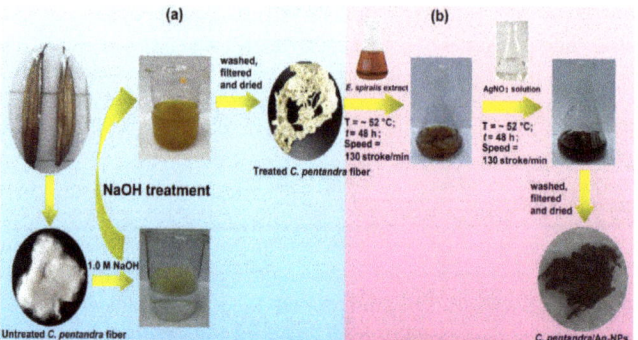

Figure 2. (a) Alkaline treatment of *C. pentandra* fiber and (b) in-situ biofabrication of Ag-NPs using *E. spiralis* extract and AgNO$_3$ solution steps of preparation.

2.3. In-Situ Biofabrication of Treated C. pentandra Fiber with Ag-NPs

This in-situ process was done using two steps of the loading process by following the method of Ravindra et al. [11] and Sivaranjana et al. [13] with some modification as shown in Figure 2b. Firstly, the treated *C. pentandra* fiber was immersed in the *E. spiralis* extract. The treated *C. pentandra* fiber was immersed in the 30 mL of *E. spiralis* extract (2.5 g) in a 150 mL conical flask. The *E. spiralis* extract was prepared based on the previous study [14]. The mixture was then shaken at ~52 °C using water bath shaker at 130 strokes/min for 48 h. Then, the fiber was filtered using filter paper and kept for the next step. Secondly, the immersed treated *C. pentandra* fiber in *E. spiralis* extract was then immersed in 3 mL of 0.1 M AgNO$_3$ solution as a silver precursor. The mixture was shaken in a water bath shaker at 130 stroke/min and temperature of ~52 °C for 48 h. After the shaking process, the fiber was filtered from the solution and washed with deionized for two times to remove any excess of AgNO$_3$ solution before being dried in an oven at 60 °C overnight. The treated *C. pentandra* fiber loaded with Ag-NPs was abbreviated as *C. pentandra*/Ag-NPs hereafter.

As a control, the treated *C. pentandra* fiber was immersed only in AgNO$_3$ solution in the absence of *E. spiralis* extract to determine the significant of *E. spiralis* extract. A mass of 1.0 g of treated *C. pentandra* fiber was immersed into the 30 mL of 0.1 M AgNO$_3$ in different conical flasks. The mixture of fiber was shaken in a waterbath shaker (Memmert, Germany) at 130 stroke/min and temperature of 52 °C for 48 h. The fiber was then filtered and washed with 100 mL of deionized water two times to remove any excess of AgNO$_3$ solution before dried in the oven overnight at 60 °C. The treated *C. pentandra* fiber immersed only in the AgNO$_3$ solution was then stored in the plastic container for further usage and abbreviated as *C. pentandra*/Ag-NO$_3$ hereafter.

2.4. Characterization Studies of Untreated C. pentandra Fiber, Treated C. pentandra Fiber and C. pentandra/Ag-NPs

The UV-vis spectroscopy analysis was started by loading the sample into a solid sample holder. The samples then were scanned from the 300 to 900 nm with a UV-vis spectrophotometer (UV-2600, Shimadzu, Kyoto, Japan) at a medium rate based on transmittance (%) measurement. The XRD analysis was determined using XRD (PANalytical X'pert PRO, Amsterdam, The Netherlands) at 45 kV and a current of 30 mA with Cu-Kα radiation. The fiber sample was cut into small pieces and put on a solid sample holder. The XRD pattern was initiated to scan from 10 to 90° at a 2θ angle. The FETEM analysis was determined using FETEM (JEOL, JEM-2100F, Tokyo, Japan). The fiber samples were prepared by sonicating a small piece of fiber in the ethanol solution for 10 min. The samples were then dropped on the copper grate surface using a dropper. The dropped sample was then air-dried completely before running the analysis. The average size of Ag-NPs was measured using image J followed by plotting the histogram of particle size diameter distribution using SPSS software. The particle size distribution histogram is designed based on the counted 100 Ag-NPs incorporated in the *C. pentandra* fiber. The SEM and EDX analyses were observed using Focused Ionized Beam Scanning Electron Microscope (FIBSEM) coupled with EDX using Helios NanoLab G3 UC, FEI, Hillsboro, Oregon, OR, USA. The fiber sample was prepared by placing it on the aluminum holder. The fiber samples were then coated with platinum to increase the electron conductivity of the sample. TGA analysis was studied using a thermogravimetric analyzer (TA Instruments, TGA 55, New castles, Delaware, DE, USA). A known weight of the sample was placed onto platinum crucible and the analysis was carried out under nitrogen flow at the heating rate of 20 °C/min at a temperature from 50 to 700 °C. The surface area of untreated *C. pentandra* fiber and treated *C. pentandra* fiber was determined using surface area analyzer (NOVA touch LX3, Quantachrome Instruments, Palm Beach County, Florida, FL, USA). The analysis was begun by degassing the adsorbents at 50 °C for 180 min at rate 10 °C/min to remove any physisorbed gas. The FTIR analysis was investigated using Attenuated Transmittance Reflectance-Fourier Transform Infrared (ATR-FTIR) spectrometer (Perkin Elmer, Frontier, Waltham, Massachusetts, MA, USA). The small sample of fiber was put on the ATR-FTIR sample holder. The sample was then scanned from 4000 to 650 cm^{-1} wavenumber.

2.5. Silver Content Analysis and Silver Ions Release of *C. pentandra*/Ag-NPs

The amount of silver (Ag) content in the *C. pentandra*/Ag-NPs was determined using the method proposed by Rehan et al. [15]. The Ag content in *C. pentandra*/Ag-NPs was extracted by immersing 0.2 g dried *C. pentandra*/Ag-NPs with 20 mL of 15% aqueous nitric acid in a conical flask. The mixture was immersed for 2 h in a water bath shaker at 80 °C. After immersed, the filtrate was filtered on Whatman No. 42 filter paper and the Ag$^+$ ions concentration was measured using Inductively Coupled Plasma Optical Emissions Spectrophotometer (ICP-OES) (Avio 500, Perkin Elmer, Medtech Park, Singapore) at 328.1 nm wavelength. The Ag content in the *C. pentandra*/fiber sample was calculated using Equation (1):

$$\frac{C \times V}{\left[W \times \left(1 - \frac{MC}{1000}\right)\right]} = X \qquad (1)$$

where X is the Ag content in the fiber (g/kg), C is the Ag$^+$ ions concentration (mg/L) in extracted solution; V is the volume of the extracted solution (L); W is the weight of dried *C. pentandra*/Ag-NPs (g); MC is the moisture content in dried *C. pentandra*/Ag-NPs (%). The MC of *C. pentandra*/Ag-NPs was measured using an oven drying method (method No. 44-15A) as followed by Hussain et al. [16]. The *C. pentandra*/Ag-NPs sample was conditioned at ambient temperature for 24 h. The conditioned sample was then dried in the oven at 105 °C for 2 h. Equation (2) was used to calculate the percentage of moisture content as shown below:

$$\text{Moisture (\%)} = \frac{W_b - W_d}{W_b} \times 100 \qquad (2)$$

where W_b is mass of the sample and W_d is mass of the *C. pentandra*/Ag-NPs after dried in the oven.

The release rate of silver ions from *C. pentandra*/Ag-NPs was investigated by following the method by Zhang et al. [17] and Liu et al. [18]. A mass of 0.05 g of each sample of *C. pentandra*/Ag-NPs at different stirring reaction times (6–144 h) was put into 50 mL of deionized water in the different conical flasks. The mixture was shaken in a water bath shaker at 105 stroke/min and at room temperature. During the shaking time process, 10 mL solution was withdrawn from the release media and another 10 mL of fresh deionized water was added at time intervals of 6, 12, 24, 48, 72 and 96, 120, 144 h. The amount of released Ag$^+$ ions was measured using ICP-OES at 328.1 nm wavelength. The procedure was repeated for the sample of *C. pentandra*/Ag-NPs and the results were compared. The experiments were conducted in duplicate and the results were reported in average value. The percentage of Ag$^+$ ions release rate was calculated using Equation (3) as below:

$$\text{Ions release rate (\%)} = \frac{C_b - C_a}{C_b} \times 100 \qquad (3)$$

where C_b and C_a are Ag$^+$ ions concentration before and after adsorption (mg/L), respectively.

2.6. Antibacterial Application

2.6.1. Antibacterial Disk Diffusion Assay

The in-vitro antibacterial activities of C. pentandra/Ag-NPs was evaluated qualitatively using the Kirby-Bauer technique [19], which conformed to the recommended standards of Clinical and Laboratory Standards Institute (CLSI). Two Gram-positive bacteria (S. aureus and E. faecalis), including two Gram-negative bacteria (E.coli and P. vulgaris) were used in this study. Gentamicin antibiotic disk standard (10 µg), plain disk and E. spiralis extract were used as positive and negative controls, respectively. All the glassware, apparatus and culture media were sterilized in an autoclave at 0.1 MPa and 121 °C for 15 min. The agar plate was prepared by solidifying 20 mL of liquid Mueller Hinton agar (MHA) into disposable sterilized petri dishes. The inoculum was prepared by subculturing 100 µL of stock culture bacteria into new sterile Mueller Hinton broth (MHB). The bacterial suspension was incubated overnight at 37 °C in the incubator before adjusted their optical density OD$_{600}$ to 0.10 absorbance (1.5 × 10^6 CFU/mL) using UV spectrophotometer (Secomam, Champigny sur Marne, France). The different masses of fibers (1, 2 and 4 mg) with the diameter around ~3 mm were applied directly on the MHA plate streaked with adjusted inoculum by following the method by Ravindra et al. [11]. The experiment was carried out in triplicate and the diameter of the inhibition zone was measured after 24 h of incubation at 37 °C. The data were reported in the mean ± standard error of the mean (S.E.) of three experiments.

2.6.2. Percentage of Bacterial Growth Inhibition

The percentage of bacterial growth inhibition in the presence of the C. pentandra/Ag-NPs was evaluated quantitatively by following the method of Shameli et al. [20] with some modification. This analysis is based on spectrophotometrically OD value measurements to evaluate bacterial growth. The different masses of fibers (1, 2 and 4 mg) were placed into a sterile 96-well plate. The inoculum was prepared by subculturing 100 µL of stock culture bacteria into new sterile MHB. The inoculum was incubated overnight at 37 °C in the incubator. Afterward, the optical density OD$_{600}$ of the bacterial suspension was adjusted to 1.0 absorbance using UV spectrophotometer (Secomam, Champigny sur Marne, France). This OD$_{600}$ value corresponds to 8 × 10^8 CFU/mL. The adjusted inoculum was then diluted to 10^5 (1:1000 dilution) CFU/mL using sterile MHB. The volume of 100 µL of adjusted inoculum (10^5 CFU/mL) was added to each 96-well plate containing the C. pentandra/Ag-NPs. The final volume of each 96-well plate ensures 140 µL by adding sterile MHB. The inoculum of C. pentandra/Ag-NPs free medium under the same condition and volume was used as a blank control. The blank control of C. pentandra/Ag-NPs sample in MHB media in the absence of inoculum was used. The ampicillin standard (8 µg/mL) was used as positive controls. All the 96-well plates were then sealed using parafilm to avoid the evaporation from each well followed by incubating at 37 °C for 18 h. After the incubation process, the OD$_{600}$ value of the inoculum in each well was determined using a microplate reader (Infinite 200, Tecan, Männedorf, Switzerland) at 600 nm wavelength. The data were reported in the mean ± standard error of the mean (S.E.) of three experiments. The percentage of bacterial growth inhibition rate was calculated using Equation (4) as below:

$$\text{Bacterial growth inhibition (\%)} = \left(\frac{OD_{control} - OD_{sample}}{OD_{control}}\right) \times 100 \qquad (4)$$

where, $OD_{control}$ is inoculum only, and OD_{sample} is the differences between $OD_{C.\ pentandra/Ag\text{-}NPs}$ with bacteria and $OD_{C.\ pentandra/Ag\text{-}NPs}$ without bacteria (blank).

2.6.3. Statistical Analysis

The statistical analysis was done using ANOVA (one way) analysis to compare the statistical difference among the groups. The analysis was further analyzed the post hoc Tukey HSD test to see which pairs are different between the groups using SPSS version 22. Significant p values <0.05 were considered statistically significant.

2.7. Catalytic Dye Reduction Application

The catalytic reduction of rhodamine B (RhB) and methylene blue (MB) dye by $NaBH_4$ as a model of the reaction has followed a method of Joseph and Mathew [21] and Vidhu and Philip [22] with some modification. Prior to the experiment, a mass of 0.1 g of C. pentandra/Ag-NPs was added into 100 mL of dye aqueous solution (20 mg/L). Thereafter, the suspension was magnetically stirred in the dark for 6 h for MB and 1 h for RhB dye, respectively. This step is important to establish the adsorption/desorption equilibrium between dye molecules and the surface of the Ag-NPs. After achieved the equilibrium, the freshly prepared of 10 mL of 0.1 M $NaBH_4$ solution was added to start the reaction. An amount of solution was withdrawn every 1 min for RhB dye and every 5 min for MB dye. The solution was then centrifuged and subjected to UV–vis spectrophotometer to measure the absorbance at 554 nm for RhB dye and 664 nm for MB dye. The percentage of dye reduction was calculated using Equation (5) as below:

$$\text{Dye reduction (\%)} = \frac{(C_0 - C_t)}{C_0} \times 100 \tag{5}$$

where C_0 and C_t are the concentration of the dye solution at a time corresponding to 0 and t at the characteristic wavelength, respectively [23].

The kinetics of the dye reduction reaction by C. pentandra/Ag-NPs was studied by following the pseudo-first-order and pseudo-second-order kinetic model. The equation of the pseudo-first-order model was described in Equation (6) [21] as below:

$$\ln[C_t]/[C_0] = kt \tag{6}$$

where, $[C_0]$ is the concentration of dye at time $t = 0$, $[C_t]$ is the concentration at time t, t is reaction time and k is pseudo-first-order rate constant. The plot of $\ln[C_t]$ against t was plotted to get the k constant value.

Moreover, the equation of the pseudo-second-order model was described in Equation (7) [23] as below:

$$\frac{1}{C_t} - \frac{1}{C_0} = kt \tag{7}$$

where, C_t and C_0 are the concentration of the dye solution at times t and 0 min, respectively, k is the pseudo-second-order rate constant. The plot of t/C_t against t was plotted to get the k constant value.

3. Results and Discussion

3.1. Characterization Studies of Alkaline Treated C. pentandra Fiber

The surface morphology of untreated C. pentandra fiber was observed using SEM analysis. The smooth surface of untreated C. pentandra fiber in the SEM images at different magnification is observed in Figure 3a,b. After alkaline treatment, it clearly showed the treated C. pentandra fiber have rougher, more flaky or grooved surface and less attached as seen in Figure 3c,d, respectively. The plant fiber surface becomes rougher and compressed due to the collapse of the lumen structure and removal of the hemicellulose and lignin covered on the cellulose region [24,25]. It is assumed that in the absence of hemicellulose and lignin-containing compositions on the fiber surface enhances the compatibility between fiber and matrix for the deposition of metal nanoparticles [26].

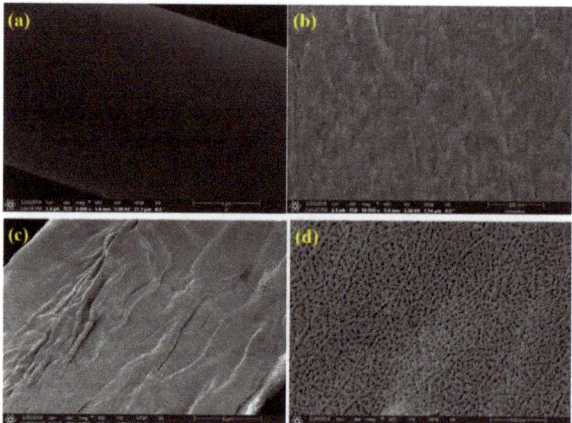

Figure 3. SEM images of (**a,b**) untreated *C. pentandra* fiber and (**c,d**) treated *C. pentandra* fiber at 6000× and 50,000× magnification, respectively.

The EDX spectra of untreated *C. pentandra* fiber show the major peak of Carbon (C) and Oxygen (O) elements with a percentage of 57.9% and 36.9%, respectively as shown in Figure 4a. These elements are attributed to the hemicellulose and cellulose as the main compositions in the untreated *C. pentandra* fiber. For the EDX spectra of treated *C. pentandra* fiber, besides the C (47.6%) and O (47.4%) as the major element, Na peak appeared at 1.0 KeV with a percentage of 3.8% as shown in Figure 4b. This peak was due to the treatment of *C. pentandra* fiber with NaOH solution. The peak of platinum (Pt) (1.2%) also appeared for both untreated and treated *C. pentandra* fiber due to the fiber was coated with the platinum for the analysis. The percentage of oxygen was increased from 36.9% to 47.4% after alkaline treatment proved that the increased of oxygen density after alkaline treatment. This was due to the disruption of the fiber clusters, removing the hemicellulose and lignin covered on the cellulose region [9,27].

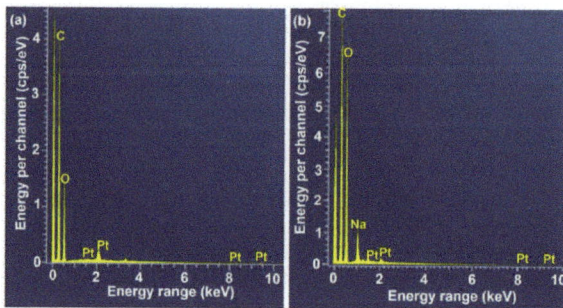

Figure 4. EDX spectra of (**a**) untreated *C. pentandra* fiber and (**b**) treated *C. pentandra* fiber.

The porosity of the treated *C. pentandra* fiber was further confirmed using surface area analysis based on Langmuir plots. The values of S_L surface area obtained for untreated *C. pentandra* fiber was 33.96 m^2/g. However, after treated with the alkaline solution, the treated *C. pentandra* fiber showed the values of S_L surface area was increased to 49.65 m^2/g. This result proved that the porosity of treated *C. pentandra* fiber was increased after treatment and also increased the surface area of *C. pentandra* fiber. The large surface area of treated *C. pentandra* fiber assisted the deposition of Ag-NPs in the fiber surface.

The decomposition profile of absorbed water, hemicellulose, cellulose and lignin-containing in *C. pentandra* fiber are depending on their weight compositions. The initial decomposition peak of fibers at a lower temperature (25 to 150 °C) is corresponding to the vaporization of absorbed water in the samples [7,25]. According to [28], hemicellulose starts to decompose at 220–315 °C, while the temperature range of 315–400 °C corresponds to the cellulose decomposition. However, lignin is decomposed at a wider temperature range (200 to 720 °C) [29]. The TGA and derivative thermogravimetry DTG curves of untreated *C. pentandra* fiber and treated *C. pentandra* fiber as a function of temperature are shown in Figure 5. The initial decomposition peak of untreated *C. pentandra* fiber approximately at ~100 °C (5%) is corresponding to vaporization of absorbed water in the samples as shown in Figure 5a. The main *C. pentandra* fiber decomposition occurred at perature around 200–370 °C. This peak region is corresponding to the peak of hemicellulose and lignin [25]. The weight loss of treated *C. pentandra* fiber was slightly decreased than untreated *C. pentandra* fiber from 71% to 69%, respectively. The DTG curve also showed the main *C. pentandra* fiber decomposition occurred in the region from 200–370 °C. The DTG peak was shifted from 320 to 341 °C for untreated and treated *C. pentandra* fiber, respectively corresponding to the cellulose decomposition. This result proved that the base treatment removed the hemicellulose and lignin in the *C. pentandra* fiber and exposed cellulose crystalline region for the attachment of Ag-NPs. The DTG curves of untreated *C. pentandra* fiber also show the small peak of decomposition at 221 °C. This peak is corresponding to the hemicellulose decomposition of untreated *C. pentandra* fiber. This peak is in line with the invisible peak at this region suggesting the removal of hemicellulose of the treated *C. pentandra* fiber during the alkaline treatment. In addition, a more intense peak was observed at 320 °C was due to the decomposition of hemicellulose and lignin. This finding proved that the removal of these compositions during the alkaline treatment to increase the roughness of *C. pentandra* fiber surface and increased the reactive site exposed on the surface for loading of Ag-NPs. The same observation was also reported by Fiore et al. [7], who reported that the removal of hemicellulose from the fiber after treated with NaOH solution. In Figure 5b, the degradation at 390–628 °C show slightly increased to 23% weight loss in comparison with untreated *C. pentandra* fiber corresponding to the increasing number of the macromolecules of *C. pentandra* fiber making it difficult to degrade at a higher temperature only and increased the thermal stability of treated *C. pentandra* fiber. A similar finding was reported by Komal et al. [30] proved that the effective removal of hemicellulose and waxes present on the surface of plant fiber resulted in the enhancement of the thermal stability of plant fiber after alkaline treatment.

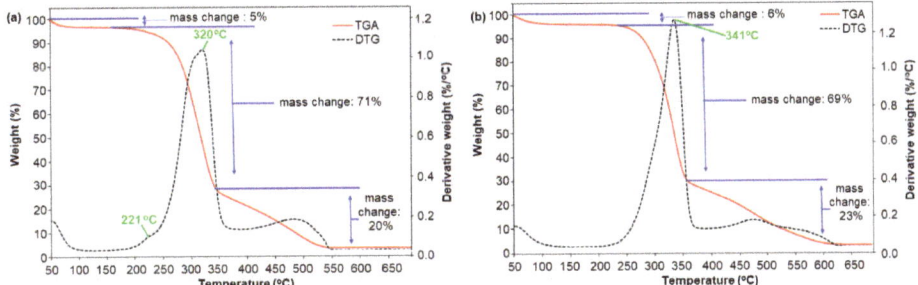

Figure 5. TGA and DTG curves of (**a**) untreated *C. pentandra* fiber and (**b**) treated *C. pentandra* fiber.

3.2. In-Situ Biofabrication of Ag-NPs in C. pentandra Fiber(C. pentandra/Ag-NPs)

The success of treated *C. pentandra* fiber incorporated with Ag-NPs can be preliminarily determined visually based on the color of the fiber. The photograph showed that the color of treated *C. pentandra*/Ag-NPs was changed to brown after the bio-fabrication process as shown in Figure 6. The schematic illustration of predicted mechanisms of Ag-NPs got in-situ deposited in the *C. pentandra* fiber also shown in Figure 6. This happened might be due to the interaction of Ag^+ ions with the functional groups like hydroxyl, carbonyl, ether, aldehyde and acetyl groups that is present in the cellulose of *C. pentandra* fiber and terpenoidal saponin compound of *E. spiralis* extract. The addition of *E. spiralis* extract in the bio-fabrication process help to control the size, shape and stability of Ag-NPs loaded into treated *C. pentandra* fiber.

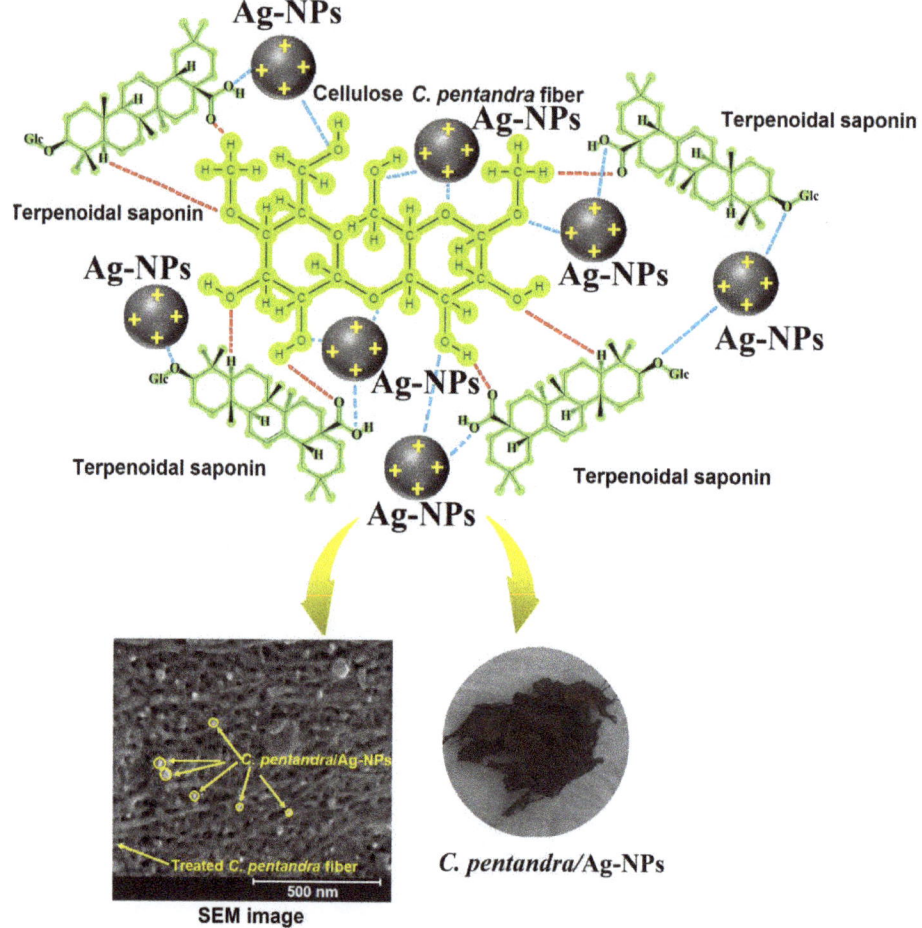

Figure 6. Schematic illustration predicted the formation of in-situ bio-fabrication of Ag-NPs using *E. spiralis* extract in *C. pentandra* fiber.

3.3. Characterization Studies of C. pentandra/Ag-NPs

3.3.1. UV-vis Spectroscopy Analysis

The UV-vis spectra of untreated *C. pentandra* fiber, treated *C. pentandra* fiber, *C. pentandra*/Ag-NPs are shown in Figure 7. The Ag peak in UV-vis spectra appeared around 400 to 450 nm. However, no Ag peak was observed in the UV-vis spectra of untreated and treated *C. pentandra* fiber alone. The highest intensity of Ag peak of *C. pentandra*/Ag-NPs appeared around 400–450 nm confirmed the success of Ag-NPs produced in *C. pentandra* fiber in the presence of *E. spiralis* extract [31].

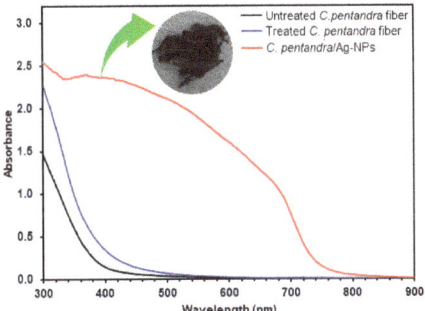

Figure 7. UV–vis spectra of untreated *C. pentandra* fiber, treated *C. pentandra* fiber and *C. pentandra*/Ag-NPs.

3.3.2. XRD Analysis

The crystalline structure of Ag-NPs incorporated in *C. pentandra* fiber can be determined using XRD analysis. The XRD pattern of treated *C. pentandra* fiber and *C. pentandra*/Ag-NPs is shown in Figure 8. The peak at 15.89°, 22.70° and 34.95° are corresponding to the amorphous peaks of treated *C. pentandra* fiber as shown in Figure 8a. However, the five diffraction peaks of *C. pentandra*/Ag-NPs appeared at 38.48°, 43.44°, 64.76°, 77.74° and 81.76° of 2θ value corresponding to (111), (200), (220), (311) and (222) of indexed of FCC plane of Ag, respectively as shown in Figure 8b. This crystallographic plane is based on ICDD/ICSD X'Pert High Score Plus (Ref. No. 01-087-0719). These peaks show the crystalline structure of Ag-NPs in *C. pentandra* fiber.

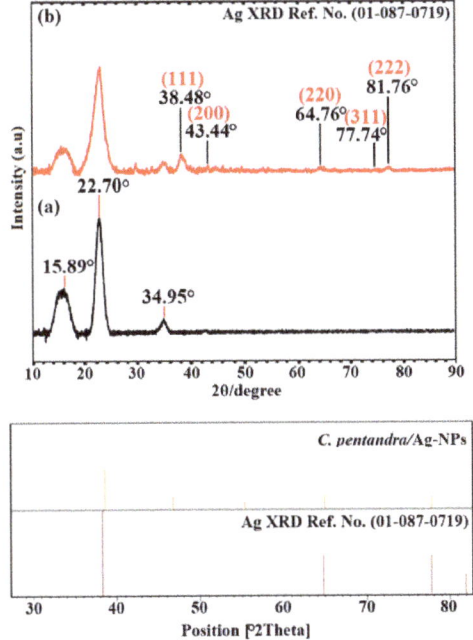

Figure 8. X-ray Diffraction (XRD) patterns of (**a**) treated *C. pentandra* fiber and (**b**) Ag-NPs in *C. pentandra* fiber.

3.3.3. FETEM and SAED Pattern Analyses

The FETEM image of C. pentandra/AgNO$_3$ is shown in Figure 9a. This result showed that the C. pentandra fiber itself also can act as a reducing agent by donating the electron and hydrogen atom from the negatively charged functional groups in the cellulose of fiber. However, the FETEM image observed the big size and aggregation of Ag-NPs were formed. The particle size distribution histogram measured the average size of Ag-NPs incorporated in C. pentandra fiber is 37.86 nm as shown in Figure 9b. Figure 9c showed the results of the SAED pattern and lattice d-spacing of C. pentandra/AgNO$_3$. The two rings around the SAED pattern at (111) and (311) is in line with the FCC plane of Ag-NPs of (111), (200), (220) and (222). Figure 9d showed the image of Ag-NPs with a latticed-spacing of ~0.14 nm correspond to the (220) cubic plane of Ag.

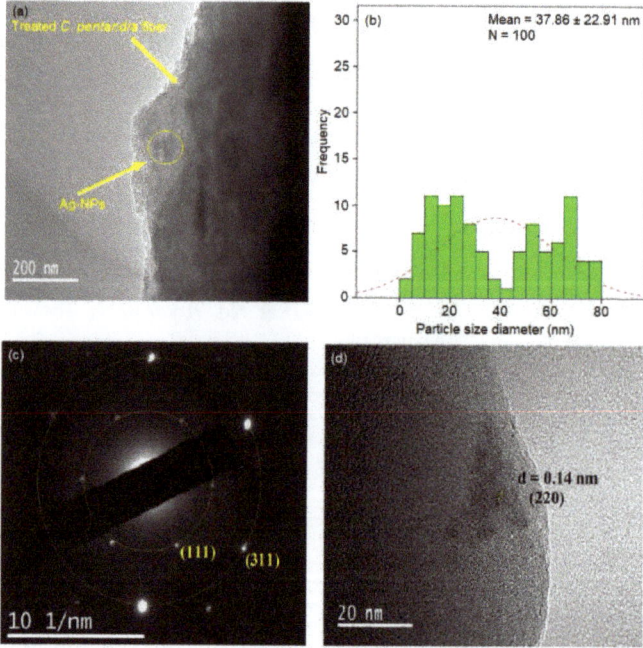

Figure 9. (a) Field Emission Transmission Electron Microscope (FETEM) image (b) particle size distribution histogram (c) SAED pattern and (d) lattice d-spacing parameter of C. pentandra/AgNO$_3$.

However, after the addition of E. spiralis extract in the process of incorporation of Ag-NPs in C. pentandra fiber, the smaller size average size of Ag-NPs was observed as shown in Figure 10a. The shape of Ag-NPs is a spherical shape. The average size of Ag-NPs incorporated in C. pentandra/Ag-NPs was decreased to 4.74 nm as shown in Figure 10b. The E. spiralis extract was introduced into the C. pentandra fiber to act as the reducing agent to reduce Ag$^+$ to Ag-NPs and also as stabilizing agent from its negatively charged functional groups in the E. spiralis extract. This result proved that the importance and novelty of using E. spiralis extract help to control the size, shape and stability of Ag-NPs with a simple technique, nontoxic and no additional of any chemical binding agent. Figure 10c,d showed the results of the SAED pattern and lattice d-spacing of C. pentandra/Ag-NPs, respectively. It clearly showed that the two rings around the SAED pattern at (200) and (222) are attributed to the FCC plane of Ag. This pattern is in line with the XRD pattern of the FCC plane of Ag-NPs of (111), (200), (220) and (222) of Ag-NPs. Figure 10c shows the image of C. pentandra/Ag-NPs with a latticed-spacing of ~0.23 nm correspond to the (111) FCC plane of Ag. This plane is consistent with the appearance of the highest intensity of XRD peak at angle 38.48° (111) cubic plane of Ag as shown in Figure 8b.

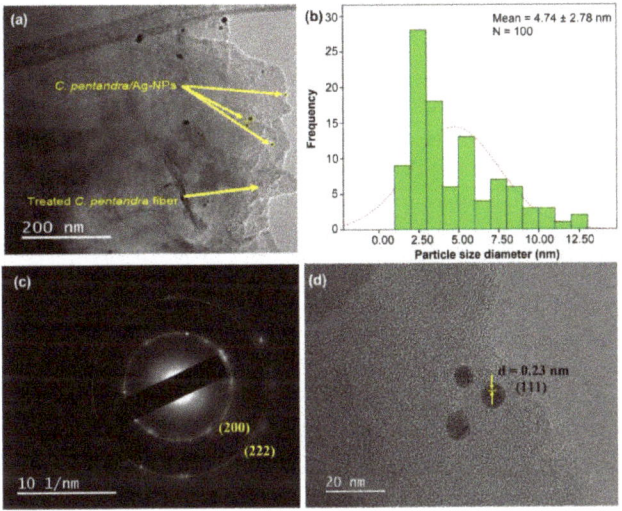

Figure 10. (a) FETEM image (b) particle size distribution histogram (c) SAED pattern and (d) latticed-spacing parameter of C. pentandra/Ag-NPs.

3.3.4. SEM and EDX Analyses

The SEM image of C. pentandra/Ag-NPs is shown in Figure 11a. From the image, it shows that the attachment of C. pentandra /Ag-NPs distributed on the rough surface of treated C. pentandra fiber. The smaller size of C. pentandra /Ag-NPs in a spherical shape surface showing that the significant of E. spiralis extract as reducing and stabilizing agent for loading of Ag-NPs in the C. pentandra fiber surface. In the EDX spectrum, the Ag peak was detected at 3.0 KeV with a percentage of 5.1% as shown in Figure 11b. The appearance peak of C and O elements with the percentage of 75.6% and 19.3% respectively are corresponding to the cellulose compositions in the treated C. pentandra fiber.

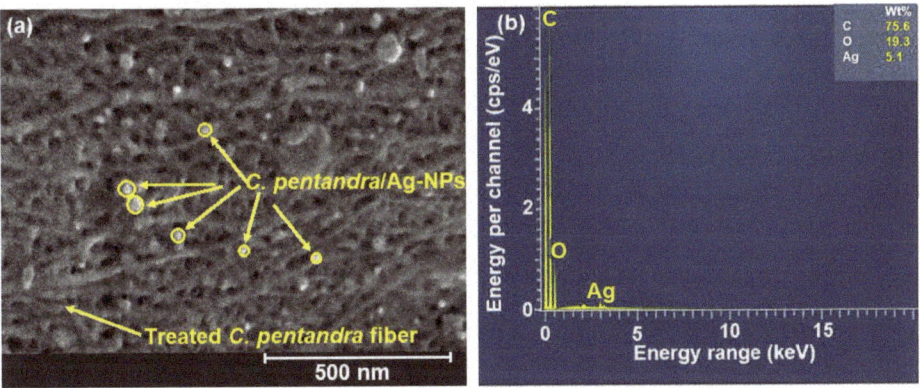

Figure 11. (a) SEM image and (b) EDX spectra of C. pentandra/Ag-NPs.

3.3.5. TGA Analysis

The TGA and DTG curves of *C. pentandra*/Ag-NPs as a function of temperature are shown in Figure 12. The initial peak decomposition of *C. pentandra* /Ag-NPs occurred approximately at ~100 °C (5% weight loss) corresponded to the vaporization of absorbed water in the fiber. The DTG curves show the small peak of *C. pentandra*/Ag-NPs decomposition occurred at 188 °C (1%). This peak corresponded to the peak of NO_3^- that is derived from $AgNO_3$ solution. The small peak of NO_3^- decomposition indicates the Ag^+ ions were reduced to Ag^0. The major DTG curve peak decompositions of *C. pentandra*/Ag-NPs occurred at 349 °C (75% of weight loss) corresponding to the cellulose region of the treated *C. pentandra* fiber. This result also shows that the possible mechanism of loading of Ag-NPs into treated *C. pentandra* fiber occurred at the cellulose region. This phenomenon suggests that the Ag-NPs were successfully loaded into the treated *C. pentandra* fiber using $AgNO_3$ as Ag precursor.

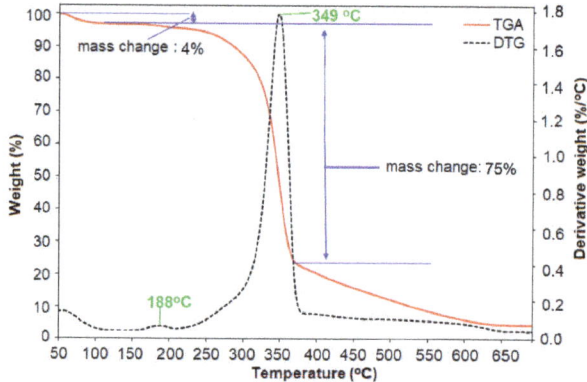

Figure 12. DTG curves of *C. pentandra*/Ag-NPs a function of temperature.

3.3.6. FTIR Analysis

The functional groups of cellulose, hemicellulose and lignin in the *C. pentandra* fiber can be analyzed using FTIR analysis. Generally, the cellulose fiber structure consists of carbonyl, carboxyl and aldehyde groups [32]. These compositions untreated and alkaline treated on *C. pentandra* fiber were investigated based on the peak shifting of the related functional groups in the FTIR spectra. The FTIR spectra of untreated *C. pentandra* fiber appeared its absorption bands were at 3346, 2918, 1736, 1314, 1238, 1037 and 604 cm^{-1} as shown in Figure 13a. The peak at 3346 cm^{-1} is responsible for the hydroxyl group stretching of the hydrogen bonding network. At the peak of 2918 cm^{-1} is related to the functional groups of C–H stretching vibration of methyl and methylene groups in cellulose or hemicellulose structure [33]. The peak at 1736 cm^{-1} is corresponding to the C=O stretching vibration of hemicellulose [25]. The peak at 1314 cm^{-1} is corresponding to the C–H bending of aldehyde groups of cellulose structure. The peak at 1238 cm^{-1} is corresponding to the C–O stretching of the acetyl groups in the hemicellulose. The peak at 1037 cm^{-1} is responsible for due to the presence of xylane and the glycosidic linkages of hemicellulose [25]. The peak at 604 cm^{-1} related to the bonding of oxygen from the hydroxyl groups.

After alkaline treatment of *C. pentandra* fiber, the FTIR spectrum showed the shift in wavenumber or changes in peak intensity explains the types of functional groups involved in the fiber as shown in Figure 13b. The treated *C. pentandra* fiber showed the peak shifted from 3346 to 3337 cm^{-1} suggests the hydroxyl group stretching of the hydrogen bonding network in the treated *C. pentandra* fiber. The peak at 2899 cm^{-1} was shifted from 2918 cm^{-1} for untreated *C. pentandra* fiber suggests the C–H stretching vibration of methyl and methylene groups in the cellulose structure [25]. The peak 1735 cm^{-1} in the untreated *C. pentandra* fiber was disappeared in the treated *C. pentandra* fiber spectra was due to the removal of hemicellulose after alkaline treatment. The peak 1314 cm^{-1} of untreated *C. pentandra* fiber was shifted to 1321 cm^{-1} suggesting C–H bending of aldehyde groups of cellulose structure of treated *C. pentandra* fiber. The intensity of the peak at 1280 cm^{-1} was decreased after alkaline treatment suggesting that the C–O stretching of the acetyl groups. The peak at 1037 cm^{-1} of untreated fiber was shifted to 1027 cm^{-1} with strong peak intensity relate to the presence of xylane and the glycosidic linkages. This major peak shifted can be related to the removal of the hemicellulose structure of treated *C. pentandra* fiber after alkaline treated. This result supported the finding in TGA analysis asserted that the hemicellulose of *C. Pentandra* fiber was removed after alkaline treatment. The peak shifted at 560 cm^{-1} is related to the bonding of oxygen from the hydroxyl groups.

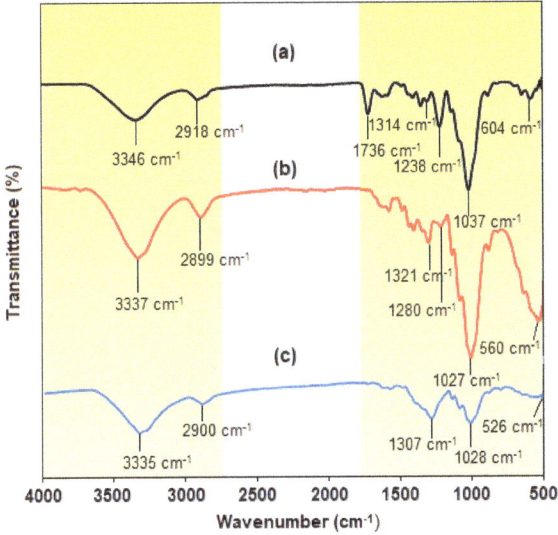

Figure 13. Fourier Transform Infrared (FTIR) spectra of (**a**) untreated *C. pentandra* fiber, (**b**) treated *C. pentandra* fiber and (**c**) *C. pentandra*/Ag-NPs.

The FTIR spectrum of *C. pentandra*/Ag-NPs showed the absorption bands at 3335, 2900, 1307, 1028 and 526 cm^{-1} as shown in Figure 13c. After loaded with Ag-NPs, the peak shifted to the 3335 cm^{-1} suggesting to the hydroxyl group stretching of the hydrogen bonding network. The peak shifted to the 2899 cm^{-1} suggesting the C–H stretching vibration of methyl and methylene groups in cellulose and hemicellulose structure. The cellulose structure has an aldehyde group (–CHO) which was oxidized to carboxylic acid, while Ag$^+$ ion was reduced to Ag-NPs. This mechanism caused the incorporation of Ag-NPs in *C. pentandra* fiber by strong attachment between Ag-NPs and *C. pentandra* fiber. The peak at 1280 cm^{-1} in the treated *C. pentandra* fiber was disappeared suggesting that the involvement of C–O stretching of the acetyl groups in the hemicellulose for loading Ag-NPs into *C. pentandra* fiber. The peak intensity at 1028 cm^{-1} was decreased after loaded with Ag-NPs suggesting the C–OH of a primary group of the gluco–pyranose ring. The peak shifted at 526 cm^{-1} is related to the bonding of oxygen from the hydroxyl groups in the *C. pentandra* fiber. The FTIR analysis shows the functional groups of *C. pentandra* fiber cellulose structures which consist of carbonyl, carboxyl and aldehyde groups. These functional groups are responsible for the reduction of Ag$^+$ ions to Ag-NPs.

3.4. Silver Content Analysis in C. pentandra/Ag-NPs

The amount of Ag-NPs deposited in *C. pentandra*/Ag-NPs was determined quantitatively using ICP-OES analysis. The amount of Ag-NPs calculated from *C. pentandra*/Ag-NPs was 40.19 g/kg while for C. pentandra/AgNO$_3$, the amount of Ag-NPs calculated was only 35.47 g/kg. In the presence of E. spiralis extract, increased the reducing agent to the C. pentandra fiber for the reduction of Ag$^+$ to Ag^0. Thus, increased the amount of Ag-NPs incorporated in C. pentandra fiber.

3.5. Silver Ions Release of C. pentandra/Ag-NPs

The antibacterial activity of Ag-NPs is related with the release of Ag$^+$ ions from Ag-NPs. In this study, the percentage of Ag$^+$ ions release rate was observed from 0 to 144 h. In 6 h, the percentage of Ag$^+$ ions release rate is 90% and increased to 97% after 144 h as shown in Figure 14. This result supports the potential of C. pentandra/Ag-NPs as an antibacterial activity over a long time and highly diffusive of Ag$^+$ ions to diffuse in the media and inhibit the bacteria growth. This Ag$^+$ ions release caused toxic to the cell of bacteria by generating reactive oxygen species (ROS) and finally caused death of bacteria [34]. Besides that, by supporting Ag-NPs in C. pentandra fiber can control the aggregation of the colloidal Ag-NPs which resulted to no bioactivity and bioavailability of Ag-NPs in the media and reduced their antibacterial activity. The usage of Ag-NPs is widely applied due to their slower dissolution rate which led to a continuous release of Ag$^+$ ions from Ag-NPs [35]. In addition, the smaller size of Ag-NPs gives advantages by releasing more Ag$^+$ ions to the media and inhibits the bacteria growth. The Ag-NPs also are highly diffusive ions into the culture growth medium which are influenced by the oxidation and dilution process from Ag-NPs to Ag$^+$ ions [36]. In addition, Ag-NPs also easily dissociate into Ag$^+$ ions after contact with water.

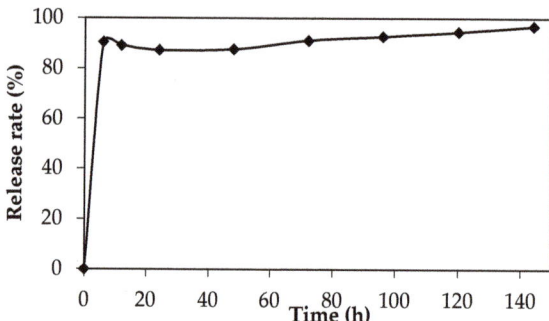

Figure 14. The release rate of Ag$^+$ ions from 6 to 144 h of C. pentandra/Ag-NPs.

3.6. Antibacterial Application

3.6.1. Antibacterial Disk Diffusion Assay

The qualitative analysis of the antibacterial activity of C. pentandra/Ag-NPs was evaluated based on the diameter of growth inhibition zone against the tested bacteria and the results are shown in Figure 15. The C. pentandra/Ag-NPs inhibited the growth of all tested bacteria species in a dose-dependent manner. The results showed that the diameter of the growth inhibition zone increased with an increasing amount of C. pentandra/Ag-NPs from 1 to 4 mg as shown in Table 1. The significant differences in the diameter of the growth inhibition zone were also observed between the amounts of C. pentandra/Ag-NPs used ($p < 0.05$). The multiple comparison post hoc test value showed no significant difference in the diameter of the growth inhibition zone between the mass from 1 to 2 mg of C. pentandra/Ag-NPs ($p > 0.05$). By increasing the mass of C. pentandra/Ag-NPs up to 4 mg, the diameter of the growth inhibition zone increased significantly ($p < 0.05$). The finding can be explained due to the more Ag-NPs accumulated on the bacterial surface which can enter the cell and damage the nuclei and eventually causing bacterial death [37]. The suppression of bacterial growth increased with the increase in the amount of Ag-NPs is in agreement with the finding from the research by Sowmyya and Lakshmi [38].

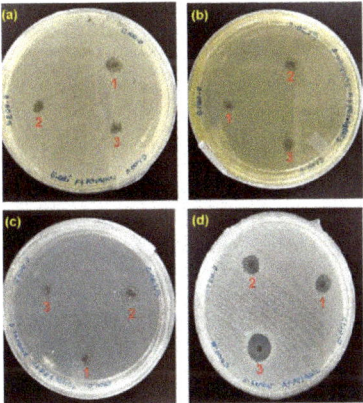

Figure 15. The images of inhibition zones growth against (**a**) *E. coli*, (**b**) *P. vulgaris*, (**c**) *E. faecalis* and (**d**) *S. aureus* around the different mass of *C. pentandra* incorporated with Ag-NPs at 1 (1 mg), 2 (2 mg), and 3 (4 mg).

Table 1. The diameter of the growth inhibition zone of *C. pentandra*/Ag-NPs against different bacteria species.

Sample	The Diameter of Growth Inhibition Zone (mm) [a]			
	Bacteria Species			
	E. coli	*P. vulgaris*	*E. faecalis*	*S. aureus*
Mass of *C. pentandra*/Ag-NPs (mg)				
a) 1	7.25 ± 0.20	6.00 ± 0.82	6.75 ± 0.61	8.25 ± 0.20
b) 2	8.00 ± 0.41	6.50 ± 0.41	7.50 ± 1.22	8.75 ± 1.02
c) 4	9.50 ± 0.41	7.50 ± 0.71	8.25 ± 0.20	9.75 ± 0.20
Control				
Gentamicin (positive control) (10 µg)	19.50 ± 0.71	23.50 ± 0.41	15.50 ± 0.41	21.75 ± 0.20
E. spiralis extract (negative control)	NA	NA	NA	NA
Treated fiber (negative control)	NA	NA	NA	NA
Untreated fiber (negative control)	NA	NA	NA	NA

NA means no activity; [a] is mean of the triplicate experiment, ±Standard Error (S.E).

For the bacteria species, the order of the strongest antibacterial activity of *C. pentandra*/Ag-NPs was *S. aureus*. The less antibacterial activity of *C. pentandra*/Ag-NPs against *P. vulgaris* might be due to the presence of capsule on the bacterial cell wall and the negatively charged of the outer lipid membrane (lipopolysaccharide) cover [39]. The electrostatic repulsion between the nanoparticles and Gram-negative bacteria hinders particles attachment and penetration into the cells [4]. However, the negatively charged of *C. pentandra*/Ag-NPs can bind electrostatically with the negatively charged of teichoic acid present in Gram-positive bacteria cell leading to the enhancement of cell permeability, cytoplasmic leakage and cell death [4,40].

Further analysis was tested on the significant differences in antibacterial activity between Gram-positive and Gram-negative bacteria. Surprisingly, the difference between these bacteria is not significant ($p > 0.05$). This result approved that the *C. pentandra*/Ag-NPs possessed antibacterial activity against both types of bacteria. According to Pollini et al. [41], a diameter of more than 1.0 mm of the microbial growth inhibition zone can be considered as a good antibacterial product. In this study, the *C. pentandra*/Ag-NPs which exhibited more than 1.0 mm of growth inhibition zone has potential antibacterial application, especially in biomedical, textile, wastewater treatment and food packaging areas. The performance of antibacterial activities of *C. pentandra*/Ag-NPs with other Ag-NPs is shown in Table 2. From the Table 2, it showed that the *C. pentandra*/Ag-NPs have comparable antibacterial activities compare to other Ag-NPs. This result showed *C. pentandra*/Ag-NPs have good antibacterial activities for both Gram-positive and Gram-negative bacteria. Yet, the good dispersion of Ag-NPs on the *C. pentandra* surface can contact well with bacteria and releasing more Ag^+ ions for the effective antibacterial mechanisms.

Table 2. The comparison on the performance of antibacterial activities based on the zone of growth inhibition by *C. pentandra*/Ag-NPs with other Ag-NPs loaded in supporting materials reported in the literature.

Supporting Material	Bacteria	The Zone of Growth Inhibition (mm)	Ref.
Ag-NPs loaded in *C. pentandra* fiber	E. coli	6.5 ± 0.4	This study
	P. vulgaris	4.3 ± 0.7	
	E. faecalis	5.3 ± 0.2	
	S.aurues	6.8 ± 0.2	
Ag-NPs loaded in cotton pad	E. coli	6.2 ± 1.4	[1]
	L. monocytogens	3.1 ± 1.1	
	S.aureus	3.3 ± 1.2	
	S. epidermis	3.3 ± 1.2	
ZnO loaded in cotton	S.aureus	3.1 ± 0.1	[42]
	E. coli	3.3 ± 0.1	
Ag-NPs loaded in Jute fiber	B. subtillus	1.0 ± 0.9	[33]
	E. coli	2.5 ± 0.8	
Ag-NPs loaded in cotton	E. coli	1.5	[11]

3.6.2. Percentage of Bacterial Growth Inhibition

The inhibition of bacterial growth was further determined quantitatively based on the OD_{600} value measurements. The percentage of bacterial growth inhibition of *C. pentandra*/Ag-NPs against the tested bacteria is summarized in Table 3. The percentage of bacterial growth inhibition showed high inhibitory activity against all tested bacteria which supported the results obtained by using antibacterial disk diffusion assay analysis. Surprisingly, the percentage of inhibition of bacterial growth by ampicillin antibiotic standard is lower than that of *C. pentandra*/Ag-NPs. However, there is no significant difference in the percentage of inhibition of bacterial growth between the bacteria species used ($p > 0.05$). The percentage of inhibition of bacterial growth of Gram-positive bacteria (*S. aureus* and *E. faecalis*) is lower than Gram-negative bacteria (*E.coli* and *P. vulgaris*). However, there is no significant difference in the percentage of inhibited bacterial growth between the species used ($p > 0.05$). This might be due to the less structural difference in cell wall compositions between Gram-positive and Gram-negative bacteria [43]. The high percentage of bacterial growth inhibition was observed for *C. pentandra*/Ag-NPs at the highest dosage (4 mg) against all tested bacteria (>90%). Conversely, there is no significant difference with the increasing mass of *C. pentandra*/Ag-NPs used from 1 to 4 mg. This can be explained due to the Ag-NPs deposited on the *C. pentandra* fiber surface are randomly distributed on the *C. pentandra* fiber surface.

Table 3. The percentage of bacterial growth inhibition of *C. pentandra*/Ag-NPs against different bacteria species.

Sample Mass of *C. pentandra*/Ag-NPs (mg)	The Percentage of Bacterial Growth Inhibition (%) [a]			
	Bacteria Species			
	E. coli	P. vulgaris	E. faecalis	S. aureus
a) 1	80.91	93.23	93.87	88.76
b) 2	95.45	93.69	97.96	89.28
c) 4	96.61	97.40	99.60	92.50
Ampicillin (positive control) (8 µg/mL)	81.31	50.27	96.00	97.63

NA means no activity; [a] is mean of the triplicate experiment, ±Standard Error (SE).

3.7. Catalytic Dye Reduction Application

3.7.1. Rhodamine B Dye

The catalytic properties of *C. pentandra*/Ag-NPs on the reduction of RhB dye with $NaBH_4$ is shown in Figure 16. The decrease in absorbance peak intensity at 554 nm as a function of time reflects the decrease in the concentration of RhB in the system. A controlled experiment was performed on RhB dye in the presence of NaBH$_4$ only. The result indicates that in the absence of C. pentandra/Ag-NPs, the peak at 554 nm slightly decreased in absorbance of RhB dye solution (20 mg/L) even after 120 min of reaction time (4%) as shown in Figure 16a. This result also displays the reduction of organic dyes by NaBH$_4$ is possible but not kinetically favorable due to the kinetic barriers differences in the thermodynamic potential of electron donor (NaBH$_4$) and acceptor (RhB dye) [44]. After the addition of C. pentandra/Ag-NPs under the same condition, the RhB dye peak–peak at 554 nm decreased quickly and reaches an equilibrium reaction time within 4 min (94%). A new peak was observed around 402 nm corresponding to the peak of Ag as shown in Figure 16b.

This indicates that the ability of C. pentandra/Ag-NPs which can act as nanocatalyst and accelerate the reaction. According to Ganguly et al. [45], the reduction of dye molecules generally obeys two stages pathway; initially adsorption of dye molecules onto the Ag-NPs catalyst surface followed by electron transfer phenomenon among catalyst, BH$_4^-$ ions and dye molecules. The peak observed around 400 to 450 nm at all concentrations of RhB tested corresponding to the peak of Ag as evidence of electron relay process between BH$_4^-$ ions and RhB dye during the reduction reaction process. This peak was shifted to the blue shift and less intensity than observed in the case of RhB dye reduction. This was due to the fact that the λ_{max} of RhB is detached from the SPR absorption of Ag-NPs and reduces the possibility of interaction between these two peaks [21]. The Ag peak was increased with decreasing reduction time until the completed reaction shows that more Ag-NPs involved as electron relay transfer process and RhB is detached during the reduction reaction.

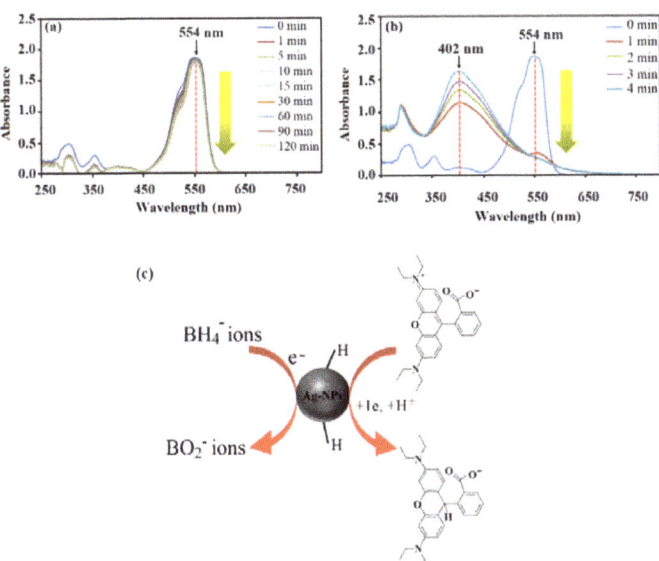

Figure 16. UV–vis spectra of reduction of RhB dye by (**a**) NaBH$_4$ alone, (**b**) in the presence of C. pentandra/Ag-NPs at 20 mg/L RhB and (**c**) the proposed mechanism of C. pentandra/Ag-NPs as nanocatalyst for the reduction of RhB dye.

The proposed mechanism of catalytic reaction by C. pentandra/Ag-NPs on the RhB dye reduction can be illustrated in Figure 16c. The redox potential of Ag-NPs is in between the RhB dye (−0.48 V) and NaBH$_4$ (−1.33 V) [46]. Thus, can act as electron transfer agents and relay electron from the donor NaBH$_4$ to the acceptor RhB dye. Upon the addition of C. pentandra/Ag-NPs, the BH$_4^-$ ions dissociate from NaBH$_4$ and donate the electrons as well as transfer it to C. pentandra/Ag-NPs. The RhB dye on the surface of C. pentandra/Ag-NPs will be accepted that electrons and reduced dye molecules. The negatively charged of C. pentandra/Ag-NPs surface brings the RhB dye molecules closer to the surface of C. pentandra/Ag-NPs via electrostatic attraction.

3.7.2. Methylene Blue Dye

The aqueous solution of MB dye appeared strong absorption peak at 664 nm (λ_{max}) and reduction of MB dye with time by C. pentandra/Ag-NPs was monitored at this peak. The decreasing of absorbance peak at 664 nm with times reflects the decrease in the concentration of MB in the system. This peak was reduced to leucomethylene blue [47]. The reduction of MB dye by NaBH$_4$ in the absence of C. pentandra/Ag-NPs as nanocatalyst is shown in Figure 17a. From the figure, it shows that a similar trend was observed as in RB dyes where there are no significant changes observed after 120 min. This proved that the reduction of MB dye by NaBH$_4$ is not kinetically favorable [48]. However, after the addition of C. pentandra/Ag-NPs, the fast reduction time occurred within 20 min (99%) as shown in Figure 17b. The fastest reduction time was achieved at 20 mg/L MB using C. pentandra/Ag-NPs due to good distribution of Ag-NPs on the C. pentandra fiber surface to be contacted with the MB dye molecule and BH_4^- ions effectively [45]. The peak observed at 425 nm is corresponding to the peak of Ag. However, a lower intensity of the Ag peak was obtained suggesting that the release of Ag in the solution was controlled by the attachment of Ag-NPs on the C. pentandra fiber surface. The amount of Ag detected in all solutions was less than 5%. This result showed that the Ag-NPs loaded in C. pentandra/Ag-NPs can limit the release of Ag-NPs in the environment at only low concentrations of Ag. This is happened due to the Ag-NPs after loaded in C. pentandra fiber are strongly attached to the C. pentandra fiber. This result suggests that the C. pentandra/Ag-NPs increase the stability and avoid the agglomeration of Ag-NPs from the attachment on the C. pentandra fiber surface without decreasing the catalytic performance of Ag-NPs besides controlling the release of Ag-NPs into the solution.

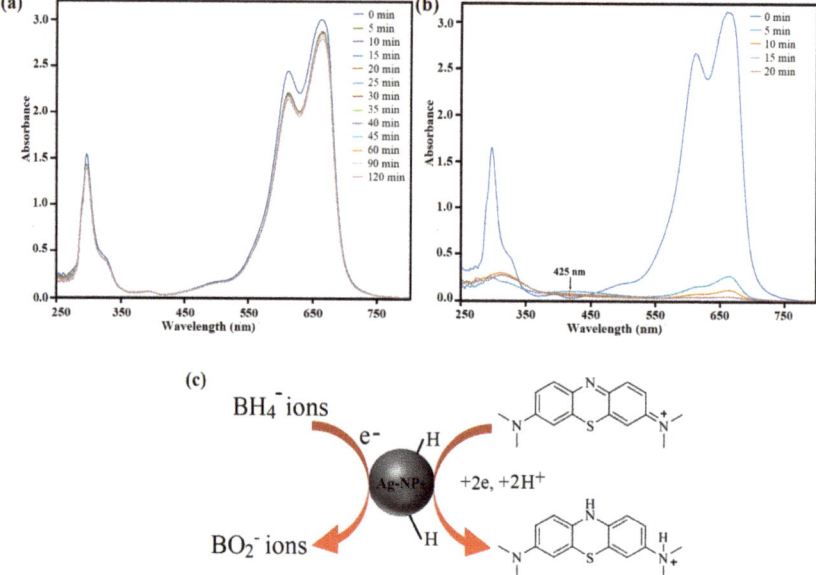

Figure 17. UV–vis spectra of reduction of MB dye by (a) NaBH$_4$ alone, (b) in the presence of C. pentandra/Ag-NPs and (c) the proposed mechanism of C. pentandra/Ag-NPs as nanocatalyst for the reduction of MB dye.

The proposed mechanism of catalytic reaction by C. pentandra/Ag-NPs on the MB dye reduction can be illustrated in Figure 17c. The catalytic reduction by C. pentandra/Ag-NPs followed electron transfer process from Ag-NPs catalyst to MB dye molecules. This electron transfer is depending on the small size of Ag-NPs to make contact with the dye molecules. Then, the MB dye molecules earn the electron from the catalyst surface to reduce its colorless and product.

3.7.3. Kinetic Study

The kinetic study was studied using a pseudo-first-order and pseudo-second-order model. The applicability of the kinetic models was determined based on the correlation coefficient (R^2) value of a particular model. The pseudo-first-order kinetic model can be described as the diffusion control process through a boundary [49]. The pseudo-second-order kinetic model is based on the assumption that the rate-determining step is due to chemisorption [50,51]. The pseudo-second-order kinetic process is greatly affected by the number of metal ions on the Ag-NPs [52]. The rate constant (k) of the RhB and MB dye reduction process by C. pentandra/Ag-NPs can be determined from the slope of the plot for both models as shown in Table 4. Based on the correlation coefficients value (R^2), the reduction of both RhB and MB dye by C. pentandra/Ag-NPs is fitted well with pseudo-first-order model for both RhB and MB dye suggest that the diffusion control process through a boundary was occurred [49]. Diffused BH_4^- ions produced hydrogen that was attached over the Ag-NPs surface together with dye molecules. Then, the electron transfer between Ag-NPs donated by BH_4^- ions to the dye molecules were occurred to degrade dye [48].

Table 4. The results of pseudo-first-order and pseudo-second-order kinetic model of RhB and MB dye reduction by C. pentandra/Ag-NPs.

Dye	Pseudo-First-Order		Pseudo-Second-Order	
	k (min^{-1})	R^2	k (min^{-1})	R^2
RhB	0.7475	0.9912	1.5101	0.8284
MB	0.3582	0.9765	1.8653	0.8767

The performance of C. pentandra/Ag-NPs for the catalytic reduction of RhB and MB dye was compared with other reported Ag-NPs catalyst as shown in Table 5. It can be concluded, the reduction rate recorded from this work can be considered as the good nanocatalyst to reduce dyes using an environmentally benign method, simple method, efficient, easy to separate, stable nanoparticles, difficult to swelling and no need to add a binding agent.

Table 5. Comparison of the catalytic reduction performance of MB and RhB dye by AgNPs nanocatalyst synthesized from another method of preparation.

Method	Catalyst	Dye	Concentration (mg/L)	Reduction Time (min)	k (min^{-1})	Ref.
NaBH$_4$	Ag-NPs loading on C. pentandra fiber	MB RhB	20	10 5	0.75 0.36	This study
NaBH$_4$	Ag-NPs	MB RhB	0.001	12 10	0.18 0.22	[38]
NaBH$_4$	Ag-NPs loading on polypyrrole coated	MB RhB	1.5	10 10	- -	[53]
NaBH$_4$	Ag-NPs	MB	5	30	-	[54]
Photocatalytic	Ag-NPs	MB	5	60	0.007	[55]
Photocatalytic	Ag-NPs	MB	15	80	-	[56]

4. Conclusions

As a conclusion, in-situ bio-fabrication of Ag-NPs in alkaline treated *C. pentandra* fiber as supporting materials were successfully assembled using *E. spiralis* extract and AgNO$_3$ solution. This method also is significant to control the bioavailability and bioactivity of Ag-NPs in the antibacterial and dye reduction catalytic application. In addition, the incorporation of Ag-NPs in the *C. pentandra* fiber can control the adverse effect of nanoscale of Ag-NPs by strong association of Ag-NPs with the negatively charged of functional group in the cellulose of *C. pentandra* fiber. The TGA analysis also shows that the possible mechanism of loading of Ag-NPs into treated *C. pentandra* fiber occurred at cellulose region and alkaline treatment helped to expose more cellulose region for loading of Ag-NPs into *C. pentandra* fiber. The characterization studies clearly showed the significant of *E. spiralis* extract as reducing and stabilizing agents added for loading of Ag-NPs on the *C. pentandra* fiber surface. The prepared *C. pentandra*/Ag-NPs also exhibited good antibacterial activity towards both Gram-positive and Gram-negative bacteria *S. aureus*, *E. faecalis*, *E. coli* and *P. vulgaris*. *C. pentandra*/Ag-NPs also display the ability as catalytic activity towards the Rhodamine B and methylene blue dyes. The *C. pentandra*/Ag-NPs have potential as a promising nanomaterial for biomedical applications such as for wound healing and coating of biomaterials, wastewater treatment, food packaging and textile in the wide range of microorganism.

Author Contributions: Synthesis, experimental works and writing original draft, W.K.A.W.M.K.; supervision, review and editing, K.S.; dye catalytic analysis or interpretation of data, review and editing, N.W.C.J.; Sample characterization, N.A.O.; antibacterial analysis or interpretation of data, review and editing, N.M.H. and S.D.J. All authors have read and agreed to the published version of the manuscript.

Funding: This research received no external funding.

Acknowledgments: The authors would like to express sincere gratitude to the Universiti Teknologi Malaysia for financial support under research university grants (Grants No. #4B422, #15H73, #20H33 and #20H55). All authors are thankful to Malaysia–Japan International Institute of Technology (MJIIT) of UTM for providing an excellent research environment to complete this work.

Conflicts of Interest: The authors declare no conflict of interest.

References

1. Shankar, S.; Rhim, J.W. Facile approach for large-scale production of metal and metal oxide nanoparticles and preparation of antibacterial cotton pads. *Carbohydr. Polym.* **2017**, *163*, 137–145. [CrossRef]
2. Jeong, S.H.; Yeo, S.Y.; Yi, S.C. The effect of filler particle size on the antibacterial properties of compounded polymer/silver fibers. *J. Mater. Sci.* **2005**, *40*, 5407–5411. [CrossRef]
3. Ahmed, M.A.; Messih, M.F.A.; El-Sherbeny, E.F.; El-Hafez, S.F.; Khalifa, A.M.M. Synthesis of metallic silver nanoparticles decorated mesoporous SnO2 for removal of methylene blue dye by coupling adsorption and photocatalytic processes. *J. Photochem. Photobiol. A Chem.* **2017**, *346*, 77–88. [CrossRef]
4. Ahmad, A.; Wei, Y.; Syed, F.; Tahir, K.; Rehman, A.U.; Khan, A.; Ullah, S.; Yuan, Q. The effects of bacteria-nanoparticles interface on the antibacterial activity of green synthesized silver nanoparticles. *Microb. Pathog.* **2017**, *102*, 133–142. [CrossRef]
5. Chouhan, N.; Ameta, R.; Meena, R.K. Biogenic silver nanoparticles from Trachyspermum ammi (Ajwain) seeds extract for catalytic reduction of p-nitrophenol to p-aminophenol in excess of NaBH$_4$. *J. Mol. Liq.* **2017**, *230*, 74–84. [CrossRef]
6. Varadavenkatesan, T.; Selvaraj, R.; Vinayagam, R. Phyto-synthesis of silver nanoparticles from Mussaenda erythrophylla leaf extract and their application in catalytic degradation of methyl orange dye. *J. Mol. Liq.* **2016**, *221*, 1063–1070. [CrossRef]
7. Fiore, V.; Scalici, T.; Nicoletti, F.; Vitale, G.; Prestipino, M.; Valenza, A. A new eco-friendly chemical treatment of natural fibres: Effect of sodium bicarbonate on properties of sisal fibre and its epoxy composites. *Compos. Part B Eng.* **2016**, *85*, 150–160. [CrossRef]
8. Ramesh, M.; Palanikumar, K.; Reddy, K.H. Plant fibre based bio-composites: Sustainable and renewable green materials. *Renew. Sustain. Energy Rev.* **2017**, *79*, 558–584. [CrossRef]

9. Dong, B.H.; Hinestroza, J.P. Metal nanoparticles on natural cellulose fibers: Electrostatic assembly and in situ synthesis. *ACS Appl. Mater. Interfaces* **2009**, *1*, 797–803. [CrossRef]
10. Xu, S.; Chen, S.; Zhang, F.; Jiao, C.; Song, J.; Chen, Y.; Lin, H.; Gotoh, Y.; Morikawa, H. Preparation and controlled coating of hydroxyl-modified silver nanoparticles on silk fibers through intermolecular interaction-induced self-assembly. *Mater. Des.* **2016**, *95*, 107–118. [CrossRef]
11. Ravindra, S.; Murali Mohan, Y.; Narayana Reddy, N.; Mohana Raju, K. Fabrication of antibacterial cotton fibres loaded with silver nanoparticles via "Green Approach". *Colloids Surf. A Physicochem. Eng. Asp.* **2010**, *367*, 31–40. [CrossRef]
12. Tye, Y.Y.; Lee, K.T.; Wan Abdullah, W.N.; Leh, C.P. Potential of Ceiba pentandra (L.) Gaertn. (kapok) fiber as a resource for second generation bioethanol: Parametric optimization and comparative study of various pretreatments prior enzymatic saccharification for sugar production. *Bioresour. Technol.* **2012**, *116*, 536–539. [CrossRef]
13. Sivaranjana, P.; Nagarajan, E.R.; Rajini, N.; Jawaid, M.; Rajulu, A.V. Cellulose nanocomposite films with in situ generated silver nanoparticles using Cassia alata leaf extract as a reducing agent. *Int. J. Biol. Macromol.* **2017**, *99*, 223–232. [CrossRef] [PubMed]
14. Wan Mat Khalir, W.K.A.; Shameli, K.; Miyake, M.; Othman, N.A.N.A. Efficient one-pot biosynthesis of silver nanoparticles using Entada spiralis stem powder extraction. *Res. Chem. Intermed.* **2018**, *44*, 7013–7028. [CrossRef]
15. Rehan, M.; Barhoum, A.; Van Assche, G.; Dufresne, A.; Gätjen, L.; Wilken, R. Towards multifunctional cellulosic fabric: UV photo-reduction and in-situ synthesis of silver nanoparticles into cellulose fabrics. *Int. J. Biol. Macromol.* **2017**, *98*, 877–886. [CrossRef]
16. Hussain, M.; Zahoor, T.; Akhtar, S.; Ismail, A.; Hameed, A. Thermal stability and haemolytic effects of depolymerized guar gum derivatives. *J. Food Sci. Technol.* **2018**, *55*, 1047–1055. [CrossRef]
17. Zhang, M.; Lin, H.; Wang, Y.; Yang, G.; Zhao, H.; Sun, D. Fabrication and durable antibacterial properties of 3D porous wet electrospun RCSC/PCL nanofibrous scaffold with silver nanoparticles. *Appl. Surf. Sci.* **2017**, *414*, 52–62. [CrossRef]
18. Liu, G.; Haiqi, G.; Li, K.; Xiang, J.; Lan, T.; Zhang, Z. Fabrication of silver nanoparticle sponge leather with durable antibacterial property. *J. Colloid Interface Sci.* **2018**, *51*, 4338–4348. [CrossRef]
19. Bauer, A.W.; Kirby, W.M.; Sherris, J.C.; Turck, M. Antibiotic susceptibility testing by a standardized single disk method. *Am. J. Clin. Pathol.* **1966**, *45*, 493–496. [CrossRef]
20. Shameli, K.; Ahmad, M.B.; Al-Mulla, E.A.J.; Shabanzadeh, P. Antibacterial effect of silver nanoparticles on talc composites. *Res. Chem. Intermed.* **2015**, *41*, 251–263. [CrossRef]
21. Joseph, S.; Mathew, B. Facile synthesis of silver nanoparticles and their application in dye degradation. *Mater. Sci. Eng. B Solid-State Mater. Adv. Technol.* **2015**, *195*, 90–97. [CrossRef]
22. Vidhu, V.K.; Philip, D. Catalytic degradation of organic dyes using biosynthesized silver nanoparticles. *Micron* **2014**, *56*, 54–62. [CrossRef]
23. Qing, W.; Chen, K.; Wang, Y.; Liu, X.; Lu, M. Green synthesis of silver nanoparticles by waste tea extract and degradation of organic dye in the absence and presence of H_2O_2. *Appl. Surf. Sci.* **2017**, *423*, 1019–1024. [CrossRef]
24. Ridzuan, M.J.M.; Abdul Majid, M.S.; Afendi, M.; Aqmariah Kanafiah, S.N.; Zahri, J.M.; Gibson, A.G. Characterisation of natural cellulosic fibre from Pennisetum purpureum stem as potential reinforcement of polymer composites. *Mater. Des.* **2016**, *89*, 839–847. [CrossRef]
25. Kabir, M.M.; Wang, H.; Lau, K.T.; Cardona, F. Applied surface science effects of chemical treatments on hemp fibre structure. *Appl. Surf. Sci.* **2013**, *276*, 13–23. [CrossRef]
26. Asim, M.; Jawaid, M.; Abdan, K.; Ishak, M.R. Effect of alkali and silane treatments on mechanical and fibre-matrix bond strength of kenaf and pineapple leaf fibres. *J. Bionic Eng.* **2016**, *13*, 426–435. [CrossRef]
27. Zhou, Y.; Fan, M.; Chen, L. Interface and bonding mechanisms of plant fibre composites: An overview. *Compos. Part B Eng.* **2016**, *101*, 31–45. [CrossRef]
28. Yang, H.; Yan, R.; Chen, H.; Lee, D.H.; Zheng, C. Characteristics of hemicellulose, cellulose, and lignin pyrolysis. *Fuel* **2007**, *86*, 1781–1788. [CrossRef]
29. Williams, P.T.; Besler, S. The influence of temperature and heating rate on the slow pyrolysis of biomass. *Renew. Energy* **1996**, *3*, 233–250. [CrossRef]

30. Komal, U.K.; Verma, V.; Aswani, T.; Verma, N.; Singh, I. Effect of chemical treatment on mechanical behavior of banana fiber reinforced polymer composites. *Mater. Today Proc.* **2018**, *5*, 16983–16989. [CrossRef]
31. Dong, C.; Zhang, X.; Cai, H.; Cao, C. Green synthesis of biocompatible silver nanoparticles mediated by Osmanthus fragrans extract in aqueous solution. *Optik (Stuttg)* **2016**, *127*, 10378–10388. [CrossRef]
32. Emam, H.E.; Saleh, N.H.; Nagy, K.S.; Zahran, M.K. Functionalization of medical cotton by direct incorporation of silver nanoparticles. *Int. J. Biol. Macromol.* **2015**, *78*, 249–256. [CrossRef] [PubMed]
33. Lakshmanan, A.; Chakraborty, S. Coating of silver nanoparticles on jute fibre by in situ synthesis. *Cellulose* **2017**, *24*, 1563–1577. [CrossRef]
34. Kędziora, A.; Speruda, M.; Krzyżewska, E.; Rybka, J.; Łukowiak, A.; Bugla-Płoskońska, G. Similarities and differences between silver ions and silver in nanoforms as antibacterial agents. *Int. J. Mol. Sci.* **2018**, *19*, 444. [CrossRef]
35. Greulich, C.; Braun, D.; Peetsch, A.; Diendorf, J.; Siebers, B.; Epple, M.; Köller, M. The toxic effect of silver ions and silver nanoparticles towards bacteria and human cells occurs in the same concentration range. *RSC Adv.* **2012**, *2*, 6981–6987. [CrossRef]
36. Kourmouli, A.; Valenti, M.; Van Rijn, E.; Beaumont, H.J.E.; Kalantzi, O.I.; Schmidt-Ott, A.; Biskos, G. Can disc diffusion susceptibility tests assess the antimicrobial activity of engineered nanoparticles. *J. Nanopart. Res.* **2018**, *20*, 2–7. [CrossRef]
37. Alsammarraie, F.K.; Wang, W.; Zhou, P.; Mustapha, A.; Lin, M. Green synthesis of silver nanoparticles using turmeric extracts and investigation of their antibacterial activities. *Colloids Surf. B Biointerfaces* **2018**, *171*, 398–405. [CrossRef]
38. Sowmyya, T.; Lakshmi, G.V. Spectroscopic investigation on catalytic and bactericidal properties of biogenic silver nanoparticles synthesized using Soymida febrifuga aqueous stem bark extract. *J. Environ. Chem. Eng.* **2018**, *6*, 3590–3601. [CrossRef]
39. Patil, M.P.; Singh, R.D.; Koli, P.B.; Patil, K.T.; Jagdale, B.S.; Tipare, A.R.; Do Kim, G. Antibacterial potential of silver nanoparticles synthesized using Madhuca longifolia flower extract as a green resource. *Microb. Pathog.* **2018**, *121*, 184–189. [CrossRef]
40. Nithya, A.; Jeeva Kumari, H.L.; Rokesh, K.; Ruckmani, K.; Jeganathan, K.; Jothivenkatachalam, K. A versatile effect of chitosan-silver nanocomposite for surface plasmonic photocatalytic and antibacterial activity. *J. Photochem. Photobiol. B Biol.* **2015**, *153*, 412–422. [CrossRef]
41. Pollini, M.; Russo, M.; Licciulli, A.; Sannino, A.; Maffezzoli, A. Characterization of antibacterial silver coated yarns. *J. Mater. Sci. Mater. Med.* **2009**, *20*, 2361–2366. [CrossRef] [PubMed]
42. Ghayempour, S.M. Montazer, Ultrasound irradiation based in-situ synthesis of star-like Tragacanth gum/zinc oxide nanoparticles on cotton fabric. *Ultrason. Sonochem.* **2017**, *34*, 458–465. [CrossRef] [PubMed]
43. Saravanan, M.; Barik, S.K.; Mubarak Ali, D.; Prakash, P.; Pugazhendhi, A. Synthesis of silver nanoparticles from Bacillus brevis (NCIM 2533) and their antibacterial activity against pathogenic bacteria. *Microb. Pathog.* **2018**, *116*, 221–226. [CrossRef]
44. Arya, G.; Sharma, N.; Ahmed, J.; Gupta, N.; Kumar, A.; Chandra, R.; Nimesh, S. Degradation of anthropogenic pollutant and organic dyes by biosynthesized silver nano-catalyst from Cicer arietinum leaves. *J. Photochem. Photobiol. B Biol.* **2017**, *174*, 90–96. [CrossRef] [PubMed]
45. Ganguly, S.; Mondal, S.; Das, P.; Bhawal, P.; Kanti Das, T.; Bose, M.; Choudhary, S.; Gangopadhyay, S.; Das, A.K.; Das, N.C. Natural saponin stabilized nano-catalyst as efficient dye-degradation catalyst. *Nano-Struct. Nano-Objects* **2018**, *16*, 86–95. [CrossRef]
46. Ismail, M.; Khan, M.I.; Khan, S.B.; Akhtar, K.; Khan, M.A.; Asiri, A.M. Catalytic reduction of picric acid, nitrophenols and organic azo dyes via green synthesized plant supported Ag nanoparticles. *J. Mol. Liq.* **2018**, *268*, 87–101. [CrossRef]
47. Saha, J.; Begum, A.; Mukherjee, A.; Kumar, S. A novel green synthesis of silver nanoparticles and their catalytic action in reduction of methylene blue dye. *Sustain. Environ. Res.* **2017**, *27*, 245–250. [CrossRef]
48. Naseem, K.; Begum, R.; Wu, W.; Irfan, A.; Al-Sehemi, A.G.; Farooqi, Z.H. Catalytic reduction of toxic dyes in the presence of silver nanoparticles impregnated core-shell composite microgels. *J. Clean. Prod.* **2019**, *211*, 855–864. [CrossRef]
49. Ofomaja, A.E.; Naidoo, E.B.; Modise, S.J. Kinetic and pseudo-second-order modeling of lead biosorption onto pine cone powder. *Ind. Eng. Chem. Res.* **2010**, *49*, 2562–2572. [CrossRef]

50. Ho, Y.S.; McKay, G. The kinetics of sorption of divalent metal ions onto sphagnum moss peat. *Water Res.* **2000**, *34*, 735–742. [CrossRef]
51. Senthil Kumar, P.; Ramalingam, S.; Sathyaselvabala, V.; Kirupha, S.D.; Sivanesan, S. Removal of Copper(II) ions from aqueous solution by adsorption using cashew nut shell. *Desalination* **2011**, *266*, 63–71. [CrossRef]
52. Ho, Y.S.; McKay, G. Pseudo second order model for sorption process. *Process Biochem.* **1999**, *76*, 451–465. [CrossRef]
53. Yihan, S.; Mingming, L.; Guo, Z. Ag nanoparticles loding of polypyrrole-coated superwetting mesh for on-demand separation of oil-water mixtures and catalytic reduction of aromatic dyes. *J. Colloids Interface Sci.* **2018**, *527*, 187–194. [CrossRef] [PubMed]
54. Rajegaonkar, P.S.; Deshpande, B.A.; More, M.S.M.S.; Waghmare, S.S.; Sangawe, V.V.; Inamdar, A.; Shirsat, M.D.; Adhapure, N.N. Catalytic reduction of p-nitrophenol and methylene blue by microbiologically synthesized silver nanoparticles. *Mater. Sci. Eng. C* **2018**, *93*, 623–629. [CrossRef]
55. Choudhary, M.K.; Kataria, J.; Sharma, S. Evaluation of the kinetic and catalytic properties of biogenically synthesized silver nanoparticles. *J. Clean. Prod.* **2018**, *198*, 882–890. [CrossRef]
56. Tahir, K.; Nazir, S.; Li, B.; Ullah, A.; Ul, Z.; Khan, H.; Ahmad, A. An efficient photo catalytic activity of green synthesized silver nanoparticles. *Sep. Purif. Technol.* **2015**, *150*, 316–324. [CrossRef]

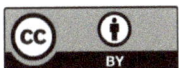

© 2020 by the authors. Licensee MDPI, Basel, Switzerland. This article is an open access article distributed under the terms and conditions of the Creative Commons Attribution (CC BY) license (http://creativecommons.org/licenses/by/4.0/).

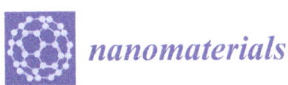

Article

Sensitive SQUID Bio-Magnetometry for Determination and Differentiation of Biogenic Iron and Iron Oxide Nanoparticles in the Biological Samples

Martin Škrátek [1,*], Andrej Dvurečenskij [1], Michal Kluknavský [2], Andrej Barta [2], Peter바́liš [2], Andrea Mičurová [2], Alexander Cigáň [1], Anita Eckstein-Andicsová [3], Ján Maňka [1,*] and Iveta Bernátová [2]

1. Institute of Measurement Science, Slovak Academy of Sciences, 841 04 Bratislava, Slovakia; andrej.dvurecenskij@savba.sk (A.D.); alexander.cigan@savba.sk (A.C.)
2. Institute of Normal and Pathological Physiology, Centre of Experimental Medicine, Slovak Academy of Sciences, 813 71 Bratislava, Slovakia; michal.kluknavsky@savba.sk (M.K.); andrej.barta@savba.sk (A.B.); peter.balis@savba.sk (P.B.); andrea.micurova@savba.sk (A.M.); iveta.bernatova@savba.sk (I.B.)
3. Polymer Institute, Slovak Academy of Sciences, 845 41 Bratislava, Slovakia; anita.andicsova@savba.sk
* Correspondence: martin.skratek@savba.sk (M.Š.); jan.manka@savba.sk (J.M.)

Received: 30 August 2020; Accepted: 2 October 2020; Published: 9 October 2020

Abstract: This study aimed to develop the method for determination of the ultra-small superparamagnetic iron oxide nanoparticle (USPION)-originated iron (UOI) in the tissues of rats on the basis of the magnetic characteristics (MC) in the liver, left heart ventricle (LHV), kidneys, aorta and blood of Wistar-Kyoto (WKY). Rats were treated intravenously by USPIONs dispersed in saline (transmission electron microscope (TEM) mean size ~30 nm, hydrodynamic size ~51 nm, nominal iron content 1 mg Fe/mL) at the low iron dose of 1 mg/kg. MC in the form of the mass magnetisation (M) versus the magnetic field (H) curves and temperature dependences of M (determined using the SQUID magnetometer), histochemical determination of iron (by Perl's method) and USPION-induced superoxide production (by lucigenin-enhanced chemiluminescence) were investigated 100 min post-infusion. USPIONs significantly elevated superoxide production in the liver, LHV, kidney and aorta vs. the control group. Histochemical staining confirmed the presence of iron in all solid biological samples, however, this method was not suitable to unequivocally confirm the presence of UOI. We improved the SQUID magnetometric method and sample preparation to allow the determination of UOI by measurements of the MC of the tissues at 300 K in solid and liquid samples. The presence of the UOI was confirmed in all the tissues investigated in USPIONs-treated rats. The greatest levels were found in blood and lower amounts in the aorta, liver, LHV and kidneys. In conclusion, we have improved SQUID-magnetometric method to make it suitable for detection of low amounts of UOI in blood and tissues of rats.

Keywords: SQUID; magnetic properties; iron content; magnetite nanoparticles; superoxide; aorta; heart

1. Introduction

Biogenic iron is present in all biological systems. Detail regulation of iron metabolism was described previously [1–3]. Nanomaterials, including iron nanoparticles (NPs), are widely used in various industrial applications. However, the fast development of nanotechnologies and nanomaterials may pose a serious health hazard for humans and animals [4]. Ultrasmall superparamagnetic iron oxide nanoparticles of γ-Fe_2O_3 (maghemite) and Fe_3O_4 (magnetite) with the size of 10–50 nm (ultra-small superparamagnetic iron oxide nanoparticles (USPIONs)) can be used in various biomedical and medical applications [5–7]. The advantage of the USPIONs lies in the possibility to use them for targeted drug delivery in the presence of the magnetic field [8]. Stability of USPIONs depends on the local microcellular environment (chemical composition, pH, etc.). Intraendosomal degradation of nanoparticles poses a risk of iron overload, which may be dangerous mainly locally as they can modulate innate iron metabolism on systemic or cellular levels. There is an increasing number of studies that documented intracellular toxicity of iron NPs showing NP-induced inflammation, apoptosis, mitochondrial disorders and oxidative damage [9,10]. Recently, a correlation between exposure to iron oxide NPs and metabolism is of particular concern in nanotoxicology related fields, as NPs can potentially enter to iron metabolism and, thus, to affect its physiological roles. Iron NPs may also increase reactive oxygen species production and to produce oxidative stress, which can further induce adverse effects on DNA, proteins as well as membrane lipids [9,11] and to induce inflammation, changes in blood pressure (BP) regulatory systems via modulation of vascular function. Yet, there is still limited information on the uptake of the USPIONs to the individual organs and tissues and their possible effects on metabolism and physiological functions.

From the methodological point of view, iron content in the tissues can be determined using colorimetric, spectrophotometric, histochemical methods or by the technique of atomic absorption spectrometry depending on the purpose [12,13]. However, these methods do not allow to distinguish clearly between the biogenic iron and USPION-originating iron. Both biogenic nanoparticles (e.g., ferritin) and USPIONs are superparamagnetic, however, usually with the different blocking temperature [14,15].

SQUID magnetometry is a novel approach to quantify different iron forms in biological samples with high sensitivity that may provide new information for the investigation of iron NPs effects on living organism as well as for the understanding of the pathomechanisms of various diseased states. SQUID magnetometry is one of the methods enabling to determine the blocking temperature (e.g., so-called zero field cooled—ZFC, field cooled—FC and alternating current (AC) measurements) [16,17] and in such a way to identify the presence of applied USPIONs. In previous experimental research, SQUID magnetometry was widely used as a tool for determination of the various form of iron. Measurements were done using iron nanoparticles, namely in cell cultures [18–20], after in vivo treatment in mice [21,22] and also in embryos of Xenopus Laevis [23]. Using SQUID magnetometry, Janus et al. [24] showed that blood of patients with atherosclerosis was characterised by a higher concentration of ferrimagnetic particles such as Fe_3O_4 and γ-Fe_2O_3 (associated with the elevated values of the magnetic saturation (M_s)) and significant changes in the superparamagnetic behaviour characterised with changes in the remnant magnetisation (M_r) and the magnetic coercivity (H_c).

The question of the measurement of biogenous iron content is also very important. SQUID magnetometric determination of biogenic iron was performed in various tissues of mice (duodenum, liver, spleen, kidney, heart or brain) [21,25] and rat blood [26]. In addition, iron content was also determined by SQUID magnetometry in human brain [27]. The authors of the above-mentioned studies used various techniques to characterise and determine the amount of iron. Measurement of the $M(H)$ dependences is the standard method of iron determination by magnetometry, however, more information can be obtained by measurement of the temperature dependences of magnetisation, e.g., the ZFC and FC magnetisation characteristics. Another way is the determination of the isothermal remnant magnetisation (IRM) or using the AC susceptometry.

SQUID magnetometry, in combination with biomedical research, can provide a better understanding of iron metabolism in various diseased states as well as to distinguish biogenic iron from that originating from USPIONs. However, the investigation can be difficult, when NPs are used in very low doses which are diffusely distributed in the human or animal body.

Thus the aim of our study was to develop the method for determination of the amount of the USPION-originated iron in the tissues of rats and to investigate the magnetic characteristics of the liver, left heart ventricle, kidneys, aorta and blood of WKY rats after i.v. application of the low dose of USPIONs.

2. Materials and Methods

2.1. Nanoparticles

Commercially available water dispersion of polyethylene glycol (PEG)-coated USPIONs were purchased from Sigma-Aldrich (Bratislava, Slovakia, cat. No. 747408). USPIONs' concentration was 1 mg Fe/mL and they were dispersed in water. The size of USPIONs confirmed by the transmission electron microscope was 28–32 nm, the zeta potential was −12 mV, polydispersity index was 0.1, and the hydrodynamic size was about 45 nm (all parameters declared by the manufacturer). Before i.v. administration to rats, USPIONs were autoclaved at 121 °C for 30 min and mixed with sterile saline to reach a final dose of 1 mg of Fe/kg of body weight.

2.2. Determination of the Iron Core Size, Polydispersity Index and Hydrodynamic Size

USPIONs iron core size was checked using transmission electron microscope (TEM) Jeol-1200FX (JEOL Ltd., Tokyo, Japan). As indicated in Figure 1, the average size of USPIONs was 29.8 ± 0.2 nm (mean ± standard error of the mean—SEM), which was in the expected range.

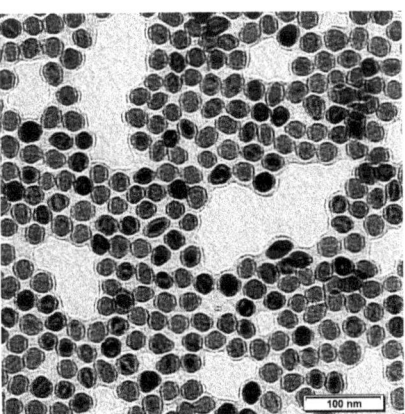

Figure 1. Transmission electron microscope (TEM) figure of polyethylene glycol (PEG)-coated ultra-small superparamagnetic iron oxide nanoparticle (USPION) dispersion. Size of nanoparticles iron core was 29.8 ± 0.2 nm (mean ± standard error of the mean—SEM), and no aggregation of nanoparticles was found.

Dynamic light scattering (DLS) measurements were performed using Zetasizer Nano-ZS (Malvern Instruments, Malvern, UK) equipped with a helium/neon laser (λ = 633 nm) and thermoelectric temperature controller at a scattering angle of 173° and 25 °C. All of the data analyses were made in automatic mode. The measured size was presented as the average value of 20 runs, with triplicate measurements within each run.

For the hydrodynamic size analysis, diluted USPIONs (0.01 mg/1 mL) were used. As indicated in Figure 2, the particle size calculated from the number average was 51.3 ± 16.3 d.nm with a dispersity of 0.147. During the measurement, no formation of NPs aggregates was observed.

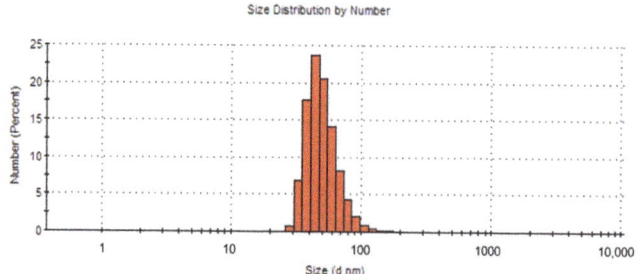

Figure 2. Distribution of USPIONs according to their size.

2.3. Animals

All of the procedures used in this study were approved by the State Veterinary and Food Administration of the Slovak Republic in accordance with the European Union Directive 2010/63/EU.

Rats were divided into two groups: control (Cont.) and the group treated with PEG-coated ultra-small superparamagnetic iron oxide (Fe_3O_4) nanoparticles (USPIONs). Control rats were given 10-min infusions of saline, starting approximately 30 min from the beginning of the experiment. USPION-treated rats were given 10-min infusions of USPIONs at the dose of 1 mg Fe/kg.

Wistar-Kyoto (WKY) male rats, 12–16 weeks old, were used in this study. Rats were housed under standard conditions at 22–24 °C in a 12-h light/dark cycle and fed with pelleted diet Altromin formula 1324, variant P (Altromin Spezialfutter, Lage, Germany) and tap water ad libitum.

One day before the experiment, all of the rats had two catheters implanted under 2.5–3.5% isoflurane anaesthesia, as described previously [26]. All of the rats were also pre-treated with meloxicam (Meloxidolor, Le Vet Beheer B.V., Oudewated, Nederland) at 2 mg/kg intramuscularly before surgery to prevent post-surgical pain. Fine-bore polyethylene catheters (Smiths Medical International Ltd., Kent, UK) were inserted into the left carotid artery (internal diameter 0.28 mm) for i.v. administration of USPIONs (suspended in saline) or saline (in control), respectively. Catheters were exteriorised in the interscapular region, and rats were allowed to recover from anaesthesia for approximately 20–24 h. During the experiments, the conscious rats were placed into a plastic box with dark walls and transparent lid (27 cm × 14 cm × 9 cm in size), which allowed the rats free movement. At the end of the experiment, rats were exposed to brief CO_2 anaesthesia and decapitated 100 min post USPION-infusion. The samples of the liver, left heart ventricle, kidney, aorta and blood were collected for the determination of the magnetic characteristics, histochemical determination of the iron and superoxide production. Tissues were dissected using ceramic scissors and ceramic or plastic forceps. After dissection, the tissues were cleaned out of the connecting tissue, washed in the saline solution and dried of saline solution using filtration paper. Trunk blood was collected into Eppendorf test tubes. Fresh tissues were collected for determination of superoxide and for histochemical analyses. For determination of USPIONs by SQUID, the tissues and blood were frozen in the liquid nitrogen and kept at −80 °C until further analyses.

2.4. Superoxide Production

The production of superoxide was measured in the 15–20 mg fresh samples of the tissues using lucigenin (50 µmol/L)-enhanced chemiluminescence using a TriCarb 2910TR liquid scintillation analyser (TriCarb, Perkin Elmer, Waltham, MA, USA), as described previously by Kluknavsky et al. [26]. The results are expressed in the form of cpm/mg of wet tissue.

2.5. Histochemical Determination of Iron in the Tissues

Tissues of the liver, left heart ventricle, kidneys and aorta of control and USPION-treated rats were collected and routinely fixed at 10% buffered neutral formalin. Samples were routinely fixed in paraffin and then cut into 5 μm slices. Slices were deparaffinised and the Perl's method for iron staining was used for determination of iron in the tissues of USPION-treated and control rats as described previously [28]. Iron was converted to ferric ion with acid solutions of ferrocyanides. Ferric iron in the tissue react with the ferrocyanide, resulting in the formation of a blue pigment called Prussian blue. Nuclei are stained in red by safranine method.

2.6. Statistical Analysis

Statistical analysis was performed by Student's t-test. The values were found to significantly differ when $p < 0.05$. The data were presented as mean ± SEM. GraphPad Prism 5.0 (GraphPad Software, Inc., San Diego, CA, USA) was used for the statistical analyses.

2.7. Method for Determination of the USPIONs Content in the Tissues

Determination of USPION content in tissue and blood samples was done by measuring their magnetic properties. A Quantum Design (San Diego, CA, USA) SQUID magnetometer MPMS-XL 7AC was used. Magnetic characterisation of USPIONs was done by measuring the temperature dependence of the mass magnetisation M in both the ZFC (zero field cooled) and FC (field cooled) conditions (at the applied magnetic field of 50 Oe), in the temperature range from 1.8 to 300 K and the isothermal magnetisation curves (M vs. H dependence) measured at the temperatures of 2 and 300 K and the applied field up to 7 T.

2.7.1. The Problems of the Proper Sample Preparing for Magnetic Measurements

At first, we solved the problems of incorrect mounting of the sample. The example of such problematic measurement due to improper sample mounting could be seen in Figure 3a. A sample (103 mg) of the fresh liver of 7-week WKY rat was inserted into standard capsule used in magnetic measurements, and the capsule was fixed by cotton into the straw. $M(H)$ curve was measured at 300 K. A reciprocating sample option (RSO) was used with a scan length of 4 cm through the 2nd order gradiometer, and the number of averaged scans per measurement was 5. The centring procedure was performed by application of the small magnetic field. The magnet was not quenched, so the start of the measurement was with non-zero magnetisation (Figure 3a, point A). Scan through the gradiometer and voltage output are shown in Figure 3b. Relatively good voltage output was obtained. As the field was increasing (Figure 3a, point B) the magnetisation was changed to the negative values and this way, it was fitted by the MPMS (Figure 3b). Then the maximum field was reached (Figure 3a, point C), this leads to a good fit of the output voltage (Figure 3b) but with unbalanced output on the borders (maximum at 0.5 and 3.5 cm). This unbalanced output results from the position of the sample in capsule and from the cover of capsule and cotton. Then the field decreased to the point D, and its voltage output (Figure 3c) was not properly fitted, giving positive voltage fit of the curve from the sample holder instead of negative one from the sample alone. These false measurements added a hysteresis to the measured $M(H)$ curve. Point E showed (Figure 3a) no problem with fitting at all, the signal from the sample mounting is again neglected, due to higher output of the sample alone (voltage outputs at the points C and E were rescaled down to be shown with the other signals). There is also a visible problem with sample instability, as the water from the sample was evaporating, the final point of $M(H)$ curve was not overlapping with the point C.

Unsuitable sample holder could also affect the measurement of the temperature dependence of the magnetisation (Figure 4a). When the mass magnetisation goes close to zero, there is significant "jump" to the opposite value, for both ZFC and FC curves. In some cases, the presence of sudden changes in the values of the magnetisation could be observed for higher applied magnetic field too (Figure 4b). Here, the heart from a 9-week old WKY rat was measured. Another example of improper use of a capsule as a sample holder is in Figure 4c. Corrupted measurement occurs in the low magnetic field region, but the overall appearance of the curve is acceptable.

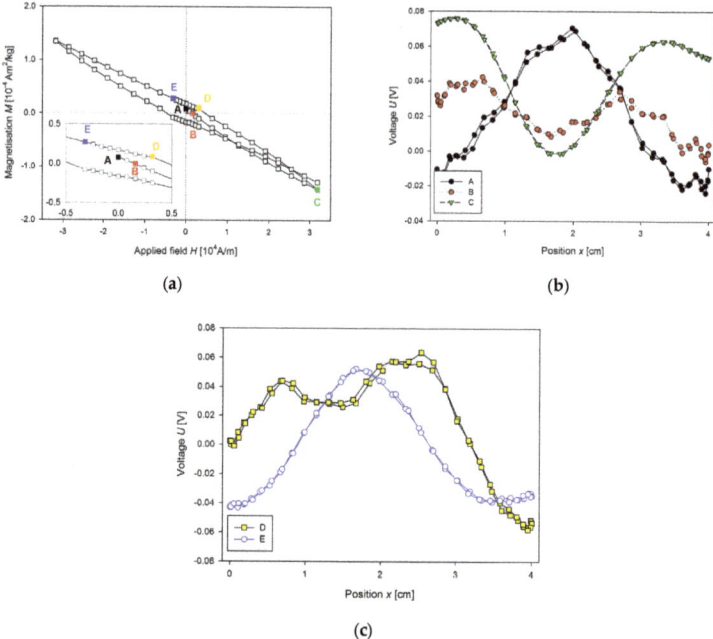

Figure 3. (a) M(H) dependence of the fresh sample of the liver of Wistar-Kyoto (WKY) rat, (b) the voltage output of longitudinal SQUID scan for marked points (A–C) of the M(H) dependence presented in Figure 3a, (c) the voltage output of the longitudinal SQUID scan for marked points (D–E) of the MH dependence shown in Figure 3a.

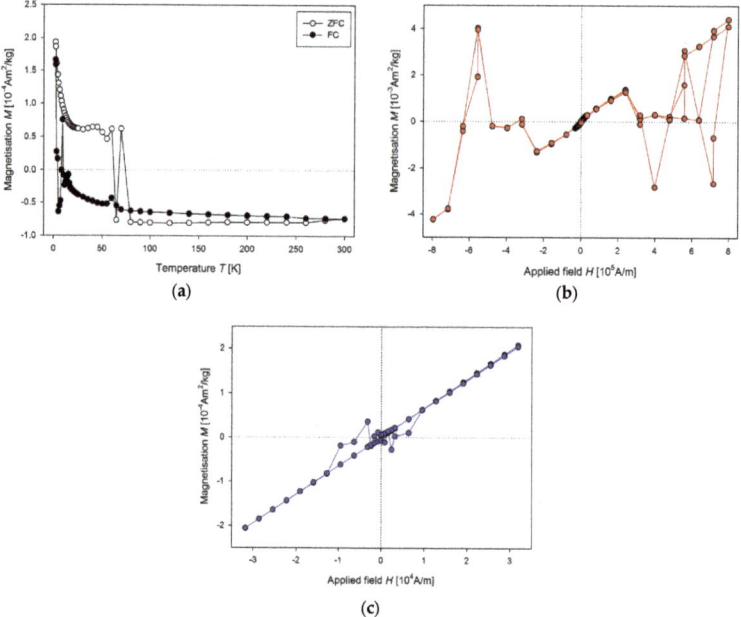

Figure 4. (a) Temperature dependence of the mass magnetisation of the same sample as in Figure 3, (b) M(H) dependence of the WKY rat heart at 300 K, (c) M(H) dependence of WKY rat liver at 300 K.

2.7.2. Polyethylene Holder for Powder and Liquid Samples

Considering all the problems and restrictions in the sample preparation for the magnetic measurement, the plastic sample holder (Figure 5) was developed. It is created from high-density polyethylene (HDPE; specification: ultra-high molecular weight polyethylene, Tivar 1000 natural, developed by Quadrant EPP (now Mitsubishi Chemical Advanced Materials Composites, Nitra, Slovakia)). This material shows a relatively small change of magnetic properties with the temperature in the range of 2–300 K, the diameter of the holder is 6 mm and the length of 210 mm was chosen to be as long as a standard plastic straw for MPMS with the end caps. These dimensions were chosen to minimise the weight, possible problems with thermal stability and to minimise the time needed for changes in temperature during cooling and heating. According to [29], the sample space was chosen to be 3 mm in diameter and 5 mm of length.

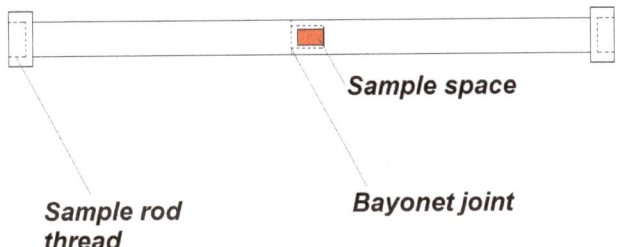

Figure 5. Schematics of high-density polyethylene sample holder configuration.

If the sample holder was without a cavity for the sample, its length ensures that no signal is created on the output of 2nd order gradiometer. HDPE is diamagnetic, so the cavity for the sample creates proportional signal to its dimensions, but with reciprocal value attributable to paramagnetic material. Magnetic properties of this sample holder with a cavity filled with He gas to minimise the possible paramagnetic output of air are in Figure 6.

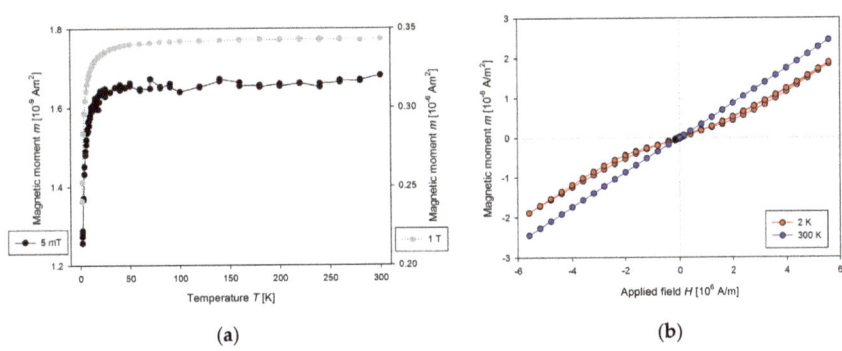

Figure 6. (a) The temperature dependence of the magnetic moment for presented plastic sample holder with the cavity filled with He gas measured at 5 mT (left axis) and 1 T (right axis) and (b) the magnetic field dependence of the magnetic moment for presented plastic sample holder measured at 2 and 300 K.

The measured data show a strong dependence of the magnetic moment of the cavity on temperature, mainly below 50 K. There is a need to measure corrections for each sample holder before measurement of the samples, which should be later subtracted. The sample holder proved to be temperature stable during measurements, so there is no visible shift in position in the temperature range from 1.8 to 350 K. It is used for measurement of the powder samples and liquids. When measuring such samples, one should be aware of the evaporation of liquid samples during long measurements, as there is often significant change in the magnetic moment of the sample.

2.7.3. Holder and Stabilisation of the Liquid Samples

For determination of magnetic properties of liquid samples, we use pre-weighted 18 cm long and 6 mm narrow strip of standard office paper (80 g/m^2), which was bent over the long side to the shape of V (Figure 7), which prevented the sample in the form of drop of 10 µL to spread to sides of the paper. Then the sample was dried in the vacuum for one hour or dried on air for 24 h at room temperature. After drying, the paper with the dry sample was weighted to obtain the actual dry weight of the sample knowing the weight of the paper without the sample. Type of the paper used for measurements of the liquid samples may differ, depending on the experiment, it can be laboratory filtration paper or standard office paper. For nanoparticle dispersion measurement, a strip of transparent foil was used, due to its ability to hold the drop of liquid in the desired shape. After this procedure, the sample was inserted to the plastic straw and attached to the sample rod.

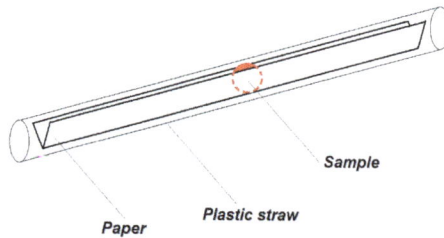

Figure 7. Schematics of sample configuration with V-shaped paper and a standard plastic straw.

2.7.4. Holder and Stabilisation of the Tissue Samples

For measurements of the small tissue samples with the fresh tissue weights about 15–60 mg or even less in case of the aorta (about 10 mg), a method for their stabilisation in the straw holder was derived. Defrosted tissues were cut with cylindrical-shaped instrument with a diameter of 5.5 mm (3.5 mm for kidney) and was mounted on pre-weighted, 18 cm long copper wire with 0.2 mm diameter (Figure 8). The aorta was not cut, it was mounted by a wire embedded via the lumen of the artery. The sample was then vacuum dried for 1 h. During drying the sample shrunk and adhered to the wire. Diameter of the dried sample was then ~4.5 mm (~3 mm for kidney) and the sample attached to the wire was weighted, so we obtained the dry weight of the sample. The Cu wire itself is diamagnetic, long enough again to have negligible output signal to a magnetic moment of the sample.

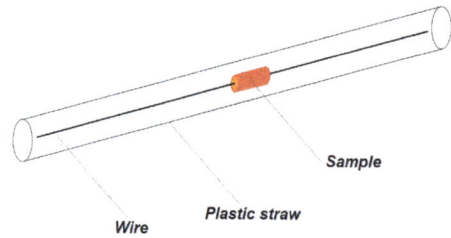

Figure 8. Schematics of the sample configuration in holder with copper wire and a plastic straw.

3. Results

3.1. Magnetic Characteristics of USPION Dispersion per Se

To determine USPIONs uptake during the experiment with animals, one need to characterise USPIONs dispersion. A volume of 10 µL of the dispersion was dropped to the transparent foil (18 cm long and 4 mm wide) vacuum dried for 1 h and inserted into the straw as described above. The hysteresis curves were measured (Figure 9a) at 2 and 300 K. The curves show no difference in total magnetisation at 2 K compared to 300 K, and the USPIONs dispersion is superparamagnetic with no hysteresis at 300 K, but the tendency to saturation is present. The temperature dependence (Figure 9b) showed that the ZFC curve has a peak with maximum at 260 K, indicating that at room temperature the NPs are superparamagnetic. The FC curve exhibits maximum at 240 K and a plateau at low temperature, which can be ascribed to interparticle interactions.

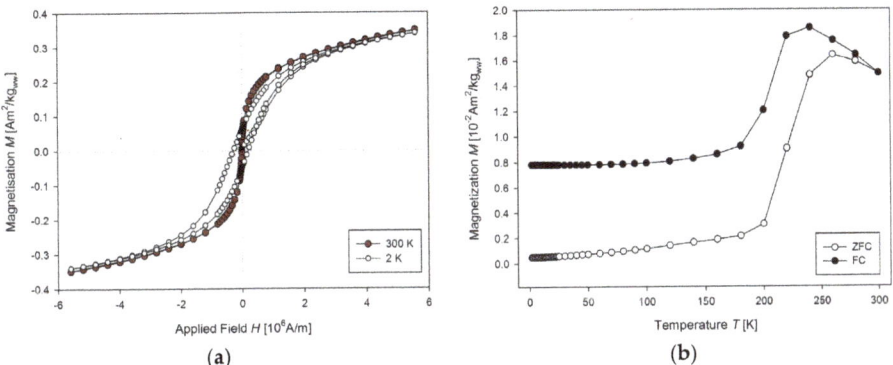

Figure 9. Properties of USPION dispersion per se. (**a**) The mass magnetisation vs. the applied magnetic field measured at 2 and 300 K. (**b**) The mass magnetisation vs. the temperature measured at 4000 A/m applied magnetic field.

3.2. Magnetic Characteristics of USPION-Treated Tissues

Samples of the liver, left heart ventricle, kidneys, aorta, and whole arterial blood were prepared according to the procedures described above (Section 2). Magnetisation (M) measurements were realised similarly to the measurement of USPION dispersion. Hysteresis curves measured at 2 K for control and USPION-treated group, respectively (Figure 10a) showed almost no differences between these two groups, the saturation magnetisation (M_s) and the magnetic coercivity (H_c) were almost the same. However, the measurement of the temperature dependence of M (Figure 10b) showed considerable differences between control and USPION-treated group. ZFC and FC curves for the liver of USPION-treated rats were similar to that determined in the USPION dispersion per se at the higher temperature values and confirmed the presence of the USPIONs in the liver. There is also clearly visible maximum for the ZFC curve at 10 K (Inset of Figure 10b), which is characteristic for ferritin and confirms its presence in the liver. Liver of the control group showed only a contribution of naturally occurring ferritin and diamagnetism at the higher temperature (Figure 10b). As the temperature dependence measurement is time and liquid helium (used for cooling the MPMS) consuming, it was decided to measure the contribution of USPIONs at 300 K by measuring shortened $M(H)$ dependence.

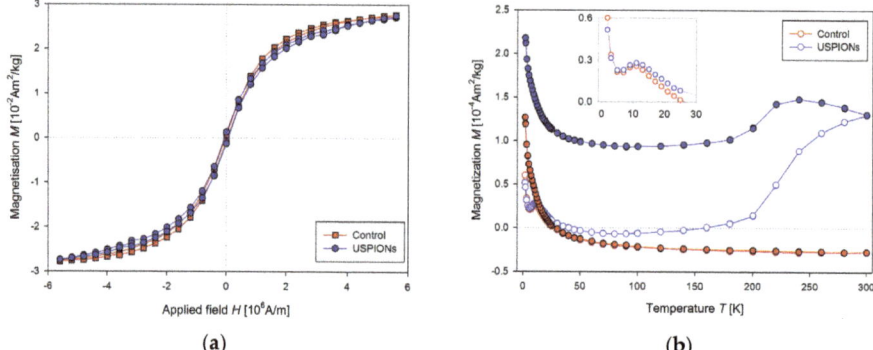

Figure 10. Magnetic properties of the liver of control and USPION-treated rats. (a) The mass magnetisation vs. applied magnetic field measurement at a temperature of 2 K, (b) the mass magnetisation vs. the temperature at the applied magnetic field of 4000 A/m. The inset shows the peak at the ZFC (zero field cooled) curve both for control and USPIONs group. Curves are the average of 5 measurements per group.

Parameters of sequence used for measurement are: RSO, scan length 4 cm, 2 × 5 scans per measurement, corresponding to every single point in the figures, frequency 1.5 Hz, measurement length of the partial M(H) dependences was 20 min, the applied field increased one-way only from 0 to 1 T. This setup, together with improved sample mounting, allows us to perform rapid and precise measurements of magnetic properties of the samples. Result of the measurements of liver samples is shown in Figure 11a. The presented data are averaged of control ($n = 11$) and USPION-treated ($n = 9$) group. In the control group, M decreases with the applied magnetic field linearly, which is caused by prevailing diamagnetism of the investigated samples. Data from USPION-treated rats showed initial curvature at low fields, which originated from the USPIONs. After this curvature the slope of the curve goes similar to the control group, indicating the still prevailing diamagnetism in the tissue samples over the contribution of the USPIONs, whose magnetisation saturates at the higher applied magnetic field.

Determination of USPIONs content in the treated tissue was done by subtracting of the averaged value of the mass magnetisation of control group values ($M_{control}$) from each of the USPION samples values (Figure 11b):

$$M'_{sample} = M_{sample} - M_{control} \quad (1)$$

and comparing M'_{sample} with the mass magnetisation of the USPION ($M_{USPIONs}$) dispersion measured at 300 K and 1 T field. The iron content in the USPIONs treated samples was determined using the following relation:

$$c\left[\frac{\mu g_{Fe}}{g}\right] = \frac{M'_{sample} \times m_{Fe}}{M_{USPIONs} \times m_{sample}} \times 10^6 \quad (2)$$

where c is the USPIONs content in the sample (in µg of Fe per gram of the sample dry weight), m_{Fe} is the mass of iron in USPION dispersion (in our case: $m_{Fe} = 10$ µg) and m_{sample} is the mass of the dried sample.

The same procedure of the measurement as for the liver was used for the samples from left heart ventricle (Figure 12) and kidney (Figure 13). In the case of kidney, the smaller cutting tool was used, with a diameter of 3.5 mm.

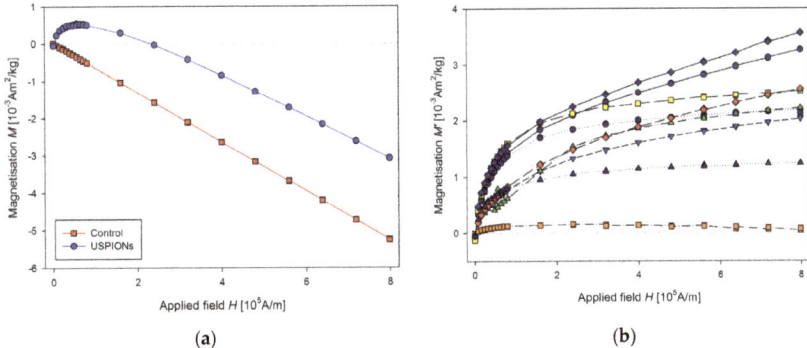

Figure 11. Magnetic properties of the liver of control and USPION-treated rats. (**a**) The partial $M(H)$ dependences at 300 K. Data are presented as the averaged curve from the control group ($n = 11$) and USPION-treated group ($n = 9$). The mass of dry samples was in the range of 12–30 mg. (**b**) Corresponding M' data for individual rats of the USPION-treated group after subtraction of the control group average.

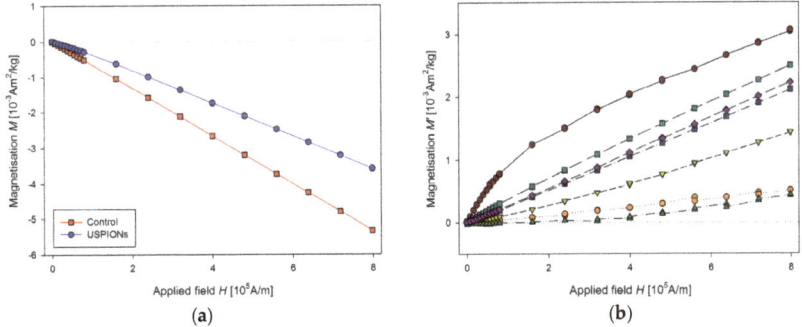

Figure 12. Magnetic properties of the left heart ventricle of control and USPION-treated rats. (**a**) The partial $M(H)$ dependences at 300 K and (**b**) corresponding M' data for individual rats of the USPION-treated group after subtraction of the control group average. Data (**a**) are presented as the averaged curve from the control group ($n = 10$) and USPION-treated group ($n = 7$). The mass of dry samples was in the range of 14–25 mg.

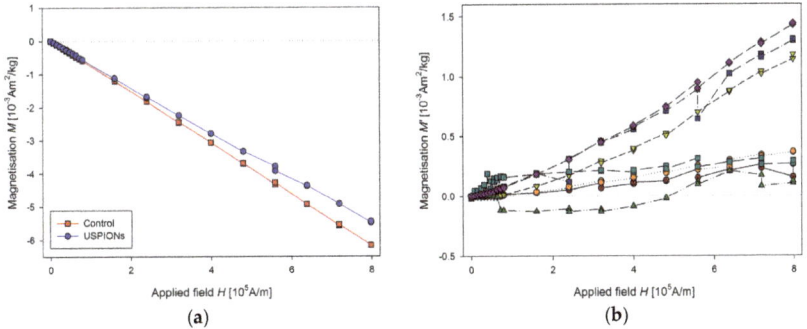

Figure 13. Magnetic properties of the kidney of control and USPION-treated rats. (**a**) The partial $M(H)$ dependences at 300 K, (**b**) corresponding M' data for individual rats of the USPION-treated group after subtraction of the control group average. Data (**a**) are presented as the averaged curve from the control group ($n = 6$) and USPION-treated group ($n = 7$). The mass of dry samples was in the range of 3–6 mg. The smaller cutting tool was used (diameter of 3.5 mm).

Samples of the aorta were cut to a length of 5 mm and prepared similarly to tissue samples. The measured mass magnetisation is presented in Figure 14.

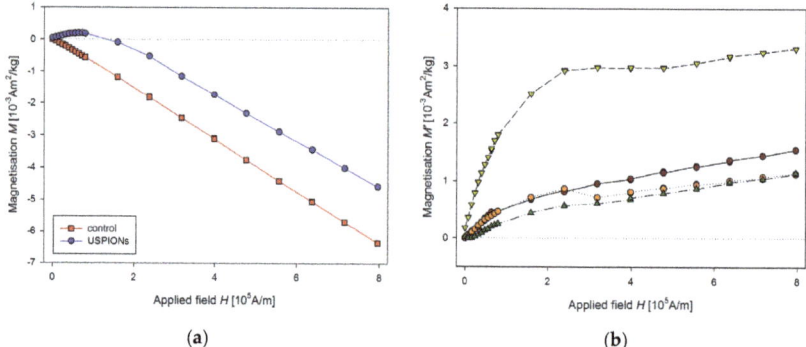

(a) (b)

Figure 14. Magnetic properties of the aorta of control and USPION-treated rats. (a) The partial $M(H)$ dependences at 300 K, (b) corresponding M' data for individual rats of the USPION treated group after subtraction of the control group average. Data (a) are presented as the averaged curve from the control group ($n = 4$) and USPION-treated group ($n = 4$). The mass of dry samples was in the range of 1.8–2.5 mg.

Samples of blood were prepared according to Section 2.7, before preparation the blood was defrosted and homogenised using an ultrasonic bath for 60 s (50 kHz, 30 W). Measured mass magnetisation is presented in Figure 15.

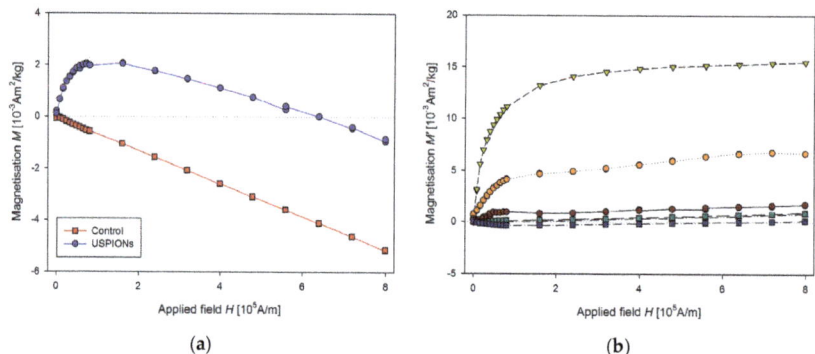

(a) (b)

Figure 15. Magnetic properties of the blood of control and USPION-treated rats. (a) The partial $M(H)$ dependences at 300 K and (b) corresponding M' data for individual rats of the USPION treated group after subtraction of the control group average (b). Data (a) are presented as the averaged curve from the control group ($n = 4$) and USPION-treated group ($n = 6$). The mass of dry samples was in the range of 1.3–2.3 mg.

From measurements of M of the control groups, we derived the sensitivity of our method of determination of USPION-originated iron content as a variance of measurement changes with the magnetic field (Figure 16). Therefore, a line to the data was fitted by the weighted regression. In particular, we supposed $var(\epsilon_i) = \sigma^2 x^2$, i.e., the weights $w_i = 1/x_i^2$. Then, a confidence band around the fitted line $\hat{y}$ is determined as $\hat{y} \pm 2\hat{\sigma}x_i$, where the parameters of $\hat{y}$ and $\hat{\sigma}$ were estimated by the weighted least squares procedure. Then the upper border of the band around should be considered as a minimum value of M for a sample with USPION content. Value of this minimal iron content was determined using the same procedure as for the USPION treated samples. Determined sensitivity is presented in the Table 1 for each type of samples. The samples with the lower USPION content than the determined sensitivity were omitted and final mean USPION content (for dry and wet sample) is presented in the Table 1 together with number of averaged samples. Presented are also dry and wet weights of the samples of each measured tissue and blood. For better clarity, the data for the USPION content in tissues presented also in the Figure 17.

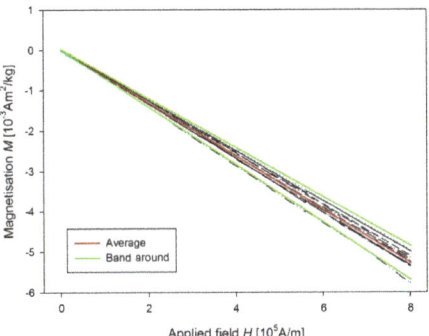

Figure 16. Confidence band around (green lines) of M data of the liver control group (black lines for individual samples) and their mean value (red line).

Table 1. Summary of USPION-originated iron content in the tissues and whole blood of rats treated with USPIONs (1 mg/kg i.v., 100 min post-infusion). Mean sample mass is presented as dry and wet weight. Sensitivity of the measurement method is expressed in µg of USPION iron per g of dry sample weight. n is the number of samples where USPION content was determined. Results are presented as mean ± SEM.

	Sample Wet Weight (ww) [mg]	Sample Dry Weight (dw) [mg]	Fe Content [µg/g$_{dw}$]	Fe Content [µg/g$_{ww}$]	Sensitivity [µg/g$_{dw}$]	n
Liver	41.3 ± 2.3	15.9 ± 0.9	2.1 ± 0.4	0.8 ± 0.2	0.6	8
LHV	60.1 ± 4.0	19.2 ± 1.3	1.6 ± 0.3	0.5 ± 0.1	1.1	4
Kidney	13.6 ± 1.7	4.0 ± 0.5	1.5 ± 0.3	0.4 ± 0.1	0.9	3
Aorta	8.5 ± 0.7	2.4 ± 0.2	9.4 ± 1.3	2.6 ± 0.3	1.6	4
Blood	9.6 ± 1.1	1.8 ± 0.2	45.9 ± 21.8	8.4 ± 4.1	1.6	5

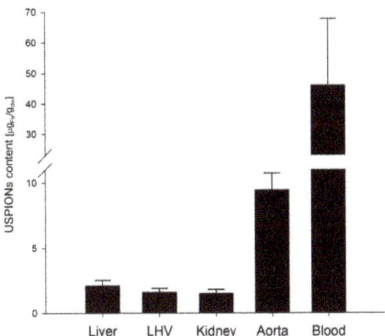

Figure 17. Mean USPION-originated iron content determined in the tissues of liver, left heart ventricle (LHV), kidney, aorta and whole arterial blood. Results are presented as mean ± SEM.

3.3. Histochemical Staining of Iron in the Tissues

The samples of the liver, left heart ventricle, kidneys and aorta of control and USPION-treated rats stained using the Perl's method confirmed the presence of iron in the tissues of control and USPION-treated rats. However, it is not possible to unequivocally confirm that iron content in USPION-treated samples is due to USPIONs presence in these tissues (Figure 18).

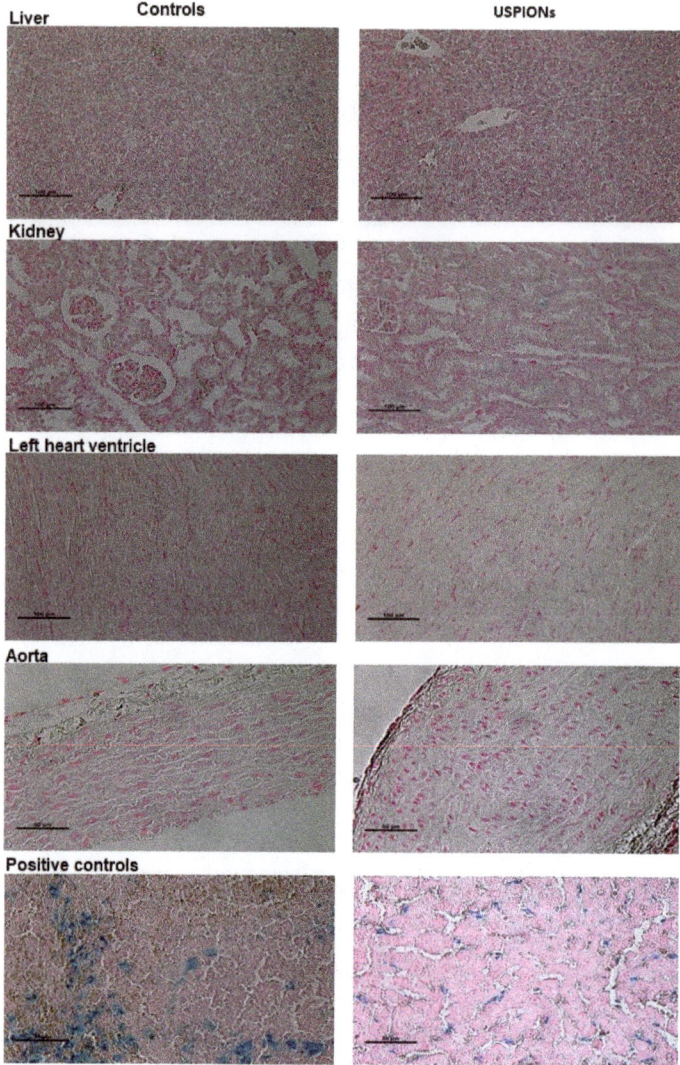

Figure 18. Iron staining in the liver, left heart ventricle, kidneys and aorta of control (left column) and USPION-treated (right column) rats. Staining of iron in the spleen of control rat (bottom left, positive control of biogenic iron) and positive staining of iron in the liver of rats treated with USPIONs at the dose of 20 mg Fe/kg (bottom right, positive control of USPION-originated iron). Prussian blue pigment determines iron. Nuclei are stained in red.

3.4. Superoxide Production

Intravenous administration of USPIONs resulted in the significant increase of superoxide production in the liver, LHV, kidneys and aorta by approximately 110%, 101%, 54% and 66%, respectively, compared to the control group ($p < 0.05$ in all groups) as shown in Figure 19.

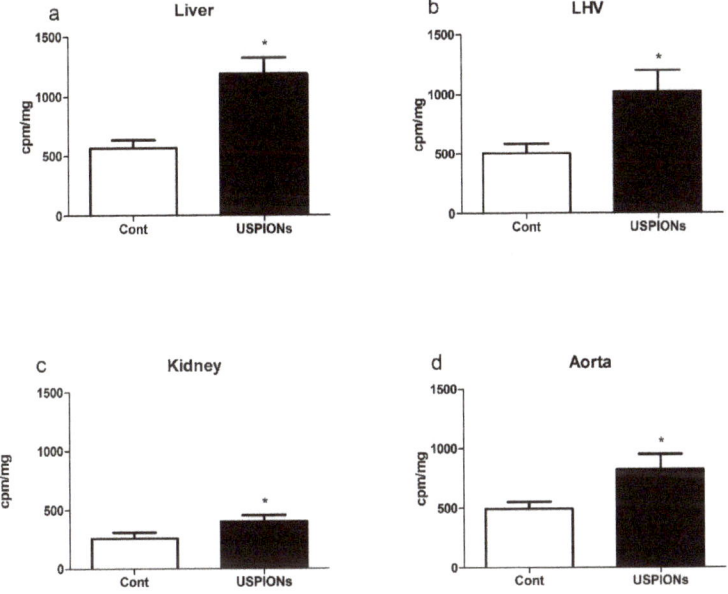

Figure 19. Superoxide production (a) in the liver, (b) left heart ventricle (LHV), (c) kidney and (d) aorta. The values represent the mean ± SEM. * $p < 0.05$ vs. control (Cont) group.

4. Discussion

In this study, we focused on the determination of USPION-originated iron content and its distinction from the naturally present iron in the tissues. For that purpose, we developed the method for determination of the presence of iron originated from USPIONs in the tissues of rats after i.v. administration of a low dose of NPs. We showed that the SQUID magnetometry is able to determine and to distinguish USPION-originated iron even if it is in low amount and not clearly detectable by Perl's histochemical method.

We have dealt with the application of USPIONs, and we investigated their effects on various organs of the WKY rats. As bare iron oxide nanoparticles administered in higher doses were previously shown to be toxic as they produce the development of oxidative stress [9,11], we used a low dose of PEG-coated magnetite USPIONs. PEG is a neutral, hydrophilic and biocompatible polymer which improves the dispersion of NPs in water, it improves their bio-distribution and increases blood circulation time [30]. However, despite the PEG-coating and administration of a low dose of USPIONs, we found elevated production of the superoxide, which was increased in all tissues and organs investigated in this study, similarly as it was found using various types of NPs [31]. On the other hand, we were unable to unequivocally confirm elevated iron content in the tissues using the histochemical method. Thus, we used SQUID magnetometry for determination of the distribution and content of USPION-originated iron in the samples of the organs as well as in the blood of rats and for differentiation of USPIONs from the biogenic iron and determination of it content.

However, due to extremely weak magnetic signals (with changing polarity), it was necessary to analyse and adjust the measurement conditions in the MPMS measuring system. Special attention was paid to preparing and mounting of the samples and to the design of the sample holders. As the magnetic moment of the samples was extremely weak, close to the value of standard holders/capsules, it was necessary to design such a configuration, where the material in vicinity of the measured sample is homogeneous in the whole operating space. In such a way, it is possible to subtract the background from the total measured signal.

We found that the proper mounting of the sample into the MPMS system is extremely important. The frequently used configuration for measurements of biological samples is to use standard plastic or gelatine capsules which are inserted into the drinking-straw and fixed by a cotton stopper [19,21,23,27,32]. However, this configuration leads to several problems. Firstly, there is a need to subtract the background signal generated by the capsule and the cotton. Secondly, when the value of the magnetic moment of the sample is close to that of the capsule, but in the opposite direction, this often leads to instability of scan through gradiometer coils, the usually centred peak is shifted, and the system is not able to properly fit the measured values (as shown in Figure 3). Similar problems were observed in previous studies [33,34], but the authors ascribed them mistakenly as a sort of hardware problem. In some studies, the authors have similar issues with the proper sample mounting. The problem of sample geometry and proper mounting for inorganic samples has been discussed previously in the article of Sawicki et al. [29]. The authors recommended to glue the sample to the long silicone rod attached at the end of the measuring rod for MPMS instead of using a plastic straw. In the study of [25], freeze-drying of the samples and mounting to a straw without capsule was used. In another study [18], the authors described the mounting of cancer cell samples treated with nanoparticles to the long strip of filtration paper.

Another problem which we have to solve is the attachment of the small samples into the measurement straw. We have solved this problem by the development of the cylindrical shaped instrument to obtain repeatedly the samples of the same shape, because we observed differences in the results if the shapes of the samples were different. Our method with the cutting of the biological samples of the same shape and their attachment during the vacuum drying worked well for samples from the muscles, kidneys or heart, which retain its shape after cutting. The rings of the aorta can also be used when the wire is embedded via the lumen of the artery. However, the samples of the liver or brain were more difficult to be prepared as a cylindrical sample due to their soft structure. In this study, we used a higher mass of the liver to ensure a suitable shape of the sample. With specific caution to the preparation of the sample (cut from the bigger mass of the "crude" sample), our method can also be used for the liver. However, we were unable to perform the measurements successfully in the brain tissues due to their soft structure. We assume that for samples of the brain, their homogenisation in proper buffer and manipulation similar to that for the liquid samples would be more suitable than the procedure for solid tissue samples.

For the liquid samples, such as blood or its derivatives, which need to be prepared differently from solid tissues, we developed a procedure which was inspired with the work of Hashimoto et al. [18]. Liquid samples (10 µL) were pipetted on the suitable type of paper. The type of paper used for the measurement of liquid samples may differ. The laboratory filtration paper can be used for the cell cultures measurement. For blood samples measurement, we used the standard white V-shaped strip of the office (80 g/m^2) paper, which we found more suitable than laboratory filtration paper. When filtration paper was used, the sample was soaked into it and spread on a relatively big area, which produced inconsistent results. Thus, to keep a small area of the dried sample is essential. Such a preparing of the samples has several advantages: (a) fine localised sample; (b) the sample is time-stable; (c) sample can be stored at room temperature and (d) it is ready for repeated measurements. In addition, as the paper is longer than the base length of gradiometer, the paper has a negligible additional signal to the magnetic moment of the sample. We also assume that this procedure can be used for determination of the presence of the USPIONs in homogenates of the soft tissues that cannot be measured in the solid state.

In the conditions used in our study, we set the detection limit of SQUID magnetometry to 0.6 µg Fe/g of the sample dry weight using PEGylated NPs. Another way of iron NPs determination in rodent tissues has recently been described by Poller at al., who used magnetic particle spectroscopy [35] to analyse fate and metabolic processing of very small iron oxide NPs in atherosclerotic mice after injection of 300 µmol of iron NPs.

It is worthy to note that we observed a relatively high variability of the results during experiment, mainly in blood. This may result from individual metabolic differences between rats. We also found that the amount of USPIONs in blood and tissues can be affected by stress, which significantly alters blood circulation and can also potentially affect the stability of USPIONs [36]. Thus, our experience has shown that caution is needed when manipulating experimental subjects and ensuring the best possible stress-free conditions is needed to reduce the variability of results.

In conclusion, we have improved the SQUID magnetometric method for determination of the low content of nanoparticle-originated iron in the solid and liquid samples of the animal tissues at 300 K, which allows distinguishing the low dose of USPION-originated iron from the biogenic iron naturally present in the tissues and blood. This method is more cost-effective and less time-consuming then measurements at 2 K, which requires liquid He for cooling of the system. Furthermore, the once-prepared sample is stable, and it can be stored at room temperature and repeatedly measured. This method also allows for the determination of the USPIONs in the tissues after administration of the low doses of NPs when standard methods are unable to determine USPION-originated iron in the tissues.

Author Contributions: Conceptualization, M.Š. and I.B.; Data curation, M.Š.; Formal analysis, M.Š., A.D., A.M., J.M. and I.B.; Funding acquisition, J.M. and I.B.; Investigation, M.Š., A.D., M.K., A.B., P.B., A.M., A.E.-A. and J.M.; Methodology, M.Š., M.K., A.B., P.B., A.C., J.M. and I.B.; Project administration, J.M. and I.B.; Visualization, M.Š., A.B., A.E.-A. and I.B.; Writing—original draft, M.Š. and I.B.; Writing—review & editing, M.Š., A.D., A.C., J.M. and I.B. All authors have read and agreed to the published version of the manuscript.

Funding: This research was funded by the Slovak Research and Development Agency under Contract No. APVV-16-0263 and by the grants VEGA 2/0160/17 and VEGA 2/164/17.

Acknowledgments: The authors thank R. Kurjakova, J. Petova, B. Bolgacova and R. Tanglmajer for their excellent technical assistance.

Conflicts of Interest: The authors declare no conflict of interest.

References

1. Hentze, M.W.; Muckenthaler, M.; Galy, B.; Camaschella, C. Two to Tango: Regulation of Mammalian Iron Metabolism. *Cell* **2010**, *142*, 24–38. [CrossRef] [PubMed]
2. Chen, C.; Paw, B.H. Cellular and mitochondrial iron homeostasis in vertebrates. *Biochim. Biophys. Acta (BBA)-Bioenerg.* **2012**, *1823*, 1459–1467. [CrossRef] [PubMed]
3. Moroishi, T.; Nishiyama, M.; Takeda, Y.; Iwai, K.; Nakayama, K.I. The FBXL5-IRP2 Axis Is Integral to Control of Iron Metabolism In Vivo. *Cell Metab.* **2011**, *14*, 339–351. [CrossRef] [PubMed]
4. Nel, A.; Xia, T.; Mädler, L.; Li, N. Toxic Potential of Materials at the Nanolevel. *Science* **2006**, *311*, 622–627. [CrossRef]
5. Estelrich, J.; Escribano-Ferrer, E.; Queralt, J.; Busquets, M.A. Iron Oxide Nanoparticles for Magnetically-Guided and Magnetically-Responsive Drug Delivery. *Int. J. Mol. Sci.* **2015**, *16*, 8070–8101. [CrossRef]
6. Bietenbeck, M.; Florian, A.; Sechtem, U.; Yilmaz, A. The diagnostic value of iron oxide nanoparticles for imaging of myocardial inflammation—Quo vadis? *J. Cardiovasc. Magn. Reson.* **2015**, *17*, 54. [CrossRef]
7. Gonzales-Weimuller, M.; Zeisberger, M.; Krishnan, K.M. Size-dependant heating rates of iron oxide nanoparticles for magnetic fluid hyperthermia. *J. Magn. Magn. Mater.* **2009**, *321*, 1947–1950. [CrossRef]
8. Škrátek, M.; Šimáček, I.; Dvurečenskij, A.; Majerová, M.; Maňka, J. Magnetometric Measurements of Low Concentration of Coated Fe_3O_4 Nanoparticles. *Acta Phys. Pol. A* **2014**, *126*, 396–397. [CrossRef]
9. Singh, N.; Jenkins, G.J.S.; Asadi, R.; Doak, S.H. Potential toxicity of superparamagnetic iron oxide nanoparticles (SPION). *Nano Rev.* **2010**, *1*, 5358. [CrossRef]
10. Fröhlich, E. The role of surface charge in cellular uptake and cytotoxicity of medical nanoparticles. *Int. J. Nanomed.* **2012**, *7*, 5577–5591. [CrossRef]
11. Gaharwar, U.S.; Meena, R.; Rajamani, P. Iron oxide nanoparticles induced cytotoxicity, oxidative stress and DNA damage in lymphocytes. *J. Appl. Toxicol.* **2017**, *37*, 1232–1244. [CrossRef] [PubMed]

12. NiedzielskiiD, P.; Zielińska-Dawidziak, M.; Kozak, L.; Kowalewski, P.; Szlachetka, B.; Zalicka, S.; Wachowiak, W. Determination of Iron Species in Samples of Iron-Fortified Food. *Food Anal. Methods* **2014**, *7*, 2023–2032. [CrossRef]
13. Borzoei, M.; Zanjanchi, M.A.; Sadeghi-Aliabadi, H.; Saghaie, L. Optimization of a methodology for determination of iron concentration in aqueous samples using a newly synthesized chelating agent in dispersive liquid-liquid microextraction. *Food Chem.* **2018**, *264*, 9–15. [CrossRef] [PubMed]
14. Bruvera, I.J.; Zélis, P.M.; Calatayud, M.P.; Goya, G.F.; Sánchez, F.H. Determination of the blocking temperature of magnetic nanoparticles: The good, the bad, and the ugly. *J. Appl. Phys.* **2015**, *118*, 184304. [CrossRef]
15. Lee, T.H.; Choi, K.-Y.; Kim, G.-H.; Suh, B.J.; Jang, Z.H. Exponential blocking-temperature distribution in ferritin extracted from magnetization measurements. *Phys. Rev. B* **2014**, *90*, 184411. [CrossRef]
16. Zheng, R.; Gu, H.-W.; Zhang, B.; Liu, H.; Zhang, X.; Ringer, S. Extracting anisotropy energy barrier distributions of nanomagnetic systems from magnetization/susceptibility measurements. *J. Magn. Magn. Mater.* **2009**, *321*, L21–L27. [CrossRef]
17. Hansen, M.F.; Mørup, S. Estimation of blocking temperatures from ZFC/FC curves. *J. Magn. Magn. Mater.* **1999**, *203*, 214–216. [CrossRef]
18. Hashimoto, S.; Oda, T.; Yamada, K.; Takagi, M.; Enomoto, T.; Ohkohchi, N.; Takagi, T.; Kanamori, T.; Ikeda, H.; Yanagihara, H.; et al. The measurement of small magnetic signals from magnetic nanoparticles attached to the cell surface and surrounding living cells using a general-purpose SQUID magnetometer. *Phys. Med. Biol.* **2009**, *54*, 2571–2583. [CrossRef]
19. Levy, M.; Wilhelm, C.; Devaud, M.; Levitz, P.; Gazeau, F. How cellular processing of superparamagnetic nanoparticles affects their magnetic behavior and NMR relaxivity. *Contrast Media Mol. Imaging* **2012**, *7*, 373–383. [CrossRef]
20. Rojas, J.M.; Gavilán, H.; Del Dedo, V.; Lorente-Sorolla, E.; Sanz-Ortega, L.; Da Silva, G.B.; Costo, R.; Perez-Yagüe, S.; Talelli, M.; Marciello, M.; et al. Time-course assessment of the aggregation and metabolization of magnetic nanoparticles. *Acta Biomater.* **2017**, *58*, 181–195. [CrossRef]
21. Gutiérrez, L.; Spasic, M.V.; Muckenthaler, M.; Lázaro, F.J. Quantitative magnetic analysis reveals ferritin-like iron as the most predominant iron-containing species in the murine Hfe-haemochromatosis. *Biochim. Biophys. Acta (BBA)-Mol. Basis Dis.* **2012**, *1822*, 1147–1153. [CrossRef] [PubMed]
22. Zysler, R.D.; Lima, J.E.; Mansilla, M.V.; Troiani, H.E.; Mojica-Pisciotti, M.L.; Gurman, P.; Lamagna, A.; Colombo, L. A New Quantitative Method to Determine the Uptake of SPIONs in Animal Tissue and Its Application to Determine the Quantity of Nanoparticles in the Liver and Lung of Balb-c Mice Exposed to the SPIONs. *J. Biomed. Nanotechnol.* **2013**, *9*, 142–145. [CrossRef] [PubMed]
23. Marín-Barba, M.; Gavilán, H.; Gutiérrez, L.; Lozano-Velasco, E.; Rodriguez-Ramiro, I.; Wheeler, G.N.; Morris, C.J.; Morales, M.P.; Ruiz, A. Unravelling the mechanisms that determine the uptake and metabolism of magnetic single and multicore nanoparticles in aXenopus laevismodel. *Nanoscale* **2018**, *10*, 690–704. [CrossRef] [PubMed]
24. Janus, B.; Bućko, M.; Chrobak, A.; Wasilewski, J.; Zych, M. Magnetic characterization of human blood in the atherosclerotic process in coronary arteries. *J. Magn. Magn. Mater.* **2011**, *323*, 479–485. [CrossRef]
25. Hautot, D.; Pankhurst, Q.A.; Dobson, J. Superconducting quantum interference device measurements of dilute magnetic materials in biological samples. *Rev. Sci. Instrum.* **2005**, *76*, 045101. [CrossRef]
26. Kluknavsky, M.; Balis, P.; Škrátek, M.; Maňka, J.; Bernátová, I. (−)-Epicatechin Reduces the Blood Pressure of Young Borderline Hypertensive Rats During the Post-Treatment Period. *Antioxidants* **2020**, *9*, 96. [CrossRef]
27. Kumar, P.; Bulk, M.; Webb, A.; Van Der Weerd, L.; Oosterkamp, T.H.; Huber, M.; Bossoni, L. A novel approach to quantify different iron forms in ex-vivo human brain tissue. *Sci. Rep.* **2016**, *6*, 38916. [CrossRef]
28. John Bancroft, M.G. *Theory and Practice of Histological Techniques*, 6th ed.; Churchill Livingstone: London, UK, 2008; ISBN 9780443102790.
29. Sawicki, M.; Stefanowicz, W.; Ney, A. Sensitive SQUID magnetometry for studying nanomagnetism. *Semicond. Sci. Technol.* **2011**, *26*, 26. [CrossRef]
30. Yoffe, S.; Leshuk, T.; Everett, P.; Gu, F.X. Superparamagnetic Iron Oxide Nanoparticles (SPIONs): Synthesis and Surface Modification Techniques for use with MRI and Other Biomedical Applications. *Curr. Pharm. Des.* **2012**, *19*, 493–509. [CrossRef]
31. Yu, Z.; Li, Q.; Wang, J.; Yu, Y.; Wang, Y.; Zhou, Q.; Li, P. Reactive Oxygen Species-Related Nanoparticle Toxicity in the Biomedical Field. *Nanoscale Res. Lett.* **2020**, *15*, 115. [CrossRef]

32. Gutiérrez, L.; Lázaro, F.J. Comparative study of iron-containing haematinics from the point of view of their magnetic properties. *J. Magn. Magn. Mater.* **2007**, *316*, 136–139. [CrossRef]
33. Dlháň, Ľ.; Kopani, M.; Boča, R. Magnetic properties of iron oxides present in the human brain. *Polyhedron* **2019**, *157*, 505–510. [CrossRef]
34. Kopani, M.; Hlinkova, J.; Ehrlich, H.; Valigura, D.; Boca, R. Magnetic Properties of Iron Oxides in the Human Globus pallidus. *J. Bioanal. Biomed.* **2017**, *9*, 080–090. [CrossRef]
35. Poller, W.C.; Pieber, M.; Boehm-Sturm, P.; Ramberger, E.; Karampelas, V.; Möller, K.; Schleicher, M.; Wiekhorst, F.; Löwa, N.; Wagner, S.; et al. Very small superparamagnetic iron oxide nanoparticles: Long-term fate and metabolic processing in atherosclerotic mice. *Nanomed. Nanotechnol. Biol. Med.* **2018**, *14*, 2575–2586. [CrossRef] [PubMed]
36. Líšková, S.; Bališ, P.; Mičurová, A.; Kluknavský, M.; Okuliarová, M.; Puzserová, A.; Škrátek, M.; Sekaj, I.; Maňka, J.; Valovič, P.; et al. Effect of Iron Oxide Nanoparticles on Vascular Function and Nitric Oxide Production in Acute Stress-Exposed Rats. *Physiol. Res.* **2020**, under review.

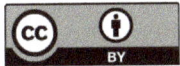

© 2020 by the authors. Licensee MDPI, Basel, Switzerland. This article is an open access article distributed under the terms and conditions of the Creative Commons Attribution (CC BY) license (http://creativecommons.org/licenses/by/4.0/).

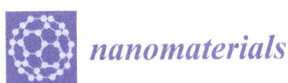

Review

Comprehensive Survey on Nanobiomaterials for Bone Tissue Engineering Applications

Pawan Kumar [1,*], Meenu Saini [1], Brijnandan S. Dehiya [1], Anil Sindhu [2], Vinod Kumar [3], Ravinder Kumar [4,*], Luciano Lamberti [5], Catalin I. Pruncu [6,7,*] and Rajesh Thakur [3]

1. Department of Materials Science and Nanotechnology, Deenbandhu Chhotu Ram University of Science and Technology, Murthal 131039, India; meenu.rschmsn@dcrustm.org (M.S.); drbrijdehiya.msn@dcrustm.org (B.S.D.)
2. Department of Biotechnology, Deenbandhu Chhotu Ram University of Science and Technology, Murthal 131039, India; sindhu.biotech@gmail.com
3. Department of Bio and Nanotechnology, Guru Jambheshwar University of Science and Technology, Hisar 125001, India; indoravinod2@gmail.com (V.K.); rtnano@gmail.com (R.T.)
4. School of Mechanical Engineering, Lovely Professional University, Phagwara 144411, India
5. Dipartimento di Meccanica, Matematica e Management, Politecnico di Bari, 70125 Bari, Italy; luciano.lamberti@poliba.it
6. Department of Design, Manufacturing & Engineering Management, University of Strathclyde, Glasgow G1 1XJ, UK
7. Department of Mechanical Engineering, Imperial College London, London SW7 2AZ, UK
* Correspondence: pawankamiya@yahoo.in (P.K.); rav.chauhan@yahoo.co.in (R.K.); catalin.pruncu@strath.ac.uk (C.I.P.)

Received: 1 September 2020; Accepted: 9 October 2020; Published: 13 October 2020

Abstract: One of the most important ideas ever produced by the application of materials science to the medical field is the notion of biomaterials. The nanostructured biomaterials play a crucial role in the development of new treatment strategies including not only the replacement of tissues and organs, but also repair and regeneration. They are designed to interact with damaged or injured tissues to induce regeneration, or as a forest for the production of laboratory tissues, so they must be micro-environmentally sensitive. The existing materials have many limitations, including impaired cell attachment, proliferation, and toxicity. Nanotechnology may open new avenues to bone tissue engineering by forming new assemblies similar in size and shape to the existing hierarchical bone structure. Organic and inorganic nanobiomaterials are increasingly used for bone tissue engineering applications because they may allow to overcome some of the current restrictions entailed by bone regeneration methods. This review covers the applications of different organic and inorganic nanobiomaterials in the field of hard tissue engineering.

Keywords: nano-biomaterials; nanotechnology; scaffolds; hard tissue engineering

1. Introduction

Nanobiomaterials denote nanometer-sized materials whose structures and constituents have significant and novel characteristics with a strong impact on healing and medicine [1,2]. They include metals, ceramics, polymers, hydrogels, and novel self-assembled materials [3]. Rapid developments in nanotechnology not only led to create new materials and tools for biomedical applications, but also changed the way of using these materials in science and technology [4,5].

Human bone is a dynamic tissue that can rebuild and remodel in the body throughout life [6]. The human bone is a hierarchical assembly of nano- to macro-scale organic and inorganic components involved in transmitting physio-chemical and mechano-chemical cues [7,8]. The schematic of Figure 1 shows that normal human bone contains 30% organic collagen fibrils and 70% inorganic minerals [9–12], while 2% of the total volume is occupied by bone cells, osteoblasts, osteoclasts, lining cells, progenitor cells, and adipocytes [13,14]. Crystalline phases form 65% of the dry weight of the mineral matrix and most part of calcined fraction in calcium phosphate [15,16].

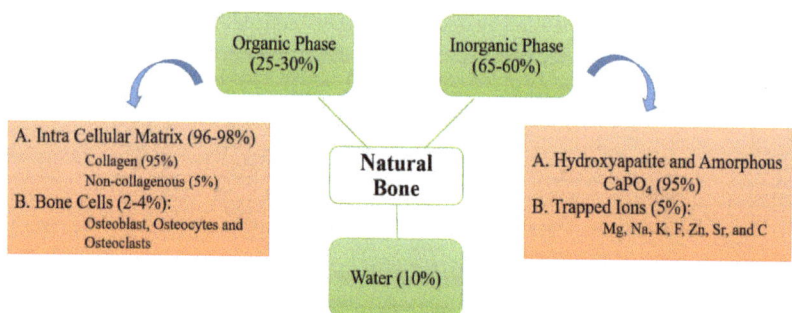

Figure 1. Composition of natural bone.

The continuously growing population and the higher complexity of human interactions have generated new bone-related diseases (e.g., bone tumors, bone infections, and bone loss). This requires effective handling and treatment for bone regeneration [17,18]. Tissue engineering has revolutionized orthopedic and surgical studies, providing a new direction in the field based on nanoscale surface modification to simulate properties of extracellular matrix (ECM) and new foundations of structural variables of autologous tissue [19,20]. Tissue engineering is used to generate, restore, and/or replace tissues and organs by using biomaterials and helps to produce similar native tissue or organ [21].

Nanotechnology solved many questions in tissue engineering by modifying regenerative strategies [22]. Biomedical applications of nanotechnology became a hot subject because different nanomaterials are utilized for the synthesis of scaffolds or implants [23,24]. These nanomaterials may be metallic [25], ceramic, or polymeric [26] with different structural forms such as tubes, rods, fibers, and spheres [27]. Various properties of materials such as physiochemical, electrical, mechanical, optical, catalytic, and magnetic properties can be improved at the nanoscale [28] and tailored to specific applications. Nanomaterials synthesized through top-down or bottom-up approaches [29] (Figure 2) have outstanding properties, which are used for biomedical applications particularly in tissue engineering [22].

Existing biomaterials often do not integrate with host tissue completely. This may cause infection and foreign body reactions that lead to implant failure [30]. Indeed, nanostructured biomaterials imitate the natural bone's extracellular matrix (ECM), producing an artificial microenvironment that promotes cell adhesion, proliferation and differentiation [31]. The specific biological, morphological, and biochemical properties of nanobiomaterials attract researchers to use them for the hard tissue engineering [32]. Nanostructured biomaterials can be used to fabricate high-performance scaffolds or implants with tailored physical, chemical, and biological properties. Several natural and synthetic nanostructured biomaterials are now available for the fabrication of scaffolds with decent bioactivity [33].

This survey article presents the most relevant applications of nanobiomaterials to bone tissue engineering, trying to highlight how organic and inorganic nanobiomaterials can deal with the above mentioned requirements on bone regeneration and the multiple challenges entailed by such a complicated subject. A broad overview of the various types of nanobiomaterials and their applications in the field of hard tissue engineering is provided.

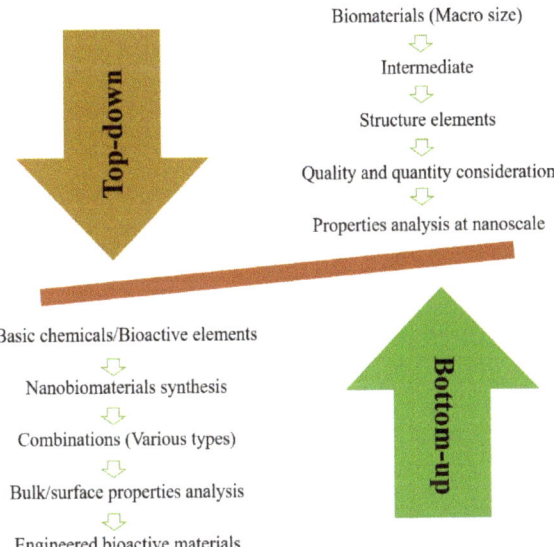

Figure 2. Design of bioactive materials based on top-down and bottom-up approaches.

Besides the introductory articles mentioned above and other general articles on topics related to nanomaterials and the different contexts where they operate, the present survey covers some 550 technical papers focusing on types, fabrication, and applications of nanobiomaterials. These articles have been selected using three widely used academic search engines: Scopus, Web of Science, and Google Scholar. For that purpose, keywords such as "tissue engineering", "bone tissue engineering", "tissue regeneration", "scaffolds", "nanomaterials", and "nanobiomaterials" as well as their combinations have been used as input for the search process. High priority is given to peer-reviewed journal articles with respect to book chapters and conference proceedings, which count for some 10 papers, less than 1.75% of the total number of surveyed articles. More detailed statistics on the articles surveyed for each topic will be reported at the end of the corresponding subsections.

The paper is structured as follows. Sections 2 and 3 describe the various types of organic and inorganic nanobiomaterials and their applications in bone tissue engineering/regenerative medicines, drug/gene delivery, anti-infection properties, coatings, scaffold fabrication, and cancer therapy; generalizing conclusions are given at the end of each section. The conclusion section summarizes the main findings of this survey.

2. Nanobiomaterials

Nanobiomaterials cover a wide variety of biomaterials including natural and artificial materials, used for various applications in tissue engineering [34–36]. These materials can be classified into two categories, i.e., organic nanobiomaterials and inorganic nanobiomaterials, where the former is characterized by the presence of carbon-containing constituents. Organic–inorganic hybrids are much more effective biomaterials than pure polymers, bioglasses, metals, alloys, and ceramics [37] as they try to combine best properties of constituents following the general concept of composite material. Section 2.1 will review the different types of organic nanobiomaterials, while Section 2.2 will review the different types of inorganic nanobiomaterials.

2.1. Organic Nanobiomaterials

Nanostructured materials have characteristics like biocompatibility, nontoxicity, and non-carcinogenicity. When used for replacement or restoration of body tissue, they are regarded as organic nanobiomaterials [38].

Several research groups have shifted their attention from metallic to organic nanomaterials, such as lipids, liposomes, dendrimers, and polymers including chitosan, gelatin, collagen, or other biodegradable polymers [39]. Organic materials are combinations of a few of the lightest elements, particularly hydrogen, nitrogen and oxygen, and carbon-containing chemical compounds located within living organisms [40]. Proteins, nucleic acids, lipids, and carbohydrates (the polysaccharides) are the basic types of organic materials [41].

Table 1 presents a general classification of organic nanobiomaterials and summarizes representative applications of each material in tissue engineering. The following subsections present a general description of each nanomaterial type listed in Table 1 and a detailed literature survey on the corresponding developments for tissue engineering.

Table 1. Types of organic nanobiomaterials with their applications.

Types of Nanomaterials	Size (nm)	Applications	References
Lipid	<100	Nanocarriers for anticancer drug doxorubicin Osteoblastic bone formation Osteoporosis treatment	[42–45]
Liposome	>25	High encapsulation of hydrophilic drug (drug delivery) Growth factor delivery Therapeutic gene delivery Used as a template	[46–48]
Dendrimers	<10	Multidrug delivery system	[46,49,50]
Chitosan	20–200	Nano/microparticles or fiber-based scaffolds Drug delivery Support chondrocyte adhesion Implant coating	[51–55]
Collagen	–	Drug Delivery Scaffolds	[56]
Gelatin	<200	Bone scaffold systems formation Drug-loaded gelatin nanoparticles (DGNPs) Promote cell growth	[24,57,58]
Poly(lactic-co-glycolic acid) PLGA	100–250	Drug delivery Scaffold system Nanostructured Film Enhanced cell attachment and growth	[59–62]
Carbon Nanotubes	20–100	Drug delivery Biosensing Mechanically improved scaffold fabrication Enhanced rat brain neuron response	[63–66]

2.1.1. Lipids

Lipids are small hydrophobic or amphiphilic molecules [67]. They can be classified as fatty lipids of acylglycerol, phospholipids such as glycerides, seduction lipids, sterols, demonstrations of lipids played, lipids, and polylactide Kane [68]. Lipids are essential agents for the physiological and pathophysiological functioning of cells [69]. Generally, 10–1000 nm sized spherical lipid nanoparticles are synthesized [70]. All organisms consist of lipids as basic components, among other ingredients. The use of these lipids in pharmaceutical and biomedical fields can solve the problem of biocompatibility and biodegradation [71]. Besides liposomes (lipids arranged in the formation), other unique structures (e.g., hexagonal, spongy, solid structure, etc.) resulting from lipid polymorphisms also are available [72,73]. The latter have better stability and production efficiency than liposomes [48]. Lipid nanocarriers are better than polymeric nanoparticles (NPs) in terms of biocompatibility and lower toxicity, production cost and scalability, and encapsulation efficiency of highly lipophilic actives [74,75]. Lipid nanocarriers such as solid lipid nanoparticles (SLN) [76], nanostructured lipid carriers (NLC) [77], lipid nanocapsules

(LNC) [78], and drug–lipid conjugates [79] are used for various administration routes (i.e., parenteral, oral, and topical ones) [80]. Lipid polymer hybrid nanoparticles (LPHNs) can also be used in the area of bioimaging agents for medicinal diagnostics as delivery vehicles like iron oxide, quantum dots (QDs) fluorescent dyes, and inorganic nanocrystals [81].

2.1.2. Liposomes

Liposomes were discovered in the mid-1960s by A. D. Bangham [82]. The vesicle of the liposome is easily fabricated in a laboratory and made of one or more phospholipid bilayers [83] (Figure 3). These are self-assembled versatile particles with diameters ranging from nanometer to micrometer scale [84]. Resembling lipid cell membranes, the nature of phospholipid depends on the length of fatty acid chains [48]. They have the ability to encapsulate and carry hydrophobic aqueous agents [82]. They exhibit many advantages over other carrier systems [85,86].

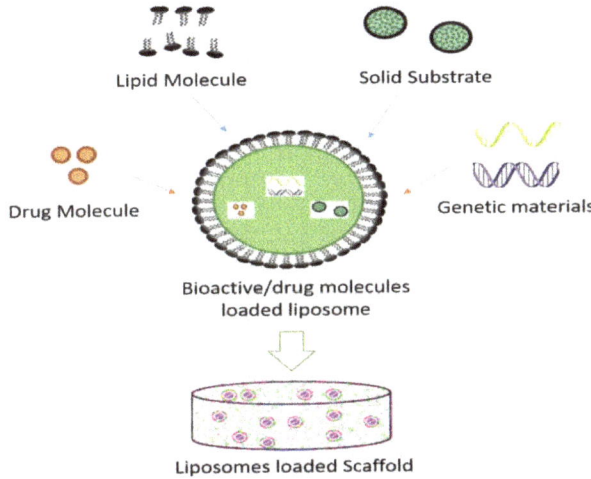

Figure 3. Fabrication of liposome loaded scaffold.

Bone morphogenetic protein-2 (BMP-2) is one of the most potent proteins in bone regeneration [87]. For this reason, encapsulation of BMP-2 in nanomaterials has attracted great interest. BMP-2-loaded liposomal-based scaffolds may possess better osteoinductivity and bone formation ability [88].

Liposomes can carry drugs directly to the site of action and sustain their levels without causing toxicity for long periods [89]. By changing the composition of lipids, liposome properties can change. Some liposome preparations for anticancer drugs have successfully released on the market by acquiring FDA's approval [83]. Gentamycin- and vancomycin-integrated liposome-loaded particles are employed for manufacturing of scaffolds [90]. The integration of bioactive aspirin into a liposome delivery system would have a beneficial impact on stem cell osteoblast differentiation [91]. The initial drug amount and the chemical and physical drug properties are considerable factors for the encapsulation efficiency [92]. DOXIL®, the first FDA-approved nanodrug, which consists of liposomes encapsulating doxorubicin, was prepared by this remote loading method [93]. This method can also be used for preparing liposomes encapsulating other drugs such as daunorubicin and vincristine [94]. Liposomal systems are highly used despite being the oldest of the non-viralgene-delivery vehicles [95]. Scaffolds used as delivery vehicles for bioactive agents offer many advantages such as enhanced and extended gene expression, and the ability to control a localized delivery of cargo [96] (see Figures 3 and 4).

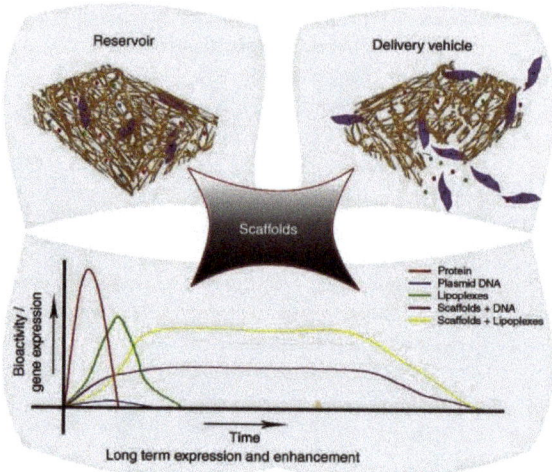

Figure 4. Schematic depiction of the role of tissue-engineered scaffolds in gene delivery [96] (adapted with permission from Elsevier © 2009).

2.1.3. Dendrimers

Dendrimers are the newest class of highly-defined macromolecules, which differs from simple polymers by branching at each repeating unit [97]. Their step-by-step controlled synthesis is used worldwide for molecular chemistry, while their repeating structure made of monomers relate them to the world of polymers [98,99]. The repetitively branched nanometer-scale dimension of dendrimers is an ideal candidate for a variety of tissue engineering [100], molecular imaging [101], and drug delivery [102] applications. Dendrimers can be a main component of scaffolds mimicking cross-linkers, chemical surface modifiers, and charge modifiers, as well as natural extracellular matrices [103].

The combination of dendrimers with other conventional structural polymers, such as proteins, carbohydrates and linear synthetic polymers, leads to obtain new physical, mechanical and biochemical properties of hybrid structures [100,104]. The center of dendrimer may be composed of polypropylimine (PPI), di-aminobutyl (DAB), polyamidoamine (PAMAM), and ethylenediamine (EDA), along with various surface residues such as amine, carboxyl, and alcoholic groups [105]. A dendrimer can be synthesized for particular use in different parts with controlled properties like solubility and thermal stability [106].

Dendrimer–drug conjugation is a better approach to the encapsulation of cytotoxic pharmaceuticals. In this way, numerous cytotoxic and anticancer drugs, and targeted individuals such as monoclonal antibodies, peptides, and folic acid, can be conjugated to a single dendrimer molecule [107]. The drug is covalently conjugated to the dendrimer rather than complexed (Figure 5) [108] and these conjugates are relatively more stable.

Dendrimers are a good choice for hydrophobic moieties and poorly water-soluble drugs [109]. PAMAM dendrimer/DNA complexes were employed to encapsulate functional fast biodegradable polymer films used for substrate-mediated gene delivery [110].

The physicochemical characteristics, such as solubility and pharmacokinetics, of dendrimers are better than those of linear polymers. Therefore, dendrimers are ideal candidates for incorporation into scaffolds used for tissue engineering applications [111,112]. A few scaffolds were fabricated with dendrimers such as poly(caprolactone) chains conjugated to a poly(L-lysine) dendritic core to fabricate an HA-composite [113], linear PCL/n-HA hybrids [114], N-hydroxy succinimide/1-ethyl-3-(3-dimethyl aminopropyl) carbodiimide (NHS/EDC) cross-linked scaffold [115], and dexamethasone carboxymethyl chitosan/PAMAM [116] for in vitro bone regeneration.

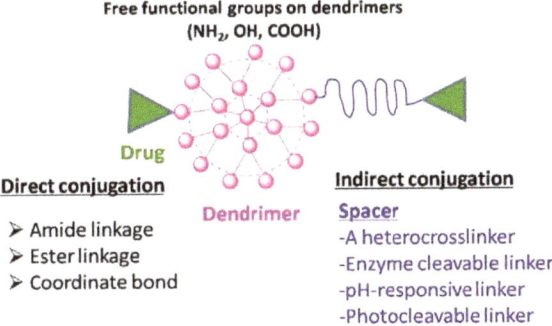

Figure 5. Structure of a typical dendrimer–drug conjugate (Reused with permission from Elsevier [108].)

2.1.4. Polymeric Nanomaterials

Polymeric nanoparticles of size range 10 nm to 1 µm are the most advanced noninvasive approaches to tissue engineering and drug delivery applications [117]. They are comprised of repeating units of chain-like macromolecules with multiple structures and compositions [118]. In general, polymeric nanoparticles can be used for different applications by changing the physicochemical properties of nanoparticles. Polymers are differently processed to produce nanofibers [119], spherical nanoparticles [120] and polymeric micelles [121] for specific applications.

There are several techniques to synthesize polymer-based nanoparticles, applied in tissue engineering [122]. Gelation [123], emulsion–solvent evaporation [124], nanoprecipitation [125], salting-out [122], and desolvation process [126] are generally preferred for natural polymers, like proteins and polysaccharides. Similar to other nanoparticle systems, polymer-based nanoparticles or nanocomposites can be functionalized to perform active targeting [127].

Polymeric nanoparticles alter and may enhance the pharmacokinetic and pharmacodynamic properties used for various drug types because they show controlled and sustained release properties [128]. They offer a variety of benefits ranging from the administration of non-soluble drugs to protection of unstable compounds [129]. These nanoparticles can be loaded with therapeutic or bioactive molecules (Figure 6) either by dispersion or adsorption within the polymer matrix, or encapsulation [130,131].

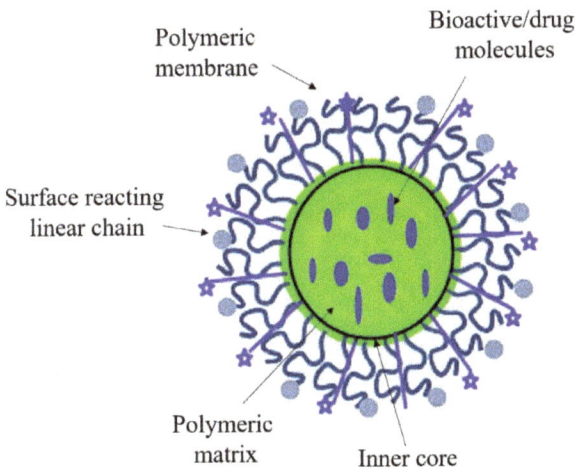

Figure 6. Bioactive/drug molecules loaded polymeric nanoparticles.

Drug release may occur directly from nanoparticles through diffusion and polymeric nanoparticles may dissociate into monomers [132]. Polymers used for nanoparticle fabrication should be degradable via enzymatic or non-enzymatic routes under common metabolic pathways [133,134]. Drug-containing polymeric nanoparticles must be stable during migration to the plasma, that is, at almost neutral pH [135].

Chitosan, collagen, gelatin, hyaluronic acid, alginate, and albumin are representative examples of natural biopolymers [136,137]. Polymeric nanoparticles are one of the fastest-growing platforms for the applications in tissue engineering because of their biocompatibility, biodegradability, low cytotoxicity, high permeation, ability to deliver poorly soluble drugs, and retaining bioactivity after degradation [117]. Some newly designed polymeric nanoparticles are sensitive to pH, temperature, oxidizing/reducing agents, and magnetic field which support a high efficiency and specificity for tissue engineering applications [138,139]. Due to good biocompatibility and adjustable chemical composition, and their ability to reorganize, polymeric nanoparticles are very promising as nanobiomaterials for the fabrication of scaffolds or bone substitutes [140]. Plasma protein-based nanoparticles have shown high biodegradability, bioavailability, long in vivo half-lives, and long shelf lives without any toxicity. Blood plasma is a complex mixture of 100,000 proteins, but only two of these proteins have been used in drug administration and tissue regeneration [141,142].

Chitosan

Chitosan is a natural and nontoxic linear biopolymer synthesized from alkaline N-deacetylation of chitin [143]. It can be extracted from exoskeleton of crustacean shells (i.e., crabs and shrimps) some microbes, yeast, and fungi [144]. It has different molecular weights and is soluble in various organic solutions at pH 6.5 and below. The shape of the chitosan nanoparticles is affected by the degree of deacetylation [145,146]. The presence of amine and hydroxyl group leads the use of these compounds in many research areas [147,148]. Chitosan has outstanding biochemical properties, making it very attractive for applications in many areas including tissue engineering and/or regenerative medicine (Figure 7) [149]. Chitosan nanoparticles carry well therapeutic agents and biomolecules because of their high biocompatibility and biodegradability. Because of their small size, they can pass through biological barriers in vivo and deliver the drugs at the targeted site [150].

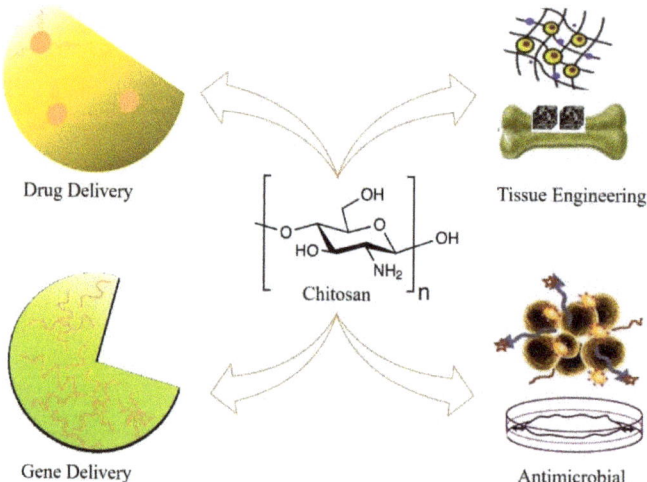

Figure 7. Prospective applications of chitosan.

Applications of Chitosan: Scaffolds prepared from chitosan and ceramics, especially hydroxyapatite, may have superior osteoconductive properties [151]. Bone morphogenetic protein-2 (BMP-2)-loaded chitosan nanoparticles used for the coating of Ti implants were selected in order to examine bone regeneration in mice [55]. Chitosan and growth factor (BMP-7) were used to functionalize a thick electrospun poly(ε-caprolactone) nanofibrous implant (from 700 µm to 1 cm thick), which produced a fish scale-like chitosan/BMP-7 nano-reservoir. This nanofibrous implant mimicked the extracellular matrix and enabled in vitro colonization and bone regeneration [152]. There, the polycationic nature of chitosan entails an antimicrobial behavior at nanoscale [153]. Besides the orthodontic field, there are relevant applications of chitosan in skin healing, nerve regeneration, and oral mucosa [39]. Nanobioglass incorporated chitosan-gelatin scaffolds showed excellent cytocompatibility and ability to accelerate the crystallization of bone-like apatite in vitro [154,155]. The nanocomposite of chitosan/hydroxyapatite-zinc oxide (CTS/HAp-ZnO) supporting organically modified montmorillonite clay (OMMT) was synthesized and used for hard tissue engineering applications [156]. BMP-2 and BMP-7 loaded poly(3-hydroxybutyrate-co3-hydroxyvalerate) nanocapsules were used for the fabrication of chitosan-poly(ethylene oxide) scaffolds [157]. Mili et al. [158] used nerve growth factor (NGF) loaded chitosan nanoparticles for neural differentiation of canine mesenchymal stem cells. Freeze-dried nano-TiO$_2$/chitosan scaffolds showed high biocompatibility and antibacterial effects [159]. Chitosan-poly(vinyl alcohol)-gum tragacanth (CS/PVA/GT) hybrid nanofibrous scaffolds showed 20 MPa ultimate tensile strength and supported L929 fibroblast cells growth [160]. Collagen–chitosan–calcium phosphate microsphere scaffolds fused with glycolic acid did not show relevant differences in their degradation, cytocompatibility, porosity, and Young's modulus [160,161].

Collagen

The main constituents of living human bone are collagen type-1 (protein) and calcium phosphate or hydroxyapatite (mineral) [162]. Collagen is the major structural protein of the soft and hard tissues in living organisms [163]. It can have a significant role in preserving biological and structural integrity of extracellular matrix (ECM) [164]. It is a versatile material that is widely used in the biomedical field (Figure 8) due to advantages including high biocompatibility and biodegradability [165]. Collagen is mainly used as a carrier for drug delivery as well as osteogenic and bone filling material [166]. Collagen matrix was also used to deliver gene promoting bone synthesis [167]. Collagen with recombinant human bone morphogenetic protein-2 was used to monitor bone formation [168].

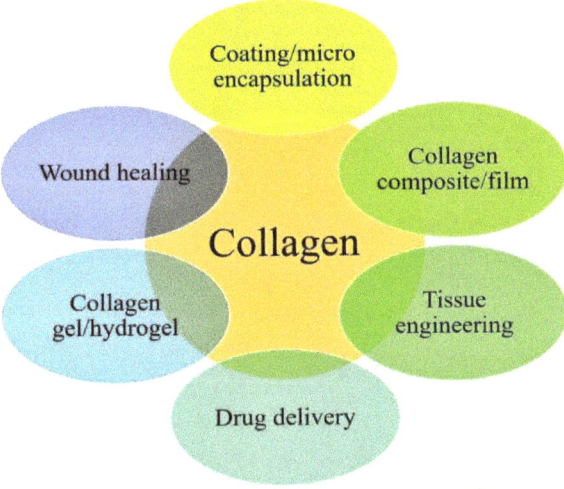

Figure 8. Biomedical applications of collagen.

Bone morphogenic protein (BMP)-loaded collagen activates osteoinduction in the host tissue [169]. Collagen-based nanospheres/nanoparticles can be used as a systematic delivery carrier for various therapeutic agents or biomolecules [166]. As collagen type-I and hydroxyapatite are a basic part of the bone, hydroxyapatite and collagen were used to fabricate scaffolds that enhance osteoblast differentiation and accelerate osteogenesis [170].

Collagen-based biomaterials in various formats such as 3-D scaffolds have been employed for tissue engineering [171]. The combination of collagen with elastin was successfully fabricated and in vitro tests proved the adhesion and proliferation of cells without any cytotoxicity [172]. Collagen-based inks were used for 3D bioprinting employed for tissue repairing and scaffold fabrication. The collagen-based ink was extruded with a temperature stage of −40 °C, followed by freeze-drying and cross-linking by using 1-ethyl-(3-3-dimethylaminopropyl) hydrochloride solution [173].

Gelatin

Gelatin represents a derivative of collagen, extracted by collagen hydrolysis from the skin, bones, and/or connective tissues of animals. It is a cost effective, biocompatible, and biodegradable polymer, which supports cross-linking of functional groups. Gelatin is a versatile polymer that is known for his wealth merits [174]. Pharmaceutical or medical grade gelatin has fragility and transparency for tablet coatings, suspensions, capsule formulations, and nano-formulations (Figure 9).

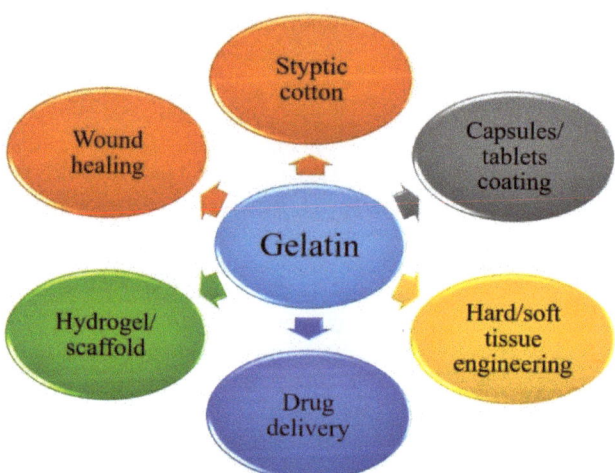

Figure 9. Biomedical and pharmaceutical uses of gelatin.

Because of their great biocompatibility, the injected gelatin-loaded nanoparticles have been reported in the skeletal system [24,175,176]. It is a polyampholyte at pH 9 (gelatin A) and pH 5 (gelatin B). Gelatin nanoparticles are used as a biomaterial for the delivery of biomolecules and therapeutic agents [177]. However, digestive process of gelatin showed low antigenicity, with the formation of harmless metabolic products. In order to prevent infectious disease transmission, genetic engineering approaches were used for the production of human recombinant gelatin [178,179].

At the nanoscale, gelatin shows high biocompatibility, biodegradability, and low immunogenicity [180]. The presence of a higher number of functional groups on polymer backbone helps with crosslinking and chemical modification [181]. The cross-linking is necessary to stabilize the macromolecular structure of gelatin is not stable at normal body temperature due to the low melting temperature [182,183].

Gelatin methacryloyl (GelMA) hybrid hydrogel demonstrated a wide range of tissue engineering applications. When exposed to light irradiation, GelMA scaffolds convert into hydrogels with tunable mechanical properties [184]. Gelatin enables therapeutic cell adhesion without comprising cell phenotypes [185]. Porous HA-gelatin microparticles (1 to 100 μm) support human osteoblast-like Saos-2 cells growth and cell delivery [186]. A mechanically strong gelatin–silk hydrogel composite was prepared by direct blending of gelatin with amorphous Bombyxmori silk fibroin (SF) [187]. Gelatin coated polyamide (PA) scaffold showed good biomechanical, cell attachment, and wound healing characteristics while being transplanted to nude rats [188]. Poly(lactide-co-glycolide) (PLGA)–gelatin fibrous scaffolds possess the highest Young's modulus (770 ± 131 kPa) and tensile strength (130 ± 7 kPa) [189]. Methacrylamide-modified gelatin (GelMOD) 3D CAD scaffolds showed excellent stability in culture medium and support porcine mesenchymal stem cell adhesion and subsequent proliferation [190].

Gelatin-based microcarriers used embryonic stem cell delivery for the applications in tissue engineering [191]. The magnetic nanoparticles were assembled with magnetic gelatin membranes to produce 3D multilayered scaffolds (Figure 10), which are used for controlled distribution of magnetically labeled stem cells [192].

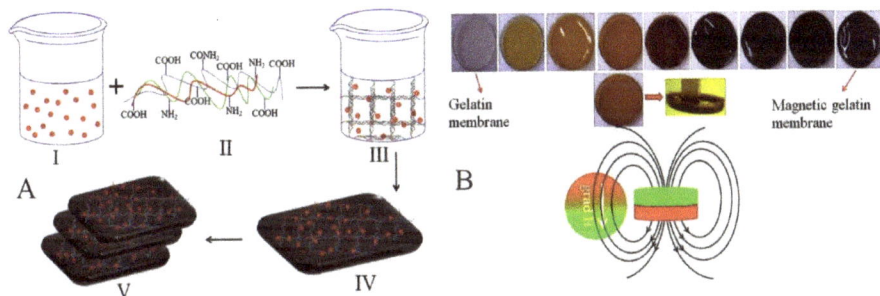

Figure 10. (**A**) Fabrication of a multilayered magnetic gelatin scaffold. (**B**) Magnetic gelatin membranes with increasing MNPs concentration from left to right as well as a representation of the properties of the magnetic gradient. (Adapted with permission from © 2015 American Chemical Society [192]).

Poly (Lactic-co-glycolic) acid (PLGA)

PLGA is considered as one of the most efficient tissue engineering materials due to its (i) high biocompatibility, (ii) biodegradability, (iii) potential to interact with biological materials, and (iv) clinical use approved by FDA [193]. Biodegradable biomolecule-loaded PLGA nanoparticles can be used for the preparation of a drug delivery system, which can be further utilized in scaffold fabrications [194–196]. These nanoparticles may increase the mechanical properties of the scaffolds but decrease swelling behavior without changing the morphology of the scaffold [197]. Afterward, this system is effective to prepare a controlled release platform for model drugs that favors the bio-distribution and development of clinically relevant therapies [198]. Different methods such as gas foaming [199], porogen leaching [200], solid freedom fabrication [201], and phase separation [202] can be used for PLGA scaffolds fabrication.

2.1.5. Carbon Nanostructures

Carbon nanomaterials are great candidate materials for bone tissue engineering due to their conductivity, lightweight, stability and strength [203]. Nanostructures such as fullerenes, carbon nanotubes, carbon nanofibers, and graphene are the most common structures (Figure 11) [204,205].

Han et al. [205] pointed out that carbon is biocompatible and can be used in many clinical applications, such as prosthetic heart valves. However, a pure form of carbon nanomaterials cannot be used as a substrate for bone tissue [206]. Therefore, carbon-based materials are used in combined form to fabricate scaffolds [207]. Carbon nanostructures doped or reinforced compositions became more popular due to their high performance and compatibility with bone tissues [203].

Carbon nanofibers (CNF) are cylindrical or conical structures of various diameters and lengths. The interior structure of the CNF contains an improved layout of graphene sheets. Graphene is a single-layer two-dimensional material composed of long-edged reactive carbon atoms. Graphene leaves are characterized by stable dispersion and orientation of nanofillers [208–210].

Carbon nanotubes (CNT) enhance mechanical and electrical properties, which helps to generate innovative products. CNTs are one of the ideal and favorable materials used for designing novel polymer composites [211]. Many authors focused on the progress of composite materials fabrication-integrating CNTs to enhance its applications in biomedical field [212–216].

Nanodiamonds (4–10 nm) are typically different from other nanostructures as they are sp^3 hybridized [203]. They show admirable protein binding ability and can be used as a carrier for some biomolecules such as BMP-2 [217]. The carbon nanotube/gold hybrids are employed commonly for the delivery of the anticancer drug doxorubicin hydrochloride into A549 lung cancer cell line [218].

Nanoscaffolds can be produced by electrospinning poly(ε-caprolactone) (PCL) and different types of carbon nanomaterials such as carbon nanotubes, graphene, and fullerene [219]. Mesoporous silica (mSiO$_2$) decorated carbon nanotubes (CNTs) hybrid composite were used for the simultaneous applications of gentamicin and protein cytochrome C delivery and imaging [220]. Single-walled carbon nano-horns encapsulated with positively charged lipids complex were used for targeted drug and protein delivery [221].

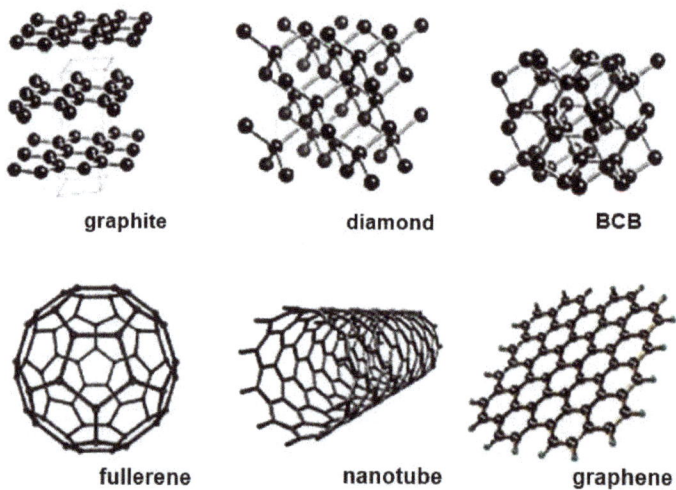

Figure 11. Structure of various allotropes of carbon (adapted with permission from Royal Society of Chemistry [205]). In the figure, "BCB" stands for "benzocyclobutene".

2.1.6. Summary and Statistical Analysis of the Survey on Organic Nanobiomaterials

The survey on organic nanobiomaterials presented in Section 2.1 regarded some 200 articles. Polymeric nanomaterials, carbon nanostructures, and nanocomposite materials are the most widely investigated subject (60.8% of the studies), followed by dendrimers (21.1%) and lipids/liposomes (18.1%). While dendrimers and lipid/liposomes are mainly utilized as nanocarriers, the other nanomaterials cover a much broader spectrum of applications. The development of new nanomaterials (especially carbon nanomaterials or materials including natural bone constituents such as, for example, collagen) that can improve tissue regeneration, cell growth, and drug/protein delivery currently represents the main research area in the field of organic nanobiomaterials with a strong tendency to design hybrid materials and improve fabrication techniques of the resulting nanocomposite materials/scaffolds/structures. Such a trend has become very clear in the last 5–6 years. However, much work remains to be done in order to fully understand interactions between different phases of nanocomposite materials and cell/tissues to be repaired/treated. Another important issue strictly related to the above mentioned one is how to "optimize" the composition of the nanocomposite for the specific purposes on which the material itself is designed.

2.2. Inorganic Nanobiomaterials

Inorganic biomaterials are those lacking carbon element and they are widely employed for in vivo and in vitro biomedical research [222]. These crystalline or glass structured nanomaterials are used to replace or restore a body tissue [36]. The main applications of inorganic biomaterials, including bioceramics and bioglasses, are for orthopedics and dentistry. Modifications in composition and fabrication techniques may produce a range of biocompatible materials such as bioceramics [223]. Natural bone also includes inorganic materials like calcium (Ca) and phosphorus (P) in the form of hydroxyapatite (HA) crystals, as well as carbonate (CO_3^{2-}), potassium (K), fluoride (F), chlorine (Cl), sodium (Na), magnesium (Mg), and some trace elements including copper (Cu), zinc (Zn), strontium (Sr), iron (Fe), and silicon (Si) [224]. Therefore, it is very logical to investigate on nanomaterials based on these inorganic constituents.

Table 2 presents a general classification of inorganic nanobiomaterials and summarizes representative applications of each material in tissue engineering. The following subsections present a general description of each nanomaterial type listed in Table 2 and a detailed literature survey on the corresponding developments for tissue engineering.

Table 2. Types of inorganic nanomaterials with their applications.

Types of Nanomaterials	Size (nm)	Applications	References
Nano Silica	10–100	Composite-based scaffold Bio-imaging Drug delivery Enhanced osteogenic differentiation	[225–227]
Gold nanostructured materials	5–50	Bioinorganic hybrid nanostructures Thin film scaffold Bio-imaging	[228–230]
Magnetic nanomaterials and nanoparticles	10	Drug and gene delivery Improved cell adhesion Cell tracking	[21,231,232]
Bioactive Glasses	20–500	Improved scaffolds performance Drug and gene delivery	[233,234]
Silver nanoparticles	1–100	Tissue repair and regeneration Antibacterial action	[235–237]
Nanostructured Titanium	<300	Nano tubular anodized titanium Improved mechanical properties Enhanced chondrocyte adhesion Support osteoblast adhesion and proliferation Orthopedic coating	[238–243]
Hydroxyapatite	20–80 ~200–500	Enhanced osteoblast functioning Increase bone apatite formation	[244,245]
Zirconia nanoparticles	<100	Enhanced osteointegration Antibacterial implants formation	[246,247]
Alumina nanoparticles	<80	Enhanced bone cells adhesion and proliferation Calcium phase deposition	[245,248]
Copper nanoparticles	<100	Antimicrobial implant fabrication	[25]

2.2.1. Nano Silica

A huge amount of investigations on biomedical applications of silica nanostructures have been carried out in the past decade [249]. The ability to synthesize uniform, porous and dispersible nanoparticles, together with the fact that particles' size and shape can be easily controlled [226], certainly favored the variety of applications of silica in tissue engineering [250]. Furthermore, as silica is biocompatible and chemically stable [251,252], it has been used also for biomedical imaging and medication administration [225], either itself or as a coating of other compounds [251].

Mesoporous silica nanoparticles (MSNPs) have been used as a drug delivery vehicle [253] and to improve mechanical properties of biological materials. It was noted their use as well as for sustained and prolonged release or administration of intracellular genes in bone tissue engineering [226]. MSNPs work as efficient biocompatible nanocarriers due to (i) high visibility, (ii) dispersibility, (iii) binding capability to a target tissue, (iv) ability to load and deliver large concentrations of cargos, and (v) triggered or controlled release of cargos [250]. The functioning of MSNPs can be tailored by modifying the silanol group present within the pore interiors and on the outer surface. These positive chemical moieties are adsorbed by negatively charged SiO^- groups at neutral pH, through electrostatic interactions (Figure 12).

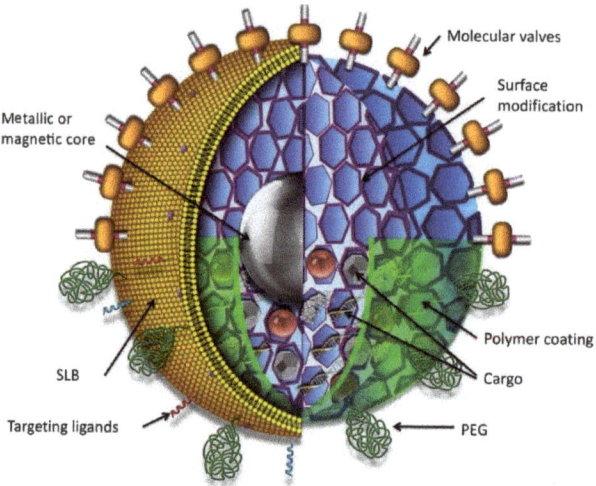

Figure 12. Schematic of a multifunctional mesoporous silica nanoparticle showing possible core/shell design, surface modifications, and multiple types of cargos. (Adapted with permission from © 2013 American Chemical Society [250]).

Anitha et al. [254] reported a composite matrix containing crystalline rod-shaped core with uniform amorphous silica sheath (Si–n HA), which showed good biocompatibility, osteogenic differentiation, vascularization, and bone regeneration potential. Silicate containing hydroxyapatite stimulates cell viability of human mesenchymal stem cells for extended proliferation [255]. Zhou et al. [256] synthesized PLGA–SBA15 composite membranes with different silica contents by electrospinning method; these membranes showed better osteogenic initiation then the pure PLGA membranes. Ding et al. [257] successfully fabricated levofloxacin (LFX)-loaded polyhydroxybutyrate/poly(ε-caprolactone) (PHB/PCL) and PHB/PCL/sol–gel-derived silica (SGS) scaffolds, which support the growth of MG-63 osteoblasts. A microfluidic device was used to generate photo-cross-linkable gelatin microgels (GelMA), coupled with providing a protective silica hydrogel layer for applications in injectable tissue constructs [258]. Dexamethasone (DEX)-loaded aminated mesoporous silica nanoparticles (MSNs-NH2) were prepared via electrophoretic deposition (EPD) and successfully incorporated within poly(l-lactic acid)/poly(ε-caprolactone) (PLLA/PCL) matrix to fabricate composite nanofibrous scaffolds for bone tissue engineering applications [259].

2.2.2. Nano Bioglass

Bioglasses (BG) have been intensively investigated as biomaterials since their discovery in 1969 and first developments in the 1970s made by L. Hench [260]. Compared to common glass, bioglass contains less silica and higher amounts of calcium and phosphorous. As a biomaterial for tissue engineering, bioglass is applied independently or in combination with a number of polymers [261] (Figure 13). BG can arouse fibroblasts with higher bioactivity by accelerating bioactive growth factors and proteins as compared to untreated fibroblasts [262].

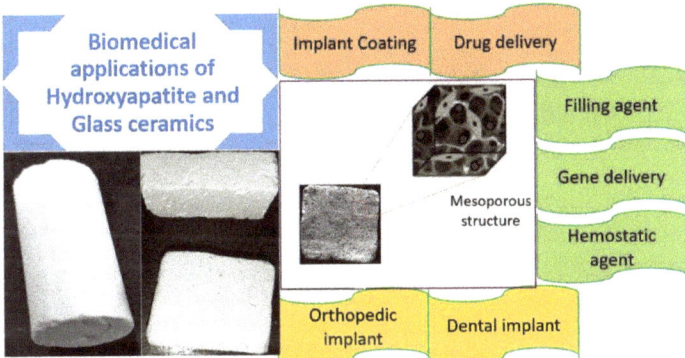

Figure 13. Biomedical applications of hydroxyapatite and glass ceramics.

BG degrade slowly when implanted into the targeted patient's site and release ions, which favors the biosynthesis of hydroxyapatite [263]. The silica-rich surface of bioglass promotes the exchange of Ca^{2+} and PO_4^{3-} with physiological fluid, which leads to the generation of a Ca–P layer [264,265]. This biodegradation may be enhanced by the presence of a SiO_2 network, which forms non-bridging silicon-oxygen bonds [266]; the low connectivity of the SiO_2 network enhances dissolution of bioglass while the presence of Na and Ca forms Si–O–Si bonds and reduces dissolution rate. Mesoporous BG can be fabricated using the sol-gel method, which can be a good carrier for targeted drug delivery [267]. The sol–gel method was also used by Kumar et al. [268] to develop bioglass nanoparticles with a higher content of silica, which are suited for bone tissue applications.

Bioglass nanoparticles show high biocompatibility and surface area, which can enhance in vitro osteoconductivity as compared to layer and microsized particles of bioglass [269]. The size of the particles can be modified by changing the synthesis parameters and techniques. However, because of its brittleness, the glass alone cannot be used to heal large bone defects [270]. In order to solve this issue, Bioglass 45S5 was used with poly(D,L-lactide) (PDLLA), a biodegradable polymer, to form a composite scaffold with enhanced biomechanical characteristics [271]. The early failure of a bioglass composite at the interface occurs because of nonuniform mechanical strength, phase separation, nonhomogeneous mixture, and different degradation properties of two compounds. A hybrid composite of poly(methyl methacrylate) (PMMA) and bioactive glass was manufactured via the sol-gel method (Figure 14) to enhance physicochemical and mechanical properties [272].

An elastin-like polypeptidic and bioglass (ELP/BG) hydrogel was also fabricated that is mechanically robust, injectable, and self-healable. This ELP/BG biocomposite can be useful for drug delivery and tissue engineering purposes [273]. A 3D construct of type-I collagen and 45S5 Bioglass meets the basic requirements of a scaffold including biocompatibility, osteoconductivity, osteoinductivity, and biodegradability [274]. Bioglass nanoparticles were also used with bacterially derived poly(3-hydroxybutyrate) to fabricate bioactive composite film using a fermentation technique [275]. Different glass modifiers (Mg^{2+}, Ca^{2+}, and Sr^{2+}) were used to prepare borosilicate bioactive glasses through a melt-quenching technique which showed good antibacterial properties [276].

Poly(propylene fumarate) (PPF) was used to functionalize bioglass particles that enhance the bioactivity and cell adhesion, proliferation, and bone regeneration [277].

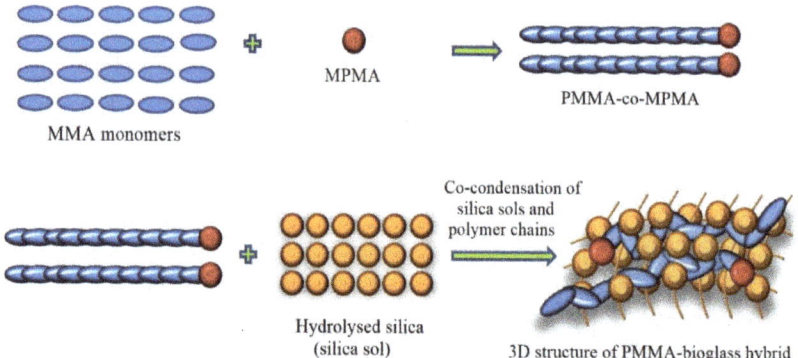

Figure 14. Schematic procedure for the fabrication of a PMMA-bioglass class II hybrid (Adapted with permission from © 2013 American Chemical Society [272]).

2.2.3. Nano Hydroxyapatite

Hydroxyapatite ($Ca_{10}(PO_4)_6(OH)_2$) is a significant natural mineral constituent of bones (70% wt.) and teeth (96% wt.) [278,279]. Synthetic HA is a biocompatible ceramic material, used for biomedical applications (Figure 13) because it may replicate the behavior of mineral part of the bone [280,281]. It shows outstanding biocompatibility with bones, teeth, skin, and muscles, both in vitro and in vivo [282,283]. The stoichiometric molar ratio Ca/P in synthetic HA of 1.67 is not the actual ratio in the hydroxyapatite of normal bones, because of the presence of other elements such as C, N, Fe, Mg, and Na [284]. Hydroxyapatite (HA) can be easily synthesized by using different methods such as hydrothermal, sol–gel, and co-precipitation methods [285]. The comparison of mineral compositions of hydroxyapatite, bone and teeth is shown in Table 3 [286,287].

Table 3. Mineral composition of hydroxyapatite, bone, and teeth.

Types	Ca	P	Ca/P	Total Inorganic (%)	Total Organic (%)	Water (%)
HA	39.6	18.5	1.67	100	-	-
Dentine	35.1	16.9	1.61	70	20	10
Bone	34.8	15.2	1.71	65	25	10
Enamel	36.5	17.1	1.63	97	1.5	1.5

HA shows such excellent biocompatibility, bio-inertia and bioactivity without toxicity, immunogenicity [288,289]. It has a good ability to make bonds with bone directly and it is primarily used in therapeutic applications such as implants and fillers for bones and teeth in different forms [290]. To overcome the low mechanical strength of hydroxyapatite scaffolds, a large number of natural and synthetic polymers were combined with HA such as collagen, polyethylene, polylactic acid, alginates, poly(methyl methacrylate), and polycaprolactone [136].

Woodard et al. [291] compared the activity of nano- and microsized ceramic materials in the body. Their studies demonstrated a substantial increase in osteoblast adhesion and protein adsorption in nanomaterials. The major components of the inorganic nanostructure can have a higher biological activity than micro-components [245]. Polydopamine (pDA)-templated hydroxyapatite (tHA) was introduced into polycaprolactone (PCL) matrix to make bioactive tHA/PCL composite based fibrous scaffold; in vitro and in vivo investigations (Figure 15) showed a favorable cytocompatibility at a given concentration of tHA (0–10% wt.) [292].

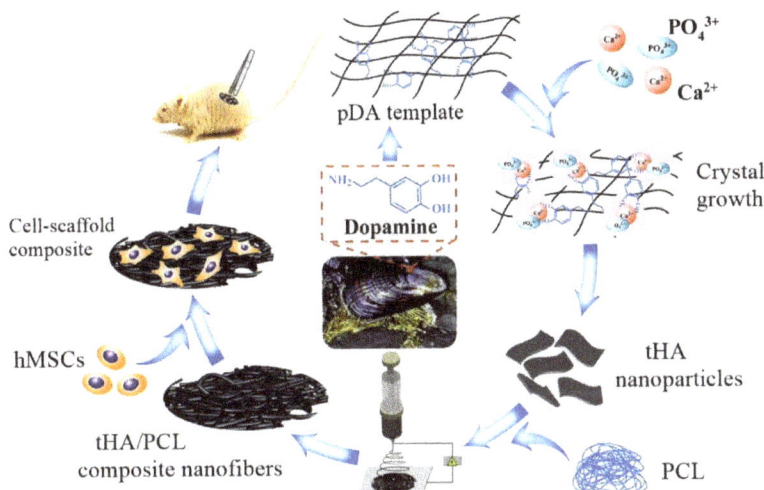

Figure 15. Schematic illustration of preparation and evaluation of tHA/PCL composite nanofibers. (Adapted with permission from © 2016 American Chemical Society [292].)

A new type of scaffold with bamboo fiber (5%) incorporated nano-hydroxyapatite/poly(lactic-co-glycolic) (30%) was fabricated via freeze-drying; bamboo fibers improved biomechanical properties of n-HA/PLGA composite scaffolds thus developing a superior potential for bone tissue engineering [293]. Sol–gel synthesized hydroxyapatite–TiO_2-based nanocomposites synthesized in supercritical CO_2 have better Young's and flexural moduli than PCL/HAp composites [294]. A set of techniques including molding/particle leaching and plasma-treated surface deposition were used to fabricate bilayered PLGA/PLGA-HAp composite scaffold [295]; the in vivo rat model experiment proved that the new composite is suitable for osteochondral tissue engineering applications. Electrospinning mediated poly(ε-caprolactone)–poly(ethylene glycol)–poly(ε-caprolactone) (PCL–PEG–PCL, PCEC) and nano-hydroxyapatite (n-HA) composite scaffolds showed good biocompatibility and nontoxicity [296]. Hydroxyapatite/Na(Y/Gd)F_4:Yb^{3+}, Er^{3+} composite fibers [297], and gadolinium-doped mesoporous strontium hydroxyapatite nanorods [298] were successfully used in drug storage/release applications.

2.2.4. Silver Nanoparticles

Silver proved its bactericidal activities against many bacteria since 1000 B.C. Now silver is used as an antiseptic, antibacterial, and antitumor agent [299]. Because of their strong antibacterial activity against both Gram-positive and Gram-negative bacterial strains, silver nanoparticles were widely used for fabricating antibacterial nanocomposite-based scaffolds and coated implants [235,237]. Furthermore, silver may be combined with different materials such as CNT [300], chitosan, HA [301], and manganite [302] to get a specific function. Ag-doped or coated implants allow reducing the number of bacterial infections without interfering with bone cell growth in the body (Figure 16 [303]). The antimicrobial activity of Ag has been reported against *Escherichia coli* [304], *Candida albicans* [11], *Vibrio cholera* [305], and *Staphylococcus aureus* [306].

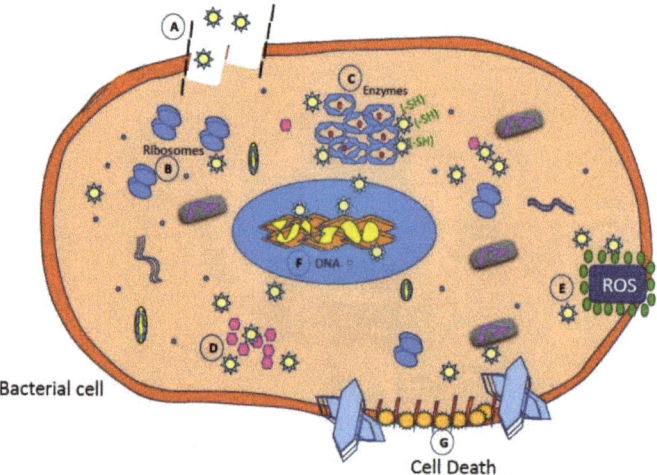

Figure 16. Schematic diagram representing mechanisms of action of Ag nanoparticles for antibacterial action (adapted with permission from Elsevier © 2018 [303]). (**A**) AgNP diffusion and uptake into the bacterial cell. (**B**) Destabilization of ribosomes. (**C**) Enzyme interaction. (**D**) Interruption of electron transfer chain. (**E**) Reactive oxygen species (ROS). (**F**) DNA damage. (**G**) Cell death.

In addition to antibacterial activity, Ag nanoparticles promote wound healing, reduce scar formation, and reduce inflammation [307]. Silver nanoparticles have many applications as antimicrobial agents when combined with different biological substances [308]. A micrometer-sized surface-enhanced Raman spectroscopy (SERS) substrate, core–shell microparticles composed of solid carbonate core coated with silver nanoparticles, and polyhedral multishell fullerene-like structure were developed for biomedical applications [309]. Soft poly(vinyl alcohol) (PVA) hydrogel films containing silver particles prepared on solid biodegradable poly(l-lactic acid) (PLLA) exhibit both antibacterial and reduced cell adhesion properties [310]. Biocompatible maleimide-coated silver nanoparticles (Ag NPs) can be used as co-cross-linkers for the preparation of a nanocomposite gelatin-based hydrogel. Covalently bound Ag nanoparticles support swelling and drug release properties of composite hydrogel without producing toxicity [311]. In situ fabricated Ag NPs (4-19 nm) and immobilized on titanium by using a plasma immersion ion implantation process motivated osteoblast differentiation in rat bone marrow stem cells (BMSCs) [312]. Patrascu et al. [313] fabricated collagen/hydroxyapatite-silver nanoparticles (COLL/HA-Ag)-based antiseptic composite for biomedical applications.

2.2.5. Gold Nanoparticles

Gold nanoparticles (GNPs) are defined as a colloid of nanometer-sized particles with better properties than bulk gold. They are produced in different shapes such as spheres [314], rods [315], star-like [316], and cages [317]. GNPs possess unique characteristics, such as easy-to-control, nanoscale size, easy preparation, high surface area, easy functionalization, and excellent biocompatibility, that make them highly suited for many tissue engineering and more in general for biotechnology applications [318,319]. GNPs are definitely superior over other types of nanoparticles in terms of low toxicity and colloidal stability. Furthermore, they present an outstanding physicochemical behavior, which is related to local plasmon resonance phenomena.

Gold nanoparticles were utilized for biosensing [320], bioimaging [321–323], cancer therapy [324], gene delivery to enhance osteogenic differentiation [325], and photo-thermal therapy [229,314,316,323]. Gold nanoparticles were also combined with other materials such as silica (to produce core and shell nanoparticles) [318,323] as well as natural polymers (to improve mechanical properties) and synthetic polymers (to enhance biocompatibility) [318].

Due to their excellent biocompatibility and chemical inertness, gold nanoparticles became the ideal choice for the preparation of scaffolds in many cases [318]. The mission of GNPs in tissue engineering and regenerative medicine is to act as a multimodal tool in order to improve scaffold properties, cell differentiation and intracellular growth factor delivery (Figure 17), while monitoring cellular events in real-time [326].

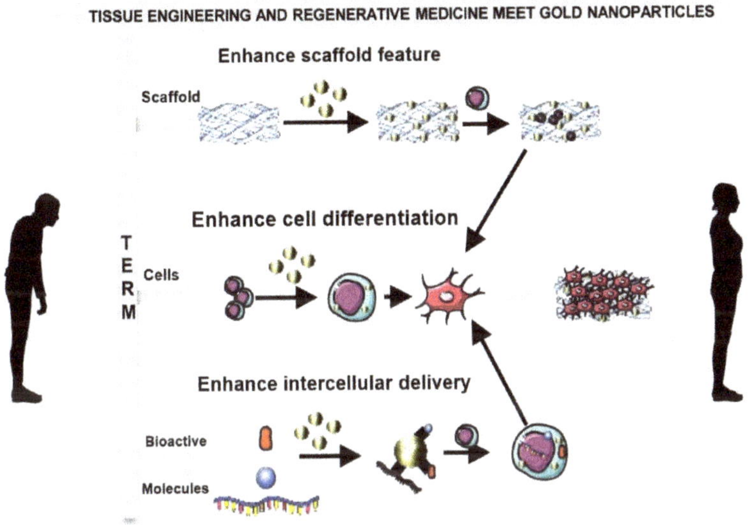

Figure 17. Scheme representing the importance of introducing GNPs in tissue engineering and the regenerative medicine (TERM) realm [326]. (Adapted with permission from Elsevier © 2017).

2.2.6. Titanium Dioxide

Titanium is widely used in many surgical applications (e.g., prostheses and implants) because of its excellent biocompatibility, good mechanical properties, and lower mass density than steel [327]. The low density and high specific strength of titanium results in lightweight implants with good mechanical properties [238,239]. Furthermore, the smooth surface of Ti mesh prevents bacterial contamination instead of adsorbate materials. Therefore, titanium mesh provides an excellent solution to guide bone regeneration [243].

Nanostructured TiO_2 materials of various morphologies such as nanoparticles, nanorods, nanowires, nanotubes, and other hierarchical nanostructures can be produced using different techniques such as, for example, microwaves [328,329], hydrothermal/solvothermal processes [330,331], sol–gel [332,333], anode oxidation [334,335], chemical vapor deposition [336,337], sonochemical processes [338,339], and green synthesis [340–342].

As can be seen from Figure 18, nanostructured TiO_2 is a multifunctional material for a wide range of applications in engineering and biomedical areas. Interestingly, TiO_2 nanoparticles represent a miniature of electrochemical cells capable of light-induced redox chemistry. This quality can be used for manipulating biomolecules and cell metabolic processes. TiO_2 nanoparticles prove to have a higher affinity for binding proteins and other cellular components when used within cellular environment [343,344]. TiO_2 nanoparticles can also be used to enhance photodynamic therapy (PDT) and sonodynamic therapy (SDT) [345].

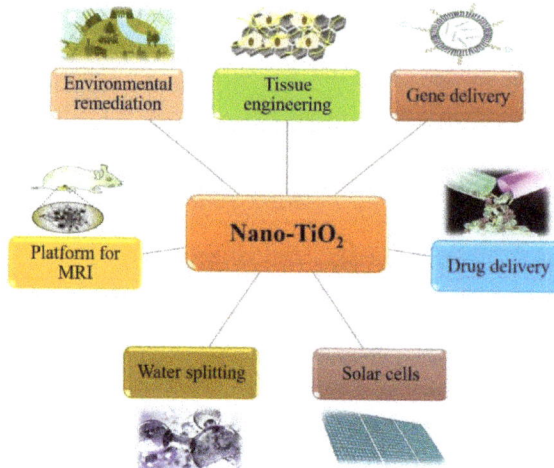

Figure 18. Schematic representation of the many fields of applications of nanostructured TiO$_2$.

Titanium nanotubes (TNTs) possess excellent biocompatibility and drug-releasing performance. Furthermore, they can be generated on the surface of the existing medical implants [346,347]. The physical adsorption of the drugs promotes the anti-inflammatory properties of the TNTs, and with improved osteoblast adhesion, the drug-eluting technique is extended [348].

TiO$_2$ based scaffolds are biocompatible, have good osteoconductive performance and antibacterial properties [349], and show high porosity, excellent interconnectivity, and sufficient mechanical strength [350,351]. Nanostructured TiO$_2$ can be combined with several polymers including polylactic acid (PLA) [352]; poly(ether-ether ketone) (PEEK) [353]; poly(lactic-co-glycolic acid) (PLGA) [354]; and inorganic materials such as SiO$_2$ [355], Al$_2$O$_3$ [356], bioglass [357], hydroxyapatite [358], graphene [359], and calcium phosphate [360].

Nano-TiO$_2$ surface coated implants can limit autoimmune reactions between the underlying bone tissue surfaces and the implant [361]. However, material deterioration or generation of chronic inflammation in the implanted tissues may reduce success rate [361,362]. Various TiO$_2$ nanostructures were used for loading and eluting cefuroxime as an antibiotic on orthopedic implants [363].

2.2.7. Zirconia

Zirconia was first recognized by M.H. Klaproth in 1789 and used as a pigment for ceramics for a long time [364]. Since the 1970s, zirconia received massive consideration as a biomedical material in association to its chemical and biological inertness [365]. Consequently, zirconia was also used to overcome the brittleness of alumina and the consequent failure of implants [366], and as a material for the repair and replacement of bones due to its unique biomechanical properties [367].

Investigations on zirconia biomaterials began in the 1960s. Classical orthopedics studied for many years have used zirconia in the area of hip replacement [368,369]. Zirconium oxide (zirconia) possesses improved mechanical properties and has become one of the most popular ceramic materials in the field of healthcare due to its high biocompatibility and low toxicity [364,370].

Zirconia is one of the most useful structured ceramics because it provides high resistance to bending and fracture. However, zirconium oxide with a low fracture toughness due to the presence of alumina abrasive grains [371] also was introduced as an alternative to having excellent wear resistance due to the unwanted release of orthopedic alumina. Porous zirconia stents can be manufactured by cutting CAD/CAM blocks in the desired shape, and zirconia stents assembled with HA significantly increase the volume of new bone formation in vivo [372].

While it might be concluded that zirconia has one of the best combinations of mechanical strength, fracture resistance, biocompatibility, and biological activity, its performance can be further enhanced via a proper modification of material's surface or by combining the material with some other bioactive ceramics and glass [367]. In addition, as a result of the introduction of Zr into the Ca-Si system, no toxicity was observed. Previous studies confirmed that the optimum content of zirconium and strontium increases the surface energy of the magnesium alloy and enhances the ability to stimulate bone formation around the implant [373,374]. Hydroxyapatite and fluorapatite slurry coated zirconia scaffolds induce osteoconductivity and enhance bonding strength up to 33 MPa [375]. The dispersion of zirconia with alumina lead to produce ZrO_2-toughened alumina (Al_2O_3), known as zirconia-toughened alumina (ZTA) [376].

Zirconia (ZrO_2)/β-tricalcium phosphate (β-TCP) composite has shown excellent mechanical properties and supports osteoblast regeneration [377]. Silk fibroin-chitosan-zirconia (SF/CS/nano ZrO_2) and chitin–chitosan/nano ZrO_2 composites provide a suitable environment for cell infiltration and colonization [378,379]. Different temperature based hydroxyapatite-zirconium composites such as 873 K (HZ600), 923 K (HZ650), and 973 K (HZ700) demonstrated that osteoblast growth and mineralization were not influenced by any composite [380]. A new biphasic calcium phosphate (BCP) scaffold reinforced with zirconia (ZrO_2) was fabricated through the fused deposition modeling (FDM) technique. The 90% BCP and 10% ZrO_2 scaffold thus created had significantly better mechanical properties than 100% BCP and 0% ZrO_2 scaffold [381].

ZrO_2 nanoparticle (NP)-doped CTS–PVA–HAP composites (ZrCPH I–III) showed improvement in the tensile strength of ZrCPH I–III with respect to the CTS–PVA–HAP scaffold [382]. Sol–gel cum solvothermal derived mesoporous titanium zirconium (TiZr) oxide nanospheres were used for ibuprofen, dexamethasone, and erythromycin drugs loading and in vitro release studies [383]. The excellent biocompatibility of Zr makes it a good material for metal–organic frameworks (MOFs). Surface functionalization of Zr-fumarate MOF (Figure 19) was used for dichloroacetate (DCA) drug loading, which is more efficient at transporting the drug mimic calcein into HeLa cells [384].

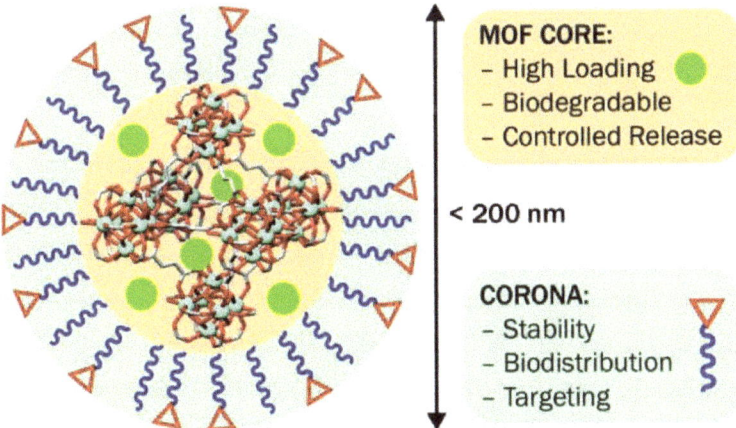

Figure 19. Schematic showing the Zr-fumarate structure with preferred properties of a metal–organic framework (MOF)-based drug delivery device (adapted with permission from © 2018 American Chemical Society [384]).

2.2.8. Alumina

Since 1975, the bio-inertness of alumina has been confirmed. Alumina has very high hardness and resistance to abrasion on the Moh scale next to diamond [385]. In addition, the crystalline nature of alumina makes it insoluble at room temperature in regular chemical reagents [386]. Alumina has been used in many fabrications of artificial implants since it was inserted into an artificial femur head in the 1970s [387]. Pure and densified alumina, α-Al$_2$O$_3$ (corundum), was the first ceramic material used in the biomedical field for dental restorations, cochlear implants, and load-bearing hip prostheses [388]. As porous alumina does not degrade under in vitro and in vivo environments, it may be used for biosensing [389], good electrical insulation [390], and immune isolation [391].

Properties such as abrasion resistance, power and chemical inertness favor the use of alumina in hard tissue engineering [392]. If the alumina is implanted in bone marrow, no toxic effects are generated in the surrounding tissue [393]. However, the high stiffness of alumina may lead to have a high elastic incompatibility between the biological tissue and the implant [394]. The tensile strength of alumina can be increased by reducing grain size and increasing its density [395]. In view of their good mechanical behavior, alumina implants are characterized by long-time survival predictions [396].

A significant feature in applications involving open and aligned porous structures, such as bone tissue scaffolds, catalysts, and membranes, is the anisotropic nature of porous alumina ceramics [397]. The α-alumina is the most stable oxide amongst transient and metastable types [398]. It should be noted that essential physico-chemical properties of alumina surface are significantly affected by the protein adsorption process. For example, the presence of liquid solutions nearby the implanted site can cause accelerated protein adsorption on the alumina's surface [399]. Piconi et al. [394] reported the in vitro biocompatibility of alumina with various cell lines such as fibroblasts and osteoblasts, and immunological cells with various cell environments.

The particle size of alumina may affect biocompatibility, particularly when using nanoparticles because of their high surface/volume ratio [400]. Alumina suspensions (70% wt.) and wheat flour (20–30% vol.) were used to synthesize different particle sized porous alumina ceramics [401]. Hydroxyapatite/alumina composite based foam was synthesized via a precipitation method under a variety of pH values that showed a good concentration of Ca^{2+} and PO$_4^{3-}$ contents [402]. The chemical modification of porous alumina surface with vitronectin and peptide (i.e., arginine-glycine-aspartic acid cysteine (RGDC)) enhanced bone cell adhesion and production of extracellular matrix [403].

Porous anodic alumina (PAA) can be fabricated on the surface of other materials through anodization process [404,405]. It can be considered a good nanocontainer to load active agents such as drugs or biomolecules [406]. Evaporation induced self-assembly derived mesoporous aluminum oxide was used for the delivery of poor-water soluble compound Telmisartan (anti-blood pressure drug) with 45% loading efficiency [407]. The drug is not loaded within the pores of the PAA completely, but the surface itself can hold some of this load, which can be quite high; this promotes another phase release [408,409].

Calcium phosphate with 20% alumina (Ca$_3$(PO$_4$)$_2$–Al$_2$O$_3$) bio-ceramic composite revealed enhanced biocompatibility and mechanical properties [410]. Using alumina nanowires reinforcement in polyhydroxy butyrate-chitosan (PHB-CTS/3% Al$_2$O$_3$) scaffolds enhanced the mechanical properties of the scaffold. The addition of alumina increased by ten times the tensile strength of PHB-CTS/3% Al$_2$O$_3$, which became higher than its counterpart for the original PHB-CTS scaffold [411].

Al$_2$O$_3$ coating was used for improving the performance of stainless steel 316L and Ti-6Al-4V implants [412]. In general, coating materials are used to protect the surface of the implant material and the interface with the biological system at hand [413]. Nanorod-like HA-coated porous Al$_2$O$_3$ was fabricated by anodic oxidation that revealed excellent biological activity in vitro [414].

2.2.9. Copper

Copper ions stimulate the proliferation of human vein endothelial cells and mesenchymal stem cells (MSCs) but not human dermal fibroblasts [415,416]. Copper nanoparticles can also act as antifungal and antibacterial agents [417]. Copper is commonly used in bone implants for its antimicrobial activity against a wide range of pathogens [418]. As copper is an essential component of the body, it may be more suitable for in vivo applications [25].

The importance of copper has been studied extensively because its deficiency can lead to osteoporosis [419]. Cu also stimulates angiogenesis and collagen deposition, which are key elements in wound healing [420]. The use of copper-based biomaterials is cost-effective compared to other vital materials based on gold and silver [421].

Copper ions were incorporated into biologically active scaffolds for controlled release to improve vascular strengthening and antimicrobial action for prolonged periods [422]. Copper-doped wollastonite (Cu–Ws) particles (1184 nm) have shown biocompatibility towards mouse mesenchymal stem cells (mMSC) up to 0.05 mg/ml concentration [423]. A freeze-dried chitosan/hydroxyapatite/copper-zinc alloy (CS/nHAp/nCu–Zn) composite-based scaffold showed lower degradation and higher protein adsorption without producing toxicity towards rat osteoprogenitor cells [422]. Collagen-copper-doped bioactive glass (CuBG-CS) scaffolds exhibited enhanced mechanical properties (up to 1.9-fold) and osteogenesis (up to 3.6-fold) than chitosan [424].

Copper nanoparticles were investigated also for wound healing applications. 1 µM concentration of 80 nm CuNPs was found not to be toxic to the cultured fibroblast, endothelial, and keratinocyte cells, and it supported endothelial cell migration and proliferation [425]. CuNPs may alter the structure of proteins and enzymes, affecting their normal functions and causing inactivation of bacterial functions at the injury site [426]. Chen et al. reported the cytotoxic effect of copper NPs towards human histolytic lymphoma (U937) and human cervical cancer cells by inducing apoptosis [427]. CuNPs were used to design a special drug delivery system for chemotherapy. For example, Figure 20 illustrates a mesoporous, upconversion, nanoparticles (mUCNPs)-based controlled-release drug carrier system exhibiting higher upconversion luminescence emission intensity [428].

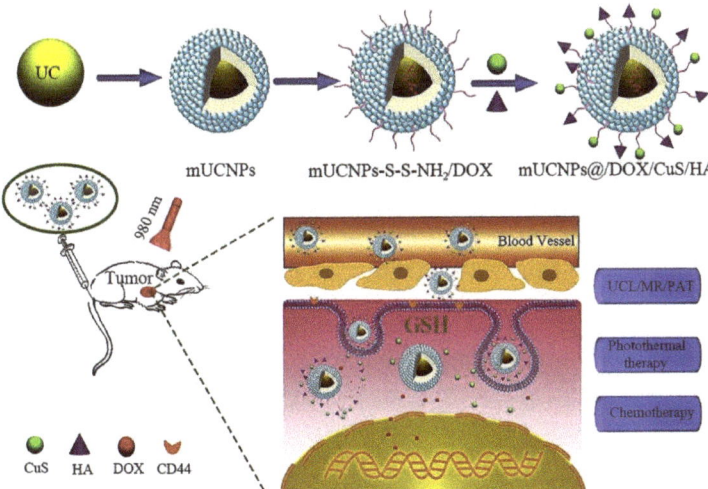

Figure 20. Schematic illustration of the mUCNPs-based redox-stimuli responsive drug delivery system for tumor diagnosis and synergetic chemo-phototherapy (adapted with permission from Elsevier © 2017 [428]).

2.2.10. Magnetic Nanoparticles

Magnetic elements (i.e., iron, nickel, cobalt, and their oxides) were utilized for the fabrication of nanomaterials for different medical applications [429,430] such as MRI, drug delivery, medical diagnostics, cancer therapy, biosensoring, and magneto-optic devices. Magnetic nanoparticles can be synthesized through different techniques including co-precipitation [431], microemulsion [432], hydrothermal synthesis [433], sol–gel process [434], polyol synthesis [435], flow injection [436], sonolysis/sonochemical methods [437], microwave irradiation [438], electrochemical synthesis [439], solvothermal method [440], chemical vapor deposition [441], laser pyrolysis [442], and green synthesis [443] using biomass or biotemplate.

Due to high magnetic flux density, magnetic nanoparticles were used for drug targeting [444] and bio-separation [445], including cell sorting [446]. Sun et al. [447] analyzed metallic, bi-metallic, magnetic cationic liposomes and superparamagnetic iron oxide nanoparticles for imaging and drug delivery. The surface of magnetic nanoparticles also needs to be functionalized to recognize specific targets (Figure 21) [448]. Polyethylene glycol (PEG) is one of the best polymers used for the functionalization of magnetic nanoparticles by surface modification [449]. Interestingly, surface modified magnetic nanoparticles reduce nonspecific interaction with biological molecules.

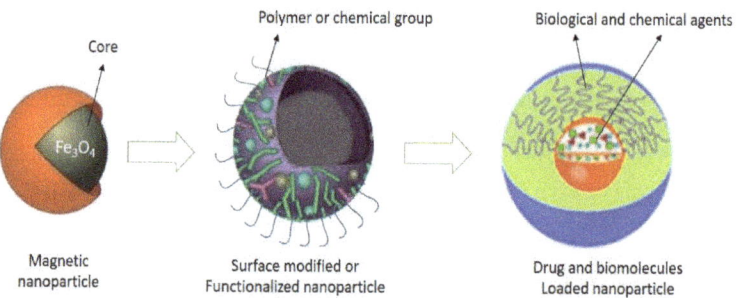

Figure 21. Surface modified magnetic nanoparticle.

Magnetic manipulation is another important advantage of magnetic nanoparticles [450]. It is done by labeling cells with magnetic nanoparticles that can easily be controlled by remote control or external magnetic field [451]. The magnetic nanoparticles, which are usually smaller than 10 nm can be easily transported through skin lipid matrix and hair follicles to the stratum granulosum, where it is condensing between corneocytes [452].

In orthopedic surgery, implant-associated infection is a serious issue, as stated in the previous sections. Infection around a bone graft can lead to serious illness or failure of surgery. Drug-loaded Fe_3O_4 composites promote cell adhesion, proliferation, and osteogenic differentiation of hBMSCs [453–455]. In stem cell therapy for bone regeneration, an application of these NPs is the magnetic targeting of stem cells to the deserved locations, known as magnetic homing of stem cells. For example, penetration of ferumoxide-labeled cells into porous hydroxyapatite ceramic implanted in a rabbit ulnar defect was significantly facilitated by this approach, which improved bone formation even in the chronic process [456].

2.2.11. Summary and Statistical Analysis of the Survey on Inorganic Nanobiomaterials

The survey on inorganic nanobiomaterials presented in Section 2.2 covered some 230 articles, practically the same as its counterpart for organic biomaterials not counting about 30 articles on fabrication techniques of silica and magnetic nanoparticles.

While the number of technical papers appears to be rather uniformly distributed among the ten types of inorganic nanomaterials considered in this survey, it should be noted that most studies focused on nanoparticles and their functionalization for drug/gene/therapy delivery, cell labeling, biosensing, and bioimaging (75%), followed by studies on development and fabrication of new composite materials and scaffolds (25%).

Gold and titania present the largest variety of nanostructures and the latter material may also be available in the form of nanotubes. Gold nanoparticles may represent the best solution for most applications in view of the possibility of controlling size and dimensions of nanostructures as well as for their special physical properties (for example, local plasmon resonance). However, massive utilization of GNPs is obviously limited by the high cost of gold. Silica and titania nanoparticles also are widely utilized as standalone materials or in combination with gold and silver nanoparticles.

Similar to what has been observed for organic nanobiomaterials, a rapidly growing research area in the field of inorganic nanobiomaterials for bone tissue engineering is to hybridize them with other materials (e.g., chitosan, PLA, PLGA, collagen, and hydroxyapatite) to enhance mechanical properties, biocompatibility and osteogenetic properties of the modified materials. Development of high-performance scaffolds comprised of multiple materials is the final stage of this complicated process.

3. Applications of Nanobiomaterials

Nanobiomaterials have outstanding mechanical, chemical, electrical and optical properties, which make them highly suited for a variety of biological applications [70]. Nanotechnologies made it possible to develop new nanoscale materials (nanobiomaterials) with upgraded surface area to volume ratio, enabling more surface interactions [457–459]. As nanobiomaterials possess very specific properties that may be tailored to specific targets (i.e., solubility (for otherwise insoluble drugs), carriers for hydrophobic entities, multifunctional capability, active and passive targeting, ligands (size exclusion), and reduced toxicity), they have tremendous potential for disease identification (as imaging tools), care delivery, and prevention in new ways [107]. Nanobiomaterials are special kinds of materials that are introduced into the body for the treatment of damaged hard tissues [460]. The huge variety of biomedical applications of nanobiomaterials are illustrated in Figure 22 [428,461–463].

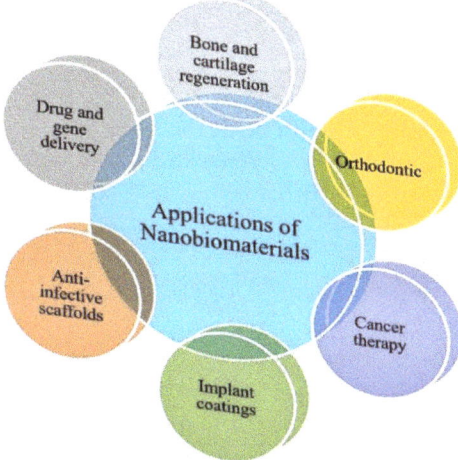

Figure 22. Applications of nanobiomaterials in the biomedical field.

Nanobiomaterials have well-defined nanostructures such as size, shape, channels, pore structure, and surface domain [464]. Nanoscale dimension enables nanobiomaterials to develop critical physical and chemical characteristics that enhance their performance [465,466]. The properties and behaviors of nanobiomaterials, therefore, allow the diagnosis, monitoring, treatment, and prevention of diseases [467]. Nano-size materials show more catalytic reactions at their surface than macro-sized or conventional materials [468]. The nanoscale biomaterials create biomimetic feature towards most of the proteins which support further biological reactions such as cell attachment, growth, proliferation and generation of new tissue [36].

3.1. Bone Regeneration

A perfect bone and cartilage repair scaffold materials should neither suppress the activity of normal cells nor induce toxicity during and after implantation [469]. Figure 23 illustrates the basic cycle of tissue regeneration using nanobiomaterials or derived scaffolds [255].

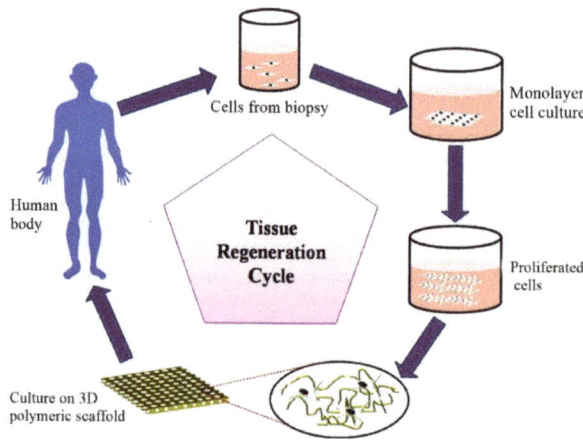

Figure 23. Basic principle procedures for tissue engineering. (Adapted with permission from ©2019 American Chemical Society [255]).

The various synthetic nanostructured matrices are able to stimulate cell differentiation with a focus on preserving the structural features, composition, and biology of natural bone tissue [470]. The main constituents used so far in this regard are nano-hydroxyapatite [471], anodized titanium [472], collagen [473], and silver-incorporated calcium silicate. Nanobiomaterials (1–100 nm) generated from polymers, metals, ceramics, and composites act as effective constituents for hard tissue and play a significant role in osteointegration on nanostructured surfaces [474].

Alumina has been widely used for the fabrication of knee and hip joint prosthesis with low wear rates [475]. Bioactive glasses were used as a prosthesis for the restoration of the ossicular chain of the middle ear and oral implant to preserve the alveolar ridge from bone resorption [476,477]. Different metal oxides such as ZnO, Fe_2O_3, TiO_2, and Al_2O_3, and polymers such as PLA, PGA, and their copolymers were used with bioactive glass systems for hard tissue engineering applications [478,479].

3.2. Drug Delivery

As mentioned above, various nanobiomaterials can be used for bone regeneration, prevention of infections, and osteointegration [480,481]. A nanoparticle that functions as carrier can stabilize the bioactive molecules through encapsulation [482], facilitating targeting cellular delivery and targeted drug release [483,484]. Nanospheres, tubes and capsules are widely accepted tools for targeted and sustained release drug delivery because of their small size and high specific surface area, which encapsulates the drug molecules and shows high reactivity to the surrounding tissues [485]. The materials selected for nanosphere fabrication depend on application principles and requirements. Some factors in this regard include size, drug characteristics, surface properties, biodegradability and biocompatibility of materials and drug release profile [486]. The 2D and 3D structures of scaffolds can be useful for the drug (poorly soluble drugs) loading purpose in tissue engineering (Figure 24).

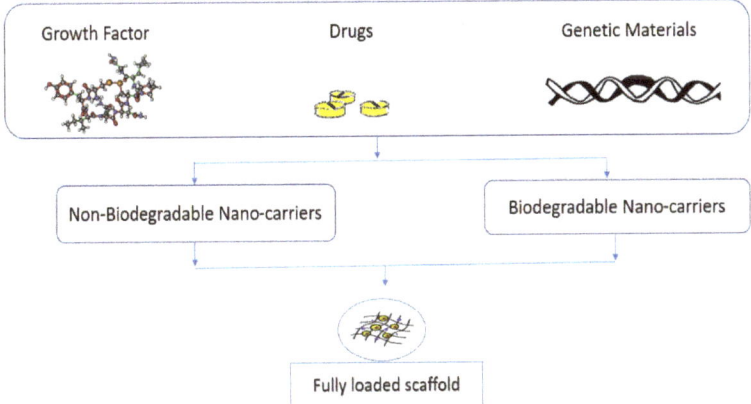

Figure 24. Drugs and biomolecules loaded scaffold for tissue engineering.

3.3. Gene Delivery

The rapid development of nanotechnology made available novel DNA and RNA delivery systems for gene therapy (Figure 25) that can be used instead of viral vectors [487]. Gene therapy collectively refers to therapies aimed at manipulating gene expression in living organisms by supplying exogenous DNA or RNA that is incorporated or not incorporated to cure or prevent diseases [488]. There is great incentive to work towards safer and targeted viral vectors and to engineer more effective non-viral systems that can achieve secure, effective gene therapy in humans because of the enormous potential for gene therapies to influence medicine.

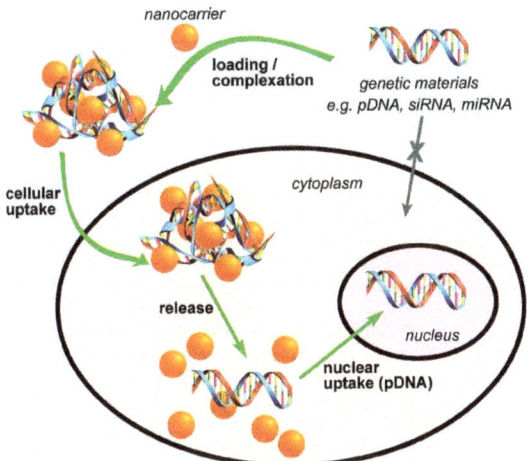

Figure 25. Fundamental steps of gene delivery by nanocarriers (orange spheres). (Adapted with permission from ©2016 Royal Society of Chemistry [489]).

There are a number of nanocarriers used for gene delivery (Figure 25) [489] applications which are based on lipids [490,491], liposomes [492–494], dendrimers [495], polymers [496,497], graphene [498,499], carbon nanotubes (CNTs) [500,501], mesoporous silica [502], gold nanoparticles [503,504], magnetic nanoparticles [505,506], and other types of inorganic nanoparticles.

The number of clinical trials for cancer [507], liver disease [508], hemophilia [509], and bone regeneration [510–512] is continuously increasing due to the promising opportunity to correct gene disorders. Nanomaterials are used for gene delivery because of their small size and superior stability [513]. Before the use of these nanomaterials, surfaces need to be functionalized with small biomolecules or polymers to adapt their physiochemical properties such as hydrophobicity, charge density, and binding affinity [514,515]. Factors including molecular weight, biodegradability, rigidity, charge density, pKa value, solubility, crystallinity, and hydrophobicity ensure effective and safe gene delivery [516,517].

Surface-modified graphene oxide through cationic polymers such as polyethylenimine (PEI) provides a large surface area for the encapsulation of DNA molecules [518]. DNA/drug molecules attached graphene oxide conjugated provide an outstanding platform for the immobilization of nucleotides on its surface [519]. Mesoporous silica nanospheres (MSNs) and functionalized single-walled carbon nanotubes (SWCNT) represent an excellent gene delivery system [520]. In Figure 26, a potential route is recorded for the use of dendrimers as vectors of gene delivery. As plasmid DNA penetrates the cell membrane, it makes (in vitro) a complex between dendrimer and DNA (called dendriplex). This complex is transported through the blood system to the specific cell. Finally, the DNA moves through the cytoplasm to reach the nucleus for gene expression in series [521,522].

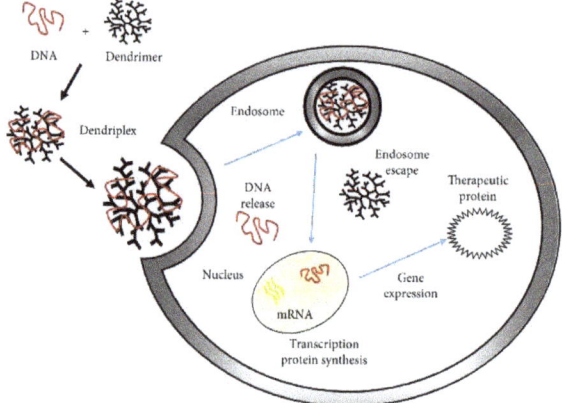

Figure 26. Schematic diagram for a possible route in the use of dendrimers as gene delivery vectors.

3.4. Anti-Infective Nanobiomaterials

Disease, injury, and trauma can lead to serious bacterial infections, which cause disease and adverse complications in host tissues and even death of patients [523]. Nanobiomaterials made from polymers, metals, and ceramics might be a potential source of infection when they are introduced into the body [524,525]. Virus and bacterial infections cause unregulated damage that leads to organ failure [526]. In polymeric biomaterials, the most common bacterial infections are powered by *Staphylococcus epidermidis (S. epidermidis)* from skin and *Staphylococcus aureus (S. aureus)*, which may identified on metallic biomaterials [527]. Ceramics and metals can represent an alternative because of their resistance to infection. However, in presence of minor imperfections on the surface or microfractures, pathogens, such as bacteria, can form a colony [528]. Biomaterials from natural sources were used as alternative as scaffolds for promoting regeneration but they carry a risk for pathogenic transmission [529].

3.5. Nanobiomaterials for Coating

Micro/nanoscale tissue engineering scaffolds play a vital role on the organization of natural extracellular matrix [530]. Nanostructured 3D scaffolds enhance cell functioning, migration, differentiation, proliferation, and extracellular matrix formation [531].

Nanobiomaterials used for coatings include silica (SiO_2), titania (TiO_2), zirconia (ZrO_2), alumina (Al_2O_3), zinc oxide (ZnO), CNT, graphene, and various combined oxides [532]. Simple calcium phosphate coating method on metals, glasses, inorganic ceramics and organic polymers (such as PLGA, PS, PP, and silicone), collagens, and silk fibers can improve biocompatibility or enhance the bioreactivity for orthopedic applications [494,533]. TiO_2 and Al_2O_3 can be used as biologically active coating agents, supporting cell adhesion, growth, osteogenic differentiation, bone matrix production, and mineralization [534]. Nanostructured TiO_2 has a positive effect on the performance of bone cells. TiO_2 is available in the form of nanocrystals [535], nanofibers [536], nanoparticles [537], also immobilized on nanotubes [538]. TiO_2 nanotube coating on any substrate enhances hydroxyapatite formation in SBF [539]. Nano silica coating on Ti-6Al-4V alloys generates apatite and supports adhesion and attachment of human osteoblast-like Saos-2 cells [540]. Nitinol coated stainless steel has shown enhanced biocompatibility but Ni ions produce an allergic response and toxicity [541]. Zirconia coated pure and yttrium-stabilized nanostructure promote deposition of apatite from SBF, which supports cell adhesion and growth [542]. Zinc oxide doped with alumina or functionalized with the silane coupling agent KH550 supports the proliferation of fibroblasts [543].

Carbon nanotubes have been used with various synthetic and natural polymers or minerals for the improvement of mechanical properties [544]. CNT and other nano-carbon forms stimulate cell adhesion and growth of osteogenic cells. Graphene-based films and composites used for biomaterial coatings can be obtained from pure or oxidized graphene. These graphene-based films improve the osteogenic differentiation manifested by collagen I and osteocalcin, high calcium phosphate deposition, and high alkaline phosphatase activity [545,546]. Due to the antimicrobial impression of graphene, graphene oxide (GO), and their derivatives, these materials can be used for implant coating [547]. Graphene oxide (GO) coating on the collagen scaffold induces morphological changes depending on GO concentration [548]. The application of GO improved physical properties like compressive strength as well as adsorption of Ca and proteins without changing porosity [549]. Graphene oxide-silk fibroin (GO-SF) composite used as an alternative to coating with collagen, showed improved biomechanical properties and proved could work in cellular environments [550].

HA can accelerate new bone formation by coating on titanium and tantalum scaffolds. It was demonstrated that after 6 weeks of implantation with titanium and tantalum scaffolds coated is possible to reach fully dense bone formation [551]. Calcium-phosphate-coated Fe foam showed better differentiation and proliferation rate of human mesenchymal stem cells than uncoated Fe foam [552]. Polymer-coated mesoporous silica nanoparticles are effective, cell-specific targeted chemotherapeutic agent delivery method [553]. In rat calvarial defects, HA-coated PLGA scaffolds alone promote bone regeneration and increased exposure to HA nanoparticles on the scaffold surface has been documented to result in accelerated bone deposition by local progenitors [554].

3.6. Nanostructured Scaffolds

Scaffolds are artificial constructs that provide support, tensile strength, and aid in tissue ingrowth [555]. They can also serve as carriers for growth factors, drugs and other required ingredients [556]. Scaffolds mimic the presence of extracellular matrix and allow the replacement of tissue without producing any harmful disturbance with respect to surrounding tissues. An ideal scaffold should be biocompatible, biodegradable, bioactive, non-toxic, mechanically stable, biodegradable, and bioresorbable (Figure 27) [557]. The amalgamation of organic and inorganic materials with scaffolds may enhance morphology and mechanical properties, thus supporting better cell attachment and proliferation [558].

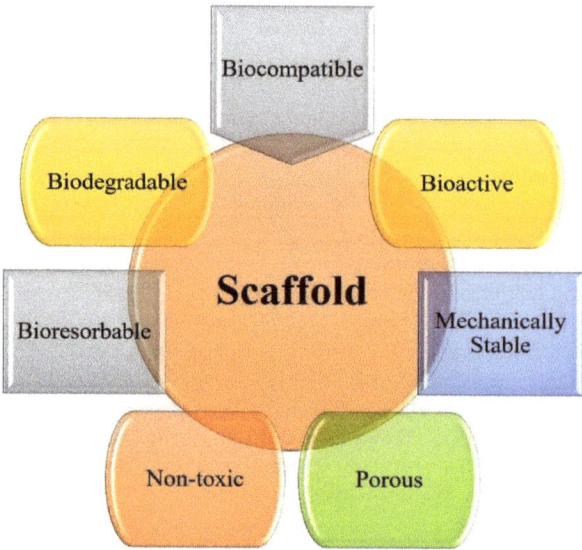

Figure 27. Desired properties of an ideal scaffold.

Scaffold properties can be improved by using nanoparticles because organic and inorganic minerals in natural bone have nanoscale structures [559]. Many studies found that the addition of titanium and iron improve biological and mechanical properties such as collagen synthesis and apatite generation [560,561]. In addition, engineered nanofibrous scaffolds are also suitable for loadbearing applications and can replace natural extracellular matrix (ECM) with artificial ECM. The nanofibrous scaffold can therefore get a much more suitable environment for cellular growth and eventual regeneration of the bone [562]. Nanofiber-based scaffolds have been fabricated by using different synthetic polymers including PCL [563–566], PLLA [567,568], copolymer [569], PLGA [61], and chitosan [569].

Different kinds of metallic nanoparticles can be used for the synthesis of composite-based scaffolds with enhanced mechanical characteristics, cell adhesion, and bone tissue generating capacity [12]. The incorporation of titanium, iron, and alumoxane in a scaffold can improve mechanical properties, collagen synthesis, calcium deposition, and alkaline phosphatase activity [561].

Graphene and its derivatives were used as reinforcement material for fibrous scaffolds, films, and hydrogels [570]. The graphene and graphene oxide incorporation into hydrogels yield enhancements in mechanical properties without producing adverse effects on encapsulated fibroblast cells [571]. Carbon-based nanomaterials can be used to improve mechanical strength of scaffolds [572]. Alumina, titania, bioglass, and hydroxyapatite support osteoblast adhesion and growth [573].

Nanobiomaterial-based composite structures are an efficient platform for the synthesis of engineered scaffolds and application in bone tissue engineering (Figure 28) [574]. Nanocomposite-based scaffolds exhibit inherent characteristics such as porous and rough surface and increased wettability, which promote fast bone regeneration. These nanocomposite-based scaffolds provide a porous structure for nutrients exchange and increased protein adsorption. Scaffolds exhibited micro/nano-scaled porous structural pathway for cell–scaffold interaction and integrin-triggered signaling pathway. The nanoscale features support bone cells (osteoblast) and bone-derived stem cells proliferation, migration, cell signaling, stem cell fate, and genetic cell fate. The nanobiomaterials based scaffold have notable mechanical and biological advantages and can induce bone tissue regeneration [531]. The nanostructured materials improve morphological characteristics of scaffolds that may enhance osteoinduction, bone cell attachment, differentiation, proliferation, and natural bone cell growth within the extracellular matrix [12].

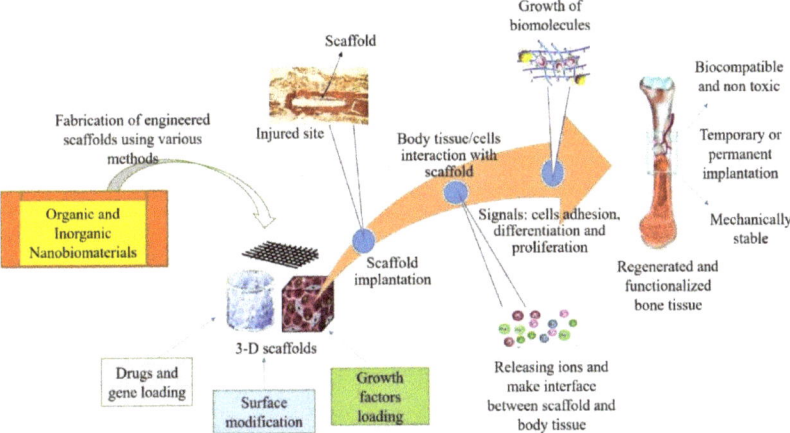

Figure 28. Engineered organic and inorganic nanobiomaterials for hard tissue engineering applications.

Hydroxyapatite (HA) has attracted attention because of its inherent biological compatibility and bone conduction as well as its similarity with bone minerals [575]. For this reason, HA was combined with a number of synthetic and natural polymers such as polycaprolactone [576], poly (lactic acid) (PLA) [577], polyethylene, poly(lactic-co-glycolic acid) (PLGA) [203], collagen [578], gelatin [148], and chitosan [579] to fabricate scaffolds. These composite based scaffolds showed improved mechanical properties, porosity and biocompatibility without or with significantly less adverse effects.

3.7. Bone Cancer Therapy

Cancer is the uncontrolled growth of tissues that could lead to invasion into other organs without proper regulation or differentiation [580]. Conventional cancer therapy is associated with multiple adverse side effects [581]. Bone metastases or "bone mets" occur when cancer cells from the primary tumor relocate to the bone and also spread in the prostate, breast, and lung, which leads to painful (75% of patients) and devastating skeletal-related events (SREs) [582,583]. Depending on the stage of the disease, history, and the overall health of the patient, disease management includes a combination of therapies as shown in Figure 29 [584].

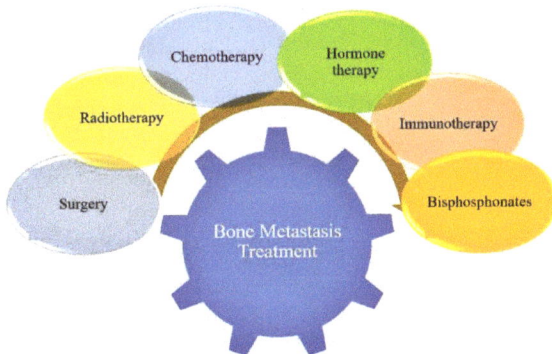

Figure 29. Bone metastasis management through combination of therapies.

The different types of nanoparticles (NPs) used as carriers for small-molecule drugs, proteins, and nucleic acids [585] can be localized to specific disease locations for the treatment of bone metastasis [586]. Nanoparticles also improve the efficiency of other methods used for treating bone metastasis [587]. The effectiveness of NPs depends on their accumulation in vascularized solid tumors via the enhanced permeability and retention (EPR) effect [588]. A wide variety of nanomaterials have been developed in the 1 to 100 nm range and include various anti-tumor drugs (Figure 30) by fine-tuning the chemical structure, scale, and shape (morphology) that can regulate the nanomaterials' functionality [589].

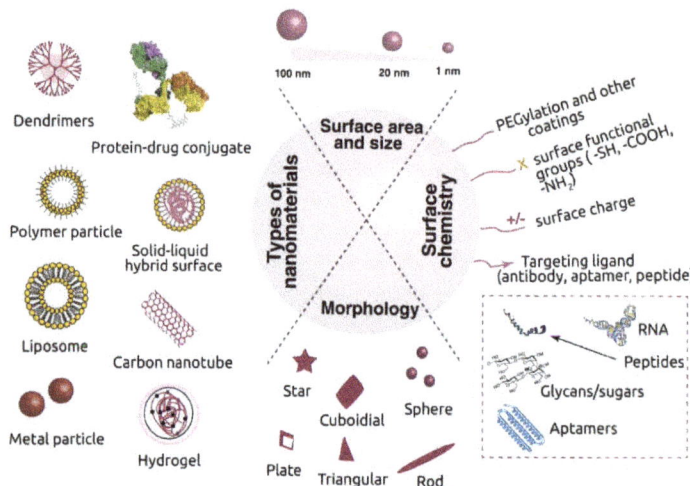

Figure 30. Schematic representation of different types of nanomaterials and their drug-loaded conjugates employed in cancer therapy. (Adapted with permission from ©2019 Springer [589]).

4. Counter-Indications

There is inevitably some sort of interaction between the organic or inorganic materials and the biological environment when individual or composite biomaterials are put in contact with the tissues and fluids of the human body. The basic clinical research may decide that the materials should not cause any local or systemic adverse reactions. Recent studies exposed that nanosized materials can easily penetrate biological membranes of normal cells and enter vascular system to facilitate redistribution in different tissues. Nanomaterials, which by themselves are not very harmful, could become toxic if are ingested in higher concentration. The toxicity of metal based biomaterials to the liver is an important basis for the safety assessment of nanosized materials. Metal based nanoparticles release ions which may enter the cells and affect the functions of organelles, leading to liver injury. Various factors including amount, composition, pH, and fabrication techniques may decide the compatibility and cytotoxicity of biomaterials. The research is ongoing to improve the existing technologies which may produce highly compatible substitutes without producing adverse effects.

5. Conclusions

This review article provided a broad overview of the various types of organic and inorganic nanobiomaterials and their applications in the field of hard tissue engineering. Besides classifying nanobiomaterials, the survey covered several key aspects like bone/cartilage regeneration, drug/gene delivery, anti-infection properties, coatings, scaffold fabrication, and cancer therapy. A total of 550 articles selected by means of web search engines widely used in science and engineering were reviewed in this study. Interestingly, the number of reviewed articles was approximately the same for organic and inorganic biomaterials.

Biomaterials science is a highly multidisciplinary area. Developments in life science and nanotechnology enabled scientists and engineers to conceive new designs and improve the existing bone structure. For example, advances in nanotechnology allowed for the development of novel methods for fabricating new nanostructured scaffolds possessing a higher efficiency in tissue regeneration.

Nanomaterials represent an excellent tool for research and therapeutic approaches in bone tissue engineering. Organic nanomaterials are more biocompatible, nontoxic, and help more with cell regeneration than inorganic nanomaterials. However, inorganic nanomaterials provide better mechanical strength and inertness to chemical agent. From the references cited in this survey it appears that nanoparticles, graphene and nanocomposites are the most diffused types of nanostructures used for hard tissue applications. An important research trend which results in a rapidly growing number of published articles is the development of new composite nanobiomaterials especially for scaffold applications.

Interactions between bone cells and nanomaterials depend on the composition of nanoparticles. Proper selection of nanoparticles may result in faster bone regeneration and recovery. Besides composition, the overall performance of a nanobiomaterial depends on porosity, microstructure, mechanical properties and functionality. Nanomaterials-based scaffolds also play a major role in three-dimensional tissue growth. Nanostructural modifications provide a favorable environment for bone regeneration.

The survey presented in the article proved that tissue engineering supports (i) application of engineering design methods to functionally engineered tissues, (ii) development of novel biomaterials for constructing scaffolds that mimic extracellular matrix, and (iii) creating artificial microenvironments. Nanobiomaterials represent an excellent tool for research and therapeutic approaches in bone tissue engineering. However, further investigations should be aimed at producing advanced nanobiomaterials suitable for hard tissue engineering that can fill the gap between biomaterial fabrication and clinical implementation.

Funding: This research received no external funding.

Conflicts of Interest: The authors declare no conflict of interest.

References

1. Patra, J.K.; Das, G.; Fraceto, L.F.; Campos, E.V.R.; Rodriguez-Torres, M.d.P.; Acosta-Torres, L.-S.; Diaz-Torres, L.A.; Grillo, R.; Swamy, M.K.; Sharma, S.; et al. Nano based drug delivery systems: Recent developments and future prospects. *J. Nanobiotechnol.* **2018**, *16*, 71. [CrossRef]
2. Parratt, K.; Yao, N. Nanostructured biomaterials and their applications. *Nanomaterials* **2013**, *3*, 242–271. [CrossRef] [PubMed]
3. Lei, Y.; Lijuan, Z.; Webster, T.J. Nanobiomaterials: State of the art and future trends. *Adv. Eng. Mater.* **2011**, *13*, B197–B217.
4. Ramos, A.P.; Cruz, M.A.E.; Tovani, C.B.; Ciancaglini, P. Biomedical applications of nanotechnology. *Biophys. Rev.* **2017**, *9*, 79–89. [CrossRef] [PubMed]
5. Capek, I.B.T.-S. *Nanocomposite Structures and Dispersions*; Elsevier: Amsterdam, The Netherlands, 2006; Chapter 1, Volume 23, pp. 1–69.
6. Florencio-Silva, R.; Rodrigues, G.; Sasso-Cerri, E.; Simões, M.J.; Cerri, P.S.; Cells, B. Biology of bone tissue: Structure, function, and factors that influence bone cells. *BioMed Res. Int.* **2015**, *2015*, 421746. [CrossRef]
7. Eliaz, N.; Metoki, N. Calcium phosphate bioceramics: A review of their history, structure, properties, coating technologies and biomedical applications. *Materials* **2017**, *10*, 334. [CrossRef]
8. McMahon, R.; Wang, L.; Skoracki, R.; Mathur, A. Development of nanomaterials for bone repair and regeneration. *J. Biomed. Mater. Res. Part B Appl. Biomater.* **2013**, *101*, 387–397. [CrossRef] [PubMed]
9. Kalenderer, Ö.; Turgut, A. Bone. In *Musculoskeletal Research and Basic Science*; Korkusuz, F., Ed.; Springer International Publishing: Cham, Switzerland, 2016; Chapter 18, pp. 303–321.

10. Farbod, K.; Nejadnik, M.R.; Jansen, J.A.; Leeuwenburgh, S.C.G. Interactions between inorganic and organic phases in bone tissue as a source of inspiration for design of novel nanocomposites. *Tissue Eng. Part B Rev.* **2013**, *20*, 173–188. [CrossRef]
11. Feng, Q.L.; Wu, J.; Chen, G.Q.; Cui, F.Z.; Kim, T.N.; Kim, J.O. A mechanistic study of the antibacterial effect of silver ions on Escherichia coli and Staphylococcus aureus. *J. Biomed. Mater. Res.* **2000**, *52*, 662–668. [CrossRef]
12. Walmsley, G.G.; Mcardle, A.; Tevlin, R.; Momeni, A.; Atashroo, D.; Hu, M.S.; Feroze, A.H.; Wong, V.W.; Lorenz, P.H.; Longaker, M.T.; et al. Nanotechnology in bone tissue engineering. *Nanomedicine* **2015**, *11*, 1253–1263. [CrossRef]
13. Mohamed, A.M. An overview of bone cells and their regulating factors of differentiation. *Malays. J. Med. Sci.* **2008**, *15*, 4–12. [PubMed]
14. Kargozar, S.; Mozafari, M.; Hamzehlou, S.; Brouki Milan, P.; Kim, H.-W.; Baino, F. Bone tissue engineering using human cells: A Comprehensive review on recent trends, current prospects, and recommendations. *Appl. Sci.* **2019**, *9*, 174. [CrossRef]
15. Combes, C.; Cazalbou, S.; Rey, C. Apatite biominerals. *Minerals* **2016**, *6*, 34. [CrossRef]
16. Glimcher, M. Bone: Nature of the calcium phosphate crystals and cellular, structural, and physical chemical mechanisms in their formation. *Rev. Miner. Geochem.* **2006**, *64*, 223–282. [CrossRef]
17. Stevens, M.M. Biomaterials for bone tissue engineering. *Mater. Today* **2008**, *11*, 18–25. [CrossRef]
18. Liu, S.; Gong, W.; Dong, Y.; Hu, Q.; Chen, X.; Gao, X. The effect of submicron bioactive glass particles on in vitro osteogenesis. *RSC Adv.* **2015**, *5*, 38830–38836. [CrossRef]
19. Cheng, C.W.; Solorio, L.D.; Alsberg, E. Decellularized tissue and cell-derived extracellular matrices as scaffolds for orthopaedic tissue engineering. *Biotechnol. Adv.* **2014**, *32*, 462–484. [CrossRef]
20. Nie, X.; Wang, D.-A. Decellularized orthopaedic tissue-engineered grafts: Biomaterial scaffolds synthesised by therapeutic cells. *Biomater. Sci.* **2018**, *6*, 2798–2811. [CrossRef]
21. Amini, A.R.; Laurencin, C.T.; Nukavarapu, S.P. Bone tissue engineering: Recent advances and challenges. *Crit. Rev. Biomed. Eng.* **2012**, *40*, 363–408. [CrossRef]
22. Zhang, L.; Webster, T.J. Nanotechnology and nanomaterials: Promises for improved tissue regeneration. *Nano Today* **2009**, *4*, 66–80. [CrossRef]
23. Kim, S.; Kim, D.; Cho, S.W.; Kim, J.; Kim, J.-S. Highly efficient RNA-guided genome editing in human cells via delivery of purified Cas9 ribonucleoproteins. *Genome Res.* **2014**, *24*, 1012–1019. [CrossRef] [PubMed]
24. Wang, C.; Shen, H.; Tian, Y.; Xie, Y.; Li, A.; Ji, L.; Niu, Z.; Wu, D.; Qiu, D. Bioactive nanoparticle—Gelatin composite scaffold with mechanical performance comparable to cancellous bones. *ACS Appl. Mater. Interfaces* **2014**, *6*, 13061–13068. [CrossRef] [PubMed]
25. Dhivya, S.; Ajita, J.; Selvamurugan, N. Metallic nanomaterials for bone tissue engineering. *J. Biomed. Nanotechnol.* **2015**, *11*, 1675–1700. [CrossRef] [PubMed]
26. Moreno-Vega, A.I.; Gómez-Quintero, T.; Nuñez-Anita, R.E.; Acosta-Torres, L.S.; Castaño, V. Polymeric and ceramic nanoparticles in biomedical applications. *J. Nanotechnol.* **2012**, *2012*, 936041. [CrossRef]
27. Kim, N.J.; Lee, S.J.; Atala, A. Biomedical nanomaterials in tissue engineering. In *Woodhead Publishing Series in Biomaterials*; Gaharwar, A.K., Sant, S., Hancock, M.J., Hacking, S.A.B.T.-N., Eds.; Woodhead Publishing: Cambridge, UK, 2013; pp. 1e–25e.
28. Gajanan, K.; Tijare, S.N. Applications of nanomaterials. *Mater. Today Proc.* **2018**, *5*, 1093–1096. [CrossRef]
29. Wang, Y.; Xia, Y. Bottom-up and top-down approaches to the synthesis of monodispersed spherical colloids of low melting-point metals. *Nano Lett.* **2004**, *4*, 2047–2050. [CrossRef]
30. Saiz, E.; Zimmermann, E.A.; Lee, J.S.; Wegst, U.G.K.; Tomsia, A.P. Perspectives on the role of nanotechnology in bone tissue engineering. *Dent. Mater.* **2013**, *29*, 103–115. [CrossRef]
31. Gardin, C.; Ferroni, L.; Favero, L.; Stellini, E.; Stomaci, D.; Sivolella, S.; Bressan, E.; Zavan, B. Nanostructured biomaterials for tissue engineered bone tissue reconstruction. *Int. J. Mol. Sci.* **2012**, *13*, 737–757.
32. España-Sánchez, B.L.; Cruz-Soto, M.E.; Elizalde-Pena, E.A.; Sabasflores-Benitez, S.; Roca-Aranda, A.; Esquivel-Escalante, K.; Luna-Barcenas, G. Trends in Tissue Regeneration: Bio-nanomaterials. In *Tissue Rigeneration*; El-Sayed Kaoud, H.A., Ed.; IntechOpen: Rijeka, Croatia, 2018.
33. Nikolova, M.P.; Chavali, M.S. Recent advances in biomaterials for 3D scaffolds: A review. *Bioact. Mater.* **2019**, *4*, 271–292. [CrossRef]

34. Zhao, Z.Y.; Liang, L.; Fan, X.; Yu, Z.; Hotchkiss, A.T.; Wilk, B.J.; Eliaz, I. The role of modified citrus pectin as an effective chelator of lead in children hospitalized with toxic lead levels. *Altern. Ther. Health Med.* **2008**, *14*, 34–38.
35. Zheng, K.; Balasubramanian, P.; Paterson, T.E.; Stein, R.; MacNeil, S.; Fiorilli, S.; Vitale-Brovarone, C.; Shepherd, J.; Boccaccini, A.R. Ag modified mesoporous bioactive glass nanoparticles for enhanced antibacterial activity in 3D infected skin model. *Mater. Sci. Eng. C* **2019**, *103*, 109764. [CrossRef]
36. Chen, F.-M.; Liu, X. Advancing biomaterials of human origin for tissue engineering. *Prog. Polym. Sci.* **2016**, *53*, 86–168. [CrossRef] [PubMed]
37. John, Ł. Selected developments and medical applications of organic–inorganic hybrid biomaterials based on functionalized spherosilicates. *Mater. Sci. Eng. C* **2018**, *88*, 172–181. [CrossRef] [PubMed]
38. Fattahi, P.; Yang, G.; Kim, G.; Abidian, M.R. Biomaterials: A review of organic and inorganic biomaterials for neural interfaces. *Adv. Mater.* **2014**, *26*, 1793. [CrossRef]
39. Virlan, M.J.R.; Miricescu, D.; Radulescu, R.; Sabliov, C.M.; Totan, A.; Calenic, B.; Greabu, M. Organic nanomaterials and their applications in the treatment of oral diseases. *Molecules* **2016**, *21*, 207. [CrossRef] [PubMed]
40. Chellan, P.; Sadler, P.J. The elements of life and medicines. *Philos. Trans. R. Soc. A Math. Phys. Eng. Sci.* **2015**, *373*, 20140182. [CrossRef] [PubMed]
41. Kiaie, N.; Aavani, F.; Razavi, M. 2—particles/fibers/bulk. In *Development and Evaluation*; Razavi, M., Ed.; Woodhead Publishing: Cambridge, UK, 2017; pp. 7–25.
42. Wang, G.; Mostafa, N.Z.; Incani, V.; Kucharski, C.; Uludağ, H. Bisphosphonate-decorated lipid nanoparticles designed as drug carriers for bone diseases. *J. Biomed. Mater. Res. Part A* **2012**, *100*, 684–693. [CrossRef] [PubMed]
43. Zhang, G.; Guo, B.; Wu, H.; Tang, T.; Zhang, B.T.; Zheng, L.; He, Y.; Yang, Z.; Pan, X.; Chow, H.; et al. A delivery system targeting bone formation surfaces to facilitate RNAi-based anabolic therapy. *Nat. Med.* **2012**, *18*, 307–314. [CrossRef] [PubMed]
44. Liu, J.; Zhang, H.; Dong, Y.; Jin, Y.; Hu, X.; Cai, K.; Ma, J.; Wu, G. Bi-directionally selective bone targeting delivery for anabolic and antiresorptive drugs: A novel combined therapy for osteoporosis? *Med. Hypotheses* **2014**, *83*, 694–696. [CrossRef]
45. Hirsjärvi, S.; Sancey, L.; Dufort, S.; Belloche, C.; Vanpouille-Box, C.; Garcion, E.; Coll, J.-L.; Hindré, F.; Benoît, J.-P. Effect of particle size on the biodistribution of lipid nanocapsules: Comparison between nuclear and fluorescence imaging and counting. *Int. J. Pharm.* **2013**, *453*, 594–600. [CrossRef]
46. Nahar, M.; Dutta, T.; Murugesan, S.; Asthana, A.; Mishra, D.; Rajkumar, V.; Tare, M.; Saraf, S.; Jain, N.K. Functional polymeric nanoparticles: An efficient and promising tool for active delivery of bioactives. *Crit. Rev. Ther. Drug Carr. Syst.* **2006**, *23*, 259–318. [CrossRef] [PubMed]
47. An, S.Y.; Bui, M.-P.N.; Nam, Y.J.; Han, K.N.; Li, C.A.; Choo, J.; Lee, E.K.; Katoh, S.; Kumada, Y.; Seong, G.H. Preparation of monodisperse and size-controlled poly(ethylene glycol) hydrogel nanoparticles using liposome templates. *J. Colloid Interface Sci.* **2009**, *331*, 98–103. [CrossRef] [PubMed]
48. Monteiro, N.; Martins, A.; Reis, R.L.; Neves, N.M. Liposomes in tissue engineering and regenerative medicine. *J. R. Soc. Interface* **2014**, *11*, 281–297. [CrossRef] [PubMed]
49. Qi, R.; Majoros, I.; Misra, A.C.; Koch, A.E.; Campbell, P.; Marotte, H.; Bergin, I.L.; Cao, Z.; Goonewardena, S.; Morry, J.; et al. Folate receptor-targeted dendrimer-methotrexate conjugate for inflammatory arthritis. *J. Biomed. Nanotechnol.* **2014**, *11*, 1370–1384. [CrossRef]
50. Duncan, R.; Izzo, L. Dendrimer biocompatibility and toxicity. *Adv. Drug Deliv. Rev.* **2005**, *57*, 2215–2237. [CrossRef]
51. De la Riva, B.; Sánchez, E.; Hernández, A.; Reyes, R.; Tamimi, F.; López-Cabarcos, E.; Delgado, A.; vora, C. Local controlled release of VEGF and PDGF from a combined brushite-chitosan system enhances bone regeneration. *J. Control. Release* **2010**, *143*, 45–52. [CrossRef]
52. Rampino, A.; Borgogna, M.; Blasi, P.; Bellich, B.; Cesàro, A. Chitosan nanoparticles: Preparation, size evolution and stability. *Int. J. Pharm.* **2013**, *455*, 219–228. [CrossRef]
53. Vedakumari, W.S.; Prabu, P.; Sastry, T.P. Chitosan-fibrin nanocomposites as drug delivering and wound healing materials. *J. Biomed. Nanotechnol.* **2015**, *11*, 657–667. [CrossRef]

54. Shim, K.; Won, H.S.; Sang, Y.L.; Sang, H.L.; Seong, J.H.; Myung, C.L.; Lee, S.J. Chitosan nano-/microfibrous double-layered membrane with rolled-up three-dimensional structures for chondrocyte cultivation. *J. Biomed. Mater. Res. Part A* **2009**, *90*, 595–602. [CrossRef]
55. Poth, N.; Seiffart, V.; Gross, G.; Menzel, H.; Dempwolf, W. Biodegradable chitosan nanoparticle coatings on titanium for the delivery of BMP-2. *Biomolecules* **2015**, *5*, 3–19. [CrossRef]
56. Nagarajan, U.; Kawakami, K.; Zhang, S.; Chandrasekaran, B. Fabrication of solid collagen nanoparticles using electrospray deposition. *Chem. Pharm. Bull.* **2014**, *62*, 422–428. [CrossRef] [PubMed]
57. Liu, Y.; Lu, Y.; Tian, X.; Cui, G.; Zhao, Y.; Yang, Q.; Yu, S.; Xing, G.; Zhang, B. Segmental bone regeneration using an rhBMP-2-loaded gelatin/nanohydroxyapatite/fibrin scaffold in a rabbit model. *Biomaterials* **2009**, *30*, 6276–6285. [CrossRef] [PubMed]
58. Jahanshahi, M.; Sanati, M.H.; Hajizadeh, S.; Babaei, Z. Gelatin nanoparticle fabrication and optimization of the particle size. *Phys. Status Solidi* **2008**, *205*, 2898–2902. [CrossRef]
59. Miller, D.C.; Thapa, A.; Haberstroh, K.M.; Webster, T.J. Endothelial and vascular smooth muscle cell function on poly(lactic-co-glycolic acid) with nano-structured surface features. *Biomaterials* **2004**, *25*, 53–61. [CrossRef]
60. Danhier, F.; Ansorena, E.; Silva, J.M.; Coco, R.; Le Breton, A.; Préat, V. PLGA-based nanoparticles: An overview of biomedical applications. *J. Control. Release* **2012**, *161*, 505–522. [CrossRef]
61. Pattison, M.A.; Wurster, S.; Webster, T.J.; Haberstroh, K.M. Three-dimensional, nano-structured PLGA scaffolds for bladder tissue replacement applications. *Biomaterials* **2005**, *26*, 2491–2500. [CrossRef]
62. Soundrapandian, C.; Mahato, A.; Kundu, B.; Datta, S.; Sa, B.; Basu, D. Development and effect of different bioactive silicate glass scaffolds: In vitro evaluation for use as a bone drug delivery system. *J. Mech. Behav. Biomed. Mater.* **2014**, *40*, 1–12. [CrossRef] [PubMed]
63. Baldrighi, M.; Trusel, M.; Tonini, R.; Giordani, S. Carbon Nanomaterials Interfacing with Neurons: An In vivo Perspective. *Front. Neurosci.* **2016**, *10*, 250. [CrossRef] [PubMed]
64. Gorain, B.; Choudhury, H.; Pandey, M.; Kesharwani, P.; Abeer, M.M.; Tekade, R.K.; Hussain, Z. Carbon nanotube scaffolds as emerging nanoplatform for myocardial tissue regeneration: A review of recent developments and therapeutic implications. *Biomed. Pharmacother.* **2018**, *104*, 496–508. [CrossRef] [PubMed]
65. Zhu, Z. An overview of carbon nanotubes and graphene for biosensing applications. *Nanomicro Lett.* **2017**, *9*, 25. [CrossRef]
66. Guo, Q.; Shen, X.; Li, Y.; Xu, S. Carbon nanotubes-based drug delivery to cancer and brain. *Curr. Med. Sci.* **2017**, *37*, 635–641. [CrossRef] [PubMed]
67. Fahy, E.; Subramaniam, S.; Murphy, R.C.; Nishijima, M.; Raetz, C.R.H.; Shimizu, T.; Spener, F.; van Meer, G.; Wakelam, M.J.O.; Dennis, E.A. Update of the LIPID MAPS comprehensive classification system for lipids. *J. Lipid Res.* **2009**, *50*, S9–S14. [CrossRef] [PubMed]
68. Vemuri, S.; Rhodes, C.T. Preparation and characterization of liposomes as therapeutic delivery systems: A review. *Pharm. Acta Helv.* **1995**, *70*, 95–111. [CrossRef]
69. Subramaniam, S.; Fahy, E.; Gupta, S.; Sud, M.; Byrnes, R.W.; Cotter, D.; Dinasarapu, A.R.; Maurya, M.R. Bioinformatics and systems biology of the lipidome. *Chem. Rev.* **2011**, *111*, 6452–6490. [CrossRef]
70. Khan, I.; Saeed, K.; Khan, I. Nanoparticles: Properties, applications and toxicities. *Arab. J. Chem.* **2019**, *12*, 908–931. [CrossRef]
71. Carbone, C.; Leonardi, A.; Cupri, S.; Puglisi, G.; Pignatello, R. Pharmaceutical and biomedical applications of lipid-based nanocarriers. *Pharm. Pat. Anal.* **2014**, *3*, 199–215. [CrossRef]
72. Bozzuto, G.; Molinari, A. Liposomes as nanomedical devices. *Int. J. Nanomed.* **2015**, *10*, 975–999. [CrossRef]
73. Puri, A.; Loomis, K.; Smith, B.; Lee, J.-H.; Yavlovich, A.; Heldman, E.; Blumenthal, R. Lipid-based nanoparticles as pharmaceutical drug carriers: From concepts to clinic. *Crit. Rev. Ther. Drug Carr. Syst.* **2009**, *26*, 523–580. [CrossRef]
74. Rai, R.; Alwani, S.; Badea, I. Polymeric nanoparticles in gene therapy: New avenues of design and optimization for delivery applications. *Polymers* **2019**, *11*, 745. [CrossRef]
75. Dolatabadi, J.E.N.; Omidi, Y. Solid lipid-based nanocarriers as efficient targeted drug and gene delivery systems. *TrAC Trends Anal. Chem.* **2016**, *77*, 100–108. [CrossRef]
76. Mukherjee, S.; Ray, S.; Thakur, R.S. Solid lipid nanoparticles: A modern formulation approach in drug delivery system. *Indian J. Pharm. Sci.* **2009**, *71*, 349–358. [CrossRef] [PubMed]

77. Tamjidi, F.; Shahedi, M.; Varshosaz, J.; Nasirpour, A. Nanostructured lipid carriers (NLC): A potential delivery system for bioactive food molecules. *Innov. Food Sci. Emerg. Technol.* **2013**, *19*, 29–43. [CrossRef]
78. Mouzouvi, C.R.A.; Umerska, A.; Bigot, A.K.; Saulnier, P. Surface active properties of lipid nanocapsules. *PLoS ONE* **2017**, *12*, e0179211. [CrossRef] [PubMed]
79. Irby, D.; Du, C.; Li, F. Lipid—Drug conjugate for enhancing drug delivery. *Mol. Pharm.* **2017**, *14*, 1325–1338. [CrossRef]
80. Talegaonkar, S.; Bhattacharyya, A. Potential of lipid nanoparticles (SLNs and NLCs) in enhancing oral bioavailability of drugs with poor intestinal permeability. *AAPS PharmSciTech* **2019**, *20*, 121. [CrossRef]
81. Dave, V.; Tak, K.; Sohgaura, A.; Gupta, A.; Sadhu, V.; Reddy, K.R. Lipid-polymer hybrid nanoparticles: Synthesis strategies and biomedical applications. *J. Microbiol. Methods* **2019**, *160*, 130–142. [CrossRef]
82. Bangham, A.D.; Standish, M.M.; Watkins, J.C. Diffusion of univalent ions across the lamellae of swollen phospholipids. *J. Mol. Biol.* **1965**, *13*, 238-IN27. [CrossRef]
83. Akbarzadeh, A.; Rezaei-Sadabady, R.; Davaran, S.; Joo, S.; Zarghami, N.; Hanifehpour, Y.; Samiei, M.; Kouhi, M.; Nejati, K. Liposome: Classification, preparation, and applications. *Nanoscale Res. Lett.* **2013**, *8*, 102. [CrossRef]
84. Daraee, H.; Etemadi, A.; Kouhi, M.; Alimirzalu, S.; Akbarzadeh, A. Application of liposomes in medicine and drug delivery. *Artif. Cells Nanomed. Biotechnol.* **2016**, *44*, 381–391. [CrossRef]
85. Fenske, D.B.; Chonn, A.; Cullis, P.R. Liposomal nanomedicines: An emerging field. *Toxicol. Pathol.* **2008**, *36*, 21–29. [CrossRef]
86. Immordino, M.L.; Dosio, F.; Cattel, L. Stealth liposomes: Review of the basic science, rationale, and clinical applications, existing and potential. *Int. J. Nanomed.* **2006**, *1*, 297–315.
87. La, W.-G.; Jin, M.; Park, S.; Yoon, H.-H.; Jeong, G.-J.; Bhang, S.; Park, H.; Char, K.; Kim, B.-S. Delivery of bone morphogenetic protein-2 and substance P using graphene oxide for bone regeneration. *Int. J. Nanomed.* **2014**, *9* (Suppl. 1), 107–116.
88. Du, G.-Y.; He, S.-W.; Sun, C.-X.; Mi, L.-D. Bone morphogenic Protein-2 (rhBMP2)-loaded silk fibroin scaffolds to enhance the osteoinductivity in bone tissue engineering. *Nanoscale Res. Lett.* **2017**, *12*, 573. [CrossRef] [PubMed]
89. Takahashi, M.; Inafuku, K.; Miyagi, T.; Oku, H.; Wada, K.; Imura, T.; Kitamoto, D. Efficient preparation of liposomes encapsulating food materials using lecithins by a mechanochemical method. *J. Oleo Sci.* **2007**, *56*, 35–42. [CrossRef]
90. Zhu, C.T.; Xu, Y.Q.; Shi, J.; Li, J.; Ding, J. Liposome combined porous β-TCP scaffold: Preparation, characterization, and anti-biofilm activity. *Drug Deliv.* **2010**, *17*, 391–398. [CrossRef]
91. Li, Y.; Bai, Y.; Pan, J.; Wang, H.; Li, H.; Xu, X.; Fu, X.; Shi, R.; Luo, Z.; Li, Y.; et al. A hybrid 3D-printed aspirin-laden liposome composite scaffold for bone tissue engineering. *J. Mater. Chem. B* **2019**, *7*, 619–629. [CrossRef]
92. Sou, K.; Inenaga, S.; Takeoka, S.; Tsuchida, E. Loading of curcumin into macrophages using lipid-based nanoparticles. *Int. J. Pharm.* **2008**, *352*, 287–293. [CrossRef]
93. Mayer, L.D.; Bally, M.B.; Cullis, P.R. Uptake of adriamycin into large unilamellar vesicles in response to a pH gradient. *Biochim. Biophys. Acta Biomembr.* **1986**, *857*, 123–126. [CrossRef]
94. Cullis, P.R.; Hope, M.J.; Bally, M.B.; Madden, T.D.; Mayer, L.D.; Fenske, D.B. Influence of pH gradients on the transbilayer transport of drugs, lipids, peptides and metal ions into large unilamellar vesicles. *Biochim. Biophys. Acta Rev. Biomembr.* **1997**, *1331*, 187–211. [CrossRef]
95. Dang, M.; Saunders, L.; Niu, X.; Fan, Y.; Ma, P.X. Biomimetic delivery of signals for bone tissue engineering. *Bone Res.* **2018**, *6*, 25. [CrossRef]
96. Kulkarni, M.; Greiser, U.; O'Brien, T.; Pandit, A. Liposomal gene delivery mediated by tissue-engineered scaffolds. *Trends Biotechnol.* **2010**, *28*, 28–36. [CrossRef] [PubMed]
97. Abbasi, E.; Aval, S.F.; Akbarzadeh, A.; Milani, M.; Nasrabadi, H.T.; Joo, S.W.; Hanifehpour, Y.; Nejati-Koshki, K.; Pashaei-Asl, R. Dendrimers: Synthesis, applications, and properties. *Nanoscale Res. Lett.* **2014**, *9*, 247. [CrossRef] [PubMed]
98. Majoral, J.-P.; Caminade, A.-M. Dendrimers containing heteroatoms (Si, P, B, Ge, or Bi). *Chem. Rev.* **1999**, *99*, 845–880. [CrossRef] [PubMed]
99. Bosman, A.W.; Janssen, H.M.; Meijer, E.W. About dendrimers: Structure, physical properties, and applications. *Chem. Rev.* **1999**, *99*, 1665–1688. [CrossRef] [PubMed]

100. Joshi, N.; Grinstaff, M. Applications of dendrimers in tissue engineering. *Curr. Top. Med. Chem.* **2008**, *8*, 1225–1236. [CrossRef] [PubMed]
101. Barrett, T.; Ravizzini, G.; Choyke, P.L.; Kobayashi, H. Dendrimers in medical nanotechnology. *IEEE Eng. Med. Biol. Mag.* **2009**, *28*, 12–22. [CrossRef] [PubMed]
102. Liu, Y.; Tee, J.K.T.; Chiu, G.N.C. Dendrimers in oral drug delivery application: Current explorations, toxicity issues and strategies for improvement. *Curr. Pharm. Des.* **2015**, *21*, 2629–2642. [CrossRef] [PubMed]
103. Courtenay, J.C.; Deneke, C.; Lanzoni, E.M.; Costa, C.A.; Bae, Y.; Scott, J.L.; Sharma, R.I. Modulating cell response on cellulose surfaces; tunable attachment and scaffold mechanics. *Cellulose* **2018**, *25*, 925–940. [CrossRef]
104. Zhou, L.; Shan, Y.; Hu, H.; Yu, B.Y.; Cong, H. Synthesis and biomedical applications of dendrimers. *Curr. Org. Chem.* **2018**, *22*, 600–612. [CrossRef]
105. Opina, A.C.; Wong, K.J.; Griffiths, G.L.; Turkbey, B.I.; Bernardo, M.; Nakajima, T.; Kobayashi, H.; Choyke, P.L.; Vasalatiy, O. Preparation and long-term biodistribution studies of a PAMAM dendrimer G5–Gd-BnDOTA conjugate for lymphatic imaging. *Nanomedicine* **2014**, *10*, 1423–1437. [CrossRef]
106. Shadrack, D.M.; Swai, H.S.; Munissi, J.J.E.; Mubofu, E.B.; Nyandoro, S.S. Polyamidoamine dendrimers for enhanced solubility of small molecules and other desirable properties for site specific delivery: Insights from experimental and computational studies. *Molecules* **2018**, *23*, 1419. [CrossRef] [PubMed]
107. Din, F.U.; Aman, W.; Ullah, I.; Qureshi, O.S.; Mustapha, O.; Shafique, S.; Zeb, A. Effective use of nanocarriers as drug delivery systems for the treatment of selected tumors. *Int. J. Nanomed.* **2017**, *12*, 7291–7309. [CrossRef] [PubMed]
108. Pooja, D.; Sistla, R.; Kulhari, H. Chapter 7—Dendrimer-drug conjugates: Synthesis strategies, stability and application in anticancer drug delivery. In *Design of Nanostructures for Theranostics Applications*; Grumezescu, A.M., Ed.; William Andrew Publishing: Norwich, NY, USA, 2018; pp. 277–303.
109. Yiyun, C.; Na, M.; Tongwen, X.; Rongqiang, F.; Xueyuan, W.; Xiaomin, W.; Longping, W. Transdermal delivery of nonsteroidal anti-inflammatory drugs mediated by polyamidoamine (PAMAM) dendrimers. *J. Pharm. Sci.* **2007**, *96*, 595–602. [CrossRef] [PubMed]
110. Fu, H.-L.; Cheng, S.-X.; Zhang, X.-Z.; Zhuo, R.-X. Dendrimer/DNA complexes encapsulated functional biodegradable polymer for substrate-mediated gene delivery. *J. Gene Med.* **2008**, *10*, 1334–1342. [CrossRef]
111. Grinstaff, M.W. Dendritic macromers for hydrogel formation: Tailored materials for ophthalmic, orthopedic, and biotech applications. *J. Polym. Sci. Part A Polym. Chem.* **2008**, *46*, 383–400. [CrossRef]
112. Grinstaff, M. Biodendrimers: New polymeric biomaterials for tissues engineering. *Chem. A Eur. J.* **2002**, *8*, 2838–2846. [CrossRef]
113. Boduch-Lee, K.A.; Chapman, T.; Petricca, S.E.; Marra, K.G.; Kumta, P. Design and synthesis of hydroxyapatite composites containing an mPEG–Dendritic Poly(l-lysine) star polycaprolactone. *Macromolecules* **2004**, *37*, 8959–8966. [CrossRef]
114. Rajzer, I. Fabrication of bioactive polycaprolactone/hydroxyapatite scaffolds with final bilayer nano-/micro-fibrous structures for tissue engineering application. *J. Mater. Sci.* **2014**, *49*, 5799–5807. [CrossRef]
115. Mintzer, M.A.; Grinstaff, M.W. Biomedical applications of dendrimers: A tutorial. *Chem. Soc. Rev.* **2011**, *40*, 173–190. [CrossRef]
116. Oliveira, J.M.; Sousa, R.A.; Kotobuki, N.; Tadokoro, M.; Hirose, M.; Mano, J.F.; Reis, R.L.; Ohgushi, H. The osteogenic differentiation of rat bone marrow stromal cells cultured with dexamethasone-loaded carboxymethylchitosan/poly(amidoamine) dendrimer nanoparticles. *Biomaterials* **2009**, *30*, 804–813. [CrossRef]
117. Fathi-Achachelouei, M.; Knopf-Marques, H.; Ribeiro da Silva, C.E.; Barthès, J.; Bat, E.; Tezcaner, A.; Vrana, N.E. Use of nanoparticles in tissue engineering and regenerative medicine. *Front. Bioeng. Biotechnol.* **2019**, *7*, 113. [CrossRef] [PubMed]
118. Jain, S.K. PEGylation: An approach for drug delivery. A review. *Crit. Rev. Ther. Drug Carr. Syst.* **2008**, *25*, 403–447. [CrossRef]
119. Yoo, H.S.; Kim, T.G.; Park, T.G. Surface-functionalized electrospun nanofibers for tissue engineering and drug delivery. *Adv. Drug Deliv. Rev.* **2009**, *61*, 1033–1042. [CrossRef] [PubMed]
120. Rao, J.P.; Geckeler, K.E. Polymer nanoparticles: Preparation techniques and size-control parameters. *Prog. Polym. Sci.* **2011**, *36*, 887–913. [CrossRef]

121. Santo, V.E.; Ratanavaraporn, J.; Sato, K.; Gomes, M.E.; Mano, J.F.; Reis, R.L.; Tabata, Y. Cell engineering by the internalization of bioinstructive micelles for enhanced bone regeneration. *Nanomedicine* **2015**, *10*, 1707–1721. [CrossRef] [PubMed]
122. Nicolas, J.; Mura, S.; Brambilla, D.; Mackiewicz, N.; Couvreur, P. Design, functionalization strategies and biomedical applications of targeted biodegradable/biocompatible polymer-based nanocarriers for drug delivery. *Chem. Soc. Rev.* **2013**, *42*, 1147–1235. [CrossRef]
123. Fàbregas, A.; Miñarro, M.; García-Montoya, E.; Pérez-Lozano, P.; Carrillo, C.; Sarrate, R.; Sánchez, N.; Ticó, J.R.; Suñé-Negre, J.M. Impact of physical parameters on particle size and reaction yield when using the ionic gelation method to obtain cationic polymeric chitosan-tripolyphosphate nanoparticles. *Int. J. Pharm.* **2013**, *446*, 199–204. [CrossRef]
124. Vaculikova, E.; Grunwaldova, V.; Kral, V.; Dohnal, J.; Jampilek, J. Preparation of candesartan and atorvastatin nanoparticles by solvent evaporation. *Molecules* **2012**, *17*, 13221–13234. [CrossRef]
125. Chung, J.W.; Lee, K.; Neikirk, C.; Nelson, C.M.; Priestley, R.D. Photoresponsive coumarin-stabilized polymeric nanoparticles as a detectable drug carrier. *Small* **2012**, *8*, 1693–1700. [CrossRef]
126. Langer, K.; Anhorn, M.G.; Steinhauser, I.; Dreis, S.; Celebi, D.; Schrickel, N.; Faust, S.; Vogel, V. Human serum albumin (HSA) nanoparticles: Reproducibility of preparation process and kinetics of enzymatic degradation. *Int. J. Pharm.* **2008**, *347*, 109–117. [CrossRef]
127. Yu, X.; Trase, I.; Ren, M.; Duval, K.; Guo, X.; Chen, Z. Design of nanoparticle-based carriers for targeted drug delivery. *J. Nanomater.* **2016**, *2016*, 1087250. [CrossRef] [PubMed]
128. Nagavarma, B.V.N.; Yadav, H.K.S.; Ayaz, A.; Vasudha, L.S.; Shivakumar, H.G. Different techniques for preparation of polymeric nanoparticles—A review. *Asian J. Pharm. Clin. Res.* **2012**, *5*, 16–23.
129. Calzoni, E.; Cesaretti, A.; Polchi, A.; Di Michele, A.; Tancini, B.; Emiliani, C. Biocompatible polymer nanoparticles for drug delivery applications in cancer and neurodegenerative disorder therapies. *J. Funct. Biomater.* **2019**, *10*, 4. [CrossRef] [PubMed]
130. Joye, I.J.; McClements, D.J. Biopolymer-based nanoparticles and microparticles: Fabrication, characterization, and application. *Curr. Opin. Colloid Interface Sci.* **2014**, *19*, 417–427. [CrossRef]
131. Ezhilarasi, P.N.; Karthik, P.; Chhanwal, N.; Anandharamakrishnan, C. Nanoencapsulation techniques for food bioactive components: A review. *Food Bioprocess Technol.* **2013**, *6*, 628–647. [CrossRef]
132. Bennet, D.; Kim, S. Polymer nanoparticles for smart drug delivery. In *Application of Nanotechnology in Drug Delivery*; Sezer, A.D., Ed.; IntechOpen: Rijeka, Croatia, 2014.
133. Makadia, H.K.; Siegel, S.J. Poly Lactic-co-glycolic acid (PLGA) as biodegradable controlled drug delivery carrier. *Polymers* **2011**, *3*, 1377–1397. [CrossRef]
134. Shoichet, M.S. Polymer scaffolds for biomaterials applications. *Macromolecules* **2010**, *43*, 581–591. [CrossRef]
135. Priya James, H.; John, R.; Alex, A.; Anoop, K.R. Smart polymers for the controlled delivery of drugs—A concise overview. *Acta Pharm. Sin. B* **2014**, *4*, 120–127. [CrossRef]
136. Kashirina, A.; Yao, Y.; Liu, Y.; Leng, J. Biopolymers as bone substitutes: A review. *Biomater. Sci.* **2019**, *7*, 3961–3983. [CrossRef] [PubMed]
137. Van Vlierberghe, S.; Dubruel, P.; Schacht, E. Biopolymer-based hydrogels as scaffolds for tissue engineering applications: A review. *Biomacromolecules* **2011**, *12*, 1387–1408. [CrossRef] [PubMed]
138. Tang, Z.; He, C.; Tian, H.; Ding, J.; Hsiao, B.S.; Chu, B.; Chen, X. Polymeric nanostructured materials for biomedical applications. *Prog. Polym. Sci.* **2016**, *60*, 86–128. [CrossRef]
139. Cheng, R.; Meng, F.; Deng, C.; Klok, H.-A.; Zhong, Z. Dual and multi-stimuli responsive polymeric nanoparticles for programmed site-specific drug delivery. *Biomaterials* **2013**, *34*, 3647–3657. [CrossRef] [PubMed]
140. Wu, S.; Liu, X.; Yeung, K.W.K.; Liu, C.; Yang, X. Biomimetic porous scaffolds for bone tissue engineering. *Mater. Sci. Eng. R Rep.* **2014**, *80*, 1–36. [CrossRef]
141. Sharma, K.; Mujawar, M.A.; Kaushik, A. State-of-art functional biomaterials for tissue engineering. *Front. Mater.* **2019**, *6*, 1–10. [CrossRef]
142. Tezcaner, A.; Baran, E.; Keskin, D. Nanoparticles based on plasma proteins for drug delivery applications. *Curr. Pharm. Des.* **2016**, *22*, 3445–3454. [CrossRef]
143. Kumar, P.; Dehiya, B.S.; Sindhu, A. Comparative study of chitosan and chitosan–gelatin scaffold for tissue engineering. *Int. Nano Lett.* **2017**, *7*, 285–290. [CrossRef]

144. Younes, I.; Rinaudo, M. Chitin and chitosan preparation from marine sources. Structure, properties and applications. *Mar. Drugs* **2015**, *13*, 1133–1174. [CrossRef]
145. Al-Qadi, S.; Grenha, A.; Carrión-Recio, D.; Seijo, B.; Remuñán-López, C. Microencapsulated chitosan nanoparticles for pulmonary protein delivery: In vivo evaluation of insulin-loaded formulations. *J. Control. Release* **2012**, *157*, 383–390. [CrossRef]
146. Berger, J.; Reist, M.; Mayer, J.M.; Felt, O.; Peppas, N.A.; Gurny, R. Structure and interactions in covalently and ionically crosslinked chitosan hydrogels for biomedical applications. *Eur. J. Pharm. Biopharm.* **2004**, *57*, 19–34. [CrossRef]
147. Agnihotri, S.A.; Mallikarjuna, N.N.; Aminabhavi, T.M. Recent advances on chitosan-based micro- and nanoparticles in drug delivery. *J. Control. Release* **2004**, *100*, 5–28. [CrossRef]
148. Kim, S.K.; Rajapakse, N. Enzymatic production and biological activities of chitosan oligosaccharides (COS): A review. *Carbohydr. Polym.* **2005**, *62*, 357–368. [CrossRef]
149. Campos, E.V.R.; Oliveira, J.L.; Fraceto, L.F. Poly(ethylene glycol) and cyclodextrin-grafted chitosan: From methodologies to preparation and potential biotechnological applications. *Front. Chem.* **2017**, *5*, 93. [CrossRef]
150. Wang, J.J.; Zeng, Z.W.; Xiao, R.Z.; Xie, T.; Zhou, G.L.; Zhan, X.R.; Wang, S.L. Recent advances of chitosan nanoparticles as drug carriers. *Int. J. Nanomed.* **2011**, *6*, 765–774.
151. Levengood, S.L.; Zhang, M. Chitosan-based scaffolds for bone tissue engineering. *J. Mater. Chem. B* **2014**, *2*, 3161–3184. [CrossRef]
152. Eap, S.; Keller, L.; Schiavi, J.; Huck, O.; Jacomine, L.; Fioretti, F.; Gauthier, C.; Sebastian, V.; Schwinté, P.; Benkirane-Jessel, N. A living thick nanofibrous implant bifunctionalized with active growth factor and stem cells for bone regeneration. *Int. J. Nanomed.* **2015**, *10*, 1061–1075.
153. Shrestha, A.; Kishen, A. The effect of tissue inhibitors on the antibacterial activity of chitosan nanoparticles and photodynamic therapy. *J. Endod.* **2012**, *38*, 1275–1278. [CrossRef]
154. Kumar, P.; Dehiya, B.S.; Sindhu, A. Synthesis and characterization of nHA-PEG and nBG-PEG scaffolds for hard tissue engineering applications. *Ceram. Int.* **2019**, *45*, 8370–8379. [CrossRef]
155. Kumar, P.; Saini, M.; Dehiya, B.S.; Umar, A.; Sindhu, A.; Mohammed, H.; Al-Hadeethi, Y.; Guo, Z. Fabrication and in-vitro biocompatibility of freeze-dried CTS-nHA and CTS-nBG scaffolds for bone regeneration applications. *Int. J. Biol. Macromol.* **2020**, *149*, 1–10. [CrossRef]
156. Bhowmick, A.; Banerjee, S.L.; Pramanik, N.; Jana, P.; Mitra, T.; Gnanamani, A.; Das, M.; Kundu, P.P. Organically modified clay supported chitosan/hydroxyapatite-zinc oxide nanocomposites with enhanced mechanical and biological properties for the application in bone tissue engineering. *Int. J. Biol. Macromol.* **2018**, *106*, 11–19. [CrossRef]
157. Yilgor, P.; Tuzlakoglu, K.; Reis, R.L.; Hasirci, N.; Hasirci, V. Incorporation of a sequential BMP-2/BMP-7 delivery system into chitosan-based scaffolds for bone tissue engineering. *Biomaterials* **2009**, *30*, 3551–3559. [CrossRef]
158. Mili, B.; Das, K.; Kumar, A.; Saxena, A.C.; Singh, P.; Ghosh, S.; Bag, S. Preparation of NGF encapsulated chitosan nanoparticles and its evaluation on neuronal differentiation potentiality of canine mesenchymal stem cells. *J. Mater. Sci. Mater. Med.* **2017**, *29*, 4. [CrossRef]
159. Kumar, P. Nano-TiO(2) doped chitosan scaffold for the bone tissue engineering applications. *Int. J. Biomater.* **2018**, *2018*, 6576157. [CrossRef]
160. Koosha, M.; Solouk, A.; Ghalei, S.; Sadeghi, D.; Bagheri, S.; Mirzadeh, H. Electrospun chitosan/gum tragacanth/polyvinyl alcohol hybrid nanofibrous scaffold for tissue engineering applications. *Bioinspired Biomim. Nanobiomater.* **2019**, *9*, 1–8.
161. Zugravu, M.; Smith, R.; Reves, B.; Jennings, J.; Cooper, J.; Haggard, W.; Bumgardner, J. Physical properties and in vitro evaluation of collagen-chitosan-calcium phosphate microparticle-based scaffolds for bone tissue regeneration. *J. Biomater. Appl.* **2012**, *28*, 566–579. [CrossRef] [PubMed]
162. Wahl, D.; Czernuszka, J. Collagen-hydroxyapatite composites for hard tissue repair. *Eur. Cell Mater.* **2006**, *11*, 43–56. [CrossRef] [PubMed]
163. Krafts, K.P. Tissue repair: The hidden drama. *Organogenesis* **2010**, *6*, 225–233. [CrossRef]
164. Dong, C.; Lv, Y. Application of collagen scaffold in tissue engineering: Recent advances and new perspectives. *Polymers* **2016**, *8*, 42. [CrossRef] [PubMed]

165. Lim, Y.-S.; Ok, Y.-J.; Hwang, S.-Y.; Kwak, J.-Y.; Yoon, S. Marine collagen as a promising biomaterial for biomedical applications. *Mar. Drugs* **2019**, *17*, 467. [CrossRef]
166. Khan, R.; Khan, M.H. Use of collagen as a biomaterial: An update. *J. Indian Soc. Periodontol.* **2013**, *17*, 539–542. [CrossRef]
167. D'Mello, S.; Atluri, K.; Geary, S.M.; Hong, L.; Elangovan, S.; Salem, A.K. Bone regeneration using gene-activated matrices. *AAPS J.* **2017**, *19*, 43–53. [CrossRef]
168. Fujioka-Kobayashi, M.; Schaller, B.; Saulacic, N.; Pippenger, B.E.; Zhang, Y.; Miron, R.J. Absorbable collagen sponges loaded with recombinant bone morphogenetic protein 9 induces greater osteoblast differentiation when compared to bone morphogenetic protein 2. *Clin. Exp. Dent. Res.* **2017**, *3*, 32–40. [CrossRef] [PubMed]
169. Nakagawa, T.; Tagawa, T. Ultrastructural study of direct bone formation induced by BMPs-collagen complex implanted into an ectopic site. *Oral Dis.* **2000**, *6*, 172–179. [CrossRef] [PubMed]
170. Xie, J.; Baumann, M.J.; McCabe, L.R. Osteoblasts respond to hydroxyapatite surfaces with immediate changes in gene expression. *J. Biomed. Mater. Res. Part A* **2004**, *71*, 108–117. [CrossRef] [PubMed]
171. Chan, E.C.; Kuo, S.-M.; Kong, A.M.; Morrison, W.A.; Dusting, G.J.; Mitchell, G.M.; Lim, S.Y.; Liu, G.-S. Three dimensional collagen scaffold promotes intrinsic vascularisation for tissue engineering applications. *PLoS ONE* **2016**, *11*, e0149799. [CrossRef]
172. Vázquez, J.J.; Martín-Martínez, E.S. Collagen and elastin scaffold by electrospinning for skin tissue engineering applications. *J. Mater. Res.* **2019**, *34*, 2819–2827. [CrossRef]
173. Marques, C.F.; Diogo, G.S.; Pina, S.; Oliveira, J.M.; Silva, T.H.; Reis, R.L. Collagen-based bioinks for hard tissue engineering applications: A comprehensive review. *J. Mater. Sci. Mater. Med.* **2019**, *30*, 32. [CrossRef]
174. Hoque, M.E.; Hutmacher, D.W.; Feng, W.; Li, S.; Huang, M.-H.; Vert, M.; Wong, Y.S. Fabrication using a rapid prototyping system and in vitro characterization of PEG-PCL-PLA scaffolds for tissue engineering. *J. Biomater. Sci. Polym. Ed.* **2005**, *16*, 1595–1610. [CrossRef]
175. Ba Linh, N.T.; Lee, K.H.; Lee, B.T. Functional nanofiber mat of polyvinyl alcohol/gelatin containing nanoparticles of biphasic calcium phosphate for bone regeneration in rat calvaria defects. *J. Biomed. Mater. Res. Part A* **2013**, *101*, 2412–2423. [CrossRef]
176. Elzoghby, A.O. Gelatin-based nanoparticles as drug and gene delivery systems: Reviewing three decades of research. *J. Control. Release* **2013**, *172*, 1075–1091. [CrossRef]
177. Santoro, M.; Tatara, A.M.; Mikos, A.G. Gelatin carriers for drug and cell delivery in tissue engineering. *J. Control. Release* **2014**, *190*, 210–218. [CrossRef]
178. Won, Y.-W.; Yoon, S.-M.; Sonn, C.H.; Lee, K.-M.; Kim, Y.-H. Nano self-assembly of recombinant human gelatin conjugated with α-tocopheryl succinate for hsp90 inhibitor, 17-AAG, delivery. *ACS Nano* **2011**, *5*, 3839–3848. [CrossRef] [PubMed]
179. Olsen, D.; Yang, C.; Bodo, M.; Chang, R.; Leigh, S.; Baez, J.; Carmichael, D.; Perälä, M.; Hämäläinen, E.-R.; Jarvinen, M.; et al. Recombinant collagen and gelatin for drug delivery. *Adv. Drug Deliv. Rev.* **2003**, *55*, 1547–1567. [CrossRef] [PubMed]
180. Su, K.; Wang, C. Recent advances in the use of gelatin in biomedical research. *Biotechnol. Lett.* **2015**, *37*, 2139–2145. [CrossRef] [PubMed]
181. Nitta, S.K.; Numata, K. Biopolymer-Based nanoparticles for drug/gene delivery and tissue engineering. *Int. J. Mol. Sci.* **2013**, *14*, 1629–1654. [CrossRef]
182. Kuijpers, A.J.; Engbers, G.H.M.; Krijsveld, J.; Zaat, S.A.J.; Dankert, J.; Feijen, J. Cross-linking and characterisation of gelatin matrices for biomedical applications. *J. Biomater. Sci. Polym. Ed.* **2000**, *11*, 225–243. [CrossRef]
183. Bigi, A.; Cojazzi, G.; Panzavolta, S.; Rubini, K.; Roveri, N. Mechanical and thermal properties of gelatin films at different degrees of glutaraldehyde crosslinking. *Biomaterials* **2001**, *22*, 763–768. [CrossRef]
184. Yue, K.; Trujillo-de Santiago, G.; Alvarez, M.M.; Tamayol, A.; Annabi, N.; Khademhosseini, A. Synthesis, properties, and biomedical applications of gelatin methacryloyl (GelMA) hydrogels. *Biomaterials* **2015**, *73*, 254–271. [CrossRef]
185. Wang, H.; Boerman, O.; Sariibrahimoglu, K.; Li, Y.; Jansen, J.; Leeuwenburgh, S. Comparison of micro- vs. nanostructured colloidal gelatin gels for sustained delivery of osteogenic proteins: Bone morphogenetic protein-2 and alkaline phosphatase. *Biomaterials* **2012**, *33*, 8695–8703. [CrossRef]

186. Perez, R.; del Valle, S.; Altankov, G.; Ginebra, M.-P. Porous hydroxyapatite and gelatin/hydroxyapatite microspheres obtained by calcium phosphate cement emulsion. *J. Biomed. Mater. Res. Part B Appl. Biomater.* **2011**, *97*, 156–166. [CrossRef]
187. Gil, E.S.; Frankowski, D.J.; Spontak, R.J.; Hudson, S.M. Swelling behavior and morphological evolution of mixed gelatin/silk fibroin hydrogels. *Biomacromolecules* **2005**, *6*, 3079–3087. [CrossRef]
188. Ulrich, D.; Edwards, S.; Su, K.; Tan, K.; White, J.; Ramshaw, J.; Lo, C.; Rosamilia, A.; Werkmeister, J.; Gargett, C. Human endometrial mesenchymal stem cells modulate the tissue response and mechanical behavior of polyamide mesh implants for pelvic organ prolapse repair. *Tissue Eng. Part A* **2013**, *20*, 785–798. [CrossRef]
189. Han, J.; Lazarovici, P.; Pomerantz, C.; Chen, X.; Wei, Y.; Lelkes, P.I. Co-Electrospun blends of PLGA, gelatin, and elastin as potential nonthrombogenic scaffolds for vascular tissue engineering. *Biomacromolecules* **2011**, *12*, 399–408. [CrossRef] [PubMed]
190. Ovsianikov, A.; Deiwick, A.; van Vlierberghe, S.; Dubruel, P.; Möller, L.; Dräger, G.; Chichkov, B. Laser fabrication of three-dimensional CAD scaffolds from photosensitive gelatin for applications in tissue engineering. *Biomacromolecules* **2011**, *12*, 851–858. [CrossRef] [PubMed]
191. Tielens, S.; Declercq, H.; Gorski, T.; Lippens, E.; Schacht, E.; Cornelissen, M. Gelatin-based microcarriers as embryonic stem cell delivery system in bone tissue engineering: An in-vitro study. *Biomacromolecules* **2007**, *8*, 825–832. [CrossRef] [PubMed]
192. Samal, S.K.; Goranov, V.; Dash, M.; Russo, A.; Shelyakova, T.; Graziosi, P.; Lungaro, L.; Riminucci, A.; Uhlarz, M.; Bañobre-López, M.; et al. Multilayered magnetic gelatin membrane scaffolds. *ACS Appl. Mater. Interfaces* **2015**, *7*, 23098–23109. [CrossRef] [PubMed]
193. Gentile, P.; Chiono, V.; Carmagnola, I.; Hatton, P.V. An overview of poly(lactic-co-glycolic) acid (PLGA)-based biomaterials for bone tissue engineering. *Int. J. Mol. Sci.* **2014**, *15*, 3640–3659. [CrossRef] [PubMed]
194. Meretoja, V.V.; Tirri, T.; Malin, M.; Seppälä, J.V.; Närhi, T.O. Ectopic bone formation in and soft-tissue response to P(CL/DLLA)/bioactive glass composite scaffolds. *Clin. Oral Implants Res.* **2014**, *25*, 159–164. [CrossRef]
195. Yang, K.; Wan, J.; Zhang, S.; Zhang, Y.; Lee, S.-T.; Liu, Z. In vivo pharmacokinetics, long-term biodistribution, and toxicology of PEGylated graphene in mice. *ACS Nano* **2011**, *5*, 516–522. [CrossRef] [PubMed]
196. Zhang, J.; Zhao, S.; Zhu, Y.; Huang, Y.; Zhu, M.; Tao, C.; Zhang, C. Three-dimensional printing of strontium-containing mesoporous bioactive glass scaffolds for bone regeneration. *Acta Biomater.* **2014**, *10*, 2269–2281. [CrossRef]
197. Padmanabhan, J.; Kyriakides, T.R. Nanomaterials, inflammation, and tissue engineering. *Wiley Interdiscip. Rev. Nanomed. Nanobiotechnol.* **2015**, *7*, 355–370. [CrossRef]
198. Lombardo, D.; Kiselev, M.A.; Caccamo, M.T. Smart nanoparticles for drug delivery application: Development of versatile nanocarrier platforms in biotechnology and nanomedicine. *J. Nanomater.* **2019**, *2019*, 3702518. [CrossRef]
199. Harris, L.D.; Kim, B.; Mooney, D.J. Open pore biodegradable matrices formed with gas foaming. *J. Biomed. Mater. Res.* **1998**, *42*, 396–402. [CrossRef]
200. Mikos, A.G.; Thorsen, A.J.; Czerwonka, L.A.; Bao, Y.; Langer, R.; Winslow, D.N.; Vacanti, J.P. Preparation and characterization of poly(l-lactic acid) foams. *Polymer* **1994**, *35*, 1068–1077. [CrossRef]
201. Zein, I.; Hutmacher, D.W.; Tan, K.C.; Teoh, S.H. Fused deposition modeling of novel scaffold architectures for tissue engineering applications. *Biomaterials* **2002**, *23*, 1169–1185. [CrossRef]
202. Zhang, R.; Ma, P.X. Poly (A-hydroxyl acids)/hydroxyapatite porous composites for bone-tissue engineering.I. Preparation and morphology. *J. Biomed. Mater. Res.* **1999**, *44*, 446–455. [CrossRef]
203. Perkins, B.L.; Naderi, N. Carbon nanostructures in bone tissue engineering. *Open Orthop. J.* **2016**, *10*, 877–899. [CrossRef]
204. Dresselhaus, M.S.; Avouris, P. Introduction to carbon materials research. *Carbon Nanotub.* **2001**, *9*, 1–9.
205. Han, Z.J.; Rider, A.E.; Ishaq, M.; Kumar, S.; Kondyurin, A.; Bilek, M.M.M.; Levchenko, I.; Ostrikov, K. Carbon nanostructures for hard tissue engineering. *RSC Adv.* **2013**, *3*, 11058–11072. [CrossRef]
206. Eivazzadeh-Keihan, R.; Maleki, A.; de la Guardia, M.; Bani, M.S.; Chenab, K.K.; Pashazadeh-Panahi, P.; Baradaran, B.; Mokhtarzadeh, A.; Hamblin, M.R. Carbon based nanomaterials for tissue engineering of bone: Building new bone on small black scaffolds: A review. *J. Adv. Res.* **2019**, *18*, 185–201. [CrossRef]
207. Geetha Bai, R.; Muthoosamy, K.; Manickam, S.; Hilal-Alnaqbi, A. Graphene-based 3D scaffolds in tissue engineering: Fabrication, applications, and future scope in liver tissue engineering. *Int. J. Nanomed.* **2019**, *14*, 5753–5783. [CrossRef]

208. Kim, H.; Macosko, C.W. Processing-property relationships of polycarbonate/graphene composites. *Polymer* **2009**, *50*, 3797–3809. [CrossRef]
209. Stankovich, S.; Dikin, D.A.; Dommett, G.H.B.; Kohlhaas, K.M.; Zimney, E.J.; Stach, E.A.; Piner, R.D.; Nguyen, S.B.T.; Ruoff, R.S. Graphene-based composite materials. *Nature* **2006**, *442*, 282–286. [CrossRef] [PubMed]
210. Bon, S.B.; Valentini, L.; Verdejo, R.; Fierro, J.L.G.; Peponi, L.; Lopez-Manchado, M.A.; Kenny, J.M. Plasma fluorination of chemically derived graphene sheets and subsequent modification with butylamine. *Chem. Mater.* **2009**, *21*, 3433–3438. [CrossRef]
211. Valentini, L.; Armentano, I.; Biagiotti, J.; Frulloni, E.; Kenny, J.M.; Santucci, S. Frequency dependent electrical transport between conjugated polymer and single-walled carbon nanotubes. *Diam. Relat. Mater.* **2003**, *12*, 1601–1609. [CrossRef]
212. MacDonald, R.A.; Voge, C.M.; Kariolis, M.; Stegemann, J.P. Carbon nanotubes increase the electrical conductivity of fibroblast-seeded collagen hydrogels. *Acta Biomater.* **2008**, *4*, 1583–1592. [CrossRef]
213. Armentano, I.; Dottori, M.; Fortunati, E.; Mattioli, S.; Kenny, J.M. Biodegradable polymer matrix nanocomposites for tissue engineering: A review. *Polym. Degrad. Stabil.* **2010**, *95*, 2126–2146. [CrossRef]
214. Armentano, I.; Fortunati, E.; Gigli, M.; Luzi, F.; Trotta, R.; Bicchi, I.; Soccio, M.; Lotti, N.; Munari, A.; Martino, S.; et al. Effect of SWCNT introduction in random copolymers on material properties and fibroblast long term culture stability. *Polym. Degrad. Stab.* **2016**, *132*, 220–230. [CrossRef]
215. Mihajlovic, M.; Mihajlovic, M.; Dankers, P.Y.W.; Masereeuw, R.; Sijbesma, R.P. Carbon nanotube reinforced supramolecular hydrogels for bioapplications. *Macromol. Biosci.* **2019**, *19*, 1800173. [CrossRef]
216. Wu, K.; Tao, J.; Qi, L.; Chen, S.; Wan, W. Intracellular microtubules as nano-scaffolding template self-assembles with conductive carbon nanotubes for biomedical device. *Mater. Sci. Eng. C* **2020**, *113*, 11971. [CrossRef]
217. Yang, Y.-L.; Ju, H.-Z.; Liu, S.-F.; Lee, T.-C.; Shih, Y.-W.; Chuang, L.-Y.; Guh, J.-Y.; Yang, Y.-Y.; Liao, T.-N.; Hung, T.-J.; et al. BMP-2 suppresses renal interstitial fibrosis by regulating epithelial–mesenchymal transition. *J. Cell. Biochem.* **2011**, *112*, 2558–2565. [CrossRef]
218. Minati, L.; Antonini, V.; Dalla Serra, M.; Speranza, G. Multifunctional branched gold–carbon nanotube hybrid for cell imaging and drug delivery. *Langmuir* **2012**, *28*, 15900–15906. [CrossRef]
219. Srikanth, M.; Asmatulu, R.; Cluff, K.; Yao, L. Material characterization and bioanalysis of hybrid scaffolds of carbon nanomaterial and polymer nanofibers. *ACS Omega* **2019**, *4*, 5044–5051. [CrossRef]
220. Singh, R.K.; Patel, K.D.; Kim, J.-J.; Kim, T.-H.; Kim, J.-H.; Shin, U.S.; Lee, E.-J.; Knowles, J.C.; Kim, H.-W. Multifunctional hybrid nanocarrier: Magnetic CNTs ensheathed with mesoporous silica for drug delivery and imaging system. *ACS Appl. Mater. Interfaces* **2014**, *6*, 2201–2208. [CrossRef]
221. Huang, W.; Zhang, J.; Dorn, H.C.; Geohegan, D.; Zhang, C. Assembly of single-walled carbon nanohorn supported liposome particles. *Bioconjug. Chem.* **2011**, *22*, 1012–1016. [CrossRef]
222. Chen, Q.; Zhu, C.; Thouas, G.A. Progress and challenges in biomaterials used for bone tissue engineering: Bioactive glasses and elastomeric composites. *Prog. Biomater.* **2012**, *1*, 2. [CrossRef]
223. Navarro, M.; Michiardi, A.; Castaño, O.; Planell, J.A. Biomaterials in orthopaedics. *J. R. Soc. Interface* **2008**, *5*, 1137–1158. [CrossRef]
224. European Centre for Disease Prevention and Control: An Agency of the European Union. Available online: http://ecdc.europa.eu (accessed on 1 September 2020).
225. Wu, X.; Wu, M.; Zhao, J.X. Recent development of silica nanoparticles as delivery vectors for cancer imaging and therapy. *Nanomed. Nanotechnol. Biol. Med.* **2014**, *10*, 297–312. [CrossRef]
226. Rosenholm, J.M.; Zhang, J.; Linden, M.; Sahlgren, C. Mesoporous silica nanoparticles in tissue engineering—A perspective. *Nanomedicine* **2016**, *11*, 391–402. [CrossRef]
227. Bitar, A.; Ahmad, N.M.; Fessi, H.; Elaissari, A. Silica-based nanoparticles for biomedical applications. *Drug Discov. Today* **2012**, *17*, 1147–1154. [CrossRef]
228. Türk, M.; Tamer, U.; Alver, E.; Çiftçi, H.; Metin, A.U.; Karahan, S. Fabrication and characterization of gold-nanoparticles/chitosan film: A scaffold for L929-fibroblasts. *Artif. Cells Nanomed. Biotechnol.* **2013**, *41*, 395–401. [CrossRef]
229. Yeh, Y.-C.; Creran, B.; Rotello, V.M. Gold nanoparticles: Preparation, properties, and applications in bionanotechnology. *Nanoscale* **2012**, *4*, 1871–1880. [CrossRef]

230. Zuber, A.; Purdey, M.; Schartner, E.; Forbes, C.; van der Hoek, B.; Giles, D.; Abell, A.; Monro, T.; Ebendorff-Heidepriem, H. Detection of gold nanoparticles with different sizes using absorption and fluorescence based method. *Sensors Actuators B Chem.* **2016**, *227*, 117–127. [CrossRef]
231. Ito, A.; Kamihira, M. *Tissue Engineering Using Magnetite Nanoparticles*, 1st ed.; Elsevier Inc.: Amsterdam, The Netherlands, 2011; Volume 104.
232. Xiong, F.; Wang, H.; Feng, Y.; Li, Y.; Hua, X.; Pang, X.; Zhang, S.; Song, L.; Zhang, Y.; Gu, N. Cardioprotective activity of iron oxide nanoparticles. *Sci. Rep.* **2015**, *5*, 8579. [CrossRef]
233. Madhumathi, K.; Sampath Kumar, T.S. Regenerative potential and anti-bacterial activity of tetracycline loaded apatitic nanocarriers for the treatment of periodontitis. *Biomed. Mater.* **2014**, *9*, 35002. [CrossRef]
234. Choi, B.; Cui, Z.-K.; Kim, S.; Fan, J.; Wu, B.M.; Lee, M. Glutamine-chitosan modified calcium phosphate nanoparticles for efficient siRNA delivery and osteogenic differentiation. *J. Mater. Chem. B* **2015**, *3*, 6448–6455. [CrossRef]
235. Ding, T.; Luo, Z.J.; Zheng, Y.; Hu, X.Y.; Ye, Z.X. Rapid repair and regeneration of damaged rabbit sciatic nerves by tissue-engineered scaffold made from nano-silver and collagen type I. *Injury* **2010**, *41*, 522–527. [CrossRef]
236. Prabhu, S.; Poulose, E.K. Silver nanoparticles: Mechanism of antimicrobial action, synthesis, medical applications, and toxicity effects. *Int. Nano Lett.* **2012**, *2*, 32. [CrossRef]
237. Saravanan, S.; Nethala, S.; Pattnaik, S.; Tripathi, A.; Moorthi, A.; Selvamurugan, N. Preparation, characterization and antimicrobial activity of a bio-composite scaffold containing chitosan/nano-hydroxyapatite/nano-silver for bone tissue engineering. *Int. J. Biol. Macromol.* **2011**, *49*, 188–193. [CrossRef]
238. Hirota, M.; Hayakawa, T.; Yoshinari, M.; Ametani, A.; Shima, T.; Monden, Y.; Ozawa, T.; Sato, M.; Koyama, C.; Tamai, N.; et al. Hydroxyapatite coating for titanium fibre mesh scaffold enhances osteoblast activity and bone tissue formation. *Int. J. Oral Maxillofac. Surg.* **2012**, *41*, 1304–1309. [CrossRef]
239. Holtorf, H.L.; Jansen, J.A.; Mikos, A.G. Ectopic bone formation in rat marrow stromal cell/titanium fiber mesh scaffold constructs: Effect of initial cell phenotype. *Biomaterials* **2005**, *26*, 6208–6216. [CrossRef]
240. Fan, X.; Lin, L.; Messersmith, P.B. Surface-initiated polymerization from TiO_2 nanoparticle surfaces through a biomimetic initiator: A new route toward polymer–matrix nanocomposites. *Compos. Sci. Technol.* **2006**, *66*, 1198–1204. [CrossRef]
241. Kevin, B.; Chang, Y.; Webster, T.J. Increased chondrocyte adhesion on nanotubular anodized titanium. *J. Biomed. Mater. Res. Part A* **2008**, *88*, 561–568.
242. Liao, D.L.; Liao, B.Q. Shape, size and photocatalytic activity control of TiO_2 nanoparticles with surfactants. *J. Photochem. Photobiol. A Chem.* **2007**, *187*, 363–369. [CrossRef]
243. Rakhmatia, Y.D.; Ayukawa, Y.; Atsuta, I.; Furuhashi, A.; Koyano, K. Fibroblast attachment onto novel titanium mesh membranes for guided bone regeneration. *Odontology* **2015**, *103*, 218–226. [CrossRef] [PubMed]
244. Shi, Z.; Huang, X.; Cai, Y.; Tang, R.; Yang, D. Size effect of hydroxyapatite nanoparticles on proliferation and apoptosis of osteoblast-like cells. *Acta Biomater.* **2009**, *5*, 338–345. [CrossRef] [PubMed]
245. Webster, T.J.; Ergun, C.; Doremus, R.H.; Siegel, R.W.; Bizios, R. Specific proteins mediate enhanced osteoblast adhesion on nanophase ceramics. *J. Biomed. Mater. Res.* **2000**, *51*, 475–483. [CrossRef]
246. Lee, J.; Sieweke, J.H.; Rodriguez, N.A.; Schüpbach, P.; Lindström, H.; Susin, C.; Wikesjö, U.M.E. Evaluation of nano-technology-modified zirconia oral implants: A study in rabbits. *J. Clin. Periodontol.* **2009**, *36*, 610–617. [CrossRef] [PubMed]
247. Opalinska, A.; Malka, I.; Dzwolak, W.; Chudoba, T.; Presz, A.; Lojkowski, W. Size-dependent density of zirconia nanoparticles. *Beilstein J. Nanotechnol.* **2015**, *6*, 27–35. [CrossRef] [PubMed]
248. Park, Y.K.; Tadd, E.H.; Zubris, M.; Tannenbaum, R. Size-controlled synthesis of alumina nanoparticles from aluminum alkoxides. *Mater. Res. Bull.* **2005**, *40*, 1506–1512. [CrossRef]
249. Ravindran Girija, A.; Balasubramanian, S. Theragnostic potentials of core/shell mesoporous silica nanostructures. *Nanotheranostics* **2019**, *3*, 1–40. [CrossRef]
250. Tarn, D.; Ashley, C.E.; Xue, M.; Carnes, E.C.; Zink, J.I.; Brinker, C.J. Mesoporous silica nanoparticle nanocarriers: Biofunctionality and biocompatibility. *Acc. Chem. Res.* **2013**, *46*, 792–801. [CrossRef]
251. Slowing, I.I.; Vivero-Escoto, J.L.; Wu, C.W.; Lin, V.S.Y. Mesoporous silica nanoparticles as controlled release drug delivery and gene transfection carriers. *Adv. Drug Deliv. Rev.* **2008**, *60*, 1278–1288. [CrossRef] [PubMed]

252. Tang, Y.; Zhao, Y.; Wang, X.; Lin, T. Layer-by-layer assembly of silica nanoparticles on 3D fibrous scaffolds: Enhancement of osteoblast cell adhesion, proliferation, and differentiation. *J. Biomed. Mater. Res. Part A* **2014**, *102*, 3803–3812. [CrossRef] [PubMed]
253. Zhou, Y.; Quan, G.; Wu, Q.; Zhang, X.; Niu, B.; Wu, B.; Huang, Y.; Pan, X.; Wu, C. Mesoporous silica nanoparticles for drug and gene delivery. *Acta Pharm. Sin. B* **2018**, *8*, 165–177. [CrossRef] [PubMed]
254. Anitha, A.; Menon, D.; Koyakutty, M.; Mohan, C.C.; Nair, S.V.; Nair, M.B. Bioinspired composite matrix containing hydroxyapatite–silica core–shell nanorods for bone tissue engineering. *ACS Appl. Mater. Interfaces* **2017**, *9*, 26707–26718.
255. Ambekar, R.S.; Kandasubramanian, B. Progress in the advancement of porous biopolymer scaffold: Tissue engineering application. *Ind. Eng. Chem. Res.* **2019**, *58*, 6163–6194. [CrossRef]
256. Zhou, P.; Cheng, X.; Xia, Y.; Wang, P.; Zou, K.; Xu, S.; Du, J. Organic/inorganic composite membranes based on poly(l-lactic-co-glycolic acid) and mesoporous silica for effective bone tissue engineering. *ACS Appl. Mater. Interfaces* **2014**, *6*, 20895–20903. [CrossRef]
257. Ding, Y.; Li, W.; Correia, A.; Yang, Y.; Zheng, K.; Liu, D.; Schubert, D.W.; Boccaccini, A.R.; Santos, H.A.; Roether, J.A. Electrospun polyhydroxybutyrate/poly(ε-Caprolactone)/sol–gel-derived silica hybrid scaffolds with drug releasing function for bone tissue engineering applications. *ACS Appl. Mater. Interfaces* **2018**, *10*, 14540–14548. [CrossRef]
258. Cha, C.; Oh, J.; Kim, K.; Qiu, Y.; Joh, M.; Shin, S.R.; Wang, X.; Camci-Unal, G.; Wan, K.; Liao, R.; et al. Microfluidics-assisted fabrication of gelatin-silica core–shell microgels for injectable tissue constructs. *Biomacromolecules* **2014**, *15*, 283–290. [CrossRef]
259. Qiu, K.; Chen, B.; Nie, W.; Zhou, X.; Feng, W.; Wang, W.; Chen, L.; Mo, X.; Wei, Y.; He, C. Electrophoretic deposition of dexamethasone-loaded mesoporous silica nanoparticles onto poly(l-Lactic Acid)/Poly(ε-Caprolactone) composite scaffold for bone tissue engineering. *ACS Appl. Mater. Interfaces* **2016**, *8*, 4137–4148. [CrossRef]
260. Jones, J.R. Reprint of: Review of bioactive glass: From Hench to hybrids. *Acta Biomater.* **2015**, *23*, S53–S82. [CrossRef]
261. Boccaccini, A.; Maquet, V. Bioresorbable and bioactive polymer/bioglass composites with tailored pore structure for tissue engineering applications. *Compos. Sci. Technol.* **2003**, *63*, 2417–2429. [CrossRef]
262. Yu, H.; Peng, J.; Xu, Y.; Chang, J.; Li, H. Bioglass activated skin tissue engineering constructs for wound healing. *ACS Appl. Mater. Interfaces* **2016**, *8*, 703–715. [CrossRef] [PubMed]
263. Fernandes, H.R.; Gaddam, A.; Rebelo, A.; Brazete, D.; Stan, G.E.; Ferreira, J.M.F. Bioactive glasses and glass-ceramics for healthcare applications in bone regeneration and tissue engineering. *Materials* **2018**, *11*, 2530. [CrossRef]
264. Fiume, E.; Barberi, J.; Verné, E.; Baino, F. Bioactive glasses: From parent 45s5 composition to scaffold-assisted tissue-healing therapies. *J. Funct. Biomater.* **2018**, *9*, 24. [CrossRef] [PubMed]
265. Islam, M.T.; Felfel, R.M.; Abou Neel, E.A.; Grant, D.M.; Ahmed, I.; Hossain, K.M.Z. Bioactive calcium phosphate-based glasses and ceramics and their biomedical applications: A review. *J. Tissue Eng.* **2017**, *8*, 2041731417719170. [CrossRef] [PubMed]
266. González, P.; Serra, J.; Liste, S.; Chiussi, S.; León, B.; Pérez-Amor, M. Raman spectroscopic study of bioactive silica based glasses. *J. Non. Cryst. Solids* **2003**, *320*, 92–99. [CrossRef]
267. Yan, X.; Yu, C.; Zhou, X.; Tang, J.; Zhao, D. Highly ordered mesoporous bioactive glasses with superior in vitro bone-forming bioactivities. *Angew. Chem. Int. Ed.* **2004**, *43*, 5980–5984. [CrossRef]
268. Kumar, P.; Dehiya, B.S.; Sindhu, A.; Kumar, V. Synthesis and characterization of nano bioglass for the application of bone tissue engineering. *J. Nanosci. Technol.* **2018**, *4*, 471–474. [CrossRef]
269. De Oliveira, A.A.R.; de Souza, D.A.; Dias, L.L.S.; de Carvalho, S.M.; Mansur, H.S.; de Magalhães Pereira, M. Synthesis, characterization and cytocompatibility of spherical bioactive glass nanoparticles for potential hard tissue engineering applications. *Biomed. Mater.* **2013**, *8*, 025011. [CrossRef]
270. Wang, W.; Yeung, K.W.K. Bone grafts and biomaterials substitutes for bone defect repair: A review. *Bioact. Mater.* **2017**, *2*, 224–247. [CrossRef] [PubMed]
271. Chen, Q.; Boccaccini, A. Poly(D,L-lactic acid) coated 45S5 Bioglass-based scaffolds: Processing and characterization. *J. Biomed. Mater. Res. Part A* **2006**, *77*, 445–457. [CrossRef] [PubMed]

272. Ravarian, R.; Zhong, X.; Barbeck, M.; Ghanaati, S.; Kirkpatrick, C.J.; Murphy, C.M.; Schindeler, A.; Chrzanowski, W.; Dehghani, F. Nanoscale chemical interaction enhances the physical properties of bioglass composites. *ACS Nano* **2013**, *7*, 8469–8483. [CrossRef] [PubMed]
273. Zeng, Q.; Desai, M.S.; Jin, H.-E.; Lee, J.H.; Chang, J.; Lee, S.-W. Self-healing elastin–bioglass hydrogels. *Biomacromolecules* **2016**, *17*, 2619–2625. [CrossRef] [PubMed]
274. Marelli, B.; Ghezzi, C.E.; Barralet, J.E.; Boccaccini, A.R.; Nazhat, S.N. Three-dimensional mineralization of dense nanofibrillar collagen–bioglass hybrid scaffolds. *Biomacromolecules* **2010**, *11*, 1470–1479. [CrossRef]
275. Misra, S.K.; Nazhat, S.N.; Valappil, S.P.; Moshrefi-Torbati, M.; Wood, R.J.K.; Roy, I.; Boccaccini, A.R. fabrication and characterization of biodegradable poly(3-hydroxybutyrate) composite containing bioglass. *Biomacromolecules* **2007**, *8*, 2112–2119. [CrossRef]
276. Fernandes, J.S.; Martins, M.; Neves, N.M.; Fernandes, M.H.V.; Reis, R.L.; Pires, R.A. Intrinsic antibacterial borosilicate glasses for bone tissue engineering applications. *ACS Biomater. Sci. Eng.* **2016**, *2*, 1143–1150. [CrossRef]
277. Xu, Y.; Luong, D.; Walker, J.M.; Dean, D.; Becker, M.L. Modification of poly(propylene fumarate)–bioglass composites with peptide conjugates to enhance bioactivity. *Biomacromolecules* **2017**, *18*, 3168–3177. [CrossRef]
278. Pepla, E.; Besharat, L.K.; Palaia, G.; Tenore, G.; Migliau, G. Nano-hydroxyapatite and its applications in preventive, restorative and regenerative dentistry: A review of literature. *Ann. Stomatol.* **2014**, *5*, 108–114. [CrossRef]
279. Leventouri, T.; Antonakos, A.; Kyriacou, A.; Venturelli, R.; Liarokapis, E.; Perdikatsis, V. Crystal structure studies of human dental apatite as a function of age. *Int. J. Biomater.* **2009**, *2009*, 698547. [CrossRef]
280. Freed, L.E.; Vunjak-Novakovic, G.; Biron, R.J.; Eagles, D.B.; Lesnoy, D.C.; Barlow, S.K.; Langer, R. Biodegradable polymer scaffolds for tissue engineering. *Nat. Biotechnol.* **1994**, *12*, 689–693. [CrossRef] [PubMed]
281. Isikli, C.; Hasirci, V.; Hasirci, N. Development of porous chitosan–gelatin/hydroxyapatite composite scaffolds for hard tissue-engineering applications. *J. Tissue Eng. Regen. Med.* **2011**, *6*, 135–143. [CrossRef] [PubMed]
282. Klein, C.; Driessen, A.A.; Degroot, K.; Vandenhooff, A. Biodegradation behavior of various calcium-phosphate materials in bone tissue. *J. Biomed. Mater. Res.* **1983**, *17*, 769–784. [CrossRef] [PubMed]
283. Rezwan, K.; Chen, Q.Z.; Blaker, J.J.; Boccaccini, A.R. Biodegradable and bioactive porous polymer/inorganic composite scaffolds for bone tissue engineering. *Biomaterials* **2006**, *27*, 3413–3431. [CrossRef] [PubMed]
284. Guzmán Vázquez, C.; Piña Barba, C.; Munguía, N. Stoichiometric hydroxyapatite obtained by precipitation and sol gel processes. *Rev. Mex. Fis.* **2005**, *51*, 284–293.
285. Li, J.; Lu, X.L.; Zheng, Y.F. Effect of surface modified hydroxyapatite on the tensile property improvement of HA/PLA composite. *Appl. Surf. Sci.* **2008**, *255*, 494–497. [CrossRef]
286. Dorozhkin, S.V. Calcium orthophosphate cements for biomedical application. *J. Mater. Sci.* **2008**, *43*, 3028–3057. [CrossRef]
287. Narasaraju, T.S.B.; Phebe, D.E. Some physico-chemical aspects of hydroxylapatite. *J. Mater. Sci.* **1996**, *31*, 1–21. [CrossRef]
288. Fathi, M.H.; Hanifi, A.; Mortazavi, V. Preparation and bioactivity evaluation of bone-like hydroxyapatite nanopowder. *J. Mater. Process. Technol.* **2008**, *202*, 536–542. [CrossRef]
289. Sopyan, I.; Singh, R.; Hamdi, M. Synthesis of nano sized hydroxyapatite powder using sol-gel technique and its conversion to dense and porous bodies. *Indian J. Chem. Sect. A* **2008**, *47*, 1626–1631.
290. Kattimani, V.S.; Kondaka, S.; Lingamaneni, K.P. Hydroxyapatite—Past, present, and future in bone regeneration. *Bone Tissue Regen. Insights* **2016**, *7*, S36138. [CrossRef]
291. Woodard, J.R.; Hilldore, A.J.; Lan, S.K.; Park, C.J.; Morgan, A.W.; Eurell, J.A.C.; Clark, S.G.; Wheeler, M.B.; Jamison, R.D.; Wagoner Johnson, A.J. The mechanical properties and osteoconductivity of hydroxyapatite bone scaffolds with multi-scale porosity. *Biomaterials* **2007**, *28*, 45–54. [CrossRef] [PubMed]
292. Gao, X.; Song, J.; Ji, P.; Zhang, X.; Li, X.; Xu, X.; Wang, M.; Zhang, S.; Deng, Y.; Deng, F.; et al. Polydopamine-templated hydroxyapatite reinforced polycaprolactone composite nanofibers with enhanced cytocompatibility and osteogenesis for bone tissue engineering. *ACS Appl. Mater. Interfaces* **2016**, *8*, 3499–3515. [CrossRef] [PubMed]
293. Jiang, L.; Li, Y.; Xiong, C.; Su, S.; Ding, H. Preparation and properties of bamboo fiber/nano-hydroxyapatite/poly(lactic-co-glycolic) composite scaffold for bone tissue engineering. *ACS Appl. Mater. Interfaces* **2017**, *9*, 4890–4897. [CrossRef] [PubMed]

294. Salarian, M.; Xu, W.Z.; Wang, Z.; Sham, T.-K.; Charpentier, P.A. Hydroxyapatite–TiO$_2$-based nanocomposites synthesized in supercritical co2 for bone tissue engineering: Physical and mechanical properties. *ACS Appl. Mater. Interfaces* **2014**, *6*, 16918–16931. [CrossRef]
295. Liang, X.; Duan, P.; Gao, J.; Guo, R.; Qu, Z.; Li, X.; He, Y.; Yao, H.; Ding, J. Bilayered PLGA/PLGA-HAp composite scaffold for osteochondral tissue engineering and tissue regeneration. *ACS Biomater. Sci. Eng.* **2018**, *4*, 3506–3521. [CrossRef]
296. Fu, S.; Wang, X.; Guo, G.; Shi, S.; Liang, H.; Luo, F.; Wei, Y.; Qian, Z. Preparation and characterization of nano-hydroxyapatite/poly(ε-caprolactone)–poly(ethylene glycol)–poly(ε-caprolactone) composite fibers for tissue engineering. *J. Phys. Chem. C* **2010**, *114*, 18372–18378. [CrossRef]
297. Liu, M.; Liu, H.; Sun, S.; Li, X.; Zhou, Y.; Hou, Z.; Lin, J. Multifunctional Hydroxyapatite/Na(Y/Gd)F$_4$:Yb^{3+},Er^{3+} composite fibers for drug delivery and dual modal imaging. *Langmuir* **2014**, *30*, 1176–1182. [CrossRef]
298. Li, Z.; Liu, Z.; Yin, M.; Yang, X.; Yuan, Q.; Ren, J.; Qu, X. Aptamer-capped multifunctional mesoporous strontium hydroxyapatite nanovehicle for cancer-cell-responsive drug delivery and imaging. *Biomacromolecules* **2012**, *13*, 4257–4263. [CrossRef]
299. Wang, L.; Hu, C.; Shao, L. The antimicrobial activity of nanoparticles: Present situation and prospects for the future. *Int. J. Nanomed.* **2017**, *12*, 1227–1249. [CrossRef]
300. Wu, C.; Lee, C.; Chen, J.; Kuo, S.; Fan, S.; Cheng, C.; Chang, F.; Ko, F. Microwave-assisted electroless deposition of silver nanoparticles onto multiwalled carbon nanotubes. *Int. J. Electrochem. Sci.* **2012**, *7*, 4133–4142.
301. Ciobanu, C.S.; Iconaru, S.L.; Coustumer, P.L.; Constantin, L.V.; Predoi, D. Antibacterial activity of silver-doped hydroxyapatite nanoparticles against gram-positive and gram-negative bacteria. *Nanoscale Res. Lett.* **2012**, *7*, 1–9. [CrossRef] [PubMed]
302. Melnikov, O.V.; Gorbenko, O.Y.; Markelova, M.N.; Kaul, A.R.; Atsarkin, V.A.; Demidov, V.V.; Soto, C.; Roy, E.J.; Odintsov, B.M. Ag-doped manganite nanoparticles: New materials for temperature-controlled medical hyperthermia. *J. Biomed. Mater. Res. A* **2009**, *91*, 1048–1055. [CrossRef] [PubMed]
303. Bapat, R.A.; Chaubal, T.V.; Joshi, C.P.; Bapat, P.R.; Choudhury, H.; Pandey, M.; Gorain, B.; Kesharwani, P. An overview of application of silver nanoparticles for biomaterials in dentistry. *Mater. Sci. Eng. C* **2018**, *91*, 881–898. [CrossRef] [PubMed]
304. Rai, M.; Yadav, A.; Gade, A. Silver nanoparticles as a new generation of antimicrobials. *Biotechnol. Adv.* **2009**, *27*, 76–83. [CrossRef]
305. Krishnaraj, C.; Jagan, E.G.; Rajasekar, S.; Selvakumar, P.; Kalaichelvan, P.T.; Mohan, N. Synthesis of silver nanoparticles using Acalypha indica leaf extracts and its antibacterial activity against water borne pathogens. *Colloids Surfaces B Biointerfaces* **2010**, *76*, 50–56. [CrossRef]
306. Jung, W.K.; Koo, H.C.; Kim, K.W.; Shin, S.; Kim, S.H.; Park, Y.H. Antibacterial Activity and Mechanism of Action of the Silver Ion in Staphylococcus aureus and Escherichia coli. *Appl. Environ. Microbiol.* **2008**, *74*, 2171–2178. [CrossRef]
307. Mihai, M.M.; Dima, M.B.; Dima, B.; Holban, A.M. Nanomaterials for Wound Healing and Infection Control. *Materials* **2019**, *12*, 2176. [CrossRef]
308. Burduşel, A.-C.; Gherasim, O.; Grumezescu, A.M.; Mogoantă, L.; Ficai, A.; Andronescu, E. Biomedical applications of silver nanoparticles: An up-to-date overview. *Nanomaterials* **2018**, *8*, 681. [CrossRef]
309. Stetciura, I.Y.; Markin, A.V.; Ponomarev, A.N.; Yakimansky, A.V.; Demina, T.S.; Grandfils, C.; Volodkin, D.V.; Gorin, D.A. New surface-enhanced raman scattering platforms: Composite calcium carbonate microspheres coated with astralen and silver nanoparticles. *Langmuir* **2013**, *29*, 4140–4147. [CrossRef]
310. Zan, X.; Kozlov, M.; McCarthy, T.J.; Su, Z. Covalently attached, silver-doped Poly(vinyl alcohol) hydrogel films on Poly(l-lactic acid). *Biomacromolecules* **2010**, *11*, 1082–1088. [CrossRef] [PubMed]
311. García-Astrain, C.; Chen, C.; Burón, M.; Palomares, T.; Eceiza, A.; Fruk, L.; Corcuera, M.Á.; Gabilondo, N. Biocompatible hydrogel nanocomposite with covalently embedded silver nanoparticles. *Biomacromolecules* **2015**, *16*, 1301–1310. [CrossRef] [PubMed]
312. Cao, H.; Zhang, W.; Meng, F.; Guo, J.; Wang, D.; Qian, S.; Jiang, X.; Liu, X.; Chu, P.K. Osteogenesis Catalyzed by Titanium-Supported Silver Nanoparticles. *ACS Appl. Mater. Interfaces* **2017**, *9*, 5149–5157. [CrossRef] [PubMed]

313. Patrascu, J.M.; Nedelcu, I.A.; Sonmez, M.; Ficai, D.; Ficai, A.; Vasile, B.S.; Ungureanu, C.; Albu, M.G.; Andor, B.; Andronescu, E.; et al. Composite scaffolds based on silver nanoparticles for biomedical applications. *J. Nanomater.* **2015**, *2015*, 587989. [CrossRef]
314. Huang, X.; Qian, W.; El-Sayed, I.H.; El-Sayed, M.A. The potential use of the enhanced nonlinear properties of gold nanospheres in photothermal cancer therapy. *Lasers Surg. Med.* **2007**, *39*, 747–753. [CrossRef]
315. Vieira, S.; Vial, S.; Maia, F.R.; Carvalho, M.R.; Reis, R.L.; Granja, P.L.; Oliveira, J.M. Gellan gum-coated gold nanorods: An intracellular nanosystem for bone tissue engineering. *RSC Adv.* **2015**, *5*, 77996–78005. [CrossRef]
316. Yuan, H.; Khoury, C.G.; Wilson, C.M.; Grant, G.A.; Bennett, A.J.; Vo-Dinh, T. In vivo particle tracking and photothermal ablation using plasmon-resonant gold nanostars. *Nanomed. Nanotechnol. Biol. Med.* **2012**, *8*, 1355–1363. [CrossRef]
317. Zhang, Q.; Uchaker, E.; Candelaria, S.L.; Cao, G. Nanomaterials for energy conversion and storage. *Chem. Soc. Rev.* **2013**, *42*, 3127–3171. [CrossRef]
318. Li, H.; Pan, S.; Xia, P.; Chang, Y.; Fu, C.; Kong, W.; Yu, Z.; Wang, K.; Yang, X.; Qi, Z. Advances in the applications of gold nanoparticles in bone tissue engineering. *J. Biol. Eng.* **2020**, *14*, 14. [CrossRef]
319. Daniel, M.-C.; Astruc, D. Gold Nanoparticles: assembly, supramolecular chemistry, quantum-size-related properties, and applications toward biology, catalysis, and nanotechnology. *Chem. Rev.* **2004**, *104*, 293–346. [CrossRef]
320. Aldewachi, H.; Chalati, T.; Woodroofe, M.N.; Bricklebank, N.; Sharrack, B.; Gardiner, P. Gold nanoparticle-based colorimetric biosensors. *Nanoscale* **2018**, *10*, 18–33. [CrossRef]
321. Morita, M.; Tachikawa, T.; Seino, S.; Tanaka, K.; Majima, T. Controlled synthesis of gold nanoparticles on fluorescent nanodiamond via electron-beam-induced reduction method for dual-modal optical and electron bioimaging. *ACS Appl. Nano Mater.* **2018**, *1*, 355–363. [CrossRef]
322. Zhang, Y.S.; Wang, Y.; Wang, L.; Wang, Y.; Cai, X.; Zhang, C.; Wang, L.V.; Xia, Y. Labeling human mesenchymal stem cells with gold nanocages for in vitro and in vivo tracking by two-photon microscopy and photoacoustic microscopy. *Theranostics* **2013**, *3*, 532–543. [CrossRef] [PubMed]
323. Khlebtsov, N.; Bogatyrev, V.; Dykman, L.; Khlebtsov, B.; Staroverov, S.; Shirokov, A.; Matora, L.; Khanadeev, V.; Pylaev, T.; Tsyganova, N.; et al. Analytical and theranostic applications of gold Na-noparticles and multifunctional nanocomposites. *Theranostics* **2013**, *3*, 167–180. [CrossRef] [PubMed]
324. Sun, T.-M.; Wang, Y.-C.; Wang, F.; Du, J.; Mao, C.; Sun, C.-Y.; Tang, R.; Liu, Y.; Zhu, J.; Zhu, Y.-H.; et al. Cancer stem cell therapy using doxorubicin conjugated to gold nanoparticles via hydrazone bonds. *Biomaterials* **2013**, *35*, 836–845. [CrossRef] [PubMed]
325. Yu, M.; Lei, B.; Gao, C.; Yan, J.; Ma, P.X. Optimizing surface-engineered ultra-small gold nanoparticles for highly efficient miRNA delivery to enhance osteogenic differentiation of bone mesenchimal stromal cells. *Nano Res.* **2017**, *10*, 49–63. [CrossRef]
326. Vial, S.; Reis, R.L.; Oliveira, J.M. Recent advances using gold nanoparticles as a promising multimodal tool for tissue engineering and regenerative medicine. *Curr. Opin. Solid State Mater. Sci.* **2017**, *21*, 92–112. [CrossRef]
327. Khorasani, A.; Goldberg, M.; Doeven, E.; Littlefair, G. Titanium in biomedical applications—Properties and fabrication: A Review. *J. Biomater. Tissue Eng.* **2015**, *5*, 593–619. [CrossRef]
328. Hong, Y.C.; Kim, J.H.; Bang, C.U.; Uhm, H.S. Gas-phase synthesis of nitrogen-doped TiO_2 nanorods by microwave plasma torch at atmospheric pressure. *Phys. Plasmas* **2005**, *12*, 114501. [CrossRef]
329. Dar, M.I.; Chandiran, A.K.; Gratzel, M.; Nazeeruddin, M.K.; Shivashankar, S.A. Controlled synthesis of TiO_2 nanospheres using a microwave assisted approach for their application in dye-sensitized solar cells. *J. Mater. Chem. A* **2014**, *2*, 1662–1667. [CrossRef]
330. Jeon, S.; Braun, P.V. Hydrothermal synthesis of er-doped luminescent TiO_2 nanoparticles. *Chem. Mater.* **2003**, *15*, 1256–1263. [CrossRef]
331. Ramakrishnan, V.M.; Natarajan, M.; Santhanam, A.; Asokan, V.; Velauthapillai, D. Size controlled synthesis of TiO_2 nanoparticles by modified solvothermal method towards effective photocatalitic and photovoltaic applications. *Mater. Res.* **2018**, *97*, 351–360.
332. Loryuenyong, V.; Angamnuaysiri, K.; Sukcharoenpong, J.; Suwannasri, A. Sol–gel derived mesoporous titania nanoparticles: Effects of calcination temperature and alcoholic solvent on the photocatalytic behavior. *Ceram. Int.* **2012**, *38*, 2233–2237. [CrossRef]

333. Maheswari, D.; Venkatachalam, P. Enhanced efficiency and improved photocatalytic activity of 1:1 composite mixture of TiO$_2$ nanoparticles and nanotubes in dye-sensitized solar cell. *Bull. Mater. Sci.* **2014**, *37*, 1489–1496. [CrossRef]
334. Cai, Q.; Paulose, M.; Varghese, O.K.; Grimes, C.A. The effect of electrolyte composition on the fabrication of self-organized titanium oxide nanotube arrays by anodic oxidation. *J. Mater. Res.* **2005**, *20*, 230–236. [CrossRef]
335. Tang, Y.; Tao, J.; Zhang, Y.; Wu, T.; Tao, H.; Bao, Z. Preparation and characterization of TiO$_2$ nanotube arrays via anodization of titanium films deposited on FTO conducting glass at room temperature. *Acta Physico Chimica Sin.* **2008**, *24*, 2191–2197. [CrossRef]
336. Ding, Z.; Hu, X.; Yue, P.; Lu, M.; Greenfield, P. Synthesis of anatase TiO$_2$ supported on porous solids by chemical vapor deposition. *Catal. Today* **2001**, *68*, 173–182. [CrossRef]
337. Lee, H.; Song, M.; Jurng, J.; Park, Y.-K. The synthesis and coating process of TiO$_2$ nanoparticles using CVD process. *Powder Technol.* **2011**, *214*, 64–68. [CrossRef]
338. Arami, H.; Mazloumi, M.; Khalifehzadeh, R.; Sadrnezhaad, S.K. Sonochemical preparation of TiO$_2$ nanoparticles. *Mater. Lett.* **2007**, *61*, 4559–4561. [CrossRef]
339. Guo, J.; Zhu, S.; Chen, Z.; Li, Y.; Yu, Z.; Liu, Q.; Li, J.; Feng, C.; Zhang, D. Sonochemical synthesis of TiO$_2$ nanoparticles on graphene for use as photocatalyst. *Ultrason. Sonochem.* **2011**, *18*, 1082–1090. [CrossRef]
340. Nasrollahzadeh, M.; Atarod, M.; Jaleh, B.; Gandomirouzbahani, M. In situ green synthesis of Ag nanoparticles on graphene oxide/TiO$_2$ nanocomposite and their catalytic activity for the reduction of 4-nitrophenol, Congo red and methylene blue. *Ceram. Int.* **2016**, *42*, 8587–8596. [CrossRef]
341. Sivaranjani, V.; Philominathan, P. Synthesize of Titanium dioxide nanoparticles using Moringa oleifera leaves and evaluation of wound healing activity. *Wound Med.* **2016**, *12*, 1–5. [CrossRef]
342. Goutam, S.P.; Saxena, G.; Singh, V.; Yadav, A.K.; Bharagava, R.N.; Thapa, K.B. Green synthesis of TiO$_2$ nanoparticles using leaf extract of Jatropha curcas L. for photocatalytic degradation of tannery wastewater. *Chem. Eng. J.* **2018**, *336*, 386–396. [CrossRef]
343. Paunesku, T.; Rajh, T.; Wiederrecht, G.; Maser, J.; Vogt, S.; Stojićević, N.; Protić, M.; Lai, B.; Oryhon, J.; Thurnauer, M.; et al. Biology of TiO$_2$–oligonucleotide nanocomposites. *Nat. Mater.* **2003**, *2*, 343–346. [CrossRef] [PubMed]
344. Paunesku, T.; Vogt, S.; Lai, B.; Maser, J.; Stojićević, N.; Thurn, K.T.; Osipo, C.; Liu, H.; Legnini, D.; Wang, Z.; et al. Intracellular distribution of TiO$_2$-DNA oligonucleotide nanoconjugates directed to nucleolus and mitochondria indicates sequence specificity. *Nano Lett.* **2007**, *7*, 596–601. [CrossRef]
345. Cesmeli, S.; Biray Avci, C. Application of titanium dioxide (TiO$_2$) nanoparticles in cancer therapies. *J. Drug Target.* **2019**, *27*, 762–766. [CrossRef]
346. Roy, P.; Berger, S.; Schmuki, P. TiO$_2$ Nanotubes: Synthesis and applications. *Angew. Chem. Int. Ed.* **2011**, *50*, 2904–2939. [CrossRef]
347. Losic, D.; Aw, M.; Santos, A.; Gulati, K.; Bariana, M. Titania nanotube arrays for local drug delivery: Recent advances and perspectives. *Expert Opin. Drug Deliv.* **2014**, *12*, 103–127. [CrossRef]
348. Wang, Q.; Huang, J.-Y.; Li, H.-Q.; Chen, Z.; Zhao, A.Z.-J.; Wang, Y.; Zhang, K.-Q.; Sun, H.-T.; Al-Deyab, S.S.; Lai, Y.-K. TiO$_2$ nanotube platforms for smart drug delivery: A review. *Int. J. Nanomed.* **2016**, *11*, 4819–4834.
349. Wu, S.; Weng, Z.; Liu, X.; Yeung, K.W.K.; Chu, P.K. Functionalized TiO$_2$ based nanomaterials for biomedical applications. *Adv. Funct. Mater.* **2014**, *24*, 5464–5481. [CrossRef]
350. Tiainen, H.; Monjo, M.; Knychala, J.; Nilsen, O.; Lyngstadaas, S.P.; Ellingsen, J.E.; Haugen, H.J. The effect of fluoride surface modification of ceramic TiO$_2$ on the surface properties and biological response of osteoblastic cells in vitro. *Biomed. Mater.* **2011**, *6*, 45006. [CrossRef] [PubMed]
351. Tiainen, H.; Lyngstadaas, S.P.; Ellingsen, J.E.; Haugen, H.J. Ultra-porous titanium oxide scaffold with high compressive strength. *J. Mater. Sci. Mater. Med.* **2010**, *21*, 2783–2792. [CrossRef]
352. Tabriz, K.R.; Katbab, A.A. Preparation of modified-TiO$_2$/PLA nanocomposite films: Micromorphology, photo-degradability and antibacterial studies. *AIP Conf. Proc.* **2017**, *1914*, 70009.
353. Wu, X.; Liu, X.; Wei, J.; Ma, J.; Deng, F.; Wei, S. Nano-TiO$_2$/PEEK bioactive composite as a bone substitute material: In vitro and in vivo studies. *Int. J. Nanomed.* **2012**, *7*, 1215–1225.

354. Eslami, H.; Azimi Lisar, H.; Jafarzadeh Kashi, T.S.; Tahriri, M.; Ansari, M.; Rafiei, T.; Bastami, F.; Shahin-Shamsabadi, A.; Mashhadi Abbas, F.; Tayebi, L. Poly(lactic-co-glycolic acid)(PLGA)/TiO$_2$ nanotube bioactive composite as a novel scaffold for bone tissue engineering: In vitro and in vivo studies. *Biologicals* **2018**, *53*, 51–62. [CrossRef] [PubMed]

355. Paušová, Š.; Krýsa, J.; Jirkovský, J.; Prevot, V.; Mailhot, G. Preparation of TiO$_2$-SiO$_2$ composite photocatalysts for environmental applications. *J. Chem. Technol. Biotechnol.* **2014**, *89*, 1129–1135. [CrossRef]

356. Liu, S.; Tao, W.; Li, J.; Yang, Z.; Liu, F. Study on the formation process of Al2O3–TiO$_2$ composite powders. *Powder Technol.* **2005**, *155*, 187–192. [CrossRef]

357. Omid-Bakhtiari, M.; Nasr-Esfahani, M.; Nourmohamadi, A. TiO$_2$-Bioactive glass nanostructure composite films produced by a sol-gel method: In vitro behavior and UV-enhanced bioactivity. *J. Mater. Eng. Perform.* **2014**, *23*, 285–293. [CrossRef]

358. Oktar, F.N. Hydroxyapatite–TiO$_2$ composites. *Mater. Lett.* **2006**, *60*, 2207–2210. [CrossRef]

359. Khalid, N.R.; Bilal Tahir, M.; Majid, A.; Ahmed, E.; Ahmad, M.; Khalid, S.; Ahmed, W. TiO$_2$-graphene-based composites: Synthesis, characterization, and application in photocatalysis of organic pollutants. In *Micro and Nanomanufacturing Volume II*; Jackson, M.J., Ahmed, W., Eds.; Springer International Publishing: Cham, Switzerland, 2018; pp. 95–122.

360. Roguska, A.; Pisarek, M.; Andrzejczuk, M.; Dolata, M.; Lewandowska, M.; Janik-Czachor, M. Characterization of a calcium phosphate–TiO$_2$ nanotube composite layer for biomedical applications. *Mater. Sci. Eng. C* **2011**, *31*, 906–914. [CrossRef]

361. Rehman, F.U.; Zhao, C.; Jiang, H.; Wang, X. Biomedical applications of nano-titania in theranostics and photodynamic therapy. *Biomater. Sci.* **2016**, *4*, 40–54. [CrossRef] [PubMed]

362. Chen, J.; Dong, X.; Zhao, J.; Tang, G. In vivo acute toxicity of titanium dioxide nanoparticles to mice after intraperitoneal injection. *J. Appl. Toxicol.* **2009**, *29*, 330–337. [CrossRef] [PubMed]

363. Chennell, P.; Feschet-Chassot, E.; Devers, T.; Awitor, K.O.; Descamps, S.; Sautou, V. In vitro evaluation of TiO$_2$ nanotubes as cefuroxime carriers on orthopaedic implants for the prevention of periprosthetic joint infections. *Int. J. Pharm.* **2013**, *455*, 298–305. [CrossRef] [PubMed]

364. Kumar, P.; Dehiya, B.S.; Sindhu, A. Bioceramics for hard tissue engineering applications: A review. *Int. J. Appl. Eng. Res.* **2018**, *13*, 2744–2752.

365. Hentrich, R.L.; Graves, G.A.; Stein, H.G.; Bajpai, P.K. An evaluation of inert and resorbale ceramics for future clinical orthopedic applications. *J. Biomed. Mater. Res.* **1971**, *5*, 25–51. [CrossRef] [PubMed]

366. Christel, P.; Meunier, A.; Heller, M.; Torre, J.P.; Peille, C.N. Mechanical properties and short-term in vivo evaluation of yttrium-oxide-partially-stabilized zirconia. *J. Biomed. Mater. Res.* **1989**, *23*, 45–61. [CrossRef] [PubMed]

367. Afzal, M.A.F.; Kesarwani, P.; Reddy, K.M.; Kalmodia, S.; Basu, B.; Balani, K. Functionally graded hydroxyapatite-alumina-zirconia biocomposite: Synergy of toughness and biocompatibility. *Mater. Sci. Eng. C* **2012**, *32*, 1164–1173. [CrossRef]

368. Cales, B.; Stefani, Y.; Lilley, E. Long-term in vivo and in vivo aging of a zirconia ceramic used in orthopaedy. *J. Biomed. Mater. Res.* **1994**, *28*, 619–624. [CrossRef] [PubMed]

369. Hu, C.Y.; Yoon, T.-R. Recent updates for biomaterials used in total hip arthroplasty. *Biomater. Res.* **2018**, *22*, 1–12. [CrossRef]

370. Vagkopoulou, T.; Koutayas, S.O.; Koidis, P.; Strub, J.R. Zirconia in dentistry: Part 1. Discovering the nature of an upcoming bioceramic. *Eur. J. Esthet. Dent.* **2009**, *4*, 130–151.

371. Tosiriwatanapong, T.; Singhatanadgit, W. Zirconia-based biomaterials for hard tissue reconstruction. *Bone Tissue Regen. Insights* **2018**, *9*. [CrossRef]

372. Aboushelib, M.N.; Shawky, R. Osteogenesis ability of CAD/CAM porous zirconia scaffolds enriched with nano-hydroxyapatite particles. *Int. J. Implant Dent.* **2017**, *3*, 21. [CrossRef] [PubMed]

373. Mushahary, D.; Sravanthi, R.; Li, Y.; Kumar, M.J.; Harishankar, N.; Hodgson, P.D.; Wen, C.; Pande, G. Zirconium, calcium, and strontium contents in magnesium based biodegradable alloys modulate the efficiency of implant-induced osseointegration. *Int. J. Nanomed.* **2013**, *8*, 2887–2902.

374. Ramaswamy, Y.; Wu, C.; Van Hummel, A.; Combes, V.; Grau, G.; Zreiqat, H. The responses of osteoblasts, osteoclasts and endothelial cells to zirconium modified calcium-silicate-based ceramic. *Biomaterials* **2008**, *29*, 4392–4402. [CrossRef]

375. Kim, H.-W.; Kim, H.-E.; Knowles, J.C. Hard-tissue-engineered zirconia porous scaffolds with hydroxyapatite sol–gel and slurry coatings. *J. Biomed. Mater. Res. Part B.* **2004**, *70*, 270–277. [CrossRef]
376. Chevalier, J.; Gremillard, L. Zirconia as a biomaterial. *Compr. Biomater.* **2011**, *1*, 95–108.
377. Alizadeh, A.; Moztarzadeh, F.; Ostad, S.N.; Azami, M.; Geramizadeh, B.; Hatam, G.; Bizari, D.; Tavangar, S.M.; Vasei, M.; Ai, J. Synthesis of calcium phosphate-zirconia scaffold and human endometrial adult stem cells for bone tissue engineering. *Artif. Cells Nanomed. Biotechnol.* **2016**, *44*, 66–73. [CrossRef]
378. Jayakumar, R.; Ramachandran, R.; Sudheesh Kumar, P.T.; Divyarani, V.V.; Srinivasan, S.; Chennazhi, K.P.; Tamura, H.; Nair, S.V. Fabrication of chitin–chitosan/nano ZrO_2 composite scaffolds for tissue engineering applications. *Int. J. Biol. Macromol.* **2011**, *49*, 274–280. [CrossRef]
379. Teimouri, A.; Ebrahimi, R.; Emadi, R.; Beni, B.H.; Chermahini, A.N. Nano-composite of silk fibroin–chitosan/Nano ZrO_2 for tissue engineering applications: Fabrication and morphology. *Int. J. Biol. Macromol.* **2015**, *76*, 292–302. [CrossRef]
380. Bermúdez-Reyes, B.; del Refugio Lara-Banda, M.; Reyes-Zarate, E.; Rojas-Martínez, A.; Camacho, A.; Moncada-Saucedo, N.; Pérez-Silos, V.; García-Ruiz, A.; Guzmán-López, A.; Peña-Martínez, V.; et al. Effect on growth and osteoblast mineralization of hydroxyapatite-zirconia (HA-ZrO_2) obtained by a new low temperature system. *Biomed. Mater.* **2018**, *13*, 035001. [CrossRef]
381. Sa, M.-W.; Nguyen, B.-N.B.; Moriarty, R.A.; Kamalitdinov, T.; Fisher, J.P.; Kim, J.Y. Fabrication and evaluation of 3D printed BCP scaffolds reinforced with ZrO_2 for bone tissue applications. *Biotechnol. Bioeng.* **2018**, *115*, 989–999. [CrossRef] [PubMed]
382. Bhowmick, A.; Pramanik, N.; Mitra, T.; Gnanamani, A.; Das, M.; Kundu, P.P. Mechanical and biological investigations of chitosan–polyvinyl alcohol based ZrO_2 doped porous hybrid composites for bone tissue engineering applications. *New J. Chem.* **2017**, *41*, 7524–7530. [CrossRef]
383. Wang, X.; Chen, D.; Cao, L.; Li, Y.; Boyd, B.J.; Caruso, R.A. Mesoporous titanium zirconium oxide nanospheres with potential for drug delivery applications. *ACS Appl. Mater. Interfaces* **2013**, *5*, 10926–10932. [CrossRef] [PubMed]
384. Abánades Lázaro, I.; Haddad, S.; Rodrigo-Muñoz, J.M.; Marshall, R.J.; Sastre, B.; del Pozo, V.; Fairen-Jimenez, D.; Forgan, R.S. Surface-functionalization of Zr-Fumarate MOF for selective cytotoxicity and immune system compatibility in nanoscale drug delivery. *ACS Appl. Mater. Interfaces* **2018**, *10*, 31146–31157. [CrossRef]
385. Milak, P.; Minatto, F.; De Noni, A., Jr.; Montedo, O. Wear performance of alumina-based ceramics—A review of the influence of microstructure on erosive wear. *Cerâmica* **2015**, *61*, 88–103. [CrossRef]
386. Gaber, A.A.A.-A.; Ibrahim, D.M.; Abd-AImohsen, F.F.; El-Zanati, M.M. Synthesis of alumina, titania, and alumina-titania hydrophobic membranes via sol–gel polymeric route. *J. Anal. Sci. Technol.* **2013**, *4*, 18. [CrossRef]
387. Elsberg, L.; Moore, M. Total hip replacement: Metal-on-metal systems. In *Clinical Performance of Skeletal Prostheses*; Hench, L.L., Wilson, J., Eds.; Springer: Dordrecht, The Netherlands, 1996; pp. 57–70.
388. Al-Sanabani, F.A.; Madfa, A.A.; Al-Qudaimi, N.H. Alumina ceramic for dental applications: A review article. *Am. J. Mater. Res.* **2014**, *1*, 26–34.
389. Lee, K.-L.; Hsu, H.-Y.; You, M.-L.; Chang, C.-C.; Pan, M.-Y.; Shi, X.; Ueno, K.; Misawa, H.; Wei, P.-K. Highly sensitive aluminum-based biosensors using tailorable fano resonances in capped nanostructures. *Sci. Rep.* **2017**, *7*, 44104. [CrossRef]
390. Bartzsch, H.; Glöß, D.; Böcher, B.; Frach, P.; Goedicke, K. Properties of SiO_2 and Al_2O_3 films for electrical insulation applications deposited by reactive pulse magnetron sputtering. *Surf. Coat. Technol.* **2003**, *174*, 774–778. [CrossRef]
391. Elisabet, X.-P.; Josep, F.-B.; Josep, P.; Marsal, F.L. Mesoporous alumina as a biomaterial for biomedical applications. *Open Mater. Sci.* **2015**, *2*, 13.
392. Mohanty, M. Medical Applications of alumina ceramics. *Trans. Indian Ceram. Soc.* **1995**, *54*, 200–204. [CrossRef]
393. Sansone, V.; Pagani, D.; Melato, M. The effects on bone cells of metal ions released from orthopaedic implants. A review. *Clin. Cases Miner. Bone Metab.* **2013**, *10*, 34–40. [CrossRef] [PubMed]
394. Piconi, C.; Condo, S.G.; Kosmac, T. Chapter 11—Alumina- and zirconia-based ceramics for load-bearing applications. In *Advanced Ceramics for Dentistry*; Shen, J.Z., Kosmač, T., Eds.; Butterworth-Heinemann: Oxford, UK, 2014; pp. 219–253.

395. Kandpal, B.C.; kumar, J.; Singh, H. Fabrication and characterisation of Al_2O_3/aluminium alloy 6061 composites fabricated by stir casting. *Mater. Today Proc.* **2017**, *4*, 2783–2792. [CrossRef]
396. Saini, M.; Singh, Y.; Arora, P.; Arora, V.; Jain, K. Implant biomaterials: A comprehensive review. *World J. Clin. Cases* **2015**, *3*, 52–57. [CrossRef] [PubMed]
397. Sarhadi, F.; Shafiee Afarani, M.; Mohebbi-Kalhori, D.; Shayesteh, M. Fabrication of alumina porous scaffolds with aligned oriented pores for bone tissue engineering applications. *Appl. Phys. A* **2016**, *122*, 390. [CrossRef]
398. Levin, I.; Brandon, D. Metastable alumina polymorphs: Crystal structures and transition sequences. *J. Am. Ceram. Soc.* **1998**, *81*, 1995–2012. [CrossRef]
399. Rahmati, M.; Mozafari, M. Biocompatibility of alumina-based biomaterials–A review. *J. Cell. Physiol.* **2019**, *234*, 3321–3335. [CrossRef]
400. Ferraz, N.; Hong, J.; Santin, M.; Ott, M. Nanoporosity of alumina surfaces induces different patterns of activation in adhering monocytes/macrophages. *Int. J. Biomater.* **2010**, *2010*, 402715. [CrossRef]
401. Gregorová, E.; Pabst, W.; Živcová, Z.; Sedlářová, I.; Holíková, S. Porous alumina ceramics prepared with wheat flour. *J. Eur. Ceram. Soc.* **2010**, *30*, 2871–2880. [CrossRef]
402. Bartonickova, E.; Vojtisek, J.; Tkacz, J.; Pořízka, J.; Masilko, J.; Moncekova, M.; Parizek, L. Porous HA/Alumina composites intended for bone-tissue engineering. *Mater. Technol.* **2017**, *51*, 631–636. [CrossRef]
403. Leary Swan, E.E.; Popat, K.C.; Desai, T.A. Peptide-immobilized nanoporous alumina membranes for enhanced osteoblast adhesion. *Biomaterials* **2005**, *26*, 1969–1976. [CrossRef] [PubMed]
404. Ding, G.; Yang, R.; Ding, J.; Yuan, N.; Zhu, Y. Fabrication of porous anodic alumina with ultrasmall nanopores. *Nanoscale Res. Lett.* **2010**, *5*, 1257. [CrossRef] [PubMed]
405. Zaraska, L.; Jaskula, M.; Sulka, G. Porous anodic alumina layers with modulated pore diameters formed by sequential anodizing in different electrolytes. *Mater. Lett.* **2016**, *171*, 315–318. [CrossRef]
406. Porta-I-Batalla, M.; Xifré-Pérez, E.; Eckstein, C.; Ferré-Borrull, J.; Marsal, L.F. 3D Nanoporous Anodic Alumina Structures for Sustained Drug Release. *Nanomaterials* **2017**, *7*, 227. [CrossRef]
407. Vishal, P. Design and fabrication of ordered mesoporous alumina scaffold for drug delivery of poorly water soluble drug. *Austin Ther.* **2015**, *2*, 1–5.
408. Kang, H.J.; Park, S.J.; Yoo, J.B.; Kim, D.J. Controlled drug release using nanoporous anodic aluminum oxide. *Solid State Phenom.* **2007**, *121*, 709–712. [CrossRef]
409. Owens, G.J.; Singh, R.K.; Foroutan, F.; Alqaysi, M.; Han, C.-M.; Mahapatra, C.; Kim, H.-W.; Knowles, J.C. Sol–gel based materials for biomedical applications. *Prog. Mater. Sci.* **2016**, *77*, 1–79. [CrossRef]
410. Kumar Panda, S.; Dhupal, D.; Kumar Nanda, B. Experimental study on $Ca_3(PO_4)_2$-Al_2O_3 bio-ceramic composite using DPSS laser. *Mater. Today Proc.* **2018**, *5*, 24133–24140. [CrossRef]
411. Toloue, E.B.; Karbasi, S.; Salehi, H.; Rafienia, M. Evaluation of mechanical properties and cell viability of poly (3-Hydroxybutyrate)-Chitosan/Al_2O_3 nanocomposite scaffold for cartilage tissue engineering. *J. Med. Signals Sens.* **2019**, *9*, 111–116.
412. Venkatesh, N.; Hanumantharaju, H.G.; Aravind, J. A Study of bio-active coating of Al_2O_3, egg and sea shell powder on Ss316l and Ti-6Al-4V. *Mater. Today Proc.* **2018**, *5*, 22687–22693. [CrossRef]
413. Mandracci, P.; Mussano, F.; Rivolo, P.; Carossa, S. Surface treatments and functional coatings for biocompatibility improvement and bacterial adhesion reduction in dental implantology. *Coatings* **2016**, *6*, 7. [CrossRef]
414. Zhao, X.; Zhang, W.; Wang, Y.; Liu, Q.; Yang, J.; Zhang, L.; He, F. Fabrication of Al_2O_3 by anodic oxidation and hydrothermal synthesis of strong-bonding hydroxyapatite coatings on its surface. *Appl. Surf. Sci.* **2019**, *470*, 959–969. [CrossRef]
415. Rodríguez, J.P.; Ríos, S.; González, M. Modulation of the proliferation and differentiation of human mesenchymal stem cells by copper. *J. Cell. Biochem.* **2002**, *85*, 92–100. [CrossRef] [PubMed]
416. Hu, G. Copper stimulates proliferation of human endothelial cells under culture. *J. Cell. Biochem.* **1998**, *69*, 326–335. [CrossRef]
417. Cioffi, N.; Torsi, L.; Ditaranto, N.; Tantillo, G.; Ghibelli, L.; Sabbatini, L.; Bleve-Zacheo, T.; D'Alessio, M.; Zambonin, P.G.; Traversa, E. Copper nanoparticle/polymer composites with antifungal and bacteriostatic properties. *Chem. Mater.* **2005**, *17*, 5255–5262. [CrossRef]
418. Gallo, J.; Holinka, M.; Moucha, C.S. Antibacterial surface treatment for orthopaedic implants. *Int. J. Mol. Sci.* **2014**, *15*, 13849–13880. [CrossRef]

419. Chaudhri, M.A.; Kemmler, W.; Harsch, I.; Watling, R.J. Plasma copper and bone mineral density in osteopenia: An indicator of bone mineral density in osteopenic females. *Biol. Trace Elem. Res.* **2009**, *129*, 94–98. [CrossRef]
420. Das, A.; Sudhahar, V.; Chen, G.-F.; Kim, H.W.; Youn, S.-W.; Finney, L.; Vogt, S.; Yang, J.; Kweon, J.; Surenkhuu, B.; et al. Endothelial antioxidant-1: A Key mediator of copper-dependent wound healing in vivo. *Sci. Rep.* **2016**, *6*, 33783. [CrossRef]
421. Nethi, S.K.; Das, S.; Patra, C.R.; Mukherjee, S. Recent advances in inorganic nanomaterials for wound-healing applications. *Biomater. Sci.* **2019**, *7*, 2652–2674. [CrossRef]
422. Tripathi, A.; Saravanan, S.; Pattnaik, S.; Moorthi, A.; Partridge, N.C.; Selvamurugan, N. Bio-composite scaffolds containing chitosan/nano-hydroxyapatite/nano-copper–zinc for bone tissue engineering. *Int. J. Biol. Macromol.* **2012**, *50*, 294–299. [CrossRef]
423. Azeena, S.; Subhapradha, N.; Selvamurugan, N.; Narayan, S.; Srinivasan, N.; Murugesan, R.; Chung, T.W.; Moorthi, A. Antibacterial activity of agricultural waste derived wollastonite doped with copper for bone tissue engineering. *Mater. Sci. Eng. C* **2017**, *71*, 1156–1165. [CrossRef] [PubMed]
424. Ryan, E.J.; Ryan, A.J.; González-Vázquez, A.; Philippart, A.; Ciraldo, F.E.; Hobbs, C.; Nicolosi, V.; Boccaccini, A.R.; Kearney, C.J.; O'Brien, F.J. Collagen scaffolds functionalised with copper-eluting bioactive glass reduce infection and enhance osteogenesis and angiogenesis both in vitro and in vivo. *Biomaterials* **2019**, *197*, 405–416. [CrossRef] [PubMed]
425. Alizadeh, S.; Seyedalipour, B.; Shafieyan, S.; Kheime, A.; Mohammadi, P.; Aghdami, N. Copper nanoparticles promote rapid wound healing in acute full thickness defect via acceleration of skin cell migration, proliferation, and neovascularization. *Biochem. Biophys. Res. Commun.* **2019**, *517*, 684–690. [CrossRef] [PubMed]
426. Michels, H.; Moran, W.; Michel, J. Antimicrobial properties of copper alloy surfaces, with a focus on hospital-acquired infections. *Int. J. Met.* **2008**, *2*, 47–56. [CrossRef]
427. Chen, Z.; Meng, H.; Xing, G.; Chen, C.; Zhao, Y.; Jia, G.; Wang, T.; Yuan, H.; Ye, C.; Zhao, F.; et al. Acute toxicological effects of copper nanoparticles in vivo. *Toxicol. Lett.* **2006**, *163*, 109–120. [CrossRef] [PubMed]
428. Khan, H.A.; Sakharkar, M.K.; Nayak, A.; Kishore, U.; Khan, A. Nanoparticles for biomedical applications: An overview. In *Nanobiomaterials: Nanostructured Materials for Biomedical Applications*, 1st ed.; Narayan, R.B.T.-N., Ed.; Woodhead Publishing: Cambridge, UK, 2017; Chapter 14, pp. 357–384.
429. Colombo, M.; Carregal-Romero, S.; Casula, M.F.; Gutiérrez, L.; Morales, M.P.; Böhm, I.B.; Heverhagen, J.T.; Prosperi, D.; Parak, W.J. Biological applications of magnetic nanoparticles. *Chem. Soc. Rev.* **2012**, *41*, 4306–4334. [CrossRef]
430. Sensenig, R.; Sapir, Y.; MacDonald, C.; Cohen, S.; Polyak, B. Magnetic nanoparticle-based approaches to locally target therapy and enhance tissue regeneration in vivo. *Nanomedicine* **2012**, *7*, 1425–1442. [CrossRef]
431. Khalil, M.I. Co-precipitation in aqueous solution synthesis of magnetite nanoparticles using iron(III) salts as precursors. *Arab. J. Chem.* **2015**, *8*, 279–284. [CrossRef]
432. Malik, M.A.; Wani, M.Y.; Hashim, M.A. Microemulsion method: A novel route to synthesize organic and inorganic nanomaterials: 1st Nano update. *Arab. J. Chem.* **2012**, *5*, 397–417. [CrossRef]
433. Daou, T.J.; Pourroy, G.; Bégin-Colin, S.; Grenèche, J.M.; Ulhaq-Bouillet, C.; Legaré, P.; Bernhardt, P.; Leuvrey, C.; Rogez, G. Hydrothermal synthesis of monodisperse magnetite nanoparticles. *Chem. Mater.* **2006**, *18*, 4399–4404. [CrossRef]
434. Takai, Z.; Mustafa, M.; Asman, S.; Sekak, K. Preparation and characterization of magnetite (Fe_3O_4) nanoparticles by sol-gel method. *Int. J. Nanoelectron. Mater.* **2019**, *12*, 37–46.
435. Hachani, R.; Lowdell, M.; Birchall, M.; Hervault, A.; Mertz, D.; Begin-Colin, S.; Thanh, N.T.K. Polyol synthesis, functionalisation, and biocompatibility studies of superparamagnetic iron oxide nanoparticles as potential MRI contrast agents. *Nanoscale* **2016**, *8*, 3278–3287. [CrossRef]
436. Salazar-Alvarez, G.; Muhammed, M.; Zagorodni, A. Novel flow injection synthesis of iron oxide nanoparticles with narrow size distribution. *Chem. Eng. Sci.* **2006**, *61*, 4625–4633. [CrossRef]
437. Hassanjani-Roshan, A.; Vaezi, M.R.; Shokuhfar, A.; Rajabali, Z. Synthesis of iron oxide nanoparticles via sonochemical method and their characterization. *Particuology* **2011**, *9*, 95–99. [CrossRef]
438. Aivazoglou, E.; Metaxa, E.; Hristoforou, E. Microwave-assisted synthesis of iron oxide nanoparticles in biocompatible organic environment. *AIP Adv.* **2017**, *8*, 48201. [CrossRef]

439. Starowicz, M.; Starowicz, P.; Zukrowski, J.; Przewoźnik, J.; Lemański, A.; Kapusta, C. Electrochemical synthesis of magnetic iron oxide nanoparticles with controlled size. *J. Nanopart. Res.* **2011**, *13*, 7167–7176. [CrossRef]
440. Huang, Y.; Zhang, L.; Huan, W.; Liang, X.; Liu, X.; Yang, Y. A study on synthesis and properties of Fe_3O_4 nanoparticles by solvothermal method. *Glas. Phys. Chem.* **2010**, *36*, 325–331. [CrossRef]
441. Wei, D.; Liu, Y.; Cao, L.; Fu, L.; Li, X.; Wang, Y.; Yu, G. A Magnetism-assisted chemical vapor deposition method to produce branched or iron-encapsulated carbon nanotubes. *J. Am. Chem. Soc.* **2007**, *129*, 7364–7368. [CrossRef]
442. Majidi, S.; Sehrig, F.Z.; Farkhani, S.M.; Goloujeh, M.S.; Akbarzadeh, A. Current methods for synthesis of magnetic nanoparticles. *Artif. Cells Nanomed. Biotechnol.* **2016**, *44*, 722–734. [CrossRef]
443. Karade, V.C.; Waifalkar, P.P.; Dongle, T.D.; Sahoo, S.C.; Kollu, P.; Patil, P.S.; Patil, P.B. Greener synthesis of magnetite nanoparticles using green tea extract and their magnetic properties. *Mater. Res. Express* **2017**, *4*, 96102. [CrossRef]
444. Kayal, S.; Bandyopadhyay, D.; Mandal, T.; Ramanujan, R. The flow of magnetic nanoparticles in magnetic drug targeting. *RSC Adv.* **2011**, *1*, 238–246. [CrossRef]
445. Safarik, I.; Safarikova, M. Magnetic techniques for the isolation and purification of proteins and peptides. *Biomagn. Res. Technol.* **2004**, *2*, 1–17. [CrossRef] [PubMed]
446. David, R.; Groebner, M.; Franz, W. Magnetic cell sorting purification of differentiated embryonic stem cells stably expressing truncated human CD4 as surface marker. *Stem Cells* **2005**, *23*, 477–482. [CrossRef] [PubMed]
447. Sun, C.; Lee, J.S.H.; Zhang, M. Magnetic nanoparticles in MR imaging and drug delivery. *Adv. Drug Deliv. Rev.* **2008**, *60*, 1252–1265. [CrossRef] [PubMed]
448. Kudr, J.; Haddad, Y.; Richtera, L.; Heger, Z.; Cernak, M.; Adam, V.; Zitka, O. Magnetic nanoparticles: From design and synthesis to real world applications. *Nanomaterials* **2017**, *7*, 243. [CrossRef]
449. Zhu, N.; Ji, H.; Yu, P.; Niu, J.; Bajwa, U.; Akram, M.W.; Udego, I.O.; Li, H.; Niu, X. Surface modification of magnetic iron oxide nanoparticles. *Nanomaterials* **2018**, *8*, 810. [CrossRef] [PubMed]
450. Akbarzadeh, A.; Samiei, M.; Davaran, S. Magnetic nanoparticles: Preparation, physical properties, and applications in biomedicine. *Nanoscale Res. Lett.* **2012**, *7*, 144. [CrossRef]
451. Pan, Y.; Du, X.; Zhao, F.; Xu, B. Magnetic nanoparticles for the manipulation of proteins and cells. *Chem. Soc. Rev.* **2012**, *41*, 2912–2942. [CrossRef]
452. Baroli, B.; Ennas, M.G.; Loffredo, F.; Isola, M.; Pinna, R.; López-Quintela, M.A. Penetration of Metallic Nanoparticles in Human Full-Thickness Skin. *J. Investig. Dermatol.* **2007**, *127*, 1701–1712. [CrossRef]
453. Li, Y.; Ye, D.; Li, M.; Ma, M.; Gu, N. Adaptive materials based on iron oxide nanoparticles for bone regeneration. *ChemPhysChem* **2018**, *19*, 1965–1979. [CrossRef]
454. Li, Y.; Liu, Y.-Z.; Long, T.; Yu, X.-B.; Tang, T.; Dai, K.-R.; Tian, B.; Guo, Y.-P.; Zhu, Z.-A. Mesoporous bioactive glass as a drug delivery system: Fabrication, bactericidal properties and biocompatibility. *J. Mater. Sci. Mater. Med.* **2013**, *24*, 1951–1961. [CrossRef] [PubMed]
455. Guo, Y.-J.; Wang, Y.-Y.; Chen, T.; Wei, Y.-T.; Chu, L.-F.; Guo, Y.-P. Hollow carbonated hydroxyapatite microspheres with mesoporous structure: Hydrothermal fabrication and drug delivery property. *Mater. Sci. Eng. C* **2013**, *33*, 3166–3172. [CrossRef] [PubMed]
456. Mahmoud, E.E.; Kamei, G.; Harada, Y.; Shimizu, R.; Kamei, N.; Adachi, N.; Misk, N.A.; Ochi, M. Cell magnetic targeting system for repair of severe chronic osteochondral defect in a rabbit model. *Cell Transplant.* **2016**, *25*, 1073–1083. [CrossRef] [PubMed]
457. Gilbertson, L.M.; Zimmerman, J.B.; Plata, D.L.; Hutchison, J.E.; Anastas, P.T. Designing nanomaterials to maximize performance and minimize undesirable implications guided by the Principles of Green Chemistry. *Chem. Soc. Rev.* **2015**, *44*, 5758–5777. [CrossRef]
458. Uskoković, V. Entering the era of nanoscience: Time to be so small. *J. Biomed. Nanotechnol.* **2013**, *9*, 1441–1470. [CrossRef]
459. Rizvi, S.A.A.; Saleh, A.M. Applications of nanoparticle systems in drug delivery technology. *Saudi Pharm. J.* **2018**, *26*, 64–70. [CrossRef]
460. Hasan, A.; Morshed, M.; Memic, A.; Hassan, S.; Webster, T.J.; Marei, H.E.-S. Nanoparticles in tissue engineering: Applications, challenges and prospects. *Int. J. Nanomed.* **2018**, *13*, 5637–5655. [CrossRef]
461. Singh, S.K.; Kulkarni, P.P.; Dash, D. Biomedical applications of nanomaterials: An overview. *Bionanotechnology* **2013**, 1–32. [CrossRef]

462. Das, S.; Mitra, S.; Khurana, S.M.P.; Debnath, N. Nanomaterials for biomedical applications. *Front. Life Sci.* **2013**, *7*, 90–98. [CrossRef]
463. Ng, C.-T.; Baeg, G.-H.; Yu, L.E.; Bay, C.-N.O. Biomedical applications of nanomaterials as therapeutics. *Curr. Med. Chem.* **2018**, *25*, 1409–1419. [CrossRef]
464. Gentile, A.; Ruffino, F.; Grimaldi, G.M. Complex-morphology metal-based nanostructures: Fabrication, characterization, and applications. *Nanomaterials* **2016**, *6*, 110. [CrossRef] [PubMed]
465. Mourdikoudis, S.; Pallares, R.M.; Thanh, N.T.K. Characterization techniques for nanoparticles: Comparison and complementarity upon studying nanoparticle properties. *Nanoscale* **2018**, *10*, 12871–12934. [CrossRef] [PubMed]
466. Jeevanandam, J.; Barhoum, A.; Chan, Y.S.; Dufresne, A.; Danquah, M.K. Review on nanoparticles and nanostructured materials: History, sources, toxicity and regulations. *Beilstein J. Nanotechnol.* **2018**, *9*, 1050–1074. [CrossRef] [PubMed]
467. Lin, P.-C.; Lin, S.; Wang, P.C.; Sridhar, R. Techniques for physicochemical characterization of nanomaterials. *Biotechnol. Adv.* **2014**, *32*, 711–726. [CrossRef] [PubMed]
468. Biener, J.; Wittstock, A.; Baumann, T.F.; Weissmüller, J.; Bäumer, M.; Hamza, A.V. Surface chemistry in nanoscale materials. *Materials* **2009**, *2*, 2404–2428. [CrossRef]
469. Williams, D.F. On the mechanisms of biocompatibility. *Biomaterials* **2008**, *29*, 2941–2953. [CrossRef]
470. Singh, A.; Elisseeff, J. Biomaterials for stem cell differentiation. *J. Mater. Chem.* **2010**, *20*, 8832–8847. [CrossRef]
471. Yang, X.; Li, Y.; Liu, X.; Zhang, R.; Feng, Q. In vitro uptake of hydroxyapatite nanoparticles and their effect on osteogenic differentiation of human mesenchymal stem cells. *Stem Cells Int.* **2018**, *2018*, 2036176. [CrossRef]
472. Lavenus, S.; Trichet, V.; Le Chevalier, S.; Hoornaert, A.; Louarn, G.; Layrolle, P. Cell differentiation and osseointegration influenced by nanoscale anodized titanium surfaces. *Nanomedicine* **2012**, *7*, 967–980. [CrossRef]
473. Somaiah, C.; Kumar, A.; Mawrie, D.; Sharma, A.; Patil, S.D.; Bhattacharyya, J.; Swaminathan, R.; Jaganathan, B.G. Collagen promotes higher adhesion, survival and proliferation of mesenchymal stem cells. *PLoS ONE* **2015**, *10*, e0145068. [CrossRef]
474. Rasouli, R.; Barhoum, A.; Uludag, H. A review of nanostructured surface and materials for dental implants: Surface coating, pattering and functionalization for improved performance. *Biomater. Sci.* **2018**, *6*, 1312–1338. [CrossRef]
475. Bertazzo, S.; Zambuzzi, W.F.; Da Silva, H.A.; Ferreira, C.V.; Bertran, C.A. Bioactivation of alumina by surface modification: A possibility for improving the applicability of alumina in bone and oral repair. *Clin. Oral Implants Res.* **2009**, *20*, 288–293. [CrossRef] [PubMed]
476. Profeta, A.C.; Huppa, C. Bioactive-glass in oral and maxillofacial surgery. *Craniomaxillofac. Trauma Reconstr.* **2016**, *9*, 1–14. [CrossRef] [PubMed]
477. Crovace, M.C.; Souza, M.T.; Chinaglia, C.R.; Peitl, O.; Zanotto, E.D. Biosilicate®—A multipurpose, highly bioactive glass-ceramic. In vitro, in vivo and clinical trials. *J. Non. Cryst. Solids* **2016**, *432*, 90–110. [CrossRef]
478. Kargozar, S.; Montazerian, M.; Fiume, E.; Baino, F. Multiple and promising applications of strontium (Sr)-containing bioactive glasses in bone tissue engineering. *Front. Bioeng. Biotechnol.* **2019**, *7*, 161. [CrossRef] [PubMed]
479. Baino, F.; Vitale-Brovarone, C. Three-dimensional glass-derived scaffolds for bone tissue engineering: Current trends and forecasts for the future. *J. Biomed. Mater. Res. Part A* **2011**, *97*, 514–535. [CrossRef]
480. Tautzenberger, A.; Kovtun, A.; Ignatius, A. Nanoparticles and their potential for application in bone. *Int. J. Nanomed.* **2012**, *7*, 4545–4557. [CrossRef]
481. Kumar, P.; Dehiya, B.S.; Sindhu, A. Ibuprofen-loaded CTS/nHA/nBG Scaffolds for the applications of hard tissue engineering. *Iran. Biomed. J.* **2019**, *23*, 190–199. [CrossRef]
482. Faraji, A.H.; Wipf, P. Nanoparticles in cellular drug delivery. *Bioorganic Med. Chem.* **2009**, *17*, 2950–2962. [CrossRef]
483. Kong, G.; Braun, R.D.; Dewhirst, M.W. Hyperthermia enables tumor-specific nanoparticle delivery: Effect of particle size hyperthermia enables tumor-specific nanoparticle delivery: Effect of particle size 1. *Cancer Res.* **2000**, *60*, 4440–4445.
484. Trewyn, B.G.; Slowing, I.I.; Chen, H.; Lin, V.S. Synthesis and functionalization of a mesoporous silica nanoparticle based on the sol-gel process and applications in controlled release. *Acc. Chem. Res.* **2007**, *40*, 846–853. [CrossRef] [PubMed]

485. Kumari, A.; Singla, R.; Guliani, A.; Yadav, S.K. Nanoencapsulation for drug delivery. *EXCLI J.* **2014**, *13*, 265–286. [PubMed]
486. Mahapatro, A.; Singh, D.K. Biodegradable nanoparticles are excellent vehicle for site directed in-vivo delivery of drugs and vaccines. *J. Nanobiotechnol.* **2011**, *9*, 55. [CrossRef] [PubMed]
487. Riley, M.K.; Vermerris, W. Recent advances in nanomaterials for gene delivery—A review. *Nanomaterials* **2017**, *7*, 94. [CrossRef]
488. Ylä-Herttuala, S. Endgame: Glybera finally recommended for approval as the first gene therapy drug in the European Union. *Mol. Ther.* **2012**, *20*, 1831–1832. [CrossRef]
489. Loh, X.J.; Lee, T.-C.; Dou, Q.; Deen, G.R. Utilising inorganic nanocarriers for gene delivery. *Biomater. Sci.* **2016**, *4*, 70–86. [CrossRef]
490. Zhao, Y.; Huang, L. Lipid nanoparticles for gene delivery. *Adv. Genet.* **2014**, *88*, 13–36.
491. Martin, B.; Sainlos, M.; Aissaoui, A.; Oudrhiri, N.; Hauchecorne, M.; Vigneron, J.-P.; Lehn, J.-M.; Lehn, P. The design of cationic lipids for gene delivery. *Curr. Pharm. Des.* **2005**, *11*, 375–394. [CrossRef]
492. Nordling-David, M.M.; Golomb, G. Gene delivery by liposomes. *Isr. J. Chem.* **2013**, *53*, 737–747. [CrossRef]
493. Ropert, C. Liposomes as a gene delivery system. *Braz. J. Med. Biol. Res.* **1999**, *32*, 163–169. [CrossRef]
494. Zylberberg, C.; Gaskill, K.; Pasley, S.; Matosevic, S. Engineering liposomal nanoparticles for targeted gene therapy. *Gene Ther.* **2017**, *24*, 441–452. [CrossRef] [PubMed]
495. Santander-Ortega, M.J.; Lozano, M.V.; Uchegbu, I.F.; Schätzlein, A.G. 6—Dendrimers for gene therapy. In *Polymers and Nanomaterials for Gene Therapy*; Narain, R., Ed.; Woodhead Publishing: Cambridge, UK, 2016; pp. 113–146.
496. Eliyahu, H.; Barenholz, Y.; Domb, A.J. Polymers for DNA delivery. *Molecules* **2005**, *10*, 34–64. [CrossRef] [PubMed]
497. Sharma, M.R.R.; Rekha, C.P. Polymers for gene delivery: Current status and future perspectives. *Recent Patents DNA Gene Seq.* **2012**, *6*, 98–107.
498. Zhao, H.; Ding, R.; Zhao, X.; Li, Y.; Qu, L.; Pei, H.; Yildirimer, L.; Wu, Z.; Zhang, W. Graphene-based nanomaterials for drug and/or gene delivery, bioimaging, and tissue engineering. *Drug Discov. Today* **2017**, *22*, 1302–1317. [CrossRef] [PubMed]
499. Imani, R.; Mohabatpour, F.; Mostafavi, F. Graphene-based nano-carrier modifications for gene delivery applications. *Carbon N. Y.* **2018**, *140*, 569–591. [CrossRef]
500. Dolatabadi, J.E.N.; Omid, Y.O.; Losic, D. Carbon nanotubes as an advanced drug and gene delivery nanosystem. *Curr. Nanosci.* **2011**, *7*, 297–314. [CrossRef]
501. Ramos-Perez, V.; Cifuentes, A.; Coronas, N.; de Pablo, A.; Borrós, S. Modification of carbon nanotubes for gene delivery vectors. In *Nanomaterial Interfaces in Biology: Methods and Protocols*; Bergese, P., Hamad-Schifferli, K., Eds.; Humana Press: Totowa, NJ, USA, 2013; pp. 261–268.
502. Keasberry, N.A.; Yapp, C.W.; Idris, A. Mesoporous silica nanoparticles as a carrier platform for intracellular delivery of nucleic acids. *Biochemistry* **2017**, *82*, 655–662. [CrossRef]
503. Mendes, R.; Fernandes, A.R.; Baptista, P.V. Gold nanoparticle approach to the selective delivery of gene silencing in cancer—The case for combined delivery? *Genes* **2017**, *8*, 94. [CrossRef]
504. Ding, Y.; Jiang, Z.; Saha, K.; Kim, C.S.; Kim, S.T.; Landis, R.F.; Rotello, V.M. Gold nanoparticles for nucleic acid delivery. *Mol. Ther.* **2014**, *22*, 1075–1083. [CrossRef]
505. Majidi, S.; Zeinali Sehrig, F.; Samiei, M.; Milani, M.; Abbasi, E.; Dadashzadeh, K.; Akbarzadeh, A. Magnetic nanoparticles: Applications in gene delivery and gene therapy. *Artif. Cells Nanomed. Biotechnol.* **2016**, *44*, 1186–1193. [CrossRef]
506. McBain, S.C.; Yiu, H.H.P.; Dobson, J. Magnetic nanoparticles for gene and drug delivery. *Int. J. Nanomed.* **2008**, *3*, 169–180.
507. Giacca, M.; Zacchigna, S. Virus-mediated gene delivery for human gene therapy. *J. Control. Release* **2012**, *161*, 377–388. [CrossRef] [PubMed]
508. Domvri, K.; Zarogoulidis, P.; Porpodis, K.; Koffa, M.; Lambropoulou, M.; Kakolyris, S.; Minadakis, G.; Zarogoulidis, K.; Chatzaki, E. Gene therapy in liver diseases: State-of-the-art and future perspectives. *Curr. Gene Ther.* **2012**, *12*, 463–483. [CrossRef] [PubMed]
509. Nienhuis, A.W.; Nathwani, A.C.; Davidoff, A.M. Gene therapy for hemophilia. *Mol. Ther.* **2017**, *25*, 1163–1167. [CrossRef]

510. Luo, J.; Sun, M.; Kang, Q.; Peng, Y.; Jiang, W.; Luu, H.; Luo, Q.; Park, J.; Li, Y.; Haydon, R. Gene therapy for bone regeneration. *Curr. Gene Ther.* **2005**, *5*, 167–179. [CrossRef]
511. Pensak, M.J.; Lieberman, J.R. Gene therapy for bone regeneration. *Curr. Pharm. Des.* **2013**, *19*, 3466–3473. [CrossRef]
512. Shapiro, G.; Lieber, R.; Gazit, D.; Pelled, G. Recent advances and future of gene therapy for bone regeneration. *Curr. Osteoporos. Rep.* **2018**, *16*, 504–511. [CrossRef]
513. De Jong, W.H.; Borm, P.J.A. Drug delivery and nanoparticles:applications and hazards. *Int. J. Nanomed.* **2008**, *3*, 133–149. [CrossRef]
514. Navya, P.N.; Daima, H.K. Rational engineering of physicochemical properties of nanomaterials for biomedical applications with nanotoxicological perspectives. *Nano Converg.* **2016**, *3*, 1. [CrossRef]
515. Sperling, R.A.; Parak, W.J. Surface modification, functionalization and bioconjugation of colloidal inorganic nanoparticles. *Philos. Trans. R. Soc. A Math. Phys. Eng. Sci.* **2010**, *368*, 1333–1383. [CrossRef]
516. Liu, C.; Zhang, N. Chapter 13—Nanoparticles in gene therapy: Principles, prospects, and challenges. In *Nanoparticles in Translational Science and Medicine*; Villaverde, A.B.T.-P., Ed.; Academic Press: Cambridge, MA, USA, 2011; Volume 104, pp. 509–562.
517. Islam, M.; Park, T.-E.; Singh, B.; Maharjan, S.; Firdous, J.; Kang, S.-K.; Yun, C.-H.; Choi, Y.; Cho, C. Major degradable polycations as carriers for DNA and siRNA. *J. Control. Release* **2014**, *193*, 74–89. [CrossRef] [PubMed]
518. Wang, Y.; Li, Z.; Weber, T.J.; Hu, D.; Lin, C.-T.; Li, J.; Lin, Y. In Situ Live Cell Sensing of multiple nucleotides exploiting DNA/RNA aptamers and graphene oxide nanosheets. *Anal. Chem.* **2013**, *85*, 6775–6782. [CrossRef] [PubMed]
519. Keles, E.; Song, Y.; Du, D.; Dong, W.-J.; Lin, Y. Recent progress in nanomaterials for gene delivery applications. *Biomater. Sci.* **2016**, *4*, 1291–1309. [CrossRef] [PubMed]
520. Radu, D.R.; Lai, C.-Y.; Jeftinija, K.; Rowe, E.W.; Jeftinija, S.; Lin, V.S.-Y. A Polyamidoamine dendrimer-capped mesoporous silica nanosphere-based gene transfection reagent. *J. Am. Chem. Soc.* **2004**, *126*, 13216–13217. [CrossRef] [PubMed]
521. Palmerston Mendes, L.; Pan, J.; Torchilin, V.P. Dendrimers as nanocarriers for nucleic acid and drug delivery in cancer therapy. *Molecules* **2017**, *22*, 1401. [CrossRef] [PubMed]
522. Kukowska-Latallo, J.F.; Bielinska, A.U.; Johnson, J.; Spindle, R.; Tomalia, D.A.; Baker, J.R. Efficient transfer of genetic material into mammalian cells using starburst polyamidoamine dendrimers. *Proc. Natl. Acad. Sci. USA* **1996**, *93*, 4897–4902. [CrossRef] [PubMed]
523. Chen, L.; Deng, H.; Cui, H.; Fang, J.; Zuo, Z.; Deng, J.; Li, Y.; Wang, X.; Zhao, L. Inflammatory responses and inflammation-associated diseases in organs. *Oncotarget* **2017**, *9*, 7204–7218. [CrossRef] [PubMed]
524. Busscher, H.J.; van der Mei, H.C.; Subbiahdoss, G.; Jutte, P.C.; van den Dungen, J.J.A.M.; Zaat, S.A.J.; Schultz, M.J.; Grainger, D.W. Biomaterial-associated infection: Locating the finish line in the race for the surface. *Sci. Transl. Med.* **2012**, *4*, 153rv10. [CrossRef]
525. Buhmann, M.T.; Stiefel, P.; Maniura-Weber, K.; Ren, Q. In vitro biofilm models for device-related infections. *Trends Biotechnol.* **2016**, *34*, 945–948. [CrossRef]
526. Lin, G.-L.; McGinley, J.P.; Drysdale, S.B.; Pollard, A.J. Epidemiology and immune pathogenesis of viral sepsis. *Front. Immunol.* **2018**, *9*, 2147. [CrossRef]
527. Oliveira, W.F.; Silva, P.M.S.; Silva, R.C.S.; Silva, G.M.M.; Machado, G.; Coelho, L.C.B.B.; Correia, M.T.S. Staphylococcus aureus and Staphylococcus epidermidis infections on implants. *J. Hosp. Infect.* **2018**, *98*, 111–117. [CrossRef] [PubMed]
528. Holzapfel, B.M.; Reichert, J.C.; Schantz, J.-T.; Gbureck, U.; Rackwitz, L.; Nöth, U.; Jakob, F.; Rudert, M.; Groll, J.; Hutmacher, D.W. How smart do biomaterials need to be? A translational science and clinical point of view. *Adv. Drug Deliv. Rev.* **2013**, *65*, 581–603. [CrossRef] [PubMed]
529. Ng, V. Risk of Disease Transmission With Bone Allograft. *Orthopedics* **2012**, *35*, 679–681. [CrossRef] [PubMed]
530. Jun, I.; Han, H.-S.; Edwards, J.R.; Jeon, H. Electrospun Fibrous scaffolds for tissue engineering: Viewpoints on architecture and fabrication. *Int. J. Mol. Sci.* **2018**, *19*, 745. [CrossRef]
531. Gong, T.; Xie, J.; Liao, J.; Zhang, T.; Lin, S.; Lin, Y. Nanomaterials and bone regeneration. *Bone Res.* **2015**, *3*, 1–7. [CrossRef]
532. Gopalu, K.; Rangaraj, S.; Venkatachalam, R.; Kannan, N. Influence of ZrO_2, SiO_2, Al_2O_3 and TiO_2 nanoparticles on maize seed germination under different growth conditions. *IET Nanobiotechnol.* **2016**, *10*, 171–177.

533. Dhandayuthapani, B.; Yoshida, Y.; Maekawa, T.; Kumar, D.S. Polymeric scaffolds in tissue engineering application: A review. *Int. J. Polym. Sci.* **2011**, *2011*, 290602. [CrossRef]
534. Mozumder, M.S.; Zhu, J.; Perinpanayagam, H. Titania-polymeric powder coatings with nano-topography support enhanced human mesenchymal cell responses. *J. Biomed. Mater. Res. Part A* **2012**, *100*, 2695–2709. [CrossRef]
535. Trentler, T.J.; Denler, T.E.; Bertone, J.F.; Agrawal, A.; Colvin, V.L. Synthesis of TiO_2 nanocrystals by nonhydrolytic solution-based reactions. *J. Am. Chem. Soc.* **1999**, *121*, 1613–1614. [CrossRef]
536. Hussian, H.A.R.A.; Hassan, M.A.M.; Agool, I.R. Synthesis of titanium dioxide (TiO_2) nanofiber and nanotube using different chemical method. *Optik* **2016**, *127*, 2996–2999. [CrossRef]
537. Shi, H.; Magaye, R.; Castranova, V.; Zhao, J. Titanium dioxide nanoparticles: A review of current toxicological data. *Part. Fibre Toxicol.* **2013**, *10*, 15. [CrossRef] [PubMed]
538. Ashkarran, A.A.; Fakhari, M.; Hamidinezhad, H.; Haddadi, H.; Nourani, M.R. TiO_2 nanoparticles immobilized on carbon nanotubes for enhanced visible-light photo-induced activity. *J. Mater. Res. Technol.* **2015**, *4*, 126–132. [CrossRef]
539. Tsuchiya, H.; Macak, J.M.; Müller, L.; Kunze, J.; Müller, F.; Greil, P.; Virtanen, S.; Schmuki, P. Hydroxyapatite growth on anodic TiO_2 nanotubes. *J. Biomed. Mater. Res. Part A* **2006**, *77*, 534–541. [CrossRef] [PubMed]
540. Inzunza, D.; Covarrubias, C.; Von Marttens, A.; Leighton, Y.; Carvajal, J.C.; Valenzuela, F.; Diaz-Dosque, M.; Méndez, N.; Martínez, C.; Pino, A.M.; et al. Synthesis of nanostructured porous silica coatings on titanium and their cell adhesive and osteogenic differentiation properties. *J. Biomed. Mater. Res. Part A* **2013**, *102*, 37–48. [CrossRef]
541. Assad, M.; Chernyshov, A.; Leroux, M.; Rivard, C. A new porous titanium-nickel alloy: Part 1. Cytotoxicity and genotoxicity evaluation. *Biomed. Mater. Eng.* **2002**, *12*, 225–237.
542. Gu, Y.W.; Khor, K.; Pan, D.; Cheang, P. Activity of plasma sprayed yttria stabilized zirconia reinforced hydroxyapatite/Ti–6Al–4V composite coatings in simulated body fluid. *Biomaterials* **2004**, *25*, 3177–3185. [CrossRef]
543. Maschhoff, P.M.; Geilich, B.M.; Webster, T.J. Greater fibroblast proliferation on an ultrasonicated ZnO/PVC nanocomposite material. *Int. J. Nanomed.* **2014**, *9*, 257–263.
544. Pei, B.; Wang, W.; Dunne, N.; Li, X. Applications of carbon nanotubes in bone tissue regeneration and engineering: Superiority, concerns, current advancements, and prospects. *Nanomaterials* **2019**, *9*, 1501. [CrossRef] [PubMed]
545. Subbiah, R.; Du, P.; Van, S.Y.; Suhaeri, M.; Hwang, M.P.; Lee, K.; Kwideok, P. Fibronectin-tethered graphene oxide as an artificial matrix for osteogenesis. *Biomed. Mater.* **2014**, *9*, 65003. [CrossRef] [PubMed]
546. Zhao, C.; Lu, X.; Zanden, Z.; Liu, J. The promising application of graphene oxide as coating materials in orthopedic implants: Preparation, characterization and cell behavior. *Biomed. Mater.* **2015**, *10*, 15019. [CrossRef] [PubMed]
547. Al-Jumaili, A.; Alancherry, S.; Bazaka, K.; Jacob, M.V. Review on the antimicrobial properties of carbon nanostructures. *Materials* **2017**, *10*, 1066. [CrossRef] [PubMed]
548. Nishida, E.; Miyaji, H.; Takita, H.; Kanayama, I.; Tsuji, M.; Akasaka, T.; Sugaya, T.; Sakagami, R.; Kawanami, M. Graphene oxide coating facilitates the bioactivity of scaffold material for tissue engineering. *Jpn. J. Appl. Phys.* **2014**, *53*, 06JD04. [CrossRef]
549. Guazzo, R.; Gardin, C.; Bellin, G.; Sbricoli, L.; Ferroni, L.; Ludovichetti, F.S.; Piattelli, A.; Antoniac, I.; Bressan, E.; Zavan, B. Graphene-based nanomaterials for tissue engineering in the dental field. *Nanomaterials* **2018**, *8*, 349. [CrossRef] [PubMed]
550. Vera-Sánchez, M.; Aznar-Cervantes, S.; Jover, E.; García-Bernal, D.; Oñate-Sánchez, R.; Hernández-Romero, D.; Moraleda, J.M.; Collado-González, M.; Rodríguez-Lozano, F.J.; Cenis, J. Silk-fibroin and graphene oxide composites promote human periodontal ligament stem cell spontaneous differentiation into osteo/cementoblast-like cells. *Stem Cells Dev.* **2016**, *25*, 1742–1754. [CrossRef] [PubMed]
551. Ghassemi, T.; Shahroodi, A.; Ebrahimzadeh, M.H.; Mousavian, A.; Movaffagh, J.; Moradi, A. Current concepts in scaffolding for bone tissue engineering. *Arch. Bone Jt. Surg.* **2018**, *6*, 90–99.
552. Farack, J.; Wolf-Brandstetter, C.; Glorius, S.; Nies, B.; Standke, G.; Quadbeck, P.; Worch, H.; Scharnweber, D. The effect of perfusion culture on proliferation and differentiation of human mesenchymal stem cells on biocorrodible bone replacement material. *Mater. Sci. Eng. B* **2011**, *176*, 1767–1772. [CrossRef]

553. Zhang, P.; Wu, T.; Kong, J.-L. In situ monitoring of intracellular controlled drug release from mesoporous silica nanoparticles coated with pH-responsive charge-reversal polymer. *ACS Appl. Mater. Interfaces* **2014**, *6*, 17446–17453. [CrossRef]
554. Kim, S.-S.; Ahn, K.-M.; Park, M.S.; Lee, J.-H.; Choi, C.Y.; Kim, B.-S. A poly(lactide-co-glycolide)/hydroxyapatite composite scaffold with enhanced osteoconductivity. *J. Biomed. Mater. Res. Part A* **2007**, *80*, 206–215. [CrossRef]
555. Rider, P.; Kačarević, Ž.P.; Alkildani, S.; Retnasingh, S.; Barbeck, M. Bioprinting of tissue engineering scaffolds. *J. Tissue Eng.* **2018**, *9*, 2041731418802090. [CrossRef]
556. Park, J.W.; Hwang, S.R.; Yoon, I.-S. Advanced growth factor delivery systems in wound management and skin regeneration. *Molecules* **2017**, *22*, 1259. [CrossRef]
557. Kleinman, H.K.; Philp, D.; Hoffman, M.P. Role of the extracellular matrix in morphogenesis. *Curr. Opin. Biotechnol.* **2003**, *14*, 526–532. [CrossRef] [PubMed]
558. Lee, E.J.; Kasper, F.K.; Mikos, A.G. Biomaterials for tissue engineering. *Ann. Biomed. Eng.* **2014**, *42*, 323–337. [CrossRef] [PubMed]
559. Sato, M.; Webster, T.J.; Sato, M.; Webster, T.J. Nanobiotechnology: Implications for the future of nanotechnology in orthopedic applications Nanobiotechnology: Implications for the future of nanotechnology in orthopedic applications. *Expert Rev. Med. Devices* **2004**, *1*, 105–114. [CrossRef] [PubMed]
560. Demais, V.; Audrain, C.; Mabilleau, G.; Chappard, D.; Baslé, M.F. Diversity of bone matrix adhesion proteins modulates osteoblast attachment and organization of actin cytoskeleton. *Morphologie* **2014**, *98*, 53–64. [CrossRef] [PubMed]
561. Tran, N.; Webster, T.J. Increased osteoblast functions in the presence of hydroxyapatite-coated iron oxide nanoparticles. *Acta Biomater.* **2011**, *7*, 1298–1306. [CrossRef] [PubMed]
562. Smith, L.A.; Ma, P.X. Nano-fibrous scaffolds for tissue engineering. *Colloids Surf. B Biointerfaces* **2004**, *39*, 125–131. [CrossRef] [PubMed]
563. Tuzlakoglu, K.; Bolgen, N.; Salgado, A.J.; Gomes, M.E.; Piskin, E.; Reis, R.L. Nano- and micro-fiber combined scaffolds: A new architecture for bone tissue engineering. *J. Mater. Sci. Mater. Med.* **2005**, *16*, 1099–1104. [CrossRef]
564. Shin, M.; Yoshimoto, H.; Vacanti, J.P. In vivo bone tissue engineering using mesenchymal stem cells on a novel electrospun nanofibrous scaffold. *Tissue Eng.* **2004**, *10*, 33–41. [CrossRef]
565. Li, W.J.; Tuli, R.; Huang, X.; Laquerriere, P.; Tuan, R.S. Multilineage differentiation of human mesenchymal stem cells in a three-dimensional nanofibrous scaffold. *Biomaterials* **2005**, *26*, 5158–5166. [CrossRef]
566. Li, W.J.; Tuli, R.; Okafor, C.; Derfoul, A.; Danielson, K.G.; Hall, D.J.; Tuan, R.S. A three-dimensional nanofibrous scaffold for cartilage tissue engineering using human mesenchymal stem cells. *Biomaterials* **2005**, *26*, 599–609. [CrossRef]
567. Woo, K.M.; Chen, V.J.; Ma, P.X. Nano-fibrous scaffolding architecture selectively enhances protein adsorption contributing to cell attachment. *J. Biomed. Mater. Res.* **2003**, *67*, 531–537. [CrossRef] [PubMed]
568. Woo, K.M.; Jun, J.H.; Chen, V.J.; Seo, J.; Baek, J.H.; Ryoo, H.M.; Kim, G.S.; Somerman, M.J.; Ma, P.X. Nano-fibrous scaffolding promotes osteoblast differentiation and biomineralization. *Biomaterials* **2007**, *28*, 335–343. [CrossRef]
569. Bhattarai, N.; Edmondson, D.; Veiseh, O.; Matsen, F.A.; Zhang, M. Electrospun chitosan-based nanofibers and their cellular compatibility. *Biomaterials* **2005**, *26*, 6176–6184. [CrossRef] [PubMed]
570. Zhang, L.; Wang, Z.; Xu, C.; Li, Y.; Gao, J.; Wang, W.; Liu, Y. High strength graphene oxide/polyvinyl alcohol composite hydrogels. *J. Mater. Chem.* **2011**, *21*, 10399–10406. [CrossRef]
571. Goenka, S.; Sant, V.; Sant, S. Graphene-based nanomaterials for drug delivery and tissue engineering. *J. Control. Release* **2014**, *173*, 75–88. [CrossRef] [PubMed]
572. Yu, M.F.; Lourie, O.; Dyer, M.J.; Moloni, K.; Kelly, T.; Ruoff, R. Strength and breaking mechanism of multiwalled carbon nanotubes under tensile load. *Science* **2000**, *287*, 637–640. [CrossRef]
573. Kim, S.-S.; Sun Park, M.; Gwak, S.-J.; Choi, C.; Kim, B.-S. Accelerated bonelike apatite growth on porous polymer/ceramic composite scaffolds in vitro. *Tissue Eng.* **2006**, *12*, 2997–3006. [CrossRef]
574. Okamoto, M.; John, B. Synthetic biopolymer nanocomposites for tissue engineering scaffolds. *Prog. Polym. Sci.* **2013**, *38*, 1487–1503. [CrossRef]
575. Hench, L.L. Bioceramics: From concept to clinic. *J. Am. Ceram. Soc.* **1991**, *74*, 1487–1510. [CrossRef]

576. Wei, B.; Yao, Q.; Guo, Y.; Mao, F.; Liu, S.; Xu, Y.; Wang, L. Three-dimensional polycaprolactone–hydroxyapatite scaffolds combined with bone marrow cells for cartilage tissue engineering. *J. Biomater. Appl.* **2015**, *30*, 160–170. [CrossRef]
577. Wei, G.; Ma, P.X. Structure and properties of nano-hydroxyapatite/polymer composite scaffolds for bone tissue engineering. *Biomaterials* **2004**, *25*, 4749–4757. [CrossRef] [PubMed]
578. Du, C.; Cui, F.-Z.; Feng, Q.; Zhu, X.D.; Groot, K. Tissue response to nano-hydroxyapatite/collagen composite implants in marrow cavity. *J. Biomed. Mat. Res.* **1998**, *42*, 540–548. [CrossRef]
579. Li, Z.; Yubao, L.; Aiping, Y.; Xuelin, P.; Xuejiang, W.; Xiang, Z. Preparation and in vitro investigation of chitosan/nano-hydroxyapatite composite used as bone substitute materials. *J. Mater. Sci. Mater. Med.* **2005**, *16*, 213–219. [CrossRef] [PubMed]
580. Jiang, W.G.; Sanders, A.J.; Katoh, M.; Ungefroren, H.; Gieseler, F.; Prince, M.; Thompson, S.K.; Zollo, M.; Spano, D.; Dhawan, P.; et al. Tissue invasion and metastasis: Molecular, biological and clinical perspectives. *Semin. Cancer Biol.* **2015**, *35*, S244–S275. [CrossRef]
581. Srinivasan, M.; Rajabi, M.A.; Mousa, S. Chapter 3—Nanobiomaterials in cancer therapy. In *Nanobiomaterials in Cancer Therapy*; Grumezescu, A.M., Ed.; William Andrew Publishing: Norwich, NY, USA, 2016; pp. 57–89.
582. Hernandez, R.K.; Wade, S.W.; Reich, A.; Pirolli, M.; Liede, A.; Lyman, G.H. Incidence of bone metastases in patients with solid tumors: Analysis of oncology electronic medical records in the United States. *BMC Cancer* **2018**, *18*, 44. [CrossRef]
583. Adjei, I.M.; Temples, M.N.; Brown, S.B.; Sharma, B. Targeted nanomedicine to treat bone metastasis. *Pharmaceutics* **2018**, *10*, 205. [CrossRef]
584. Serafini, A.N. Therapy of metastatic bone pain. *J. Nucl. Med.* **2001**, *42*, 895–906.
585. Auffinger, B.; Morshed, R.; Tobias, A.; Cheng, Y.; Ahmed, A.U.; Lesniak, M.S. Drug-loaded nanoparticle systems and adult stem cells: A potential marriage for the treatment of malignant glioma? *Oncotarget* **2013**, *4*, 378–396. [CrossRef]
586. Brannon-Peppas, L.; Blanchette, J.O. Nanoparticle and targeted systems for cancer therapy. *Adv. Drug Deliv. Rev.* **2004**, *56*, 1649–1659. [CrossRef]
587. Chu, K.F.; Dupuy, D.E. Thermal ablation of tumours: Biological mechanisms and advances in therapy. *Nat. Rev. Cancer* **2014**, *14*, 199–208. [CrossRef]
588. Nichols, J.W.; Bae, Y.H. EPR: Evidence and fallacy. *J. Control. Release* **2014**, *190*, 451–464. [CrossRef] [PubMed]
589. Navya, P.N.; Kaphle, A.; Srinivas, S.P.; Bhargava, S.K.; Rotello, V.M.; Daima, H.K. Current trends and challenges in cancer management and therapy using designer nanomaterials. *Nano Converg.* **2019**, *6*, 23. [CrossRef] [PubMed]

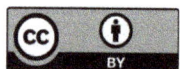

© 2020 by the authors. Licensee MDPI, Basel, Switzerland. This article is an open access article distributed under the terms and conditions of the Creative Commons Attribution (CC BY) license (http://creativecommons.org/licenses/by/4.0/).

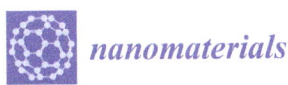

Review

A Review of Biodegradable Natural Polymer-Based Nanoparticles for Drug Delivery Applications

Humaira Idrees [1,*], Syed Zohaib Javaid Zaidi [2,*], Aneela Sabir [1], Rafi Ullah Khan [1,2], Xunli Zhang [3] and Sammer-ul Hassan [3,*]

1. Department of Polymer Engineering and Technology, University of the Punjab, Lahore 54590, Pakistan; Aneela.pet.ceet@pu.edu.pk (A.S.); Rkhan.icet@pu.edu.pk (R.U.K.)
2. Institute of Chemical Engineering and Technology, University of the Punjab, Lahore 54000, Punjab, Pakistan
3. Mechanical Engineering, Faculty of Engineering and Physical Sciences, University of Southampton, Southampton SO17 1BJ, UK; XL.Zhang@soton.ac.uk
* Correspondence: humaira.idrees212@gmail.com (H.I.); zohaib.icet@pu.edu.pk (S.Z.J.Z.); s.hassan@soton.ac.uk (S.-u.H.)

Received: 4 August 2020; Accepted: 28 September 2020; Published: 5 October 2020

Abstract: Biodegradable natural polymers have been investigated extensively as the best choice for encapsulation and delivery of drugs. The research has attracted remarkable attention in the pharmaceutical industry. The shortcomings of conventional dosage systems, along with modified and targeted drug delivery methods, are addressed by using polymers with improved bioavailability, biocompatibility, and lower toxicity. Therefore, nanomedicines are now considered to be an innovative type of medication. This review critically examines the use of natural biodegradable polymers and their drug delivery systems for local or targeted and controlled/sustained drug release against fatal diseases.

Keywords: polymers; biodegradable; nanoparticles; drug delivery; pharmaceutical

1. Introduction

Enormous amounts of research and exploration of disorders and diseases have helped us to achieve an appropriate dosage system to stabilize a patient's health [1,2]. Conventional drug delivery systems such as salting-out (salting-out agent required), supercritical fluid technology (capillary nozzle and a supercritical fluid required), dialysis (capillary nozzle and a supercritical fluid required), solvent evaporation (surfactant required), and nanoprecipitation (non-solvent for the polymer required) are also used [1]. Moreover, conventional drug delivery systems have several deficiencies such as reduced patient compliance, shorter half-life of drugs, and high peak, etc. There is, thus, increased interest amongst scientists in developing beneficial methods to improve drug delivery systems as time passes.

A hundred years ago, Paul Ehrlich proposed the idea of tiny-drug loaded magic bullets. Later, the concept of a submicron drug delivery system was conceived by Kumar and Banker in 1996. Among these carriers, liposomes and micro/nanoparticles have been the most widely considered. Liposomes present a few technological limitations, such as poor stability, poor reproducibility, and low drug encapsulation efficiency. This technology is suitable for low molecular weight drugs. Hence, the polymeric nanoparticle drug delivery system has been proposed as an effective alternative drug delivery system to the conventional system [3]. Scheme 1 illustrates the general preparation methods for nanoparticles and their applications for drug delivery systems.

Brachais et al., in 1998, prepared a solid dispersion method to synthesize an orally-controlled drug release system. They used a biodegradable hydrophobic matrix, poly (methyl glyoxylate), and a water-soluble drug, metoprolol. Jeong et al., in 1999, studied the star-shaped block copolymers using bio-degradable polyethylene oxide and poly (L-lactic acid), in which copolymers exhibit reversible sol-gel transition [4]. Avnesh Kumari et al., in 2010, reviewed biodegradable nanoparticles such as chitosan, gelatin, poly(lactic-co-glycolic acid), Polycaprolactone, PLA(Poly Lactic acid), and gelatin as having better encapsulation properties for drug release [5]. In 2014, Carlotta Marianecci et al. presented a review on surfactant vesicles, which generated interest among the scientific community in the last decades. They studied how niosomes, which are self-assembled vesicular nanocarriers for the drug delivery system, overcome the side effects of liposomes due to their less-toxic effect, are stable, and have a low cost [6]. Jeong et al., in 1999, studied star-shaped block copolymers using bio-degradable polyethylene oxide and poly (L-lactic acid); these copolymers exhibit reversible sol-gel transition.

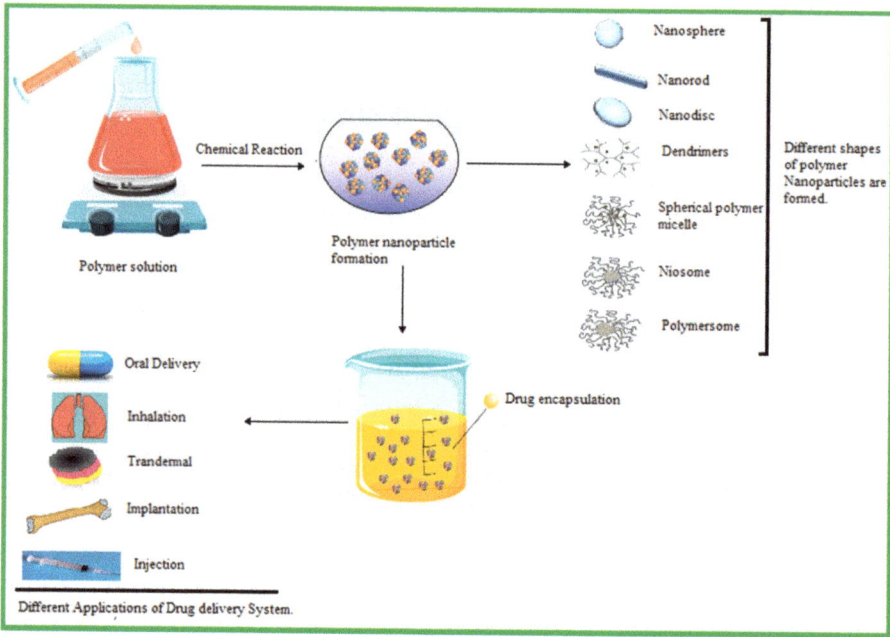

Scheme 1. Representation of the general method of synthesis/preparation of nanoparticles.

Therefore, exponential growth in the development of modified drug delivery systems is essential for dosage form improvement. Modified drug delivery systems have been considered to transport active agents in higher demand due to their delivery process, programmed target-specificity, cellular uptake, clearance, toxicity, metabolism, pharmacokinetics, excretion, greater half-life in terms of repeated administration of drugs and improved patient health [7]. The successful drug delivery systems are designed to increase the efficiency of the drug in the body by using external or internal stimuli, and nanocarrier features are modified according to the physicochemical properties of drugs [2]. Indeed, drugs essentially require highly effective, controlled release along with biocompatible encapsulation to increase patient compliance [2].

Due to the rapid increase in research in the field of polymer science, the structural backbone for the development of novel and modified drug delivery systems is considered [8]. Primarily, non-biodegradable polymeric nanoparticles, such as polymethylmethacrylate, polyacrylamide, and polystyrene, have been used for drug delivery systems; however, a huge level of toxicity and detrimental health consequences from non-biodegradable polymers have been observed. Therefore, biocompatible polymers, due to their immense properties and growth, are under discussion within the scientific community for in vivo and in vitro diagnosis and treatment of diseases [8–10].

Polymeric nanostructured materials (PNMs) have played a vital role in therapeutic diagnosis and treatment of diseases [11–14]. Through the development of PNMs as new biomaterials, significant improvement in the quality of healthcare can be achieved, due to the better accuracy and reliability in diagnostics, more effective targeting of therapeutic agents, and improved usability of scaffolds for tissue engineering and regenerative medicines [15–17]. PNMs, including micelles, polymerases, nanoparticles, nanocapsules, nanogels, nanofibers, dendrimers, brush polymers, and nanocomposites can be prepared for delivery via a variety of pathways. Their properties, such as stability, size, shape, surface charge, surface chemistry, mechanical strength, and porosity can be tailored toward specific functionalities that are required to meet the needs of the targeted biomedical application. As a result, the development of biomedical PNMs has attracted plenty of research in the field, and a vast number of recent publications can now be found in the literature.

An amalgamation of nanoparticles with polymer science has led to a new direction in the field of biomedical engineering, packaging, food processing, tissue engineering and improved treatment for water-insoluble and soluble drug delivery systems. Nanoparticles are characterized by a particle size range of 1 to 100 nm. 'Nano' is derived from the Greek word 'Nanos' which means dwarf [9–18]. The basis of the morphology, chemical and physical properties of nanoparticles relate to the different derivative materials such as ceramic, liquid, metal, semiconductors, and carbon-based nanoparticles, which may be biodegradable or non-biodegradable [19]. Nanoparticles or smart polymers are under consideration due to their advantages, including a greater surface to charge ratio, ease of characterization and ease of synthesize, the fact that they are reproducible, stable after administration, non-immunogenic, and have significant absorption properties. These unique features make them of huge interest as carriers for drugs and inexpensive formulation [20]. The effective therapeutic transformation from a macro- to a nano-drug delivery system relates to the controlled release of a drug on a target as compared to the less targeted release of conventional drug delivery systems [21]. Therefore, depending upon the method of synthesis, nanomedicines can be one of two types, i.e., nanospheres which encapsulate drugs into a smart polymeric shell (nanopolymer shell) and nanocapsules in which drugs are dispersed into the polymeric matrix [22,23]. The representation of both types of nanomedicines is shown in Figure 1. The synthesis of a nano-drug delivery system depends upon the targeted part of the body and organ. The biocompatibility and degradability of nanomedicines must be considered as they carry DNA, drugs, and proteins to the targeted area [24]. The size and surface-to-charge ratio of polymer nanoparticles play a significant role in maintaining systematic flow across the cell membrane [25,26]. The efficiency of the drugs depends upon the properties of the polymer, nanoparticles, solvent, and encapsulation method.

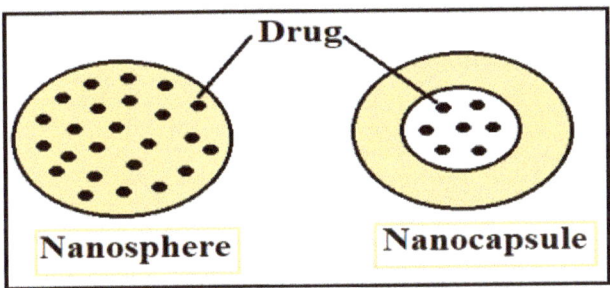

Figure 1. Schematic of nanomedicines: nanospheres and nanocapsules.

Smart polymers or nanoparticles play an essential role in the treatment of chronic diseases such as cancer, diabetes, cardiovascular and neurodegenerative disorders [27,28]. Various natural and synthetic polymers play a significant role in a targeted drug delivery system [29,30]. Some natural and synthetic polymeric materials have easy accessibility, biocompatibility, bio-decomposition properties, and easy modification. Reactive groups, such as amino, hydroxyl and carboxylic groups present on polymers, easily interact with other synthesized materials, thus endowing new modified hybrid materials with improved physical and chemical properties [31–33]. There are various types of natural polymers such as proteins, polysaccharides, peptides, collagen, albumin, gelatin, chitosan, alginate, fibroin, and synthetic polymers such as polylactic acid (PLA) and polyglycolic acid (PGA) [34]. Synthetic and natural polymers have their disadvantages and advantages. Biocompatible polymers are mostly preferred because they are economical, easily prepared, and extremely stable in the biological fluid; they show better proliferation, adhesion, and target usage with high efficiency [34]. Nanomaterials usually consist of carbon-based materials such as fullerenes, carbon dots, nanodiamonds, nano-foams, carbon nanotubes, and polymers. Inorganic nanoparticles are metals such as gold, silver and metal oxides (cerium oxide, iron oxide, silicon dioxide, titanium oxide), semiconductors and metal nanoparticles [33]. Figure 2 shows the schematic of the polymer classification.

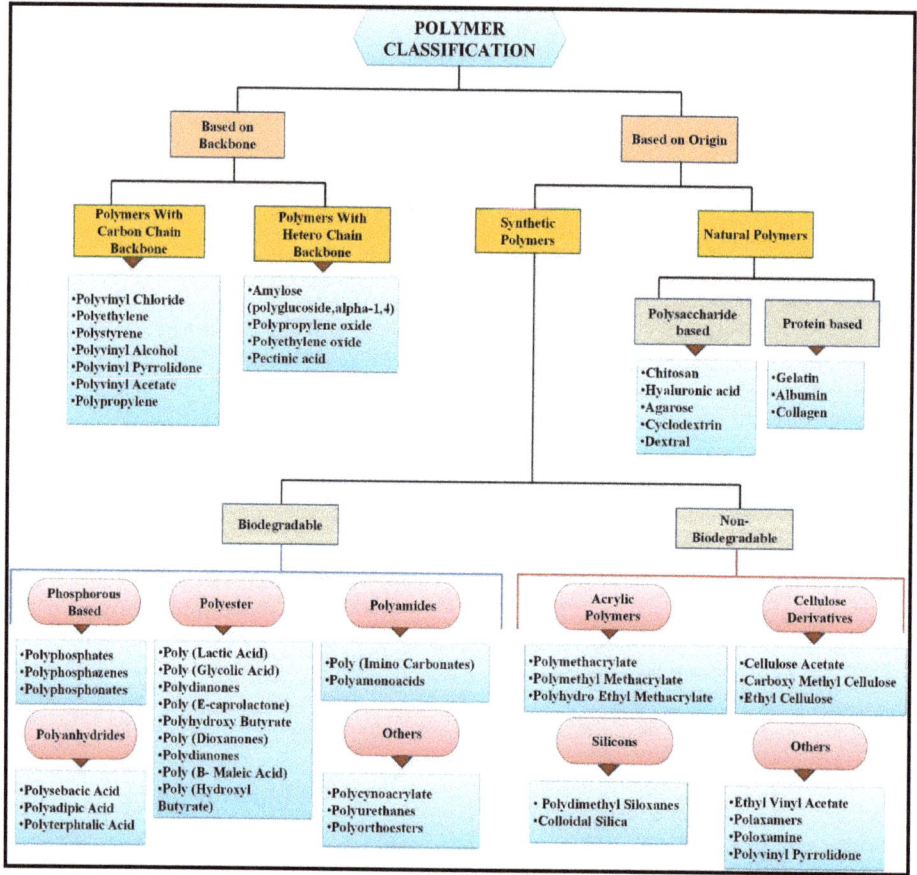

Figure 2. Schematic of polymer classification. Reference is taken from [35]. Copyright ©2019, Elsevier.

In general, the aim and specificity of the present review are highly important for some natural, biodegradable and biocompatible polymers. The present review covers some popular polymers such as chitosan, albumin, alginate, hydroxyapatite, and hyaluronic acid currently used for drug delivery systems. Furthermore, it provides information about the functionalization of the above-mentioned polymers to enhance their properties and develop an effective drug release system [36].

2. Biodegradable and Non-Biodegradable Polymer Nanomaterials (PNM): General Properties

2.1. Biodegradable Polymer Properties

Biodegradable polymers undergo degradation, non-enzymatically and enzymatically and generate a harmless, biocompatible by-product. Biodegradable polymers have a notable emphasis on the chemistry in the scheme of new molecules in targeted drug delivery applications. The use of biocompatible polymers reduces the side effects of a given drug. Biodegradable biomaterials have no constant inflammatory effect, good permeability, and good therapeutic properties. The performance of biodegradable polymers depends upon the following aspects:

(1) In situ administration of formulations
(2) On-demand delivery of the molecular targeted agent
(3) The fact that a targeted agent can be combined with radiotherapy and immunotherapy
(4) The use of FDA approved biodegradable polymers [35]

2.2. Non-Biodegradable Polymer Properties

Clinically non-biodegradable polymers are used for local injection of antibodies. Mostly non-biodegradable polymers such as acrylic polymers, cellulose derivatives, silicons, etc. are mentioned in Figure 2 in the introduction section. Polymethyl methacrylate (PMMA) is an acrylic-based non-biodegradable polymer that is mostly used for implantation as bone cement or in the form of PMMA beads. While widely used, PMMA has many disadvantages: it is a substrate for bacterial colonization, has low biocompatibility, is non-biodegradable in bead form, the release of antibiotic decreases with time, it is not heat resistant, it has fewer antibiotic elimination properties, delivery of the antibiotic, it has a variable surface area which results in uneven release rates. Due to the disadvantages of non-biodegradable polymers, scientists are interested in developing biodegradable, biocompatible polymer synthesis for a drug delivery system [37]. The main objective of this review is to study the role of five biodegradable polymers in a drug delivery system.

3. Chitosan-Based Nanoparticles

Chitosan is a polysaccharide, with 2-deoxy-2-(acetylamino) glucose units bonded by 1,4-glycosidic linkages; it is prepared by partial N-deacetylation of chitin (Figure 3). Chitin has good mechanical strength, is biocompatible, bioactive and biodegradable, but has limited utilization due to low solubility. Therefore, it is converted into chitosan by deacetylation in the presence of hydroxide at high temperatures [38]. Chitin is extracted from marine organisms such as lobsters and molluscs, and from crab shells, insects, yeast, and fungi. A long polymeric chain is composed of glycosidic linkages. Chitosan is insoluble in sulfuric acid and phosphoric acid but soluble in organic solutions with a pH lower than 6.5, such as acetic acid, citric acid, and tartaric acid. Due to its solubility, chitosan is present in films, hydrogels, pastes, nanoparticles, and nanofilms [39,40]. Chitosan has a greater degree of deacetylation and molecular weight; the variation in the size of a particle and aggregation is dependent upon the degree of deacetylation and molecular weight [3]. Recently, chitosan and its derivatives have been considered as the best vehicle in the pharmaceutical field due to their biocompatibility, and their non-carcinogenic, non-toxic, antibacterial properties. Chitosan offers a large range of options for industries and scientists for the generation of modified and novel drug delivery systems. Chitosan acts as an auxiliary agent in the therapeutic application for tissue engineering, wound dressing, and sliming. Protonation of the amino group in an acidic medium results in cation formation. Chitosan exhibits unique behavior because of its cationic nature [38,41]. Modification of chitosan and the stability of drugs delivered using chitosan decrease the adverse effects of diseases and increase the biocompatibility of drugs for various diseases [42].

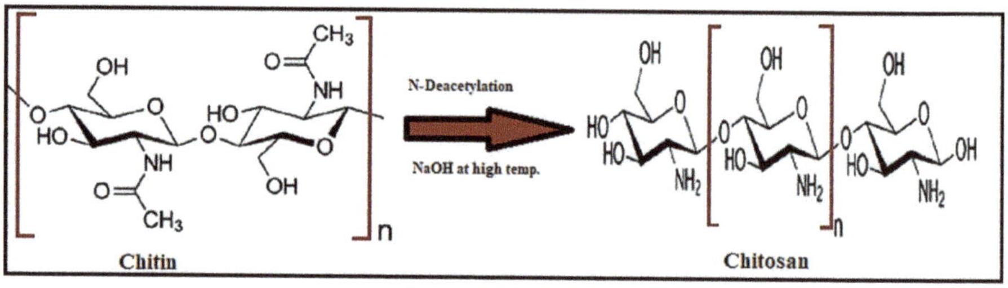

Figure 3. Structure of chitosan.

Chitosan nanoparticles widely act as a potential carrier for therapeutic applications. The cationic nature of chitosan is useful for the development of a drug delivery system. One of the major benefits of chitosan nanoparticles is their rapid uptake across the cell membrane due to the presence of amine groups. Complexation of chitosan with anionic charged polymers results in an interesting gelation property [43]. Methods generally applied for the preparation of chitosan nanoparticles include the microemulsion method, ionic gelation, and micro-emulsion solvent diffusion method [3,38]. In the microemulsion method, chitosan nanoparticles are prepared, and micellar droplets are cross-linked in the presence of glutaraldehyde. Surfactant (hexane mixture) is added to the chitosan acetic/glutaraldehyde solution. Surfactant helps in the formation of chitosan nanoparticles smaller than 100 nm under continuous stirring to complete cross-linking between the amine group of chitosan with glutaraldehyde. By applying a low pressure, the excess organic solvent is removed. The excess organic solvent used, the complexity of the washing process, and the amount of time this method takes is its main drawback [3,44]. Chitosan nanoparticles prepared using the inotropic gelation method depend upon electrostatic interaction between the amino group of chitosan and the polyanions group such as triphosphate in an aqueous medium [45–48]. Firstly, the chitosan is dissolved in acetic acid in the presence of stabilizers such as poloxamer. So, nanoparticles are formed under continuous stirring. The size of the nanoparticle depends upon the ratio of chitosan-to-stabilizer [3]. The emulsion solvent diffusion method is based on the addition of an organic phase into a chitosan solution containing a stabilizer at a higher temperature and pressure with constant stirring. Nanoparticles are formed by the addition of water to an organic solvent. This method of nanoparticle formation is better for hydrophobic-based drug delivery systems. This method also has some drawbacks, such as greater shear force and harsh process conditions [49]. Chitosan is one of the most extensively studied biopolymers because chitosan possesses some ideal properties for polymeric carriers for nanoparticles. The properties are given in Table 1.

Current studies have shown a massive variation of applications and novel modifications of chitosan, thereby increasing its overall value. Drug encapsulation using chitosan with tripolyphosphate was first reported by Bodmeier et al. [50,51] who used an inotropic gelation process, which results in the formation of chitosan nanoparticles. Chitosan (100–150 nm) nanoparticles were loaded with Rosuvastatin drug encapsulated in polyvinyl alcohol (PVA)/Sodium alginate (SA) core using an ionic gelation method. The release behavior of the drug was observed within 24 h, and chitosan particles delivered significant results in the drug release process. This biocompatible and biodegradable drug delivery system was a suitable choice for replacing the various doses of the drug Rosuvastatin [51]. In 1998, Alonso et al. synthesized the chitosan nanoparticle with the development of inter-and intra-molecular interaction between the chitosan amino group and tripolyphosphate (TPP). This method produced a high yield of chitosan nanoparticles [43]. Thandapani Gomathi et al., in 2017, synthesized chitosan nanoparticles with TPP-loaded drugs with letrozole (LTZ) for cancer treatment. Characterization techniques such as SEM, TEM, FTIR, XRD, and TGA results showed the optimum results. Additionally, the prepared formulation was evaluated in vitro to determine its biodegradability, hemocompatibility, and serum stability. The preliminary studies supported the assertion that chitosan nanoparticle synthesis had biocompatibility and hemocompatible applications, and could act as an essential pharmaceutical excipient for letrozole [52]. Synthesis techniques for chitosan nanoparticles are given in Figure 4.

Table 1. Some ideal properties of polymeric nanocarriers [3].

Nanoparticle Drug Delivery System
• Simple and low-cost to synthesize and scale-up
• High shear forces, no heat or organic solvents involved in their preparation process
• Stable and reproducible
• Appropriate for a broad classification of drugs: proteins, small molecules, and polynucleotides
• Capacity to lyophilize
• Stable after synthesis
Polymeric carriers
• Non-toxic
• Biocompatible
• Non-immunogenic
• Water-soluble
• Inexpensive
• Easy to synthesize and characterize

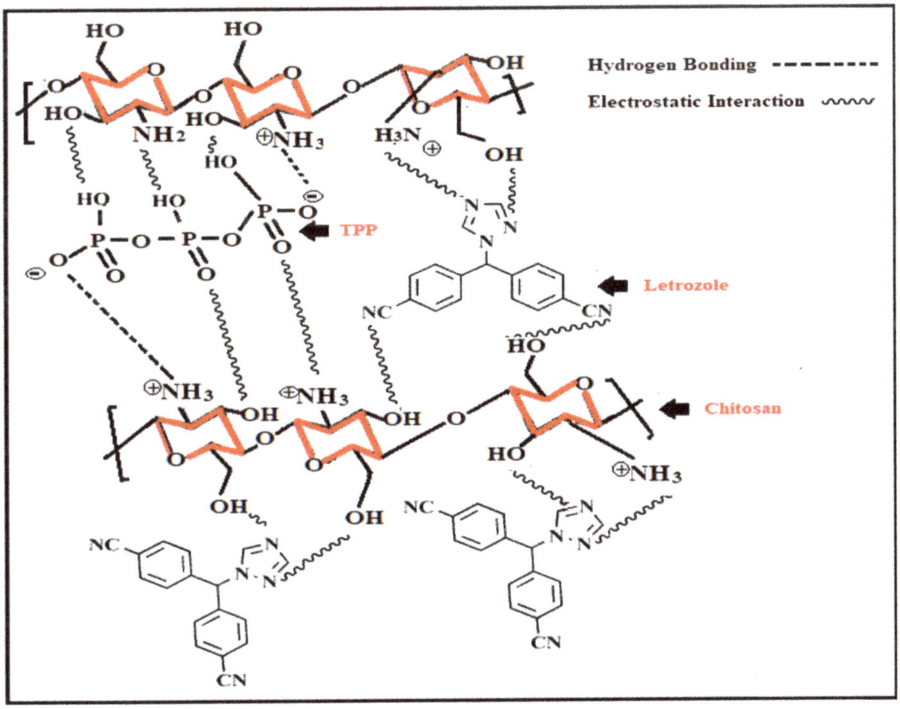

Figure 4. Shows the formation of chitosan nanoparticles modified with tripolyphosphate (TPP)-loaded letrozole [52]. Copyright ©2017, Elsevier.

The use of chitosan nanoparticles was reported by Wang et al., in 2017, for insulin delivery [53]. Zhang et al. modified chitosan by using heptamethine and folate for photodynamic treatment and tumor-imaging [54]. Kamel et al. modified chitosan by encapsulating oregano and cinnamon within chitosan in combination with 5-fluorouracil as an effective agent for tumors [55]. Lin et al. studied chitosan derivatives and found that chitosan-based nanocarriers used for co-delivery of genes and drugs were redox responsive [56]. In 2017, Gu et al. reported antibody modified nanoparticles. The delivery of drugs to the brain has always been a challenging task because the blood–brain barrier does not allow quick cellular uptake to the brain [57]. Auspicious work has been done by Par et al. for cancer treatment; the authors used glycol-modified chitosan nanoparticles for the effective release of doxorubicin [58]. In 2018, Belbekhouche et al. synthesized chitosan/polyacrylic modified nanoparticles for drug delivery systems [59]. A considerable amount of experimental work has been reported by Bernkop-Schnürch et al. [41]. The authors studied the efficiency of chitosan for different drug delivery systems: oral, gastric (for cancer treatment), nasal, buccal, intravesical, ocular, and, additionally, systems for vaccine delivery. The properties of chitosan nanoparticles vary when coupled with a hydrophilic polymer. This modified form of chitosan has shown novel susceptibility for delivering protein and interaction with the biological surface [43]. Calvo et al. examined the remarkable properties of modified chitosan using the diblock copolymer of ethylene oxide and propylene oxide as a protein carrier. The introduction of a PEG coating on the surface of chitosan decreases its cationic surface charge and, remarkably, increases its biocompatibility [60].

In 2002, Shu and Zhu [61] studied the effect of electrostatic interaction on properties of chitosan ionically crosslinked with multivalent phosphates such as tripolyphosphate, phosphate and pyrophosphate. Chitosan cross-link ionically due to the greater negative charge on the surface of phosphates. The solution pH plays a vital role in electrostatic interaction between chitosan and multivalent phosphates. Pyrophosphate/chitosan exhibits greater interaction as compared to other tripolyphosphates and phosphates. Ionically cross-linked chitosan and tripolyphosphates displayed better surface charge to size ratio for particles and showed better association with vaccines, proteins, plasmids, peptides, and oligonucleotides [61]. Recently many issues related to cancer treatment, such as hematogenous metastasis, drug resistance and local reappearance have led to the failure of treatment methods [62]. The main problem related to cancer treatment is finding a drug delivery system that fits the requirements. Shafabakhsh et al. [38] reported a review of gastric cancer treatment using chitosan nanoparticles. The authors investigated the effect of the anticancer drug norcantharidin conjugated with carboxymethyl modified chitosan.

In comparison with the simple drug, the carboxymethyl/chitosan encapsulated the drug successfully and suppressed the migration and proliferation of gastric cancer cells. This study reported that carboxymethyl chitosan could increase gene expression and may provide a favorable drug delivery system for gastric cancer treatments [38,63]. Moreover, chitosan nanoparticles used for the treatment of H. pylori infection have been shown to improve the effect of amoxicillin; chitosan nanoparticles improve the release time of the drug by preventing them from enzymatic and acidic breakdown through bonding to the mucus barrier of the stomach and drug release into the mucus barrier, thus leading to greater efficacy at the infected site [64,65].

Øilo et al. [66] suggested dental coating by using modified chitosan with other alternative antibacterial agents. The formation of biofilms causes common dental diseases that involve microbes adhering to teeth or restorative materials. Microbial adhesion is followed by bacterial growth and colonization, resulting in the formation of a compact biofilm matrix [67]. This matrix protects the underlying bacteria from the action of antibiotics and host defense mechanisms. The biofilm formed on teeth, prostheses, or implant-anchored restorations contains aciduric organisms such as *Streptococcus mutans* (*S. mutans*) and *lactobacilli* that secrete acid causing enamel and dentin demineralization. Biofilm formation on dental implants can result in a severe infection leading to dental implant failure. The formation of biofilm is reduced by different antibacterial agents such as quaternary ammonium compounds [68], inorganic nanoparticles [69], or fluoride varnish with natural products [70], which are used in the dental materials. Dental varnishes containing fluoride with natural products such as chitosan are a practical approach. Newer techniques include the use of an antibacterial polymer coating drug delivery system to prevent bacterial growth on artificial tooth surfaces in other dental materials and dental composite kits, increasing the longevity of the dental restoration [71]. Examples of such antibacterial coatings include copolymers of acrylic acid, alkyl methacrylate, and polydimethylsiloxane copolymers [72], pectin coated liposomes, and carbopol [73].

4. Alginate-Based Nanoparticles

Alginates are a group of the most important biopolymers, also known as sodium-alginates, which are unbranched polysaccharide anionic polymers (Figure 5). Alginate demonstrates a wide range of potential applications in a polymeric drug delivery system, in the food industry in the form of additives based on electrostatic interaction. A modified form of alginates has introduced a greater level of properties in the biomedical and pharmaceutical industries [74]. Alginate is made up of unbranched polysaccharides extracted from brown seaweeds and soil bacteria. Alginic acid is the resulting product extracted from seaweed which is converted into sodium alginate, currently used in the pharmaceutical industry as an effective drug carrier. Alginic acid is a linear polymer consisting of L-guluronic acid and D-mannuronic acid; these are linearly arranged in the polymer chain. Alginates from various sources differ in their extents of blocks. Hydration of alginic acid leads to the synthesis of a high-viscosity "acid gel" due to intermolecular binding. Due to gelation, water molecules are enclosed inside the alginate matrix but are still free to migrate, which has a great application in drug encapsulation and cell immobilization [74].

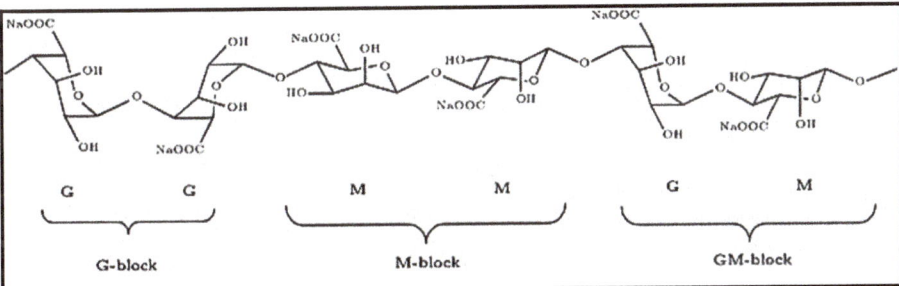

Figure 5. Types of alginate blocs: M = mannuronic acid; G = guluronic acid [75].

Alginate is a perfect polymer for chemical functionalization, due to its free carboxyl and hydroxyl groups among the backbone. Properties such as hydrophobicity and solubility, and physicochemical and biological characteristics are enhanced due to the formation of alginate derivatives based on hydroxyl and carboxylic groups. Many physical and chemical methods, such as polymer blending, grafting copolymerization with hydrophilic vinyl monomers, and compounding with other functional components, can be used to modify sodium alginate [76]. Divalent cations act as cross-linkers between the functional groups of alginate chains. Polyvalent cations such as Ca^{2+}, Sr^{2+}, or Ba^{2+} are responsible for intrachain and interchain cross-linking of alginate, forming insoluble alginate with the anionic polymer. Calcium is the main cation used because it is considered to be simply accessible, clinically safe, and cost-effective. The reaction of sodium alginate and calcium ion consists of a simple cross-linking process in which sodium-alginate is converted into calcium alginate [77].

$$2Na(Alginate) + Ca^{2+} \rightarrow Ca(Alginate)_2 + 2Na^+$$

Wandrey et al. [77] reported that, in the development of high mechanical strength and greater permeability, G alginate showed advantageous properties, and for additional properties, M alginate was suggested. Amphiphilic alginate is a current choice for drug delivery systems, and it shows properties such as low toxicity, good biocompatibility, mechanical stiffness, binding and release of drugs upon modification; it also reduces side effects and increases affinity with drugs [78,79]. Alginate-based smart polymers respond to pH [80], temperature [81], light [82], enzymes and magnetic field [81,83]. Most of the drug carriers are synthesized on the basis of an ionic complexes of alginate or its sulfate derivatives with a cationic macromolecule such as peptides or proteins. Wu et al. [84] reported on a nano-sized drug carrier for chemotherapeutic applications based on inorganic/organic hybrid alginate/CaCO$_3$ using the co-precipitation method under optimal conditions in the presence of an aqueous solution. A hydrophobic drug (paclitaxel, PTX) and hydrophilic drug (doxorubicin hydrochloride, DOX) were co-encapsulated in the alginate/CaCO$_3$ hybrid nanoparticles. Different characterization techniques were used to observe the behavior of a simple nanoparticle-encapsulated drug and a co-encapsulated one. The drug-loaded with modified nanoparticles showed greater cellular uptake and an enhanced inhibitory effect. These results showed that alginate/CaCO$_3$ hybrid nanoparticles have beneficial applications for the co-delivery of drugs with altered physicochemical properties. In another study, Jahanban-Esfahlan et al. [84] reported on an effective and drug release system for tumor treatment. They developed magnetic natural hydrogel based on alginate (Alg), Fe$_3$O$_4$ magnetic, and gelatin (Gel), nanoparticles (MNPs). Firstly, alginate was partially oxidized, then a shift-base condensation reaction was used to develop alginate-gel. Secondly, using a co-precipitation method, Fe$_3$O$_4$ nanoparticles were introduced in prepared alginate-gel. Characterization showed that this method synthesized hydrogel without any micro-phase separation. The attained Alg-Gel/Fe$_3$O$_4$ was loaded with doxorubicin hydrochloride (DOX), its drug loading, encapsulation properties and anticancer movement, were examined against Hela cells. The presence of carboxylic acid in the drug delivery system (synthesized Alg-Gel/Fe$_3$O$_4$-DOX) showed pH-dependent drug release. This modified form of alginate with magnetic nanoparticles showed promising results for a smart drug delivery system.

Moreover, Gao et al. [79] presented hydrophobic drug-based self-assembled micelles, a dual-stimuli responsive drug delivery system for hydrophobic drugs. Alginate was modified with dodecyl glycidyl as a hydrophobic group and was able to form self-assembled micelles in the aqueous solution above the critical micelle concentration. Doxorubicin (DOX) was used as an exemplary drug and successfully loaded in HMA (hydrophobic modified alginate) micelles. The enzyme and pH-stimuli release behavior of DOX from DOX-HMA micelles was such that the release of DOX was enhanced in an acidic medium. The release of drugs in the presence of a catalyst named an Alpha-Lfucosidase was effectively increased. Zhang et al. [85] synthesized graphene functionalized alginate (GO-ALG) for colon cancer treatment. This modification opened the way for many other therapeutic applications. The main issue linked with colon cancer is liver metastasis. Conventional drug delivery systems have many problems, such as failure to control the drug release ratio, poor stability, wrong targeting, and exposure to the microenvironment. This study reports the synthesis of graphene oxide (GO)-functionalized, sodium alginate (ALG) colon-targeting drug delivery system, with 5-fluorouracil (5-FU) used as the sample anticancer drug. The results showed that modified GOALG/5-FU expressively stopped tumor growth and liver metastasis and increased the life span of mice. This research opened a new route for the treatment of colon cancer liver metastasis. Nazemi et al. [86] investigated the ionic complexation of various configurations of alginate and its sulfated derivative with tetracycline hydrochloride (TCH). Remarkably, the functionalization of alginate with sulfate groups resulted in drug-polymer complex formation. Mannuronate-enriched alginate complex with TCH trapped the greater quantity of the drug. The results showed that this modification of alginate with TCH comes out as a favorable biomaterial for a cationic drug delivery system. Hügl et al. [87] entrapped the neurotrophic factor producing cell in an alginate polymer matrix. The application processes were tested for their potential in an artificial human cochlea model. Since the methods potentially affect the electrode implant capacity, the coating stability and insertion forces were analyzed on custom-made electrode arrays. Both inoculation of the alginate-cell solution into the model and a manual dip coating of electrode arrays with successive insertion into the model were promising. The filling of the model with a non-cross-linked alginate-cell solution improved the insertion forces. A good stability of the coating was examined after the first supplement. Both application schemes are a promising choice for cell-induced drug delivery to the inner ear, but an alginate-cell coating of electrodes has great potential with a reduction of insertion forces.

5. Albumin-Based Nanoparticles

Albumin is a natural, water-soluble globular protein and attractive macromolecular carrier which has a biodegradable property. Albumin is non-immunogenic, non-toxic, non-antigenic and biocompatible [88,89]. A large number of drugs can be incorporated into the nanoparticle-matrix because albumin molecules have different binding sites [90]. Albumin structure is shown in Figure 6.

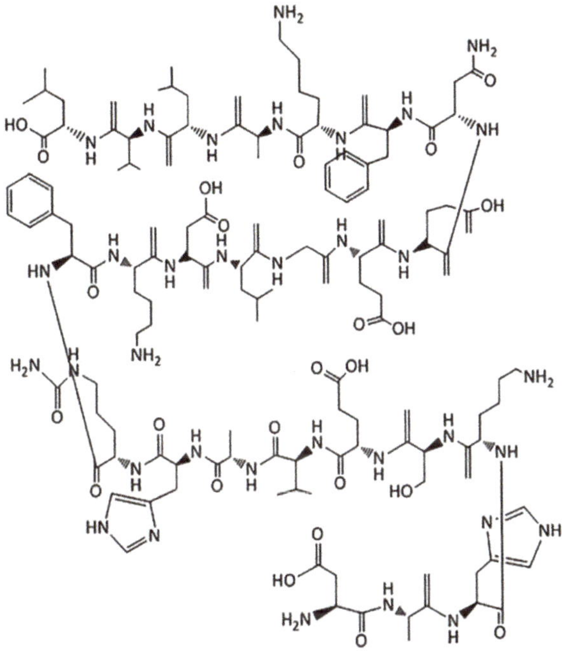

Figure 6. Structure of albumin [8]. Note that the oxygen atoms of almost all the carboxyl groups of amino acids are not shown in the structure. Copyright ©2019, Elsevier.

Albumin-based nanoparticles allow electrostatic interaction of cationic and anionic charge; drugs show non-covalent and covalent interaction with albumin nanoparticles. Figure 7 demonstrates the successful use of albumin and albumin nanoparticles for cancer treatment [89]. The presence of primary amino acid groups in albumin, such as lysine, indicates a vital role in cross-linking [91]. Albumin is prepared by controlled desolvation, coacervation, and emulsion formation. Commercially available forms of albumin are ovalbumin (egg white), human serum albumin, albumin extracted from soybeans, albumin present in bovine serum capsules, grains, and milk [92], where egg albumin has a molecular weight of up to 47,000 Da.

Furthermore, ovalbumin is non-toxic, sensitive to temperature or pH, and economical; it gives effective results in food matrix design, stabilization of foams and emulsions, and a is a good candidate for sustainable drug release [93]. A bovine serum capsule has a size of up to 69,323 Da, and due to its non-toxic behaviour, and ligand binding property it is extensively used for drug delivery applications [94]. Human serum albumin has a molecular weight of 66,500 Da and peripheral uptake, non-toxicity and biodegradability properties make it beneficial for pharmaceutical applications [95]. Albumin nanoparticles have several useful properties such as easy incorporation of various drugs and the ability to bind with proteins, due to presence of carboxylic and amino group on nanoparticle surface [96].

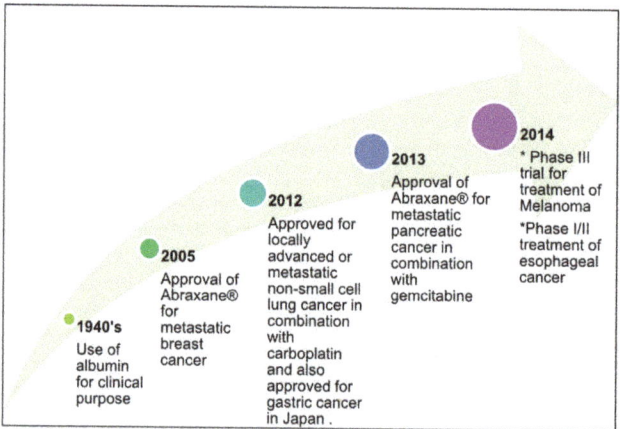

Figure 7. The successful use of albumin and an albumin nanoparticle (Abraxane) for cancer treatment [89]. Copyright ©2020, Elsevier.

Modification of albumin with PEG has not only improved the blood circulation but also provides a gateway in the pharmaceutical industry for cancer treatment drugs [97]. Albumin nanoparticles show a better affinity for cancer treatment drugs such as doxorubicin, curcumin, Abraxane, and tacrolimus [98]. Kim et al. [98] prepared HSA nanoparticles loaded with curcumin; these nanoparticles show higher solubility. Dreis et al. [99] have developed a system for the preparation of doxorubicin-loaded HSA nanoparticles. Using doxorubicin-loaded HSA nanoparticles, the toxic effect of anticancer drugs was reduced, and the multidrug resistance issue was resolved. Joshi et al. [89] discussed nanocarriers for pulmonary cancer. Surface modification of a nanoparticle helps in the effective movement of nanoparticles across the mucus layer. Surface functionalization of nanoparticles was performed using various methods such as adsorption, conjugation, and surface coating. Here, the surface of albumin modified with a neutral molecule polyethylene glycol enabled the movement through the mucus layer of the respiratory tract [89]. Surface modification based upon the required application is possible due to many reactive groups on the surface of albumin. Iwao et al. [100] presented a strategy for a site-specific drug delivery system for the cure of ulcerative colitis (UC). The authors prepared modified human serum albumin (HSA), and myeloperoxidase (MPO) and prepared nanoparticles (HSA NPs) conjugated with 5-aminosalicylic acid (5-ASA). The specific contact between 5-ASAHSANPs and MPO was examined using quartz crystal microbalance analysis.

Furthermore, Siri et al. [101] presented the effect of an albumin nanoparticle structure with its function as a drug release system. In this study, albumin nanoparticles were irradiated with gamma rays (cross-linker) by using the desolvation method. This method causes albumin nanoparticles to generate new hydrophobic pockets which make it a sound drug delivery system. The hydrophobic drug, Emodin, was used as a sample to check the release behavior. The formation of nanoparticle pockets enhanced the encapsulation property of the system. Stein et al. [102] studied the preparation of stable mTHPC-albumin nanoparticles using nanoparticle albumin-bound (nab)-technology to develop a system for drugs that are not very water-soluble. In this study, the advantages of nanotechnology and albumin with the ability of high tumor enrichment and the selective light initiation of the photosensitizer Temoporfin (mTHPC) were associated with a new delivery system for reliable tumor treatment. The nanoparticles were characterized according to size distribution and particle size, and the effect of this method on the nanoparticles as well as mTHPC stability was studied. Table 2 shows polymer/polymer modified chitosan-, alginate-, and albumin-based nano polymers for drug delivery systems.

Table 2. Shows the modified chitosan-, alginate-, and albumin-based nano polymer for drug delivery systems [8].

Polymer/Modified Polymer	Preparation Method	Model Drug
Chitosan–folic acid	Ionic gelation	5-flurouracil
Chitosan/alginate and solid lipid NPs	Ionic gelation	Ciprofloxacin
PVA/chitosan-gelation	Electrospinning method	Erythromycin
Alginate calcium carbonate	Co-precipitation	Paclitaxel
PEGylated albumin	RAFT polymerization	Lysozyme
Bovine serum albumin	Multistep process	Temozolomide
Egg albumin	Desolvation method	Curcumin
PEG-modified human serum albumin	Solid dispersion technology	Paclitaxel

6. Hydroxyapatite-Based Nanoparticles

Hydroxyapatite (HAp) has great applications in the biomedical field and is considered the best option in the pharmaceutical field due to its excellent bioactivity and biocompatibility. Hydroxyapatite is derived from the mineral compounds of human bones, teeth, and hard tissues. The basic units of HAp are calcium and phosphates (CaP) characterized as $M1_4M2_6(PO_4)6(OH)_2$, in which M1 and M2 are two crystallographic arrangements. The stability of CaP is directly related to the presence of water molecules during synthesis and the medium where it was applied [103].

Furthermore, HAp shows good mechanical strength, a porous structure, osteointegration, and osteoconductive properties. HAp can be used as an implant material due to its granular particles, porous structures, load-bearing ability and excellent biocompatibility. The combination of HAp with phosphates, such as calcium pyrophosphate and β-tricalcium phosphate (β-TCP), means that this material has a vast number of properties. The use of hydroxyapatite in the implantation, free layer of fibrous tissue composed by carbonated apatite is generated on its surface, which helps in the binding of the implant to the living bone through an osteoconduction mechanism. HAp prevents any toxicity effect during implantation, and its porous structure gives excellent diffusion properties. HAp is used in tissue engineering as a scaffold, in dental enamel repair, in medicine, for cancer cell treatment and as a bone cement [104,105]. A recent study investigated that HAp shows strong bonding due to its porous structure [106]. HAp powder was synthsized using a hydrothermal method with the use of calcium nitrate $[Ca(NO_3)_2 \cdot 4H_2O]$ for calcium and potassium dihydrogen phosphate $[(NH_4)_2HPO_4]$ and phosphorous, and it was used as a precursor. The use of HAp derivatives is in high demand in the field of orthopedics. This is undoubtedly beneficial for both commercialization and research purposes; it means that the use of composites is studied and experimented with, enhancing the performance of the previous defective bones. Li et al. [107] successfully synthesized a core–shell nanocarrier (PAA–MHAPNs) based on a grafting method. This synthesized system showed excellent results; for example, it had improved loading in terms of the quantity of anticancer drug (doxorubicin hydrochloride), electrostatic properties, and promising for application in pH-sensitive drug release systems. The loading capacity increased up to 79% at low pH. The cytotoxicity analyses designated that the PAA–MHAPNs was biocompatible. Overall, the synthesized systems have great ability as drug nanocarriers for drug delivery, excellent biocompatibility, and pH-responsive features for future intracellular drug delivery. Venkatasubbu et al. [108] presented functionalized hydroxyapatite (HAp) with folic acid (FA) modified polyethylene glycol (PEG) for therapeutic applications. In this study, in vitro analysis of anticancer drug (paclitaxel) loading in modified HAp was performed. The authors studied the initial rapid release of the drug and then the sustained release, and presented a review of three types of hydroxyapatite-based nanoparticles: magnetic HAp, luminescent HAp, and immunomagnetic HAp for bioimaging applications. Various research work on the antimicrobial property of HAp nanoparticles was presented in this study. Additionally, the silver doping particle in HAp increases its antimicrobial property by cross-linking a silver nanoparticle with a thiol group of bacteria, and HAp shows good compatibility with bone marrow stem cells [109]. Table 3 shows the advantages, disadvantages, biomedical applications and methods of synthesis of hydroxyapatite.

If we observe the bone at the microscopic level, we find the cellular composition of osteocytes and the matrix. A matrix composed of collagen fibers helps to give strength and flexibility to the bone and is associated with HAp microcrystals and mineral salts for hardness. The bone tissue is constantly replaced and remodeled, leading to the name Bone Remodeling. The stimulus from the osteocytes supports to initiate osteoclast and osteoblast for remodeling [110]. Bioactive ceramics act as an HAp layer on the fractured part, help to rise the osteoblast quickly to heal bone. Furthermore, studies proposed a combination of the HA layer with high-density polyethylene (HDPE) as a auxiliary material for bone [111–115]. This has been tested and commercially named HAPEXTM. Previously provided empirical results for osteoblast over a bioactive ceramic layer of HAp particles [112]. Composites from the bioactive ceramics joint with HAp particles and collagen fibres have possibility to act as an artificial substitute for bone [116]. The established graft have excellent mechanical properties [117]. HAp/alumina has been proposed as a bone substitute [118]. One study also concludes that mixing P_2O_5 glass with HAp achieves close to natural bone properties [119].

Table 3. Shows the advantages, disadvantages, biomedical applications, and methods of preparation for hydroxyapatite [120].

Advantages	Disadvantages	Biomedical Applications	Method of Preparation
Bioactive (hydration shell)	Strong hydration shell, ionic surface, fragile	Drug delivery system, tissue engineering' implants	Wet method, dry method, high-temperature process
Ease of modification and surface functionalization	Precipitation and turbid solution	-	-
Good attachment to polymers	Surface corona formation, aggregation	-	-
Ease of composite formation	Dispersity in chemical composition, size and shape polymorphism	-	-
Biodegradable, biocompatibility	High pH sensitivity and solubility	-	-
Self-assembly	Low stability	-	-

7. Hyaluronic Acid-Based Nanoparticles

Hyaluronic acid (HA) is an anionic polysaccharide with repeating units of N-acetyl-D glucosamine and disaccharides of D-glucuronic acid linked via β-1,4- or β-1,3-glycosidic bonds [121,122]. HA also is known as hyaluronan, present in the synovial fluids, in the extracellular matrix, in the skin and uniformly distributed in vertebrate tissues of the body [123]; the structure is shown in Figure 8. HA has good biocompatibility, greater viscoelasticity, biodegradability and the capacity to combine with the receptor cell surface. The presence of receptors such as CD44 on the surface of HA makes it a site-specific drug delivery system for anticancer drug release and its capacity for cellular uptake [124,125].

Modification of HA with hydrophobic macromolecules occurs because of hydroxyl and carboxylic functional groups and its negatively charged surface. Based on nanocarriers, HA can be divided into different drug delivery systems such as gel and cationic drug delivery systems, a polyelectrolyte microcapsule release system, a nano-emulsion delivery system, and a nano-carriers drug delivery system [126]. HA nanocarriers are not only used for cancer drug therapy but also as photosensors, for photo imaging, and gene plasmids [127]. Various modification steps can be used to enhance its properties for drug delivery systems, such as conjugation with the nanocarriers as a targeting moiety, with dendrimers, quantum dots, and graphene oxide [35,128]. Modification of HA is important due to its accumulation in the liver; hence, Choi et al. [129] synthesized polyethylene glycol-modified HA nanoparticles. By varying the degree of PEGlation, negatively charged self-assembled nanoparticles were formed. Although PEGlation of HA-NPs decreased their cellular uptake in vitro, nanoparticles having CD44HA receptor were taken in huge amount by cancer cell as compared to normal fibroblast cells. Using in vivo images, it was established that PEGlation of HA reduces the accretion of HA nanoparticles in the liver and enhances its cellular uptake. Characterization results showed the maximum accumulation of PEGylated HA nanoparticles in tumour cells. Lee and Na [130] also synthesized the sustainable drug release to reduce the toxic effect and avoid an accumulation of HA in healthy organs. The authors modified HA with a Polycaprolacton (PCL) copolymer, HA cross-linking is carried out by disulfide bond. Doxorubicin (DOX), selected as a sample anticancer drug, was successfully encapsulated into the nanoparticles with greater drug loading ability. The DOX-loaded in the modified HA significantly delayed the drug release in physiological environments. However, the drug release rate was significantly improved in the occurrence of glutathione, a thiol-containing tripeptide capable of reducing disulfide bonds in the cytoplasm. Moreover, DOX-HA-ss-NPs could efficiently transport the DOX into the tumour cell. Overall, the characterization results indicate that this modification can act as a potential carrier for a drug delivery system. In another study [131], photo-crosslinked hyaluronic acid nanoparticles (c-HANPs) were prepared for involuntary burst release of the drug into the blood. They were readily synthesized via UV-triggered chemical cross-linking with the acrylate groups in the polymer backbone. High sustainability of c-HANPs enabled their large circulation in the body. Owing to the constant discharge of the drug and improved tumour-targeting capacity, c-HANPs showed higher healing ability compared to uncrosslinked HANPs. These data imply the promising potential of c-HANP as a tumour-targeting drug carrier and have established the extraordinary effect of better stability upon the biodistribution and therapeutic ability of drug-loaded nanoparticles.

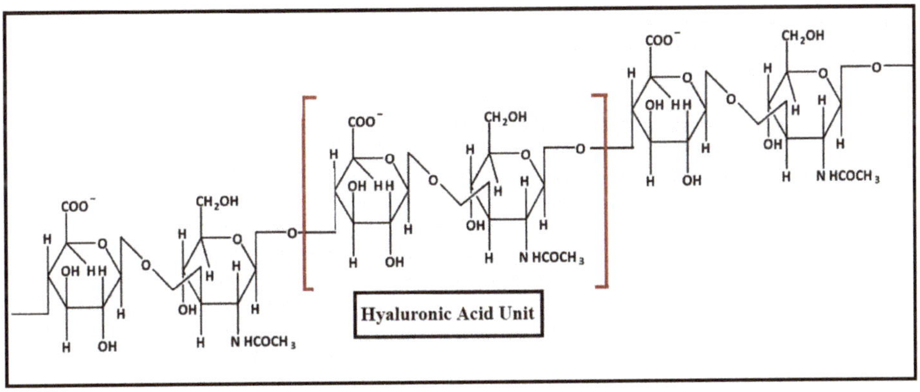

Figure 8. The structure of hyaluronic acid.

8. Conclusions

In this review, five natural biocompatible and biodegradable polymer-based nanoparticles have been critically examined for therapeutic applications. The nanoformulations are superior to macro or conventional drug delivery systems, and they can maximize dosing frequency. They can target infected areas, organs, tumor sites, and tissues in the body. Biodegradable and biocompatible polymers are appropriate materials for the development of novel drug delivery systems. Biocompatibility, mechanical properties, and low cytotoxic effects of these polymers make them an appropriate choice for drug delivery systems. It is the need of time to manipulate the system, which reduces the toxic effects of drugs on healthy organs or body parts. Still, there is room to explore more biodegradable polymers for innovative biomedical applications. With increased progress in nanotechnology, we expect progress in the area of therapeutic systems based on the development of modified nanomedicines for the proper treatment of diseases.

Funding: This research was supported by Economic and Social Research Council UK (ES/S000208/1).

Conflicts of Interest: The authors declare no conflict of interest.

References

1. Sur, S.; Rathore, A.; Dave, V.; Reddy, K.R.; Chouhan, R.S.; Sadhu, V. Recent developments in functionalized polymer nanoparticles for efficient drug delivery system. *Nano Struct. Nano Objects* **2019**, *20*, 100397. [CrossRef]
2. Tong, X.; Pan, W.; Su, T.; Zhang, M.; Domg, W.; Qi, X. Recent advances in natural polymer-based drug delivery systems. Reactive and Functional Polymers. *React. Funct. Polym.* **2020**, *148*, 104501. [CrossRef]
3. Tiyaboonchai, W. Chitosan Nanoparticles: A Promising System for Drug Delivery. *Naresuan Univ. J.* **2003**, *11*, 51–66.
4. Jeong, B.; Choi, Y.K.; Bae, Y.H.; Zentner, G.; Kim, S.W. New biodegradable polymers for injectable drug delivery systems. *J. Control. Release* **1999**, *62*, 109–114. [CrossRef]
5. Kumari, A.; Yadav, S.K.; Yadav, S.C. Biodegradable polymeric nanoparticles based drug delivery systems. *Colloids Surf. B Biointerfaces* **2010**, *75*, 1–18. [CrossRef]
6. Marianecci, C.; Di Marzio, L.; Rinaldi, F.; Celia, C.; Paolino, D.; Alhaique, F.; Esposito, S.; Carafa, M. Niosomes from 80s to present: The state of the art. *Adv. Colloid Interface Sci.* **2014**, *205*, 187–206. [CrossRef]
7. Tibbitt, M.W.; Dahlman, J.E.; Langer, R. Emerging frontiers in drug delivery. *J. Am. Chem. Soc.* **2016**, *138*, 704–717. [CrossRef]
8. George, A.; Shah, P.A.; Shrivastav, P.S. Natural biodegradable polymers based nano-formulations for drug delivery: A review. *Int. J. Pharm.* **2019**, *561*, 244–264. [CrossRef]
9. Hassan, S.; Zhang, X. Droplet-Based Microgels: Attractive Materials for Drug Delivery Systems. *Res. Dev. Mater. Sci.* **2019**, *11*, 1183–1185. [CrossRef]
10. Ramkumar, V.S.; Pugazhendhi, A.; Gopalakrishnan, K.; Sivagurunathan, P.; Saratale, G.D.; Dung, T.N.B.; Kannapiran, E. Biofabrication and characterization of silver nanoparticles using aqueous extract of seaweed Enteromorpha compressa and its biomedical properties. *Biotechnol. Rep.* **2017**, *14*, 1–7. [CrossRef]
11. Chen, M.; Yin, M. Design and development of fluorescent nanostruc-tures for bioimaging. *Prog. Polym. Sci.* **2014**, *39*, 365–395. [CrossRef]
12. Baba, M.; Matsumoto, Y.; Kashio, A.; Cabral, H.; Nishiyama, N.; Kataoka, K.; Yamasoba, T. Micellization of cisplatin (NC-6004) reduces its oto-toxicity in guinea pigs. *J. Control. Release* **2012**, *157*, 112–117. [CrossRef] [PubMed]
13. Cramer, N.B.; Standsburry, J.W.; Bowman, C.N. Recent advances and developments in composite dental restorative materials. *J. Dent. Res.* **2011**, *90*, 402–416. [CrossRef] [PubMed]
14. Mukherjee, S.; Vinugopal, J.R.; Ravichandran, R.; Ramalingam, M.; Raghunath, M.; Ramakrishna, S. Nanofiber technology for controllingstem cell functions and tissue engineering. *Micro Nanotechnol. Eng. Stem Cells Tissues* **2013**, *2*, 27–51.
15. Cheng, Z.; Zaki, A.A.; Hui, J.Z.; Muzykantov, V.R.; Tsourkas, A. Multifunctional nanoparticles: Cost versus benefit of adding targeting andimaging capabilities. *Science* **2012**, *338*, 903–910. [CrossRef] [PubMed]
16. Shi, J.; Votruba, A.R.; Farokhzad, O.C.; Langer, R. Nanotechnology in drug delivery and tissue engineering: From discovery to applications. *Nano Lett.* **2010**, *10*, 3223–3230. [CrossRef] [PubMed]
17. Liu, W.; Thomopoulos, S.; Xia, Y. Electrospun nanofibers for regenera-tive medicine. *Adv. Healthc. Mater.* **2012**, *1*, 10–25. [CrossRef]
18. De Jong, W.H.; Borm, P.J.A. Drug delivery and nanoparticles: Applications and hazards. *Int. J. Nanomed.* **2008**, *3*, 133–149. [CrossRef]
19. Pugazhendhi, A.; Prabakar, D.; Jacob, J.M.; Karuppusamy, I.; Saratale, R.G. Synthesis and characterization of silver nanoparticles using Gelidium amansii and its antimicrobial property against various pathogenic bacteria. *Microb. Pathog.* **2018**, *114*, 41–45. [CrossRef]

20. Nanotechnology for Health: Vision Paper and Basis for a Strategic Agenda for Nanomedicine. Available online: https://op.europa.eu/en/publication-detail/-/publication/60816548-e372-4216-a253c4442b527a21/language-en (accessed on 30 September 2020).
21. Kamaly, N.; Yameen, B.; Wu, J.; Farokhzad, O.C. Degradable controlled-release polymers and polymeric nanoparticles: Mechanisms of controlling drug release. *Chem. Rev.* **2016**, *116*, 2602–2663. [CrossRef]
22. Soppimath, K.S.; Aminabhavi, T.M.; Kulkarni, A.R.; Rudzinski, W.E. Biodegradable polymeric nanoparticles as drug delivery devices. *J. Control. Release* **2001**, *70*, 1–20. [CrossRef]
23. Nejati-Koshki, K.; Mesgari, M.; Ebrahimi, E.; Abbasalizadeh, F.; Aval, S.F.; Khandaghi, A.A.; Abasi, M.; Akbarzadeh, A. Synthesis and in vitro study of cisplatin-loaded Fe_3O_4 nanoparticles modified with PLGA-PEG$_{6000}$ copolymers in treatment of lung cancer. *J. Microencapsul.* **2014**, *31*, 815–823. [CrossRef] [PubMed]
24. Conde, J.; Larguinno, M.; Cordeiro, A.; Raposo, L.R.; Costa, P.M.; Santos, S.; Diniz, M.S.; Fernandes, A.R.; Baptista, P.V. Gold-nanobeacons for gene therapy: Evaluation of genotoxicity, cell toxicity, and proteome profiling analysis. *Nanotoxicology* **2013**, *8*, 521–532. [CrossRef] [PubMed]
25. Brannon-Peppas, L.; Blanchette, J.O. Nanoparticle and targeted systems for cancer therapy. *Adv. Drug Deliv. Rev.* **2012**, *56*, 1649–1659. [CrossRef]
26. Feng, S.S. Nanoparticles of biodegradable polymers for new-concept chemotherapy. *Expert Rev. Med. Devices* **2014**, *1*, 115–125. [CrossRef]
27. Yeo, W.W.Y.; Hosseinkhani, H.; Abdul Rahman, S.; Rosli, R.; Domb, A.J.; Abdullah, S. Safety Profile of Dextran-Spermine Gene Delivery Vector in Mouse Lungs. *J. Nanosci. Nanotechnol.* **2014**, *14*, 3328–3336. [CrossRef]
28. Alibolandi, M.; Abnous, K.; Ramezani, M.; Hosseinkhani, H.; Hadizadeh, F. Synthesis of AS1411-aptamer-conjugated CdTe quantum dots with high fluorescence strength for probe labeling tumor cells. *J. Fluoresc.* **2014**, *24*, 1519–1529. [CrossRef]
29. Dragan, E.S.; Bucataria, F. Design and characterization of anionic hydrogels confined in Daisogel silica composites microspheres and their application in sustained release of proteins. *Colloid. Surf. A* **2016**, *489*, 46–56. [CrossRef]
30. Farokhi, M.; Mottaghitalab, F.; Shokrgozar, M.A.; Ou, K.L.; Mao, C.; Hosseinkhani, H. Importance of dual delivery systems for bone tissue engineering. *J. Control. Release* **2016**, *225*, 152–169. [CrossRef]
31. Qi, X.; Wei, W.; Li, J.; Liu, Y.; Hu, X.; Zhang, J.; Bi, L.; Dong, W. Fabrication and Characterization of a Novel Anticancer Drug Delivery System: Salecan/Poly(methacrylic acid) Semi-interpenetrating Polymer Network Hydrogel. *ACS Biomater. Sci. Eng.* **2015**, *1*, 1287–1299. [CrossRef]
32. Dinu, M.V.; Dragan, E.S. Evaluation of Cu^{2+}, Co^{2+} and Ni^{2+} ions removal from aqueous solution using a novel chitosan/clinoptilolite composite: Kinetics and isotherms. *Chem. Eng. J.* **2010**, *160*, 157–163. [CrossRef]
33. Qi, X.; Wei, W.; Li, J.; Zuo, G.; Pan, X.; Su, T.; Zhang, J.; Dong, W. Salecan-Based pH-Sensitive Hydrogels for Insulin Delivery. *Mol. Pharmaceut.* **2017**, *14*, 431–440. [CrossRef] [PubMed]
34. Pande, V. Studies on the characteristics of zaltoprofen loaded gelatin nanoparticles by nanoprecipitation. *Inventi Rapid NDDS* **2015**, *3*, 1–7.
35. Prajapati, S.K.; Jain, A.; Jain, A. Biodegradable polymers and constructs: A novel approach in drug delivery. *Eur. Polym. J.* **2019**, *120*, 109191. [CrossRef]
36. Ossipov, D.A. Nanostructured hyaluronic acid-based materials for active delivery to cancer. *Expert Opin. Drug Deliv.* **2010**, *7*, 681–703. [CrossRef] [PubMed]
37. Kluin, O.S.; van der Mei, H.C.; Busscher, H.J.; Neut, D. Biodegradable vs. non-biodegradable antibiotic delivery devices in the treatment of osteomyelitis. *Expert Opin. Drug Deliv.* **2013**, *10*, 341–351. [CrossRef]
38. Shafabakhsh, R.; Yousefi, B.; Asemi, Z.; Nikfar, B.; Mansournia, M.A.; Hallajzadeh, J. Chitosan: A compound for drug delivery system in gastric cancer—A review. *Carbohydr. Polym.* **2020**, *242*, 116403. [CrossRef]
39. LeHoux, J.G.; Grondin, F. Some effects of chitosan on liver function in the rat. *Endocrinology* **1993**, *132*, 1078–1084. [CrossRef]
40. Peniston, Q.P.; Johnson, E.L. Process for the Manufacturer of Chitosan. U.S. Patent US4195175A, 25 March 1980.
41. Bernkop-Schnürch, A.; Dünnhaupt, S. Chitosan-based drug delivery systems. *Eur. J. Pharm. Biopharm.* **2012**, *81*, 463–469. [CrossRef]

42. Huang, G.; Liu, Y.; Chen, L. Chitosan and its derivatives as vehicles for drug delivery. *Drug Deliv.* **2017**, *24*, 108–113. [CrossRef]
43. Prabaharan, M.; Mano, J.F. Chitosan-Based Particles as Controlled Drug Delivery Systems. *Drug Deliv.* **2005**, *12*, 41–57. [CrossRef] [PubMed]
44. Maitra, A.; Kumar, P.G.; De, T.; Sahoo, S.K. Process for the Preparation of Highly Monodispersed Hydrophilicpolymeric Nanoparticles of Size Less than 100 nm. U.S. Patent US5874111A, 23 February 1999.
45. Calvo, P.; Remunan-Lopez, C.; Vila-Jato, J.L.; Alonso, M.J. Chitosan and chitosan/ethylene oxide propylene oxide block copolymer nanoparticles as novel carriers for proteins and vaccines. *Pharm. Res.* **1997**, *14*, 1431–1436. [CrossRef] [PubMed]
46. Janes, K.A.; Fresneau, M.P.; Marazuela, A.; Fabra, A.; Alonso, M.J. Chitosan nanoparticles as delivery systems for doxorubicin. *J. Control. Release* **2001**, *73*, 255–267. [CrossRef]
47. Pan, Y.; Li, Y.J.; Zhao, H.Y.; Zheng, J.M.; Xu, H.; Wei, G.; Hao, J.S.; Cui, F.D. Bioadhesive polysaccharide in protein delivery system: Chitosan nanoparticles improve the intestinal absorption of insulin in vivo. *Int. J. Pharm.* **2002**, *249*, 139–147. [CrossRef]
48. Giacone, D.V.; Dartora, V.F.; de Matos, J.K.; Passos, J.S.; Miranda, D.A.; de Oliveira, E.A.; Silveira, E.R.; Costa-Lotufo, L.V.; Maria-Engler, S.S.; Lopes, L.B. Effect of nanoemulsion modification with chitosan and sodium alginate on the topical delivery and efficacy of the cytotoxic agent piplartine in 2D and 3D skin cancer models. *Int. J. Biol. Macromol.* **2020**. [CrossRef]
49. El-Shabouri, M.H. Positively charged nanoparticles for improving the oral bioavailability of cyclosporin-A. *J. Pharm.* **2002**, *249*, 101–108. [CrossRef]
50. Bodmeier, R.; Chen, H.G.; Paeratakul, O. A novel approach to the oral delivery of micro- or nanoparticles. *Pharm. Res.* **1989**, *6*, 413–417. [CrossRef]
51. Afshar, M.; Dai, Y.-N.; Zhang, J.-P.; Wang, A.-Q.; Wei, Q. Preparation and characterization of sodium alginate/polyvinyl alcohol hydrogel containing drug-loaded chitosan nanoparticles as a drug delivery system. *J. Drug Deliv. Sci. Technol.* **2020**, *56*, 101530. [CrossRef]
52. Gomathi, T.; Sudha, P.N.; Florence, J.A.K.; Venkatesan, J.; Anil, S. Fabrication of letrozole formulation using chitosan nanoparticles through ionic gelation method. *Int. J. Biol. Macromol.* **2017**, *104*, 1820–1832. [CrossRef]
53. Wang, J.; Tan, J.; Luo, J.; Huang, P.; Zhou, W.; Chen, L.; Long, L.; Zhang, L.M.; Zhu, B.; Yang, L.; et al. Enhancement of scutellarin oral delivery efficacy by vitamin B12-modified amphiphilic chitosan derivatives to treat type II diabetes induced-retinopathy. *J. Nanobiotechnol.* **2017**, *15*, 18. [CrossRef]
54. Zhang, Y.; Lv, T.; Zhang, H.; Xie, X.; Li, Z.; Chen, H. Folate and heptamethine cyanine modified chitosan-based nanotheranostics for tumor targeted near-infrared fluorescence imaging and photodynamic therapy. *Biomacromolecules* **2017**, *18*, 2146–2160. [CrossRef] [PubMed]
55. Kamel, K.; Khalil, I.A.; Rateb, M.E.; Elgendy, H.; Elhawary, S. Chitosan-coated cinnamon/oregano-loaded solid lipid nanoparticles to augment 5-fluorouracil cytotoxicity for colorectal cancer: Extracts standardization, nanoparticles optimization and cytotoxicity evaluation. *J. Agric. Food Chem.* **2017**, *65*, 7966–7981. [CrossRef] [PubMed]
56. Lin, J.T.; Liu, Z.K.; Zhu, Q.L.; Rong, X.H.; Liang, C.L.; Wang, J. Redox-responsive nano-carriers for drug and gene co-delivery based on chitosan derivatives modified mesoporous silica nanoparticles. *Colloids Surf. B Biointerfaces* **2017**, *155*, 41–50. [CrossRef] [PubMed]
57. Gu, J.; Bayati, K.; Ho, E.A. Development of antibody-modified chitosan nanoparticles for the targeted delivery of siRNA across the blood-brain barrier as a strategy for inhibiting HIV replication in astrocytes. *Drug Deliv. Transl. Res.* **2017**, *7*, 497–506. [CrossRef] [PubMed]
58. Park, J.H.; Kwon, S.; Lee, M.; Chung, H.; Kim, J.H.; Kim, Y.S.; Park, R.W.; Kim, I.S.; Seo, S.B.; Kwon, I.C.; et al. Self-assembled nanoparticles based on glycol chitosan bearing hydrophobic moieties as carriers for doxorubicin: In vivo biodistribution and anti-tumor activity. *Biomaterials* **2006**, *27*, 119–126. [CrossRef] [PubMed]
59. Belbekhouche, S.; Mansour, O.; Carbonnier, B. Promising sub-100 nm tailor made hollow chitosan/poly(acrylic acid) nanocapsules for antibiotic therapy. *J. Colloid Interface Sci.* **2018**, *522*, 183–190. [CrossRef]
60. Calvo, P.; Remunan, C.; Jato, J.L.V.; Alonso, M.J. Novel hydrophilic chitosan-polyethylene oxide nanoparticles as protein carriers. *J. Appl. Polym.Sci.* **1997**, *63*, 125–132. [CrossRef]
61. Shu, X.Z.; Zhu, K.J. The influence of multivalent phosphate structure on the properties of ionically cross-linked chitosan films for controlled drug release. *Eur. J. Pharm. Biopharm.* **2002**, *54*, 235–243. [CrossRef]

62. Peng, Y.; Guo, J.J.; Liu, Y.M.; Wu, X.L. MicroRNA-34A inhibits the growth, invasion and metastasis of gastric cancer by targeting PDGFR and MET expression. *Biosci. Rep.* **2014**, *43*, e00112. [CrossRef]
63. Chi, J.; Jiang, Z.; Qiao, J.; Zhang, W.; Peng, Y.; Liu, W.; Han, B. Antitumor evaluation of carboxymethyl chitosan based norcantharidin conjugates against gastric cancer as novel polymer therapeutics. *Int. J. Biol. Macromol.* **2019**, *136*, 1–12. [CrossRef]
64. Gong, Y.; Tao, L.; Wang, F.; Liu, W.; Jing, L.; Liu, D.; Zhou, N. Chitosan as an adjuvant for a Helicobacter pylori therapeutic vaccine. *Mol. Med. Rep.* **2015**, *12*, 4123–4132. [CrossRef] [PubMed]
65. Arora, S.; Aggarwal, P.; Pathak, A.; Bhandari, R.; Duffoo, F.; Gulati, S.C. Molecular genetics of head and neck cancer (review). *Mol. Med. Rep.* **2012**, *6*, 19–22. [CrossRef] [PubMed]
66. Øilo, M.; Bakken, V. Biofilm and dental biomaterials. *Materials* **2015**, *8*, 2887–2900. [CrossRef]
67. Donlan, R.M. Biofilms: Microbial life on surfaces. *Emerg. Infect. Dis.* **2002**, *8*, 88–90. [CrossRef] [PubMed]
68. Schiroky, L.V.; Garcia, I.M.; Ogliari, F.A.; Samuel, S.M.W.; Collares, F.M. Triazine compound as copolymerized antibacterial agent in adhesive resins. *Braz. Dent. J.* **2017**, *28*, 196–200. [CrossRef]
69. Degrazia, F.W.; Leitune, V.C.B.; Gracia, I.M.; Arthur, R.A.; Samuel, S.M.W.; Collares, F.M. Effect of silver nanoparticles on the physicochemical and antimicrobial properties of an orthodontic adhesive. *J. Appl. Oral. Sci.* **2016**, *24*, 404–410. [CrossRef] [PubMed]
70. Wassel, M.O.; Khattab, M.A. Antibacterial activity against Streptococcus mutans and inhibition of bacterial induced enamel demineralization of propolis, miswak, and chitosan nanoparticles based dental varnishes. *J. Adv. Res.* **2017**, *8*, 387–392. [CrossRef]
71. Zhang, N.; Chen, C.; Melo, M.A.; Bai, Y.; Cheng, L.; Xu, H.H. A novel protein-repellent dental composite containing 2-methacryloyloxyethyl phosphorylcholine. *Int. J. Oral. Sci.* **2015**, *7*, 103–109. [CrossRef]
72. Fornell, A.C.; Skold-Larsoon, K.; Hallgren, A.; Bergstand, F.; Twetman, S. Effect of a hydrophobic tooth coating on gingival health, mutans streptococci, and enamel demineralization in adolescents with fixed orthodontic appliances. *Acta Odontol. Scand.* **2002**, *60*, 37–41. [CrossRef]
73. Nguyen, S.; Hiorth, M.; Rykke, M.; Smistad, G. Polymer coated liposomes for dental drug delivery—Interactions with parotid saliva and dental enamel. *Eur. J. Pharm. Sci.* **2013**, *50*, 78–85. [CrossRef]
74. Tonnesen, H.H.; Karlsen, J. Alginate in Drug Delivery Systems. *Drug Dev. Ind. Pharm.* **2002**, *28*, 621–630. [CrossRef] [PubMed]
75. Daemi, H.; Barikani, M. Synthesis and characterization of calcium alginate nanoparticles, sodium homopolymannuronate salt and its calcium nanoparticles. *Sci. Iran.* **2012**, *19*, 2023–2028. [CrossRef]
76. Yang, J.-S.; Xie, Y.-J.; He, W. Research progress on chemical modification of alginate: A review. *Carbohydr. Polym.* **2011**, *84*, 33–39. [CrossRef]
77. Ciofani, G.; Raffa, V.; Pizzorusso, T.; Menciassi, A.; Dario, P. Characterization of an alginate-based drug delivery system for neurological applications. *Med. Eng. Phys.* **2008**, *30*, 848–855. [CrossRef]
78. Lencina, M.S.; Ciolino, A.E.; Andreucetti, N.A.; Villar, M.A. Thermoresponsive hydrogels based on alginate-g-poly (N-isopropylacrylamide) copolymers obtained by low doses of gamma radiation. *Eur. Polym. J.* **2015**, *68*, 641–649. [CrossRef]
79. Gao, X.; Yu, Z.; Liu, B.; Yang, J.; Yang, X.; Yu, Y. A smart drug delivery system responsive to pH/enzyme stimuli based on hydrophobic modified sodium alginate. *Eur. Polym. J.* **2020**, *133*, 109779. [CrossRef]
80. Binauld, S.; Stenzel, M. Acid-degradable polymers for drug delivery: A decade of innovation. *Chem. Commun.* **2013**, *49*, 2082–2102. [CrossRef]
81. Liu, M.; Song, X.; Wen, Y.; Zhu, J.-L. Injectable thermoresponsive hydrogel formed by alginate-g-poly (N-isopropylacrylamide) that releases doxorubicin-encapsulated micelles as a smart drug delivery system. *ACS Appl. Mater. Interfaces* **2017**, *9*, 35673–35682. [CrossRef]
82. Luo, R.C.; Lim, Z.H.; Li, W.; Shi, P.; Chen, C.-H. Near-infrared light triggerable deformation-free polysaccharide double network hydrogels. *Chem. Commun.* **2014**, *50*, 7052–7055. [CrossRef]
83. Dong, L.; Xia, S.; Wu, K.; Huang, Z.; Chen, H.; Chen, J.; Zhang, J. A pH/enzyme-responsive tumor-specific delivery system for doxorubicin. *Biomaterials* **2010**, *31*, 6309–6316. [CrossRef]
84. Wu, J.L.; Wang, C.Q.; Zhuo, R.X.; Cheng, S.X. Multi-drug delivery system based on alginate/calcium carbonate hybrid nanoparticles for combination chemotherapy. *Colloids Surf. B Biointerfaces* **2014**, *123*, 498–505. [CrossRef] [PubMed]

85. Zhang, B.; Yan, Y.; Shen, Q.; Ma, D.; Huang, L.; Cai, X.; Tan, S. A colon targeted drug delivery system based on alginate modificated graphene oxide for colorectal liver metastasis. *Mater. Sci. Eng. C* **2017**, *79*, 185–190. [CrossRef] [PubMed]
86. Nazemi, Z.; Nourbakhsh, M.S.; Kiani, S.; Daemi, H.; Ashtiani, M.K.; Baharv, H. Effect of chemical composition and sulfated modification of alginate in the development of delivery systems based on electrostatic interactions for small molecule drugs. *Mater. Lett.* **2020**, *263*, 127235. [CrossRef]
87. Hügl, S.; Scheper, V.; Gepp, M.M.; Lenarz, T.; Rau, T.S.; Schwieger, J. Coating stability and insertion forces of an alginate-cell-based drug delivery implant system for the inner ear. *J. Mech. Behav. Biomed. Mater.* **2019**, *97*, 90–98. [CrossRef] [PubMed]
88. Rahimnejad, M.; Jahanshahi, M.; Najafpour, G.D. Production of biological nanoparticles from bovine serum albumin for drug delivery. *Afr. J. Biotechnol.* **2006**, *5*, 1918–1923.
89. Joshi, M.; Nagarsenkar, M.; Prabhakar, B. Albumin nano-carriers for pulmonary drug delivery: An attractive approach. *J. Drug Deliv. Sci. Technol.* **2020**, *56*, 101529. [CrossRef]
90. Patil, G.V. Biopolymer albumin for diagnosis and in drug delivery. *Drug Dev. Res.* **2003**, *58*, 219–247. [CrossRef]
91. Irache, J.M.; Merodio, M.; Arnedo, A.; Camapanero, M.A.; Mirshahi, M.; Espuelas, S. Albumin nanoparticles for the intravitreal delivery of anticytomegaloviral drugs. *Mini Rev. Med. Chem.* **2005**, *5*, 293–305. [CrossRef]
92. Arshady, R. Preparation of microspheres and microcapsules by interfacial polycondensation techniques. *J. Microcapsul.* **1989**, *6*, 13–28. [CrossRef]
93. Oakenfull, D.; Pearce, J.; Burley, R.W.; Damodaran, S.; Paraf, A. (Eds.) *Food Proteins and Their Applications*; Marcel Dekker: New York, NY, USA, 1997; Volume 487, p. 681.
94. Hu, Y.J.; Liu, Y.; Sun, T.Q.; Bai, A.M.; Lü, J.Q.; Pi, Z.B. Binding of anti-inflammatory drug cromolyn sodiumto bovine serumalbumin. *Int. J. Biol. Macromol.* **2006**, *39*, 280–285. [CrossRef]
95. Kratz, F. Albumin as a drug carrier: Design of prodrugs, drug conjugates and nanoparticles. *J. Control. Release* **2008**, *132*, 171–183. [CrossRef]
96. Ulbrich, K.; Hematara, T.; Herbert, E.; Kreuter, J. Transferrin- and transferrinreceptor-antibody-modified nanoparticles enable drug delivery across the blood-brain barrier (BBB). *Eur. J. Pharm. Biopharm.* **2009**, *71*, 251–256. [CrossRef]
97. Elzoghby, A.O.; Samy, W.M.; Elgindy, N.A. Albumin-based nanoparticles as potential controlled release drug delivery systems. *J. Control. Release* **2012**, *157*, 168–182. [CrossRef]
98. Kim, T.H.; Jiang, H.H.; Youn, Y.S.; Park, C.W.; Tak, K.K.; Lee, S.; Kim, H.; Jon, S.; Chen, X.; Lee, K.C. Preparation and characterization of water-soluble albuminbound curcumin nanoparticles with improved antitumor activity. *Int. J. Pharm.* **2011**, *403*, 285–291. [CrossRef]
99. Dreis, S.; Rothweiler, F.; Michaelis, M.; Cinatl, J., Jr.; Kreuter, J.; Langer, K. Preparation, characterization and maintenance of drug efficacy of doxorubicin-loaded human serum albumin (HSA) nanoparticles. *Int. J. Pharm.* **2007**, *341*, 207–214. [CrossRef]
100. Iwao, Y.; Tomiguchi, I.; Domura, A.; Mantaira, Y.; Minami, A.; Suzuki, T.; Ikawa, T.; Kimura, S.I.; Itai, S. Inflamed site-specific drug delivery system based on the interaction of human serum albumin nanoparticles with myeloperoxidase in a murine model of experimental colitis. *Eur. J. Pharm. Biopharm.* **2018**, *125*, 141–147. [CrossRef]
101. Siri, M.; Grasselli, M.; Alonso, S.d.V. Correlation between assembly structure of a gamma irradiated albumin nanoparticle and its function as a drug delivery system. *Colloids Surf. A Physicochem. Eng. Asp.* **2020**, *603*, 125176. [CrossRef]
102. Stein, N.; Mulac, D.; Fabian, J.; Herrmann, F.C.; Langer, K. Nanoparticle albumin-bound mTHPC for photodynamic therapy: Preparation and comprehensive characterization of a promising drug delivery system. *Int. J. Pharm.* **2020**, *582*, 119347. [CrossRef]
103. Gomes, D.S.; Santos, A.M.C.; Neves, G.A.; Menezes, R.R. A brief review on hydroxyapatite production and use in biomedicine. *Cerâmica* **2019**, *65*, 282–302. [CrossRef]
104. Zhao, Z.; Espanol, M.; Guillem-Marti, J.; Kempf, D.; Diez-Escudero, A.; Ginebra, M.-P. Ion-doping as a strategy to modulate hydroxyapatite nanopartilce internalization. *Nanoscale* **2016**, *8*, 1595–1607. [CrossRef]
105. Cellet, T.S.P.; Pereira, G.M.; Muniz, E.C.; Silva, R.; Rubira, A.F. Hydroxyapatite nanowhiskers embedded in chondroitin sulfate microsphere as colon targeted drug delivery system. *J. Mater. Chem. B* **2015**, *3*, 6837–6846. [CrossRef]

106. Sionkowska, A.; Kozlowsa, J. Characterization of collagen/hydroxyapatite composite sponges as a potential bone substitute. *Int. J. Biol. Macromol.* **2010**, *47*, 483–487. [CrossRef]
107. Li, D.; Huang, X.; Wu, Y.; Li, J.; Cheng, W.; He, J.; Tian, H.; Huang, Y. Preparation of pH-responsive mesoporous hydroxyapatite nanoparticles for intracellular controlled release of an anticancer drug. *Biomater. Sci.* **2016**, *4*, 272–280. [CrossRef]
108. Venkatasubbu, G.D.; Ramasamy, S.; Avadhani, G.S.; Ramakrishnan, V.; Kumar, J. Surface modification and paclitaxel drug delivery of folic acid modified polyethylene glycol functionalized hydroxyapatite nanoparticles. *Powder Technol.* **2013**, *235*, 437–442. [CrossRef]
109. Ghafarinazari, A.; Tahari, A.; Moztarzadeh, F.; Mozafari, M.; Bahroloom, M.E. Ion exchange behaviour of silver-doped apatite micro and nanoparticles as antibacterial biomaterial. *Micro Nano Lett.* **2011**, *6*, 713–717. [CrossRef]
110. Mizuno, S.; Glowacki, J. Three dimensional composite of demineralized bone powder and collagen for in vitro analysis of chondroinduction of human dermal fibroblasts. *Biomaterials* **1996**, *17*, 1819–1825. [CrossRef]
111. Ramakrishna, S.; Mayer, J.; Wintermantel, E.; Leong, K.W. Biomedical applications of polymer-composite materials: A review. *Compos. Sci. Technol.* **2001**, *61*, 1189–1224. [CrossRef]
112. Wang, M.; Joseph, R.; Bonfield, W. Hydroxyapatite-poly- ethylene composites for bone substitution: Effects of ceramic particle size and morphology. *Biomaterials* **1998**, *19*, 2357–2366. [CrossRef]
113. Bonfield, W.; Wang, M.; Tanner, K.E. Interfaces in analogue biomaterials. *Acta Mater.* **1998**, *46*, 2509–2518. [CrossRef]
114. Di Silvio, L.; Dalby, M.J.; Bonfield, W. Osteoblast behaviour on HA/PE composite surfaces with different HA volumes. *Biomaterials* **2002**, *23*, 101–107. [CrossRef]
115. Wang, M.; Bonfield, W. Chemically coupled hydroxyapatite-polyethylene composites: Processing and characterization. *Mater. Lett.* **2000**, *44*, 119–124. [CrossRef]
116. Kikuchi, M.; Itoh, S.; Ichinose, S.; Shinomiya, K.; Tanaka, J. Self-organization mechanism in a bone-like hy-droxyapatite/collagen nanocomposite synthesized in vitro and its biological reaction in vivo. *Biomaterials* **2001**, *22*, 1705–1711. [CrossRef]
117. Li, J.; Fartash, B.; Hermannson, L. Hydroxyapatite-alu-mina composites and bone-bonding. *Biomaterials* **1995**, *16*, 417–422. [CrossRef]
118. Lopes, M.A.; Silva, R.F.; Monteiro, F.J.; Santos, J.D. Microstructural dependence of Young's moduli of P_2O_5 glass reinforced hydroxyapatite for biomedical applications. *Biomaterials* **2000**, *21*, 749–754. [CrossRef]
119. Liu, Q.; de Wijn, J.R.; van Blitterswijk, C.A. Composite biomaterials with chemical bonding between hy-droxyapatite filler particles and PEG/PBT copoly-mer matrix. *J. Biomed. Mater. Res.* **1998**, *40*, 490–497. [CrossRef]
120. Ghiasi, B.; Sefidbakht, Y.; Rezaei, M. Hydroxyapatite for Biomedicine and Drug Delivery. *Nanomater. Adv. Biol. Appl.* **2019**, *104*, 85–120.
121. Choi, K.Y.; Min, K.H.; Na, J.H.; Choi, K.; Kim, K.; Park, J.H.; Kwon, I.C.; Jeong, S.Y. Self-assembled hyaluronic acid nanoparticles as a potential drug carrier for cancer therapy: Synthesis, characterization, and in vivo biodistribution. *J. Mater. Chem.* **2009**, *19*, 4102–4107. [CrossRef]
122. Schanté, C.E.; Zuber, G.; Herlin, C.; Vandamme, T.F. Chemical modifications of hyaluronic acid for the synthesis of derivatives for a broad range of biomedical applications. *Carbohydr. Polym.* **2011**, *85*, 469–489. [CrossRef]
123. Cheng, D.; Han, W.; Yang, K.; Song, Y.; Jiang, M.; Song, E. One-step facile synthesis of hyaluronic acid functionalized fluorescent gold nanoprobes sensitive to hyaluronidase in urine specimen from bladder cancer patients. *Talanta* **2014**, *130*, 408–414. [CrossRef]
124. Liu, K.; Wang, Z.Q.; Wang, S.J.; Liu, P.; Qin, Y.H.; Ma, Y.; Li, X.C.; Huo, Z.-J. Hyaluronic acidtagged silica nanoparticles in colon cancer therapy: Therapeutic efficacy evaluation. *Int. J. Nanomed.* **2015**, *10*, 6445–6454.
125. Wang, H.; Sun, G.; Zhang, Z.; Ou, Y. Transcription activator, hyaluronic acid and tocopheryl succinate multi-functionalized novel lipid carriers encapsulating etoposide for lymphoma therapy. *Biomed. Pharmacother.* **2017**, *91*, 241–250. [CrossRef] [PubMed]
126. Huang, G.; Huang, H. Hyaluronic acid-based biopharmaceutical delivery and tumor-targeted drug delivery system. *J. Control. Release* **2018**, *278*, 122–126. [CrossRef] [PubMed]

127. Zhong, W.; Pang, L.; Feng, H.; Dong, H.; Wang, S.; Cong, H.; Shen, Y.; Bing, Y. Recent advantage of hyaluronic acid for anticancer application: A review of "3S" transition approach. *Carbohydr. Polym.* **2020**, *238*, 116204. [CrossRef] [PubMed]
128. Cai, J.; Fu, J.; Li, R.; Zhang, F.; Ling, G.; Zhang, P. A potential carrier for anti-tumor targeted delivery-hyaluronic acid nanoparticles. *Carbohydr. Polym.* **2019**, *208*, 356–364. [CrossRef] [PubMed]
129. Choi, K.Y.; Min, K.H.; Yoon, H.Y.; Kim, K.; Park, J.H.; Kwon, I.C.; Choi, K.; Jeong, S.Y. PEGylation of hyaluronic acid nanoparticles improves tumor targetability in vivo. *Biomaterials* **2011**, *32*, 1880–1889. [CrossRef]
130. Na, K.; Lee, C.-S. Photochemically Triggered Cytosolic Drug Delivery Using pHResponsive Hyaluronic Acid Nanoparticles for Light-Induced Cancer Therapy. *Biomaterials* **2014**, *15*, 4228–4238.
131. Yoon, H.Y.; Koo, H.; Ki Choi, Y.; Kwon, I.C.; Choi, K.; Jae HyungPark, J.H.; Kim, K. Photo-crosslinked hyaluronic acid nanoparticles with improved stability for in vivo tumor-targeted drug delivery. *Biomaterials* **2013**, *34*, 5273–5280. [CrossRef]

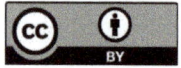

© 2020 by the authors. Licensee MDPI, Basel, Switzerland. This article is an open access article distributed under the terms and conditions of the Creative Commons Attribution (CC BY) license (http://creativecommons.org/licenses/by/4.0/).

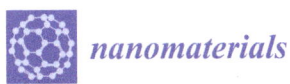

Article

rAAV-Mediated Overexpression of SOX9 and TGF-β via Carbon Dot-Guided Vector Delivery Enhances the Biological Activities in Human Bone Marrow-Derived Mesenchymal Stromal Cells

Weikun Meng [1,†], Ana Rey-Rico [2,†], Mickaël Claudel [3], Gertrud Schmitt [1], Susanne Speicher-Mentges [1], Françoise Pons [3], Luc Lebeau [3], Jagadeesh K. Venkatesan [1,‡] and Magali Cucchiarini [1,*,‡]

1. Center of Experimental Orthopaedics, Saarland University Medical Center, D-66421 Homburg, Germany; weikun.m@gmail.com (W.M.); Gertrud.Schmitt@uks.eu (G.S.); Susanne.Speicher-Mentges@uks.eu (S.S.-M.); jegadish.venki@gmail.com (J.K.V.)
2. Cell Therapy and Regenerative Medicine Unit, Centro de Investigacións Científicas Avanzadas (CICA), Universidade da Coruña, ES-15071 A Coruña, Spain; ana.rey.rico@udc.es
3. Laboratoire de Conception et Application de Molécules Bioactives, Faculty of Pharmacy, UMR 7199 CNRS—University of Strasbourg, F-67401 Illkirch, France; mickael.claudel@etu.unistra.fr (M.C.); pons@unistra.fr (F.P.); llebeau@unistra.fr (L.L.)
* Correspondence: mmcucchiarini@hotmail.com; Tel.: +49-6841-1624-987; Fax: +49-6841-1624-988
† These authors shared first authorship.
‡ These authors shared senior authorship.

Received: 31 March 2020; Accepted: 27 April 2020; Published: 28 April 2020

Abstract: Scaffold-assisted gene therapy is a highly promising tool to treat articular cartilage lesions upon direct delivery of chondrogenic candidate sequences. The goal of this study was to examine the feasibility and benefits of providing highly chondroreparative agents, the cartilage-specific sex-determining region Y-type high-mobility group 9 (SOX9) transcription factor or the transforming growth factor beta (TGF-β), to human bone marrow-derived mesenchymal stromal cells (hMSCs) via clinically adapted, independent recombinant adeno-associated virus (rAAV) vectors formulated with carbon dots (CDs), a novel class of carbon-dominated nanomaterials. Effective complexation and release of a reporter rAAV-lacZ vector was achieved using four different CDs elaborated from 1-citric acid and pentaethylenehexamine (CD-1); 2-citric acid, poly(ethylene glycol) monomethyl ether (MW 550 Da), and N,N-dimethylethylenediamine (CD-2); 3-citric acid, branched poly(ethylenimine) (MW 600 Da), and poly(ethylene glycol) monomethyl ether (MW 2 kDa) (CD-3); and 4-citric acid and branched poly(ethylenimine) (MW 600 Da) (CD-4), allowing for the genetic modification of hMSCs. Among the nanoparticles, CD-2 showed an optimal ability for rAAV delivery (up to 2.2-fold increase in lacZ expression relative to free vector treatment with 100% cell viability for at least 10 days, the longest time point examined). Administration of therapeutic (SOX9, TGF-β) rAAV vectors in hMSCs via CD-2 led to the effective overexpression of each independent transgene, promoting enhanced cell proliferation (TGF-β) and cartilage matrix deposition (glycosaminoglycans, type-II collagen) for at least 21 days relative to control treatments (CD-2 lacking rAAV or associated to rAAV-lacZ), while advantageously restricting undesirable type-I and -X collagen deposition. These results reveal the potential of CD-guided rAAV gene administration in hMSCs as safe, non-invasive systems for translational strategies to enhance cartilage repair.

Keywords: bone marrow-derived mesenchymal stromal cells; rAAV vectors; carbon dots; SOX9; TGF-β; cartilage repair

1. Introduction

Articular cartilage lesions represent serious clinical issues in orthopaedics as this specialized tissue does not fully heal on itself by lack of vascularization and of local chondroregenerative cells that may repopulate the defects [1,2]. Despite the availability of a number of clinical interventions (Pridie drilling, microfracture, cell transplantation), none can promote the generation of the original hyaline cartilage (proteoglycans, type-II collagen) in the lesions, with instead the appearance of a fibrocartilaginous repair tissue (type-I collagen) showing lesser mechanical properties and that may be prone to osteoarthritis [1–4]. Administration of chondroreparative mesenchymal stromal cells (MSCs) [5–7] in focal cartilage defects represents a valuable therapeutic alternative to activate the local healing processes [8,9], yet here again formation of the native hyaline cartilage is not observed [8,9], showing the necessity to develop improved treatments for adapted cartilage repair.

Scaffold-assisted gene transfer is an attractive therapeutic approach for cartilage repair as it has the potential to activate the intrinsic repair processes in sites of cartilage lesions by controlling the delivery of carriers coding for candidate genes [10–12], having been reported using nonviral [13–19] and lentiviral vectors [20–23]. While such gene vectors commonly support short-term transgene expression (nonviral vectors) or have the potential to activate oncogenes following genome integration (lentiviral vectors), vectors based on adeno-associated viruses (AAV) may be more adapted as they promote transgene expression over extended periods of time (some years) in a much safer manner due to the lack of viral protein coding sequences in the recombinant AAV (rAAV) backbone [10,11]. Thus far, biomaterial-assisted rAAV gene transfer for cartilage research has been described including polymeric micelles [24–27], hydrogels [28–32] and solid scaffolds [33], yet other materials may constitute valuable systems for rAAV delivery in experimental cartilage therapy. In this regard, carbon dots (CDs), a recently discovered class of carbon-dominated, biocompatible nanomaterials [34,35] used in drug delivery and theranostic approaches [35,36], may be good candidates to achieve this goal as they have been reported for their ability to intracellularly deliver nucleic acids and proteins in vitro [37] and in experimental models in vivo of cancer [38–40] and for regenerative medicine [41,42]. It remains to be seen whether CDs are capable of assisting rAAV vector transfer for cartilage repair as such vectors are more effective than nonviral vehicles to deliver genetic material in target cells [10,11].

The goal of this study was therefore to evaluate the potential of various CDs to associate with and release rAAV vectors as a means to target chondrogenically competent human MSCs (hMSCs), with a focus on transferring DNA sequences for the highly chondroreparative sex-determining region Y-type high mobility group box 9 (SOX9) transcription factor [43] and transforming growth factor beta (TGF-β) [5,6]. The data show that CDs are potent systems to efficiently vectorize and release rAAV, especially CD-2 nanoparticles, which allow hMSCs to be optimally targeted via rAAV gene transfer. Specific delivery of rAAV vectors carrying either the candidate SOX9 or TGF-β sequences assisted by CD-2 led to effective expression of the transgenes in these cells, enhancing cell proliferation and cartilage matrix deposition (glycosaminoglycans, type-II collagen) with reduced type-I and -X collagen production. These findings provide evidence on the ability of CD-assisted therapeutic rAAV gene delivery to target chondroreparative hMSCs in future non-invasive and safe applications to treat sites of cartilage injury.

2. Materials and Methods

2.1. Reagents

All reagents were purchased at Sigma (Munich, Germany) unless otherwise indicated. The anti-SOX9 (C-20) and anti-TGF-β (V) antibodies were from Santa Cruz Biotechnology (Heidelberg, Germany), the anti-type-II collagen (II-II6B3) from the NIH Hybridome Bank (University of Iowa, Ames, IA, USA), the anti-type-I collagen (AF-5610) antibody from Acris (Hiddenhausen, Germany), and the anti-type-X collagen (COL-10) antibody from Sigma. The biotinylated secondary antibodies and ABC reagent were from Vector Laboratories (Alexis Deutschland GmbH, Grünberg, Germany). The AAVanced

Concentration Reagent was from System Bioscience (Heidelberg, Germany) and the Cy3 Ab Labeling Kit from Amersham/GE Healthcare (Munich, Germany). The AAV titration ELISA was from Progen (Heidelberg, Germany). The β-gal staining kit and the Cell Proliferation Reagent WST-1 were purchased at Roche Applied Science (Mannheim, Germany), the Beta-Glo® Assay System at Promega (Mannheim, Germany), and the TGF-β Quantikine ELISA at R&D Systems (Wiesbaden, Germany).

2.2. Human Bone Marrow-Derived Mesenchymal Stromal Cells

The study was approved by the Ethics Committee of the Saarland Physicians Council (Ärztekammer des Saarlandes, reference number Ha06/08). All patients provided informed consent before being included in the study, which was performed in accordance with the Helsinki Declaration. Bone marrow aspirates (~15 mL; 0.4–1.2 × 10^9 cells/mL) were prepared from the distal femurs of patients undergoing total knee arthroplasty (n = 12, age 75 ± 3 years). Bone marrow-derived human mesenchymal stromal cells (hMSCs) were isolated by washing and centrifuging the aspirates in Dulbecco's modified Eagle's medium (DMEM) and resuspending the pellet in red blood cell lysing buffer with DMEM (1:1) [44,45]. The mixtures were washed and resuspended in DMEM, 10% fetal bovine serum, 100 U/mL penicillin, and 100 µL/mL streptomycin (growth medium) for cell plating and maintenance in T75 flasks at 37 °C under 5% CO_2. A medium change was performed after 24 h using growth medium with recombinant FGF-2 (1 ng/mL) for expansion [44,45], followed by changes every 2–3 days and replating when the cells reached a density of 85%, using cells at no more than passage 1–2.

2.3. Preparation of the Carbon Dots

The various carbon dots (CD-1 to CD-4) were generated through a bottom-up approach, using pyrolysis of citric acid (CA) as the carbon source, in the presence of various additives as passivation reagent: pentaethylenehexamine (PEHA), N,N-dimethylethylenediamine (DMEDA), branched poly(ethyleneimine) 600 Da ($bPEI_{600}$), poly(ethylene glycol) monomethyl ether 550 Da ($mPEG_{550}$), or 2 kDa ($mPEG_{2000}$) [35,38] (Figure 1 and Table 1). Pyrolysis was conducted under conventional heating or microwave irradiation, and the resulting nanoparticles were purified using extensive dialysis against HCl 0.1 N and ultrapure H_2O (MWCO 1000 Da) [35,38]. The CDs were freeze-dried, and 5.0 mg/mL stock solutions were prepared and stored at 4 °C until use [35,38]. The size and charge (zeta potential, ζ) of the nanoparticles were determined using dynamic light scattering (DLS) (NanoSizer NanoZS, Malvern UK) and transmission electron microscopy (TEM) operating at 5 kV (LVEM5, Delong Instruments, Brno, Czech Republic) [35,38] (Table 1).

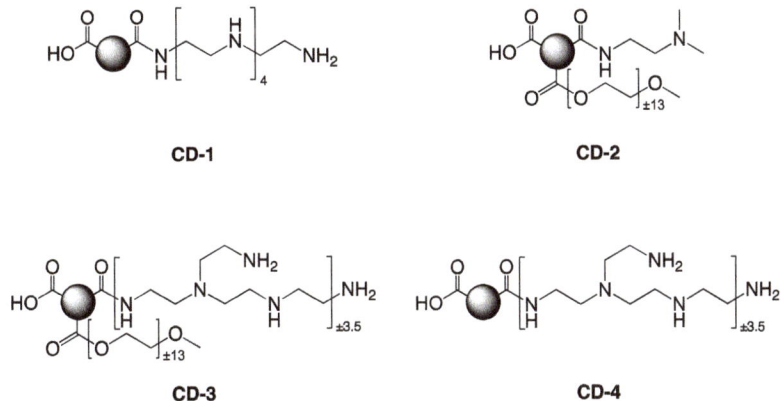

Figure 1. Structural features of the various carbon dots employed in the study. The nanoparticles CD-1 to CD-4 were generated through pyrolysis of citric acid (CA) in the presence of various passivation reagents presented in Materials and Methods and in Table 1.

Table 1. Characteristics of the various carbon dots (CD-1 to CD-4) employed in the study.

Name	Starting Material (w/w)	Activation Mode	Size (nm) [a] DLS	Size (nm) [a] TEM	Potential [a] (mV)
CD-1	CA/PEHA (1/4)	(1) 30 min at 180 °C [b] (2) 30 min at 230 °C [b]	36.4 ± 12.0	17.9	+18.6 ± 0.9
CD-2	CA/mPEG$_{550}$/DMEDA (1/3/3)	(1) 30 min at 180 °C [b] (2) 30 min at 230 °C [b]	17.7 ± 0.9	16.3	+26.9 ± 1.6
CD-3	CA/bPEI$_{600}$/mPEG$_{2000}$ (1/4/1)	MW 620 W, 190 s [c]	13.3 ± 0.4	-	+29.4 ± 0.4
CD-4	CA/bPEI$_{600}$ (1/4)	MW 620 W, 120 s [c]	11.7 ± 0.9	-	+37.6 ± 3.2

[a] Measured at 1.0 mg/mL in 1.5 mM NaCl, pH 7.4. [b] Reactions were conducted under conventional heating. [c] Reactions were conducted in a domestic microwave oven.

2.4. Preparation of the rAAV Vectors

The vectors were generated using pSSV9, a parental AAV-2 genomic clone [46,47]. rAAV-lacZ carries the E. coli β-galactosidase (lacZ) reporter gene, rAAV-FLAG-hsox9 a 1.7-kb FLAG-tagged human sox9 (hsox9) cDNA sequence, and rAAV-hTGF-β a 1.2-kb human transforming growth factor beta 1 (hTGF-β) sequence, all controlled by the cytomegalovirus immediate-early (CMV-IE) promoter [25,44,45]. Conventional packaging of not self-complementary vectors was performed using helper-free (two-plasmid) transfection in 293 cells with the packaging plasmid pXX2 and adenovirus helper plasmid pXX6 [25,45]. Vector purification was performed using the AAVanced Concentration Reagent [25], and vector titers were monitored using real-time PCR [25,44,45], averaging 10^{10} transgene copies/mL (~1/500 functional recombinant viral particles).

2.5. Cy3 Labeling

The rAAV vectors were labeled using a Cy3 Ab Labeling Kit according to the manufacturer's recommendations by mixing rAAV (1 mL) in sodium carbonate/sodium bicarbonate buffer (pH 9.3) for 30 min at room temperature, followed by labeling with Cy3 and dialysis against 20 mM HEPES (pH 7.5)/150 mL NaCl [25].

2.6. Complexation of the rAAV Vectors with the Carbon Dots and Release Studies

The various CDs (40 µL) were directly mixed with the rAAV vectors (40 µL, 8×10^5 transgene copies) and incubated for 30 min at room temperature to generate the rAAV/CD systems. Alternatively, Cy3-labeled rAAV vectors were employed for the visualization analyses of the complexation studies by mixing Cy3-labeled rAAV (40 µL, 8×10^5 transgene copies) with the CDs (40 µL) in 96-well plates in serum-free DMEM (100 µL). Cy3 labeling of the samples was monitored under live fluorescence with a rhodamine filter set (Olympus CKX41, Hamburg, Germany). For the release studies, the rAAV/CD systems as prepared above were placed in 24-well plates in 350 µL of serum-free DMEM, and rAAV was measured in aliquots of culture medium at the denoted time points using an AAV titration ELISA [25].

2.7. rAAV/CD-Mediated Gene Transfer

Monolayer cultures of hMSCs were directly incubated with the rAAV/CD systems prepared as described above in the various assays at the indicated cell densities, culture formats, and volume/multiplicity of infection (MOI) [25,44,45]. The cultures were maintained in growth medium [44,45] in a humidified atmosphere with 5% CO_2 and at 37 °C for up to 21 days for the analyses.

2.8. Transgene Expression

lacZ expression was assessed using X-Gal staining for monitoring under light microscopy (Olympus BX45) and using the Beta-Glo® Assay System to provide an estimation of the β-gal activity (values expressed as relative luminescence units—RLU—with normalization to the number of cells) [25]. Expression of SOX9 and TGF-β was monitored using immunohistochemical analysis with specific primary antibodies, a biotinylated secondary antibody, and using the ABC method with diaminobenzidine (DAB) as a chromogen for monitoring under light microscopy (Olympus BX45) [44,45]. TGF-β expression was also measured using specific ELISA [45]. All measurements were performed using a GENios spectrophotometer/fluorometer (Tecan, Crailsheim, Germany).

2.9. Cell Viability and Proliferation

Cell viability was monitored using the Cell Proliferation Reagent WST-1, with $OD^{450\,nm}$ being proportional to the number of cells [25,44,45]. Cell proliferation was provided as a direct index [44,45]. Cell viability percentage [25] was calculated as:

Cell viability (%) = (absorbance of the sample/absorbance of the negative control) × 100

All measurements were performed using a GENios spectrophotometer/fluorometer (Tecan).

2.10. Histology and Immunohistochemistry

Cells in monolayer cultures were harvested at the denoted time points for fixation in 4% formalin. Fixed cells were stained with alcian blue for glycosaminoglycans as previously reported [25], with removal of excess stain in double distilled water. The stain was quantitatively estimated using solubilization in 6 M guanidine hydrochloride overnight to measure $OD^{600\,nm}$ [25] using a GENios spectrophotometer/fluorometer. Immunohistochemical evaluations were also performed to examine the deposition of type-II, -I, and -X collagen using specific primary antibodies, biotinylated secondary antibodies, and the ABC method with DAB as a chromogen for monitoring under light microscopy (Olympus BX45) [25,44,45]. Control conditions lacking primary antibodies were also evaluated to check for secondary immunoglobulins.

2.11. Histomorphometric Analysis

The intensities of X-Gal staining and the percentages of $SOX9^+$, $TGF\textrm{-}\beta^+$, and type-$II^+/\textrm{-}I^+/\textrm{-}X^+$ collagen cells (SOX9-, TGF-β-, and type-II/-I/-X collagen-stained cells to the total cell numbers) were measured at three random sites standardized for their surface using the SIS analySIS program (Olympus) and Adobe Photoshop (Adobe Systems, Unterschleissheim, Germany) [25,45].

2.12. Statistical Analysis

Data are provided as mean ± standard deviation (SD) of separate experiments. Each condition was performed in triplicate in three independent experiments per patient. Data were obtained by two individuals blinded with respect to the groups. The t-test and the Mann-Whitney rank sum test were used where appropriate. A P value of less than 0.05 was considered statistically significant.

3. Results

3.1. Effective rAAV Association to Carbon Dots and Release

The reporter rAAV-*lacZ* gene vector was first formulated with the various CDs (CD-1 to CD-4) to examine the ability of these nanoparticles to associate with rAAV and release it over time (up to 10 days, the longest time point evaluated) using Cy labeling and fluorescent evaluation of the vectors in the systems and by measuring the rAAV concentrations in the culture medium via AAV titration ELISA.

Successful formulation of Cy3-labeled rAAV vectors with the different CDs was seen as revealed by the effective detection of live fluorescence in the samples after 24 h relative to the control conditions (CDs formulating unlabeled rAAV and CDs lacking rAAV), without visible difference between CDs or when using Cy3-labeled rAAV vectors in the absence of CD formulation (Figure 2A). Furthermore, all CDs were capable of releasing rAAV over a period of at least 10 days, with CD-2 allowing for the highest early vector release and a good maintenance of vector concentration over time (rAAV-*lacZ*/CD-2) relative to the other CDs (rAAV-*lacZ*/CD-1, rAAV-*lacZ*/CD-3, and rAAV-*lacZ*/CD-4) and versus free vector control (rAAV-*lacZ*) (Figure 2B).

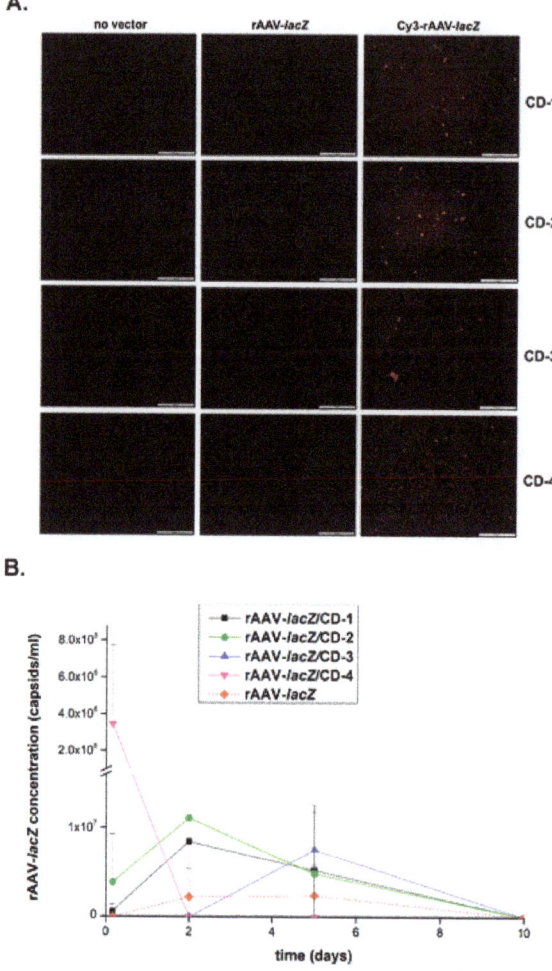

Figure 2. Complexation and release of rAAV vectors from the carbon dots. The rAAV-*lacZ* vector was labeled with Cy3 and formulated with the various CDs (40 μL rAAV, 8×10^5 transgene copies/40 μL CD) and placed in culture over time. (**A**) Cy3-labeled rAAV formulated with the various CDs were examined under live fluorescence after 24 h (magnification ×10; scale bars: 100 μm; all representative data). Control conditions included CD formulations with unlabeled rAAV, CDs lacking rAAV, and absence of CDs. (**B**) rAAV release from the various CDs was monitored by measuring the rAAV concentrations in the culture medium at the denoted time points using an AAV titration ELISA. Free vector treatment was used as a control condition.

3.2. Effective rAAV-Mediated Reporter lacZ Overexpression in hMSCs upon Delivery Assistance by Carbon Dots

The reporter rAAV-*lacZ* gene vector was next formulated with the various CDs to determine the ability of the systems to promote the safe genetic modification of hMSCs over time (up to 10 days, the longest time point evaluated) relative to control conditions (CDs lacking rAAV, i.e., -/CD; free rAAV, i.e., rAAV-*lacZ*; absence of both CDs and rAAV, i.e., -) by monitoring *lacZ* expression using X-Gal staining and via quantitative detection of the β-gal activities in the cells using a Beta-Glo® Assay and by evaluating their viability using the Cell Proliferation Reagent WST-1.

A preliminary, histomorphometric analysis of the early X-Gal staining intensities in the cells on day 1 revealed that the CD-2, CD-3, and CD-4 formulations of rAAV-*lacZ* were capable of promoting *lacZ* expression in the hMSCs without significant difference relative to free vector administration ($P \geq 0.050$) (Figure 3A). The staining intensities in the cells treated with rAAV-*lacZ*/CD-2, rAAV-*lacZ*/CD-3, and rAAV-*lacZ*/CD-4 increased on day 10, especially when using CD-2 (1.4-fold increase versus day 1; $P = 0.060$), again without difference compared with free rAAV-*lacZ* treatment ($P \geq 0.050$) (Figure 3B). In marked contrast, delivery of rAAV-*lacZ* in the cells via CD-1 promoted a significant reduction of the staining intensities in hMSCs relative to free vector administration (102.9- and 32.5-fold decrease on days 1 and 10, respectively; always $P \leq 0.040$) (Figure 3A,B). Overall, these results were supported by a comprehensive, quantitative estimation of the β-gal activities in the cells using the Beta-Glo® Assay, even showing increased activities when providing rAAV-*lacZ* via CD-2, CD-3, or CD-4 versus free vector treatment (up to 2.9- and 2.3-fold difference on days 1 and 10, respectively; always $P \leq 0.050$) and with reduced activities when using CD-1 (19- and 15.8-fold difference versus free vector administration; always $P \leq 0.020$) (Figure 3A,B).

CD-guided delivery of rAAV-*lacZ* to hMSCs using either CD-1 or CD-2 was safe, as revealed by the results of a WST-1 assay, with 100% cell viability preserved on day 1, without significant difference relative to the corresponding control conditions (-, -/CD-1, -CD-2, and free vector administration; always $P \geq 0.180$) (Figure 4A). In contrast, CD-3 and CD-4 had significantly detrimental effects on cell viability (<32%; always $P \leq 0.010$ versus all other conditions). Similar observations were noted on day 10, with 100% viability using CD-1 and CD-2, as noted in the corresponding control conditions (always $P \geq 0.050$), and about 25–30% viability using CD-3 or CD-4 (always $P \leq 0.040$ versus all other conditions) (Figure 4B).

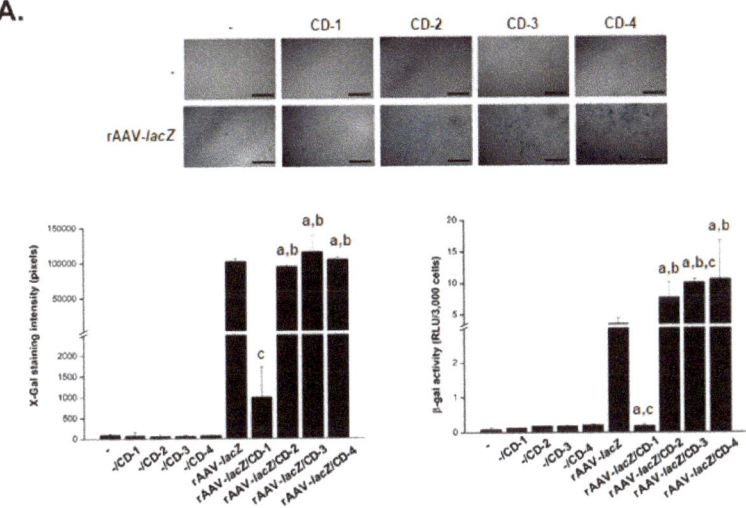

Figure 3. *Cont.*

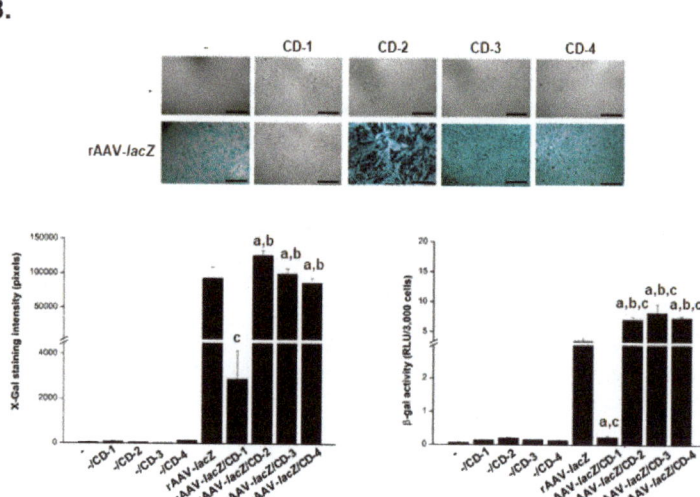

Figure 3. Detection of reporter (*lacZ*) gene overexpression in hMSCs transduced with the rAAV/CD systems. The rAAV-*lacZ* vector (20 µL, 4×10^5 transgene copies) was formulated with the various CDs (CD-1 to CD-4; 20 µL), and the resulting rAAV/CD systems (40 µL, i.e., 4×10^5 transgene copies) were incubated with hMSCs (3000 cells in 96-well plates; MOI = 133) for up to 10 days. Expression of *lacZ* was examined using X-Gal staining (top panel: magnification ×4; scale bars: 500 µm; all representative data) with corresponding histomorphometric analyses (bottom left panel) and using quantitative estimation of the β-gal activities using the Beta-Glo® Assay System (bottom right panel) after one (**A**) and 10 days (**B**). Control conditions included CDs lacking rAAV (-/CD), free rAAV (rAAV-*lacZ*), and absence of both CD and rAAV (-). Statistically significant relative to [a] -, [b] -/CD and [c] rAAV-*lacZ*.

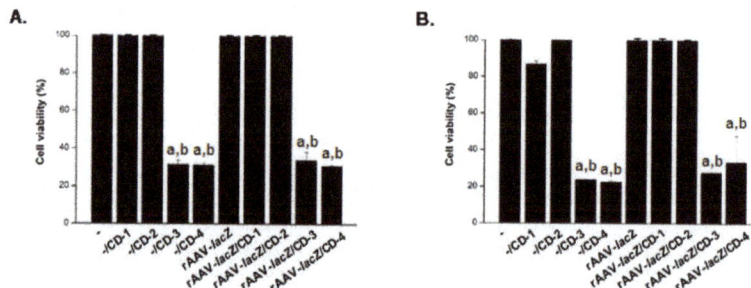

Figure 4. Cell viability in hMSCs transduced with the rAAV/CD systems. The rAAV-*lacZ* vector (20 µL, 4×10^5 transgene copies) was formulated with the various CDs (CD-1 to CD-4; 20 µL) and the resulting rAAV/CD systems (40 µL, i.e., 4×10^5 transgene copies) were incubated with hMSCs (3,000 cells in 96-well plates; MOI = 133) for up to 10 days. Cell viability was examined after one (**A**) and 10 days (**B**) using the Cell Proliferation Reagent WST-1. Control conditions included CDs lacking rAAV (-/CD), free rAAV (rAAV-*lacZ*), and absence of both CD and rAAV (-). Statistically significant relative to [a] - and [b] rAAV-*lacZ*.

3.3. Effective rAAV-Mediated SOX9 and TGF-β Overexpression in hMSCs upon Vector Delivery via Carbon Dots

In light of the efficacy and safety of CD-2, the therapeutic rAAV-FLAG-h*sox9* and rAAV-hTGF-β were next formulated independently with these nanoparticles (rAAV-FLAG-h*sox9*/CD-2 and rAAV-hTGF-β/CD-2, respectively) to determine the ability of the system to promote the overexpression of each candidate gene (SOX9, TGF-β) in hMSCs over time (up to 21 days, the longest time point evaluated) relative to control conditions (CD-2 lacking rAAV, i.e., -/CD-2, CD-2 formulating rAAV-*lacZ*, i.e., rAAV-*lacZ*/CD-2) using immunocytochemical detection of each transgene product. Therapeutic (SOX9, TGF-β) rAAV vectors without CD-2 were not included, as controls because they have been characterized in similar culture conditions in earlier studies [44,45], and in light of the quantitative estimation of the β-gal activities in the cells on day 10, significantly increased activities with rAAV-*lacZ*/CD-2 versus free rAAV-*lacZ* vector treatment were revealed (Figure 3B).

An immunocytochemical analysis of SOX9 expression in the cells revealed that administration of rAAV-FLAG-h*sox9* to hMSCs via CD-2 led to significantly higher levels of SOX9 expression relative to all other conditions after 21 days (65-, 43.3-, and 1.8-fold difference using rAAV-FLAG-h*sox9*/CD-2 versus -/CD-2, rAAV-*lacZ*/CD-2, and rAAV-hTGF-β/CD-2, respectively; always $P \leq 0.001$) (Figure 5A and Table 2). An evaluation of TGF-β expression using immunocytochemistry also showed that delivery of rAAV-hTGF-β to hMSCs via CD-2 led to significantly higher levels of TGF-β expression relative to all other conditions after 21 days (10.3-, 6.8-, and 9.4-fold difference using rAAV-hTGF-β/CD-2 versus -/CD-2, rAAV-*lacZ*/CD-2, and rAAV-FLAG-h*sox9*/CD-2, respectively; always $P \leq 0.001$) (Figure 5B and Table 2). This result was corroborated by an estimation of the levels of TGF-β production in the cells using ELISA, with up to 2.8-, 2.8-, and 3.8-fold higher TGF-β secretion levels when using rAAV-hTGF-β/CD-2 after 5, 7, and 21 days, respectively, versus all other conditions (always $P \leq 0.001$) (Figure 5B).

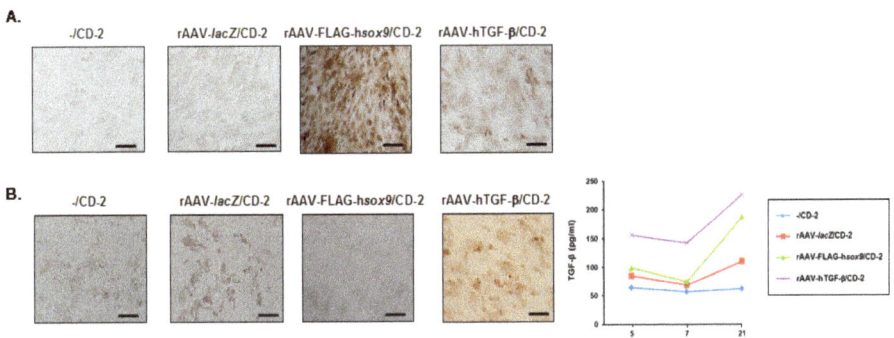

Figure 5. Detection of therapeutic (SOX9, TGF-β) gene overexpression in hMSCs transduced with the rAAV/CD-2 system. The rAAV-FLAG-h*sox9*, rAAV-hTGF-β, and rAAV-*lacZ* vectors (40 µL each vector, 8×10^5 transgene copies) were formulated with CD-2 (40 µL), and the resulting rAAV/CD systems (80 µL, i.e., 8×10^5 transgene copies) were incubated with hMSCs (10,000 cells in 48-well plates; MOI = 80) for up to 21 days. SOX9 (**A**) and TGF-β (**B**) expression was examined using immunocytochemistry (A, B; magnification ×20; scale bars: 50 µm; all representative data) and using specific (TGF-β) ELISA (B). rAAV-*lacZ*/CD-2 and CD-2 lacking rAAV were used as controls.

Table 2. Histomorphometric analyses in hMSCs transduced with the rAAV/CD-2 systems.

Parameter	-/CD-2	rAAV-*lacZ*/CD-2	rAAV-FLAG-h*sox9*/CD-2	rAAV-hTGF-/CD-2
SOX9	1.5 ± 0.6	2.3 ± 0.5	97.5 ± 1.3 [a,b]	52.8 ± 2.2 [a,b,c]
TGF-	7.8 ± 3.1	11.8 ± 2.4	8.5 ± 1.3	79.8 ± 3.9 [a,b,c]
Type-II collagen	4.8 ± 2.5	5.5 ± 2.6	84.8 ± 2.2 [a,b]	68.5 ± 4.5 [a,b,c]
Type-I collagen	85.3 ± 2.2	85.8 ± 2.6	4.3 ± 1.7 [a,b]	3.8 ± 1.0 [a,b]
Type-X collagen	73.3 ± 1.7	72.3 ± 1.7	11.8 ± 1.7 [a,b]	12.8 ± 1.7 [a,b]

Values are given as mean ± SD. All parameters are in % of positively (SOX9+, TGF-β+, type-II+/-I+/-X+ collagen) stained cells to the total cell numbers. Statistically significant relative to [a] -/CD-2, [b] rAAV-*lacZ*/CD-2 and [c] rAAV-FLAG-h*sox9*.

3.4. Effects of rAAV-Mediated SOX9 and TGF-β Overexpression on the Biological Activities in hMSCs upon Vector Delivery via Carbon Dots

The ability of the delivery systems to trigger the biological activities (cell proliferation, matrix deposition) in hMSCs over time (21 days) relative to control conditions (-/CD-2, rAAV-*lacZ*/CD-2) was then examined with the two formulations rAAV-FLAG-h*sox9*/CD-2 and rAAV-hTGF-β/CD-2 by evaluating cell viability using the Cell Proliferation Reagent WST-1 and matrix deposition via spectrophotometric detection of alcian blue staining (glycosaminoglycans) and via immunocytochemical detection of type-II, -I, and -X collagen expression.

Administration of rAAV-hTGF-β in hMSCs via CD-2 led to significantly higher levels of cell proliferation relative to all other conditions after 21 days (1.3-, 1.3-, and 1.2-fold difference using rAAV-hTGF-β/CD-2 versus -/CD-2, rAAV-*lacZ*/CD-2, and rAAV-FLAG-h*sox9*/CD-2, respectively; always $P \leq 0.001$), while no difference was seen with rAAV-FLAG-h*sox9*/CD-2 ($P \geq 0.065$ versus -/CD-2 or rAAV-*lacZ*/CD-2) (Figure 6A). Delivery of either rAAV-FLAG-h*sox9* or rAAV-hTGF-β in hMSCs via CD-2 led to significantly higher levels of glycosaminoglycans relative to all other conditions after 21 days (1.3- and 1.2-fold difference using rAAV-FLAG-h*sox9*/CD-2 versus -/CD-2 and rAAV-*lacZ*/CD-2, respectively, always $P \leq 0.002$; 1.8- and 1.7-fold difference using rAAV-hTGF-β/CD-2 versus -/CD-2 and rAAV-*lacZ*/CD-2, respectively, always $P \leq 0.001$), with a stronger effect of TGF-β relative to SOX9 (1.4-fold difference; $P \leq 0.001$) (Figure 6B). Delivery of either rAAV-FLAG-h*sox9* or rAAV-hTGF-β to hMSCs via CD-2 led to significantly higher levels of type-II collagen expression relative to all other conditions after 21 days (17.8- and 15.4-fold difference using rAAV-FLAG-h*sox9*/CD-2 versus -/CD-2 and rAAV-*lacZ*/CD-2, respectively, always $P \leq 0.001$; 14.4- and 12.5-fold difference using rAAV-hTGF-β/CD-2 versus -/CD-2 and rAAV-*lacZ*/CD-2, respectively, always $P \leq 0.001$), with a stronger effect of SOX9 relative to TGF-β (1.2-fold difference; $P \leq 0.002$) (Figure 6C and Table 2).

Interestingly, administration of rAAV-FLAG-h*sox9* or of rAAV-hTGF-β in hMSCs via CD-2 led to significantly lower levels of type-I collagen expression relative to all other conditions after 21 days (20.1- and 20.2-fold difference using rAAV-FLAG-h*sox9*/CD-2 versus -/CD-2 and rAAV-*lacZ*/CD-2, respectively, always $P \leq 0.001$; 22.7- and 22.9-fold difference using rAAV-hTGF-β/CD-2 versus -/CD-2 and rAAV-*lacZ*/CD-2, respectively, always $P \leq 0.001$), without difference between SOX9 and TGF-β ($P = 0.319$) (Figure 6D and Table 2). Similar results were noted when analyzing type-X collagen expression (6.2- and 6.1-fold difference using rAAV-FLAG-h*sox9*/CD-2 versus -/CD-2 and rAAV-*lacZ*/CD-2, respectively, always $P \leq 0.001$; 5.7-fold difference using rAAV-hTGF-β/CD-2 versus -/CD-2 or rAAV-*lacZ*/CD-2, respectively, always $P \leq 0.001$), again without difference between SOX9 and TGF-β ($P = 0.257$) (Figure 6E and Table 2).

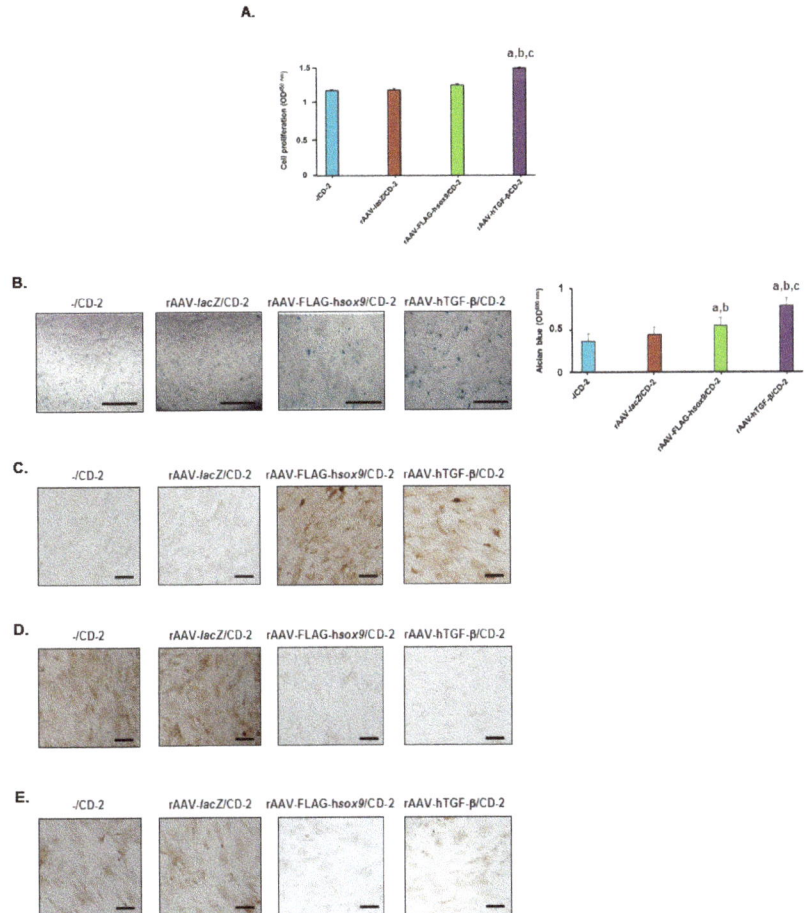

Figure 6. Biological activities in hMSCs transduced with the rAAV/CD-2 system. The rAAV-FLAG-h*sox9*, rAAV-hTGF-β, and rAAV-*lacZ* vectors (40 µL each vector, i.e., 8×10^5 transgene copies) were formulated with CD-2 (40 µL), and the resulting rAAV/CD systems (80 µL) were incubated with hMSCs (10,000 cells in 48-well plates; MOI = 80) for up to 21 days. Cell proliferation was examined using the Cell Proliferation Reagent WST-1 (**A**), glycosaminoglycans using alcian blue staining (light microscopy; magnification ×4; scale bars: 200 µm; all representative data) with spectrophotometric analysis after solubilization (histograms) (**B**), and the deposition of type-II collagen (**C**), type-I collagen (**D**), and type-X collagen (**E**) using immunocytochemistry (magnification ×20; scale bars: 50 µm; all representative data). rAAV-*lacZ*/CD-2 and CD-2 lacking rAAV were used as controls. Statistically significant relative to [a] -/CD-2, [b] rAAV-*lacZ*/CD-2, and [c] rAAV-FLAG-h*sox9*.

4. Discussion

Biomaterial-guided gene delivery using clinically adapted rAAV vectors [10,11,24–33] is an emerging, potent approach to treat focal cartilage lesions by non-invasive transfer and overexpression of chondroregenerative factors. In the present study, we examined the feasibility of providing independent rAAV constructs coding for the highly chondroreparative SOX9 transcription factor [43] and TGF-β [5,6] to hMSCs via carbon dots (CDs) as a means to stimulate the biological activities in these cells, an advantageous source of progenitor cells to enhance the intrinsic healing processes in sites of cartilage damage [5–7].

The present findings show, for the first time to our best knowledge, that CDs may be effective systems to successfully formulate and release rAAV gene transfer vectors. Among all the CDs tested here, CD-2, a carbonaceous nanoparticle prepared using pyrolysis at normal pressure of a mixture of CA, mPEG$_{550}$, and DMEDA, allowed for the highest intracellular vector release with a good over time maintenance for at least 10 days, the longest time point examined. Equally important, CD-2 was able to promote the effective and sustained modification of hMSCs when used to deliver a reporter (rAAV-*lacZ*) gene vector for at least 10 days (up to 2.2-fold increase in *lacZ* expression relative to free vector treatment) in a safe manner (100% cell viability, presumably due to the presence of the PEG protective shield around the particles), reaching levels similar to those noted with other nano-sized systems for rAAV delivery in hMSCs [24]. In contrast, the genetic modification of hMSCs using CD-3 or CD-4 was associated with decreased levels of cell viability, while CD-1 led to a reduction of gene transfer efficiency relative to free vector administration and other control conditions.

The results next demonstrate that the optimal CD-2 nanoparticles were further capable of promoting the delivery of rAAV vectors coding for the therapeutic *sox9* and TGF-β candidate genes in hMSCs, promoting a significant overexpression of each transgene in the cells over an extended period of time (about 97.5% SOX9$^+$ cells using rAAV-FLAG-h*sox9*/CD-2 and 79.8% TGF-β$^+$ cells with rAAV-hTGF-β/CD-2 after 21 days) relative to control treatments (≤7.8% and ≤11.8% transgene-expressing cells in the -/CD-2 and rAAV-*lacZ*/CD-2 conditions, respectively), higher than upon free rAAV *sox9* application (80–85%) [44] and comparable to free TGF-β gene transfer (80%) [45]. Yet, the levels of TGF-β produced via rAAV-hTGF-β/CD-2 (155–225 pg/mL) were 4- to 56-fold higher than those achieved upon free rAAV TGF-β gene transfer (17–24 pg/mL) [45]. This result is probably due to the difference of vector doses applied (MOI = 80–133 here compared with MOI = 4–20 using free vector gene administration, i.e., a 4- to 33-fold difference), but it reflects the improvement of TGF-β production via CD-2-guided rAAV gene transfer, as application of the current vector dose in a free form would have only raised 70-160 pg/mL of growth factor in cells versus 155–225 pg/mL here via CD-2 (i.e., a 1.4- to 2.2-fold difference). Interestingly, application of rAAV-hTGF-β/CD-2 resulted in the detection of 52.8% SOX9$^+$ cells, probably due to an upregulation of SOX9 expression in response to TGF-β production via rAAV/CD-2, as previously noted when using TGF-β in its recombinant form (rTGF-β) [48] or upon free rAAV TGF-β gene transfer [45], while no effects of SOX9 overexpression were seen on the levels of TGF-β. Effective SOX9 and TGF-β overexpression via CD-2-guided gene delivery led to increased levels of cartilage matrix production in the cells (glycosaminoglycan and type-II collagen expression) over time (21 days) relative to the control conditions, concordant with the respective pro-anabolic activities of SOX9 [43] and TGF-β [5–7], with observations showing short-term effects only of nonviral SOX9 gene transfer using arginine-based CDs (14 days) [42], and with our previous findings using free rAAV *sox9* or TGF-β gene transfer [44,45]. Furthermore, application of rAAV-hTGF-β/CD-2 had a significant influence on hMSC proliferation, in good agreement with the properties of the growth factor [6] and with our previous observations using free rAAV TGF-β gene transfer [45]. In contrast, rAAV-FLAG-h*sox9*/CD-2 had no impact on such a process, consistent with the activities of SOX9 [49] and with our findings via free rAAV *sox9* gene transfer [44]. Interestingly, CD-2-guided delivery of either rAAV-FLAG-h*sox9* or rAAV-hTGF-β advantageously prevented the deposition of type-I and -X collagen in hMSCs over time versus control treatments, concordant with the effects of SOX9 [49] and with results obtained using free rAAV *sox9* gene transfer [44], but in contrast to findings using rTGF-β [5] or upon free rAAV TGF-β gene delivery [45]. This might be due to differences of culture conditions and cell environment (monolayer hMSC cultures here versus three-dimensional hMSC cultures in free rAAV TGF-β gene transfer setting) [45] or to the differences between the levels of TGF-β achieved here via rAAV-hTGF-β/CD-2 (155–225 pg/mL) and the amounts of rTGF-β applied elsewhere (10 ng/mL, i.e., a 44- to 65-fold difference) [5].

In conclusion, the present work reports the possibility of transferring therapeutic rAAV (SOX9 or TGF-β) gene vectors to reparative hMSCs using optimal carbon-based nanoparticles as a novel, off-the-shelf system for cartilage repair. It will be interesting to extend the current approach in the future using adipose-derived hMSCs as these cells can be harvested at a 1000-fold higher yield in a less invasive manner than bone marrow-derived MSCs while displaying longer life-span and higher proliferative capacity and carrying micro-RNAs that regulate tissue inflammation and cell interplays [50,51]. Analyses are ongoing to test the value of the approach in a three-dimensional environment (high-density cultures) using single and combined CD-2-assisted rAAV SOX9/TGF-β gene transfer to potentiate the effects of the two factors on cell proliferation (TGF-β) and matrix deposition (glycosaminoglycans with TGF-β superiority and type-II collagen with SOX9 superiority) [52] and next in an orthotopic in vivo model of cartilage defect [14,16,53,54]. Such evaluations will provide insights into the potential benefits of CDs over other scaffolds (collagen, hyaluronic acid) or treatments like autologous platelet-rich plasma [50,55,56] for translational cartilage regeneration. Overall, this evaluation provides original evidence on the ability of CD-guided therapeutic rAAV gene transfer in regenerative hMSCs as platforms for therapy of cartilage defects in translational protocols.

Author Contributions: Conceptualization, J.K.V. and M.C. (Magali Cucchiarini); methodology, W.M., A.R.-R., M.C. (Mickaël Claudel), G.S., and S.S.-M.; software, W.M. and A.R.-R.; validation, formal analysis, investigation, data curation and visualization, W.M., A.R.-R., M.C. (Mickaël Claudel), G.S., S.S.-M., F.P., L.L., J.K.V. and M.C. (Magali Cucchiarini); writing—original draft preparation, W.M., A.R.-R., F.P., L.L., J.K.V. and M.C. (Magali Cucchiarini); writing—review and editing, W.M., A.R.-R., M.C. (Mickaël Claudel), G.S., S.S.-M., F.P., L.L., J.K.V. and M.C. (Magali Cucchiarini); resources and supervision, F.P., L.L., J.K.V. and M.C. (Magali Cucchiarini). All authors have read and agreed to the published version of the manuscript.

Funding: This research received no external funding.

Acknowledgments: We thank R. J. Samulski (The Gene Therapy Center, University of North Carolina, Chapel Hill, NC), X. Xiao (The Gene Therapy Center, University of Pittsburgh, Pittsburgh, PA), G. Scherer (Institute for Human Genetics and Anthropology, Albert-Ludwig University, Freiburg, Germany) for the human *sox9* cDNA, and E. F. Terwilliger (Division of Experimental Medicine, Harvard Institutes of Medicine and Beth Israel Deaconess Medical Center, Boston, MA, USA) for providing the genomic AAV-2 plasmid clones and the 293 cell line. We acknowledge support by the Saarland University within the funding programme Open Access Publishing.

Conflicts of Interest: The authors declare no conflicts of interest.

References

1. Buckwalter, J.A. Articular cartilage: Injuries and potential for healing. *J. Orthop. Sports Phys. Ther.* **1998**, *28*, 192–202. [CrossRef]
2. O'Driscoll, S.W. The healing and regeneration of articular cartilage. *J. Bone Jt. Surg.* **1998**, *80*, 1795–1812. [CrossRef]
3. Brittberg, M.; Lindahl, A.; Nilsson, A.; Ohlsson, C.; Isaksson, O.; Peterson, L. Treatment of deep cartilage defects in the knee with autologous chondrocyte transplantation. *N. Engl. J. Med.* **1994**, *331*, 889–895. [CrossRef] [PubMed]
4. Madry, H.; Grün, U.W.; Knutsen, G. Cartilage repair and joint preservation: Medical and surgical treatment options. *Dtsch. Arztebl. Int.* **2011**, *108*, 669–677. [PubMed]
5. Johnstone, B.; Hering, T.M.; Caplan, A.I.; Goldberg, V.M.; Yoo, J.U. In vitro chondrogenesis of bone marrow-derived mesenchymal progenitor cells. *Exp. Cell Res.* **1998**, *238*, 265–272. [CrossRef] [PubMed]
6. Mackay, A.M.; Beck, S.C.; Murphy, J.M.; Barry, F.P.; Chichester, C.O.; Pittenger, M.F. Chondrogenic differentiation of cultured human mesenchymal stem cells from marrow. *Tissue Eng.* **1998**, *4*, 415–428. [CrossRef] [PubMed]
7. Pittenger, M.F.; Mackay, A.M.; Beck, S.C.; Jaiswal, R.K.; Douglas, R.; Mosca, J.D.; Moorman, M.A.; Simonetti, D.W.; Craig, S.; Marshak, D.R. Multilineage potential of adult human mesenchymal stem cells. *Science* **1999**, *284*, 143–147. [CrossRef]
8. Slynarski, K.; Deszczynski, J.; Karpinski, J. Fresh bone marrow and periosteum transplantation for cartilage defects of the knee. *Transplant. Proc.* **2006**, *38*, 318–319. [CrossRef]
9. Gigante, A.; Cecconi, S.; Calcagno, S.; Busilacchi, A.; Enea, A. Arthroscopic knee cartilage repair with covered microfracture and bone marrow concentrate. *Arthrosc. Tech.* **2012**, *1*, e175–e180. [CrossRef]
10. Cucchiarini, M. Human gene therapy: Novel approaches to improve the current gene delivery systems. *Discov. Med.* **2016**, *21*, 495–506.

11. Cucchiarini, M.; Madry, H. Biomaterial-guided delivery of gene vectors for targeted articular cartilage repair. *Nat. Rev. Rheumatol.* **2019**, *15*, 8–29. [CrossRef] [PubMed]
12. Kelly, D.C.; Raftery, R.M.; Curtin, C.M.; O'Driscoll, C.M.; O'Brien, F.J. Scaffold-based delivery of nucleic acid therapeutics for enhanced bone and cartilage repair. *J. Orthop. Res.* **2019**, *37*, 1671–16801. [CrossRef] [PubMed]
13. Diao, H.; Wang, J.; Shen, C.; Xia, S.; Guo, T.; Dong, L.; Zhang, C.; Chen, J.; Zhao, J.; Zhang, J. Improved cartilage regeneration utilizing mesenchymal stem cells in TGF-beta1 gene-activated scaffolds. *Tissue Eng. Part A* **2009**, *15*, 2687–2698. [CrossRef]
14. Im, G.I.; Kim, H.J.; Lee, J.H. Chondrogenesis of adipose stem cells in a porous PLGA scaffold impregnated with plasmid DNA containing SOX trio (SOX-5,-6 and -9) genes. *Biomaterials* **2011**, *32*, 4385–4392. [CrossRef] [PubMed]
15. Li, B.; Yang, J.; Ma, L.; Li, F.; Tu, Z.; Gao, C. Fabrication of poly(lactide-co-glycolide) scaffold filled with fibrin gel, mesenchymal stem cells, and poly(ethylene oxide)-b-poly(L-lysine)/TGF-β1 plasmid DNA complexes for cartilage restoration in vivo. *J. Biomed. Mater. Res. A* **2013**, *101*, 3097–3108. [CrossRef] [PubMed]
16. Needham, C.J.; Shah, S.R.; Dahlin, R.L.; Kinard, L.A.; Lam, J.; Watson, B.M.; Lu, S.; Kasper, F.K.; Mikos, A.G. Osteochondral tissue regeneration through polymeric delivery of DNA encoding for the SOX trio and RUNX2. *Acta Biomater.* **2014**, *10*, 4103–4112. [CrossRef]
17. Gonzalez-Fernandez, T.; Tierney, E.G.; Cunniffe, G.M.; O'Brien, F.J.; Kelly, D.J. Gene delivery of TGF-β3 and BMP2 in an MSC-laden alginate hydrogel for articular cartilage and endochondral bone tissue engineering. *Tissue Eng. Part A* **2016**, *22*, 776–787. [CrossRef]
18. Lee, Y.H.; Wu, H.C.; Yeh, C.W.; Kuan, C.H.; Liao, H.T.; Hsu, H.C.; Tsai, J.C.; Sun, J.S.; Wang, T.W. Enzyme-crosslinked gene-activated matrix for the induction of mesenchymal stem cells in osteochondral tissue regeneration. *Acta Biomater* **2017**, *63*, 210–226. [CrossRef]
19. Park, J.S.; Yi, S.W.; Kim, H.J.; Kim, S.M.; Kim, J.H.; Park, K.H. Construction of PLGA nanoparticles coated with polycistronic SOX5, SOX6, and SOX9 genes for chondrogenesis of human mesenchymal stem cells. *ACS Appl. Mater. Interfaces* **2017**, *9*, 1361–1372. [CrossRef]
20. Brunger, J.M.; Huynh, N.P.; Guenther, C.M.; Perez-Pinera, P.; Moutos, F.T.; Sanchez-Adams, J.; Gersbach, C.A.; Guilak, F. Scaffold-mediated lentiviral transduction for functional tissue engineering of cartilage. *Proc. Natl. Acad. Sci. USA* **2014**, *111*, E798–E806. [CrossRef]
21. Glass, K.A.; Link, J.M.; Brunger, J.M.; Moutos, F.T.; Gersbach, C.A.; Guilak, F. Tissue-engineered cartilage with inducible and tunable immunomodulatory properties. *Biomaterials* **2014**, *35*, 5921–5931. [CrossRef] [PubMed]
22. Moutos, F.T.; Glass, K.A.; Compton, S.A.; Ross, A.K.; Gersbach, C.A.; Guilak, F.; Estes, B.T. Anatomically shaped tissue-engineered cartilage with tunable and inducible anticytokine delivery for biological joint resurfacing. *Proc. Natl. Acad. Sci. USA* **2016**, *113*, E4513–E4522. [CrossRef] [PubMed]
23. Rowland, C.R.; Glass, K.A.; Ettyreddy, A.R.; Gloss, C.C.; Matthews, J.R.L.; Huynh, N.P.T.; Guilak, F. Regulation of decellularized tissue remodeling via scaffold-mediated lentiviral delivery in anatomically-shaped osteochondral constructs. *Biomaterials* **2018**, *177*, 161–175. [CrossRef] [PubMed]
24. Rey-Rico, A.; Venkatesan, J.K.; Frisch, J.; Rial-Hermida, I.; Schmitt, G.; Concheiro, A.; Madry, H.; Alvarez-Lorenzo, C.; Cucchiarini, M. PEO-PPO-PEO micelles as effective rAAV-mediated gene delivery systems to target human mesenchymal stem cells without altering their differentiation potency. *Acta Biomater.* **2015**, *27*, 42–52. [CrossRef] [PubMed]
25. Rey-Rico, A.; Frisch, J.; Venkatesan, J.K.; Schmitt, G.; Rial-Hermida, I.; Taboada, P.; Concheiro, A.; Madry, H.; Alvarez-Lorenzo, C.; Cucchiarini, M. PEO-PPO-PEO carriers for rAAV-mediated transduction of human articular chondrocytes in vitro and in a human osteochondral defect model. *ACS Appl. Mater. Interfaces* **2016**, *8*, 20600–20613. [CrossRef]
26. Rey-Rico, A.; Venkatesan, J.K.; Schmitt, G.; Concheiro, A.; Madry, H.; Alvarez-Lorenzo, C.; Cucchiarini, M. rAAV-mediated overexpression of TGF-β via vector delivery in polymeric micelles stimulates the biological and reparative activities of human articular chondrocytes in vitro and in a human osteochondral defect model. *Int. J. Nanomed.* **2017**, *12*, 6985–6996. [CrossRef]
27. Rey-Rico, A.; Venkatesan, J.K.; Schmitt, G.; Speicher-Mentges, S.; Madry, H.; Cucchiarini, M. Effective remodelling of human osteoarthritic cartilage by SOX9 gene transfer and overexpression upon delivery of rAAV vectors in polymeric micelles. *Mol. Pharm.* **2018**, *15*, 2816–2826. [CrossRef]

28. Lee, H.H.; Haleem, A.M.; Yao, V.; Li, J.; Xiao, X.; Chu, C.R. Release of bioactive adeno-associated virus from fibrin scaffolds: Effects of fibrin glue concentrations. *Tissue Eng. Part A* **2011**, *17*, 1969–1978. [CrossRef]
29. Díaz-Rodríguez, P.; Rey-Rico, A.; Madry, H.; Landin, M.; Cucchiarini, M. Effective genetic modification and differentiation of hMSCs upon controlled release of rAAV vectors using alginate/poloxamer composite systems. *Int. J. Pharm.* **2015**, *496*, 614–626. [CrossRef]
30. Rey-Rico, A.; Venkatesan, J.K.; Frisch, J.; Schmitt, G.; Monge-Marcet, A.; Lopez-Chicon, P.; Mata, A.; Semino, C.; Madry, H.; Cucchiarini, M. Effective and durable genetic modification of human mesenchymal stem cells via controlled release of rAAV vectors from self-assembling peptide hydrogels with a maintained differentiation potency. *Acta Biomater.* **2015**, *18*, 118–127. [CrossRef]
31. Rey-Rico, A.; Babicz, H.; Madry, H.; Concheiro, A.; Alvarez-Lorenzo, C.; Cucchiarini, M. Supramolecular polypseudorotaxane gels for controlled delivery of rAAV vectors in human mesenchymal stem cells for regenerative medicine. *Int J Pharm* **2017**, *531*, 492–503. [CrossRef] [PubMed]
32. Madry, H.; Gao, L.; Rey-Rico, A.; Venkatesan, J.K.; Müller-Brandt, K.; Cai, X.; Goebel, L.; Schmitt, G.; Speicher-Mentges, S.; Zurakowski, D.; et al. Thermosensitive hydrogel based on PEO-PPO-PEO poloxamers for a controlled in situ release of recombinant adeno-associated viral vectors for effective gene therapy of cartilage defects. *Adv. Mater.* **2020**, *32*, 1906508. [CrossRef] [PubMed]
33. Venkatesan, J.K.; Falentin-Daudré, C.; Leroux, A.; Migonney, V.; Cucchiarini, M. Biomaterial-guided recombinant adeno-associated virus delivery from poly(sodium styrene sulfonate)-grafted poly(ε-caprolactone) films to target human bone marrow aspirates. *Tissue Eng. Part A* **2019**. [CrossRef] [PubMed]
34. Xu, X.; Ray, R.; Gu, Y.; Ploehn, H.J.; Gearheart, L.; Raker, K.; Scrivens, W.A. Electrophoretic analysis and purification of fluorescent single-walled carbon nanotube fragments. *J. Am. Chem. Soc.* **2004**, *126*, 12736–12737. [CrossRef] [PubMed]
35. Fan, J.; Claudel, M.; Ronzani, C.; Arezki, Y.; Lebeau, L.; Pons, F. Physicochemical characteristics that affect carbon dot safety: Lessons from a comprehensive study on a nanoparticle library. *Int. J. Pharm.* **2019**, *569*, 118521. [CrossRef]
36. Qiu, J.; Zhang, R.; Li, J.; Sang, Y.; Tang, W.; Rivera Gil, P.; Liu, H. Fluorescent graphene quantum dots as traceable, pH-sensitive drug delivery systems. *Int. J. Nanomedicine* **2015**, *10*, 6709–6724.
37. Zhang, J.X.; Zheng, M.; Xie, Z.G. Co-assembled hybrids of proteins and carbon dots for intracellular protein delivery. *J. Mater. Chem. B* **2016**, *4*, 5659. [CrossRef]
38. Pierrat, P.; Wang, R.; Kereselidze, D.; Lux, M.; Didier, P.; Kichler, A.; Pons, F.; Lebeau, L. Efficient in vitro and in vivo pulmonary delivery of nucleic acid by carbon dot-based nanocarriers. *Biomaterials* **2015**, *51*, 290–302. [CrossRef]
39. Giron-Gonzalez, M.D.; Salto-Gonzalez, R.; Lopez-Jaramillo, F.J.; Salinas-Castillo, A.; Jodar-Reyes, A.B.; Ortega-Munoz, M.; Hernandez-Mateo, F.; Santoyo-Gonzalez, F. Polyelectrolyte complexes of low molecular weight pei and citric acid as efficient and nontoxic vectors for in vitro and in vivo gene delivery. *Bioconjug. Chem.* **2016**, *27*, 549–561. [CrossRef]
40. Wu, Y.F.; Wu, H.C.; Kuan, C.H.; Lin, C.J.; Wang, L.W.; Chang, C.W.; Wang, T.W. Multi-functionalized carbon dots as theranostic nanoagent for gene delivery in lung cancer therapy. *Sci. Rep.* **2016**, *6*, 21170–21181. [CrossRef]
41. Chen, J.; Wang, Q.; Zhou, J.; Deng, W.; Yu, Q.; Cao, X.; Wang, J.; Shao, F.; Li, Y.; Ma, P.; et al. Porphyra polysaccharide-derived carbon dots for non-viral co-delivery of different gene combinations and neuronal differentiation of ectodermal mesenchymal stem cells. *Nanoscale* **2017**, *9*, 10820–10831. [CrossRef] [PubMed]
42. Cao, X.; Wang, J.; Deng, W.; Chen, J.; Wang, Y.; Zhou, J.; Du, P.; Xu, W.; Wang, Q.; Wang, Q.; et al. Photoluminescent cationic carbon dots as efficient non-viral delivery of plasmid SOX9 and chondrogenesis of fibroblasts. *Sci. Rep.* **2018**, *8*, 7057–7067. [CrossRef] [PubMed]
43. Bi, W.; Deng, J.M.; Zhang, Z.; Behringer, R.R.; de Crombrugghe, B. Sox9 is required for cartilage formation. *Nat. Genet.* **1999**, *22*, 85–89. [CrossRef] [PubMed]
44. Venkatesan, J.K.; Ekici, M.; Madry, H.; Schmitt, G.; Kohn, D.; Cucchiarini, M. SOX9 gene transfer via safe, stable, replication-defective recombinant adeno-associated virus vectors as a novel, powerful tool to enhance the chondrogenic potential of human mesenchymal stem cells. *Stem Cell Res. Ther.* **2012**, *3*, 22–36. [CrossRef] [PubMed]

45. Frisch, J.; Venkatesan, J.K.; Rey-Rico, A.; Schmitt, G.; Madry, H.; Cucchiarini, M. Determination of the chondrogenic differentiation processes in human bone marrow-derived mesenchymal stem cells genetically modified to overexpress transforming growth factor-β via recombinant adeno-associated viral vectors. *Hum. Gene Ther.* **2014**, *25*, 10500–10560. [CrossRef]
46. Samulski, R.J.; Chang, L.S.; Shenk, T. A recombinant plasmid from which an infectious adeno-associated virus genome can be excised in vitro and its use to study viral replication. *J. Virol.* **1987**, *61*, 3096–3101. [CrossRef]
47. Samulski, R.J.; Chang, L.S.; Shenk, T. Helper-free stocks of recombinant adeno-associated viruses: Normal integration does not require viral gene expression. *J. Virol.* **1989**, *63*, 3822–3828. [CrossRef]
48. Murphy, M.K.; Huey, D.J.; Hu, J.C.; Athanasiou, K.A. TGF-β1, GDF-5, and BMP-2 stimulation induces chondrogenesis in expanded human articular chondrocytes and marrow-derived stromal cells. *Stem Cells* **2015**, *33*, 762–773. [CrossRef]
49. Akiyama, H.; Lyons, J.P.; Mori-Akiyama, Y.; Yang, X.; Zhang, R.; Zhang, Z.; Deng, J.M.; Taketo, M.M.; Nakamura, T.; Behringer, R.R.; et al. Interactions between Sox9 and beta-catenin control chondrocyte differentiation. *Genes Dev.* **2004**, *18*, 1072–1087. [CrossRef]
50. Scioli, M.G.; Bielli, A.; Gentile, P.; Cervelli, V.; Orlandi, A.J. Combined treatment with platelet-rich plasma and insulin favours chondrogenic and osteogenic differentiation of human adipose-derived stem cells in three-dimensional collagen scaffolds. *Tissue Eng. Regen. Med.* **2017**, *11*, 2398–2410. [CrossRef]
51. Gentile, P.; Garcovich, S. Concise review: Adipose-derived stem cells (ASCs) and adipocyte-secreted exosomal microRNA (A-SE-miR) modulate cancer growth and promote wound repair. *J. Clin. Med.* **2019**, *8*, 855. [CrossRef] [PubMed]
52. Tao, K.; Frisch, J.; Rey-Rico, A.; Venkatesan, J.K.; Schmitt, G.; Madry, H.; Lin, J.; Cucchiarini, M. Co-overexpression of TGF-β and SOX9 via rAAV gene transfer modulates the metabolic and chondrogenic activities of human bone marrow-derived mesenchymal stem cells. *Stem Cell Res. Ther.* **2016**, *7*, 20–31. [CrossRef] [PubMed]
53. Cucchiarini, M.; Orth, P.; Madry, H. Direct rAAV SOX9 administration for durable articular cartilage repair with delayed terminal differentiation and hypertrophy in vivo. *J. Mol. Med.* **2013**, *91*, 625–636. [CrossRef] [PubMed]
54. Cucchiarini, M.; Asen, A.K.; Goebel, L.; Venkatesan, J.K.; Schmitt, G.; Zurakowski, D.; Menger, M.D.; Laschke, M.W.; Madry, H. Effects of TGF-β overexpression via rAAV gene transfer on the early repair processes in an osteochondral defect model in minipigs. *Am. J. Sports Med.* **2018**, *46*, 1987–1996. [CrossRef]
55. Gentile, P.; Bottini, D.J.; Spallone, D.; Curcio, B.C.; Cervelli, V.J. Application of platelet-rich plasma in maxillofacial surgery: Clinical evaluation. *J. Craniofacial Surg.* **2010**, *21*, 900–904. [CrossRef]
56. Cervelli, V.; Lucarini, L.; Spallone, D.; Palla, L.; Colicchia, G.M.; Gentile, P.; De Angelis, B. Use of platelet-rich plasma and hyaluronic acid in the loss of substance with bone exposure. *Adv. Skin Wound Care* **2011**, *24*, 176–181. [CrossRef]

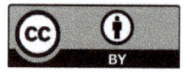

© 2020 by the authors. Licensee MDPI, Basel, Switzerland. This article is an open access article distributed under the terms and conditions of the Creative Commons Attribution (CC BY) license (http://creativecommons.org/licenses/by/4.0/).

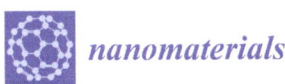

Article

Therapeutic Delivery of rAAV *sox9* via Polymeric Micelles Counteracts the Effects of Osteoarthritis-Associated Inflammatory Cytokines in Human Articular Chondrocytes

Jonas Urich [1], Magali Cucchiarini [1] and Ana Rey-Rico [2,*]

[1] Center of Experimental Orthopaedics, Saarland University Medical Center, D-66421 Homburg, Germany; jonas.urich@gmx.de (J.U.); mmcucchiarini@hotmail.com (M.C.)
[2] Cell Therapy and Regenerative Medicine Unit, Centro de Investigacións Científicas Avanzadas (CICA), Universidade da Coruña, ES-15071 A Coruña, Spain
* Correspondence: ana.rey.rico@udc.es

Received: 1 June 2020; Accepted: 22 June 2020; Published: 25 June 2020

Abstract: Osteoarthritis (OA) is a prevalent joint disease linked to the irreversible degradation of key extracellular cartilage matrix (ECM) components (proteoglycans, type-II collagen) by proteolytic enzymes due to an impaired tissue homeostasis, with the critical involvement of OA-associated pro-inflammatory cytokines (interleukin 1 beta, i.e., IL-1β, and tumor necrosis factor alpha, i.e., TNF-α). Gene therapy provides effective means to re-establish such degraded ECM compounds by rejuvenating the altered OA phenotype of the articular chondrocytes, the unique cell population ubiquitous in the articular cartilage. In particular, overexpression of the highly specialized SOX9 transcription factor via recombinant adeno-associated viral (rAAV) vectors has been reported for its ability to readjust the metabolic balance in OA, in particular via controlled rAAV delivery using polymeric micelles as carriers to prevent a possible vector neutralization by antibodies present in the joints of patients. As little is known on the challenging effects of such naturally occurring OA-associated pro-inflammatory cytokines on such rAAV/polymeric gene transfer, we explored the capacity of polyethylene oxide (PEO) and polypropylene oxide (PPO)-based polymeric micelles to deliver a candidate rAAV-FLAG-h*sox9* construct in human OA chondrocytes in the presence of IL-1β and TNF-α. We report that effective, micelle-guided rAAV *sox9* overexpression enhanced the deposition of ECM components and the levels of cell survival, while advantageously reversing the deleterious effects afforded by the OA cytokines on these processes. These findings highlight the potentiality of polymeric micelles as effective rAAV controlled delivery systems to counterbalance the specific contribution of major OA-associated inflammatory cytokines, supporting the concept of using such systems for the treatment for chronic inflammatory diseases like OA.

Keywords: osteoarthritis; human articular cartilage; rAAV vectors; SOX9; polymeric micelles; pro-inflammatory cytokines; IL-1β; TNF-α

1. Introduction

Osteoarthritis (OA) represents a prevalent, chronic, and deteriorating joint affliction that is the leading cause of impaired function and disability [1]. OA is characterized by multiple functional and structural cartilage tissue and cell shifts, such as the progressive and permanent degradation of the articular cartilage matrix (loss of type-II collagen and of proteoglycans), the restructuration of the subchondral bone, and the formation of osteophytes [2,3] due to defective homeostasis [4,5]. Of note, none of the current pharmacological options and surgical alternatives [1] for treating OA can reestablish the native cartilage quality in patients.

Current research associates the changes observed in OA disease with a complex cascade of biochemical factors, including proteolytic enzymes that promote the disruption of the cartilage macromolecules [6]. Pro-inflammatory cytokines such as interleukin 1 beta (IL-1β) and tumor necrosis factor alpha (TNF-α), produced by mononuclear cells, activated synoviocytes or by the cartilage itself, upregulate metalloproteinases gene expression, impairing chondrocyte counteracting synthetic pathways necessary to reinstate the integrity of the degenerated extracellular matrix (ECM) [6].

In this context, previous studies have shown an abolishment of type-II collagen expression from primary human articular chondrocytes via suppression of the expression of the cartilage-associated sex-determining region Y-type high mobility box 9 (SOX9) transcription factor upon treatment with IL-1β [7]. Of note, overexpression of *sox9* via lentiviral vector has already been shown to preserve chondrocytes from IL-1β-induced apoptosis and degeneration [8]. However, while efficient, lentiviral vectors are not well adapted for translational approaches, as they involve a risk of insertional mutagenesis upon integration into the genome of host cells [9]. In contrast, recombinant adeno-associated viral (rAAV) vectors mainly remain episomal in the nucleus of their targets, showing potential integration events at very low frequency (0.1–1% vide infra) [10], while also allowing for highly effective gene transfer efficiencies even in nondividing cells like articular chondrocytes (more than 70%) [11]. rAAV vectors have thus emerged as the preferred gene carriers in several regenerative medicine applications including for cartilage repair [12–16].

A high and prolonged gene transmission efficiency in articular chondrocytes both in vitro and through their compact ECM in situ has been reported via rAAV vectors (up to 80% for at least 150 days) has been reported [11]. Furthermore, gene transfer of an rAAV TGF-β vector has been shown to promote the biological activities both in human articular chondrocytes cultures in vitro and in articular cartilage explants in situ [17,18]. In addition, overexpression of *sox9* via rAAV led to increased levels of type-II collagen and proteoglycans in both normal and OA-affected articular chondrocytes in vitro [19].

Still, administration of rAAV vectors in patients may be hampered by the prevalence of anti-AAV antibodies directed against viral capsid proteins in individuals as those prevailing in synovial fluid from patients affected with joint disorders [20]. We previously described the suitability of rAAV vectors (*lacZ*) encapsulation in poly(ethylene oxide) (PEO) and poly(propylene oxide) (PPO)-based polymeric micelles from linear (poloxamers; PF68) or X-shaped copolymers (poloxamines; T908), as a way to overcome such obstacles while affording protection to the vectors in experimental settings of neutralization and increasing their gene transfer efficacy [21,22]. Interestingly, overexpression of *sox9* using such systems resulted in the effective remodeling of human OA cartilage, leading to increases in cell proliferation activities and in proteoglycan deposition relative to free vector administration [23]. Yet, it remains to be seen whether such micellar systems can also be efficient for delivering rAAV vectors and overexpressing their transgenes in an inflammatory, detrimental environment like in OA (IL-1β, TNF-α) [4,5,24].

The aim of the present study was therefore to test the ability of PF68- and T908-based polymeric micelles to deliver the therapeutic rAAV-FLAG-hsox9 candidate vector in human OA chondrocytes, the sole cell population present in the articular cartilage, in the presence of OA-associated pro-inflammatory cytokines (IL-1β, TNF-α) in a 2D environment as a preliminary proof of concept, as a means to effectively restore the chondrocyte phenotype in such cells in vitro.

2. Materials and Methods

2.1. Materials

Pluronic® F68 and Tetronic® 908 were generously provided by BASF (Ludwigshafen, Germany). The pro-inflammatory cytokines (IL-1β, TNF-α) were obtained from Prepotech (Hamburg, Germany). The anti-SOX9 (C-20) antibody was purchased at Santa Cruz Biotechnology (Heidelberg, Germany) and the anti-type-II collagen (II-II6B3) antibody at DSHB (Iowa, IA, USA). Biotinylated secondary antibodies and the ABC reagent were obtained from Vector Laboratories (Alexis Deutschland GmbH,

Grünberg, Germany). Alcian blue 8GX was from Sigma (Munich, Germany). The Cell Proliferation Reagent WST-1 was obtained from Roche Applied Science (Mannheim, Germany).

2.2. Cells

Human osteoarthritic (OA) cartilage (Mankin score 7–9) was obtained from total knee arthroplasty samples (n = 4) from patients, after informed consent signature [18] before inclusion in the study. The study was approved by the Ethics Committee of the Saarland Physicians Council (*Ärztekammer des Saarlandes*, reference number Ha06/08). All procedures were in conformity with the Helsinki Declaration. Human OA chondrocytes (passage 1–2) were isolated by collagenase digestion of cartilage slices as previously described [18,22] and cultured in DMEM, 10% FBS, 100 U/mL penicillin G, 100 μL/mL streptomycin (growth medium) prior to the studies, without cell dedifferentiation.

2.3. Plasmids and rAAV Vectors

rAAV-FLAG-h*sox9* is derived from pSSV9, an AAV-2 genomic clone [25,26], and carries a FLAG-tagged human *sox9* cDNA under the control of the cytomegalovirus immediate-early (CMV-IE) promoter [23,27–29]. The vectors were packaged using a helper-free, two-plasmid transfection system in 293 cells with the Adenovirus helper plasmid pXX6 and the packaging plasmid pXX2 [18]. The resulting vector preparations were extensively dialyzed and titrated by real-time PCR [18,30,31], averaging 10^{10} transgene copies/mL.

2.4. Preparation of Micellar Copolymer Solutions Containing rAAV-FLAG-hsox9 Vectors

Copolymer solutions (PF68 or T908) were prepared in 10% sucrose aqueous solution at 4 °C, mixed with rAAV-FLAG-h*sox9*, and maintained in ice-water bath for 30 min prior to their use as previously described [21–23]. The final micellar concentration into the culture medium was 2%. Effective interaction between the vectors and the polymeric micelles was confirmed by dynamic light scattering and electron microscopy [21–23].

2.5. Gene Transfer in Inflammatory Conditions via rAAV-FLAG-hsox9/Polymeric Micelles

Human OA chondrocytes (3000 cells/well or 40,000 cells/well for Alcian blue staining) were seeded in 96-well plates and maintained for 12 h at 37 °C under 5% CO_2 as previously described [22,23]. Monolayer cultures of OA chondrocytes were directly transduced with the rAAV-FLAG-h*sox9*/polymeric micelles (2×10^8 transgene copies, micellar concentration 2%) or after pre-incubation for 4 h with IL-1β (10 ng/mL) [32] or TNF-α (100 ng/mL) only [33], or concomitantly with IL-1β and TNF-α (10 and 100 ng/mL, respectively). Control conditions included cells cultured without vector treatment or copolymer solution (negative control) and cells transduced with free rAAV vector (positive control). Cultures were maintained for 10 days with 3 weekly medium changes.

Expression of SOX9 was monitored by immunocytochemistry using and anti-SOX9 specific primary antibody, a biotinylated secondary antibody, with the ABC method with diaminobenzidine (DAB) as previously described [23,29]. To control for secondary immunoglobulins, OA chondrocytes in monolayers cultures were assayed with exclusion of the primary antibody. All cultures were inspected under light microscopy (Olympus CKX41).

2.6. Histological and Immunocytochemical Analyses

Chondrocytes in monolayer cultures were harvested after 1 and 10 days and fixed in 4% formalin [21–23] prior to the immunocytochemical analyses. Expression of SOX9 and type-II collagen was detected using specific primary and biotinylated secondary antibodies, and the ABC method with DAB chromogen, with examination under light microscopy (Olympus CKX41) [21,22]. Alcian blue staining was involved to detect matrix proteoglycans [21,22,34,35]. Briefly, fixed monolayer cultures were stained with Alcian blue (1% in HCl 1 N) and excess stain was washed with double distilled water. The staining was solubilized by overnight incubation in 6 M guanidine hydrochloride and the absorbance at 595 nm was quantified with a GENios spectrophotometer (Tecan Crailsheim, Germany).

2.7. Histomorphometry

The mean intensities of SOX9 and type-II collagen immunostaining (ratio of positively stained surface to the total surface) were assessed at four randomized locations for each replicate condition as previously described [21–23]. Analyses were accomplished by using SIS AnalySIS (Olympus, Hamburg, Germany) and Adobe Photoshop (Adobe Systems Software CS2, Unterschleissheim, Germany) [21,23].

2.8. Evaluation of Cell Proliferation and Viability

Proliferation of chondrocytes in monolayer cultures was estimated using the Cell Proliferation Reagent WST-1, with optical density (OD) values proportional to the cell numbers [22,23,30]. Controls included the same conditions depicted in 2.5. ODs at 450 nm were registered using a GENios spectrophotometer (Tecan) and the percent's of cell viability were calculated as follows:

$$\text{Viability (\%)} = [(\text{OD sample})/(\text{OD negative control})] \times 100 \qquad (1)$$

2.9. Statistical Analysis

Each condition was tested in duplicate in four independent experiments using all patients. The values registered are depicted as mean ± standard deviation (SD). A *t*-test was employed, with $p < 0.05$ being considered statistically significant.

3. Results

3.1. Efficacy of rAAV-Mediated sox9 Overexpression in Conditions of Inflammation upon Vector Delivery via Polymeric Micelles

We first evaluated whether the presence of pro-inflammatory cytokines may alter the overexpression of SOX9 in human OA chondrocytes monolayer cultures.

In agreement with our previous observations [23], effective SOX9 overexpression was noted in the cells via rAAV-FLAG-hsox9 transduction (up to a 1.4-fold increase relative to the negative control in the absence of cytokines, $p = 0.021$) (Figure 1A,B). Similarly, supply of rAAV in polymeric micelles led to the most intense SOX9 immunoreactivity (up to a 1.8-fold increase when compared with the negative control in the absence of cytokines on day 1, $p = 0.015$), leading to more sustained levels of expression over time (up to a 1.4-fold difference with respect to the cell control in the absence of cytokines on day 10, $p = 0.009$) (Figure 1A,B).

Treatment with IL-1β did not alter the levels of SOX9 expression early on ($p = 0.450$ compared with the negative control in the absence of cytokines on day 1) (Figure 1A,B versus Figure 1C,D) while a reduction was noted after 10 days (up to a 1.1-fold difference with respect to the negative control in the absence of cytokines, $p = 0.106$) (Figure 1A,B versus Figure 1C,D). Interestingly, the treatment with rAAV-FLAG-hsox9 promoted a significant enhancement in SOX9 expression levels following IL-1β treatment (up to a 1.5-fold difference with respect to the cell control in the presence of IL-1β, $p = 0.024$), especially upon vector delivery via micellar systems (up to a 1.7-fold difference when compared with the cell control in the presence of IL-1β on day 1, $p = 0.040$) (Figure 1C,D). Such effects were also maintained over the time of evaluation (up to a 1.5-fold increase with respect to the cell control in the presence of IL-1β on day 10, $p = 0.045$) (Figure 1C,D).

Administration of TNF-α did not affect the levels of SOX9 expression, regardless of the time points evaluated ($p = 0.090$ compared with the cell control in the absence of cytokines) (Figure 1A,B versus Figure 1E,F). Overexpression of sox9 via rAAV led to increased levels of SOX9 expression (up to a 1.4-fold increase with respect to the cell control in the presence of TNF-α on day 10, $p = 0.048$) (Figure 1E,F). Notably, delivery of the vector via micellar carriers resulted in the highest levels of SOX9 expression (up to a 1.7-fold difference with respect to the cell control in the presence of TNF-α on day 1, $p = 0.021$) (Figure 1E,F).

Concomitant IL-1β/TNF-α application led to a decrease in the levels of SOX9 expression (up to a 1.2-fold difference with respect to the negative control in the absence of cytokines on day 10, $p = 0.150$) (Figure 1A,B versus Figure 1G,H). Significantly increased SOX9 levels were noted either using free rAAV-FLAG-hsox9 form (up to a 1.5-fold difference relative to the cell control in the presence of IL-1β/TNF-α on day 10, $p = 0.019$) (Figure 1G,H), or via delivery in PF68 or T908-based micelles (up to a 1.6-fold increase with respect to the cell control in the presence of IL-1β/TNF-α on day 1, $p = 0.020$) (Figure 1G,H).

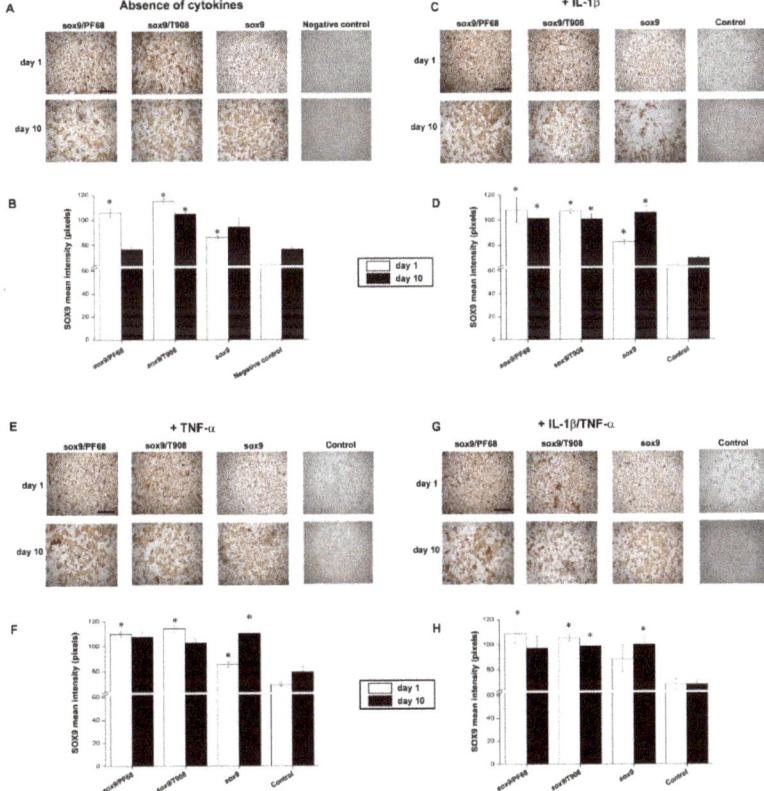

Figure 1. Transgene expression in rAAV-FLAG-hsox9-transduced human OA chondrocytes using polymeric micelles. Cells in mnolayer culture were directly transduced with the rAAV/polymeric micelles (**A,B**) or after pre-incubation for 4 h with IL-1β (10 ng/mL) (**C,D**), TNF-α (100 ng/mL) (**E,F**), or IL-1β/TNF-α (10/100 ng/mL) (**G,H**), as described in the Materials and Methods. The cultures were then processed after 1 and 10 days to detect SOX9 expression by immunocytochemistry (magnification x4, scale bar 500 µm; all representative data) (**A,C,E,G**) with corresponding histomorphometric analyses (**B,D,F,H**), as described in the Materials and Methods. Control conditions included the absence of copolymer or vector treatment (negative control) and the application of free rAAV vector (positive control). * Statistically significant compared with the negative control at similar time points.

3.2. Effects of rAAV-FLAG-hsox9/Polymeric Micelle Delivery on the Anabolic Activities of Human OA Chondrocytes in Inflammatory Conditions

We next investigated the effects of SOX9 overexpression on the deposition of type-II collagen and proteoglycans following rAAV-FLAG-hsox9 gene transfer via micellar vehicles in human OA chondrocytes monolayer cultures maintained in conditions of inflammation.

Administering of rAAV-FLAG-hsox9 significantly incremented type-II collagen deposition in the cells (up to a 1.3-fold increase with respect to the cell control in the absence of cytokines, $p = 0.017$) (Figure 2A,B). These levels increased over time, chiefly by delivery of the vectors via PF68 micelles (up to a 1.5-fold difference with respect to the negative control in the absence of cytokines on day 10, $p = 0.040$) (Figure 2A,B). Of note, these levels were higher than those achieved with free vector administration (up to a 1.2-fold difference compared with free rAAV-FLAG-hsox9 application on day 10, $p = 0.011$) (Figure 2A,B). Treatment with IL-1β decreased type-II collagen deposition (up to a 1.1-fold difference relative to the negative control in the absence of cytokines on day 1, $p = 0.300$) (Figure 2A,B versus Figure 2C,D). rAAV-FLAG-hsox9 application to IL-1β-treated chondrocytes significantly increased type-II collagen deposition, especially when using micelle-guided vector delivery (up to a 1.5-fold difference with respect to the cell control in the presence of IL-1β on day 10, $p = 0.011$; up to a 1.2-fold difference compared with free vector applying in the presence of IL-1β on day 10, $p = 0.006$) (Figure 2C,D). A similar tendency was noted when applying TNF-α alone or combined as a IL-1β/TNF-α co-treatment, showing modest decreases in type-II collagen deposition compared with cells kept in culture in the absence of cytokines ($p = 0.290$) (Figure 2A,B versus Figure 2E–H). Similarly, overexpression of SOX9 significantly increased type-II collagen deposition over time, particularly when providing rAAV-FLAG-hsox9 in micellar carriers (up to a 1.4-fold difference with respect to the cell control in the presence of TNF-α alone or as an IL-1β/TNF-α combination on day 10, $p = 0.040$) (Figure 2E–H).

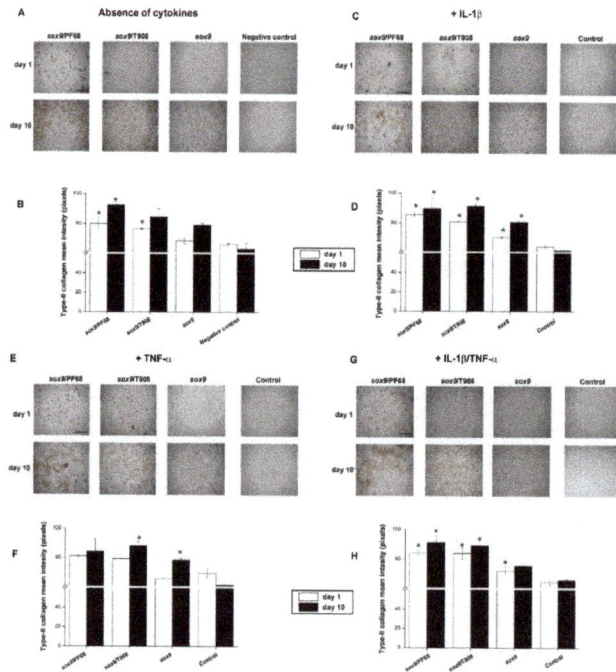

Figure 2. Remodeling activities in rAAV-FLAG-hsox9-transduced human OA chondrocytes using

polymeric micelles. Cells in monolayer culture were directly transduced with the rAAV/polymeric micelles (**A,B**) or after pre-incubation for 4 h with IL-1β (10 ng/mL) (**C,D**), TNF-α (100 ng/mL) (**E,F**), or IL-1β/TNF-α (10/100 ng/mL) (**G,H**), as described in Figure 1 and in the Materials and Methods. The cultures were processed after 1 and 10 days to detect type-II collagen deposition by immunocytochemistry (magnification x10, scale bar 200 μm; all representative data) (**A,C,E,G**) with corresponding histomorphometric analyses (**B,D,F,H**), as described in the Materials and Methods. Control conditions included the absence of copolymer or vector treatment (negative control) and the application of free rAAV vector (positive control). * Statistically significant compared with the negative control at similar time points.

Overexpression of SOX9 in rAAV-FLAG-hsox9-transduced chondrocytes significantly increased the accretion of ECM-proteoglycans compared with untransduced cells (up to an 1.8-fold difference with respect to the negative control in the absence of cytokines on day 10, $p = 0.030$) (Figure 3A,B). Of note, delivery of rAAV-FLAG-hsox9 via micellar systems led to the highest proteoglycan deposition (up to a 1.2-fold increase with respect to free vector administering on day 10, $p = 0.030$) and proliferative index (up to a 1.4-fold increase with respect to the negative control in the absence of cytokines) (Figure 3A,B). Strikingly, treatment with IL-1β significantly decreased the deposition of proteoglycans and the cell proliferation ratio (up to a 1.2-fold difference with respect to the negative control in the absence of cytokines on day 1, $p = 0.030$) (Figure 3A,B versus Figure 3C,D). Additionally, rAAV-FLAG-hsox9-mediated transduction of IL-1β-treated chondrocytes prompted the restoration of proteoglycans, an effect more marked over time (up to a 1.7-fold increase when compared to the control in the presence of IL-1β on day 10, $p = 0.038$), exhibiting higher cell proliferation. Interestingly, providing rAAV-FLAG-hsox9 in micellar carriers led to the highest proteoglycan deposition (up to a 2.1-fold increase relative to the cell control in the presence of IL-1β on day 10, $p = 0.006$), reaching values that were higher than those reached with the free vector administration (up to a 1.3-fold difference with respect to free rAAV-FLAG-hsox9 application in the presence of IL-1β on day 10, $p = 0.046$) (Figure 3C,D). Treatment with TNF-α also decreased the deposition of proteoglycans (up to a 1.2-fold difference with respect to the negative control in the absence of cytokines on day 10, $p = 0.203$) and the cell proliferation index (Figure 3A,B versus Figure 3E,F). Transduction of TNF-α-treated chondrocytes with rAAV-FLAG-hsox9 significantly increased the cell proliferation and proteoglycan deposition, especially when the vectors were delivered via micellar systems (up to a 2-fold difference compared with the cell control in the presence of TNF-α on day 10, $p = 0.010$) (Figure 3E,F). Simultaneous IL-1β/TNF-α administration significantly decreased the deposition of proteoglycans (up to a 1.1-fold difference with respect to the negative control in the absence of cytokines on day 1, $p = 0.011$) and the cell proliferation rates (Figure 3A,B versus Figure 3G,H). Again, SOX9 overexpression increased the deposition of proteoglycans following IL-1β/TNF-α treatment, especially when the vectors were transferred via micellar vehicles (up to 2-fold difference relative to the cell control in the presence of IL-1β/TNF-α on day 10, $p = 0.043$; up to a 1.5-fold difference compared with free vector administration in the presence of IL-1β/TNF-α on day 10, $p = 0.009$) (Figure 3G,H). Likewise, genetic modification of chondrocytes via rAAV-FLAG-hsox9 resulted in an increased proliferation index (up to a 1.8-fold relative to the cell control in the presence of IL-1β/TNF-α on day 10, $p = 0.001$).

3.3. Effects of rAAV-FLAG-hsox9/Polymeric Micelle Delivery on the Viability Processes in Human OA Chondrocytes in Inflammatory Conditions

We finally examined the effects of SOX9 overexpression on the cell viability processes following rAAV-FLAG-hsox9 gene transfer via micellar systems in human OA chondrocytes monolayer cultures maintained in conditions of inflammation.

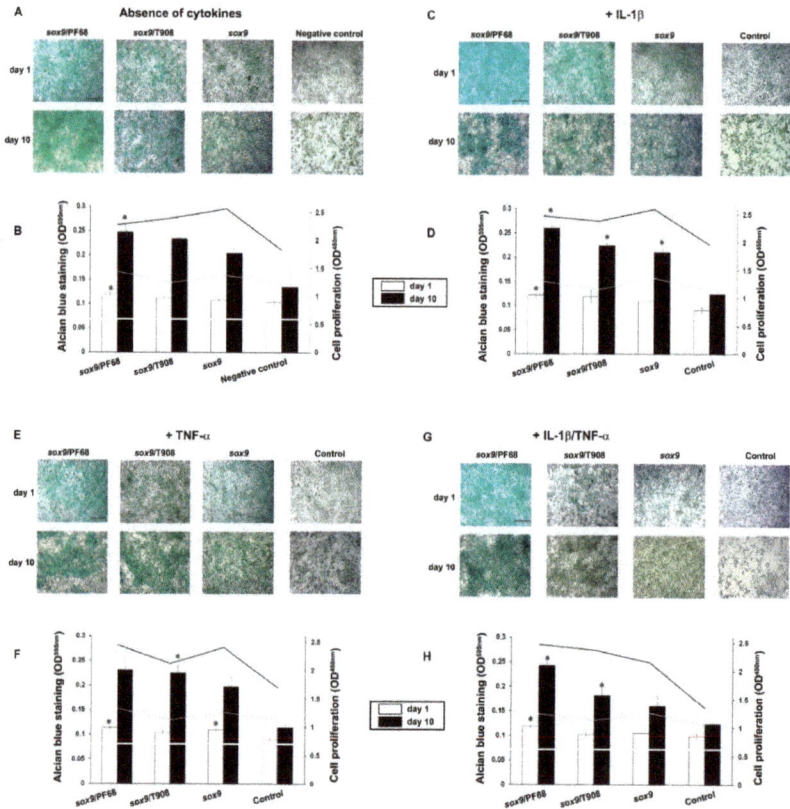

Figure 3. Biosynthetic activities in rAAV-FLAG-h*sox9*-transduced human OA chondrocytes using polymeric micelles. Cells in monolayer culture were directly transduced with the rAAV/polymeric micelles (**A,B**) or after pre-incubation for 4 h with IL-1β (10 ng/mL) (**C,D**), TNF-α (100 ng/mL) (**E,F**), or IL-1β/TNF-α (10/100 ng/mL) (**G,H**), as described in Figures 1 and 2 and in the Materials and Methods. The cultures were processed at the denoted time points for Alcian blue staining (magnification x10, scale bar 200 μm; all representative data) (**A,C,E,G**) with spectrophotometric evaluations for cell proliferation and proteoglycan deposition following solubilization in 6 M guanidine hydrochloride (**B,D,F,H**), as described in the Materials and Methods. Control conditions included the absence of copolymer or vector treatment (negative control) and the application of free rAAV vector (positive control). * Statistically significant compared with the negative control at similar time points.

In concordance with our previous observations [23], no cytotoxic effects from none of the gene transfer procedures (polymeric vehicles, free vector supply) were noticed with respect to the control condition ($p = 0.130$) (Figure 4A). A similar tendency was evidenced when providing copolymer solutions in the absence of vector treatment (not shown). Moreover, while separate cytokine treatment resulted only in slight decreases in cell viability (~90%) (Figure 4B,C), concomitant administration of both cytokines led to higher toxicity especially in untransduced cells (~75% cell viability on day 10 in the negative control in the presence of IL-1β/TNF-α) (Figure 4D). Strikingly, overexpression of SOX9 led to higher cell viability indices in the presence of both cytokines (~100% compared with the cell control in the presence of IL-1β/TNF-α on day 10, $p = 0.045$) (Figure 4D).

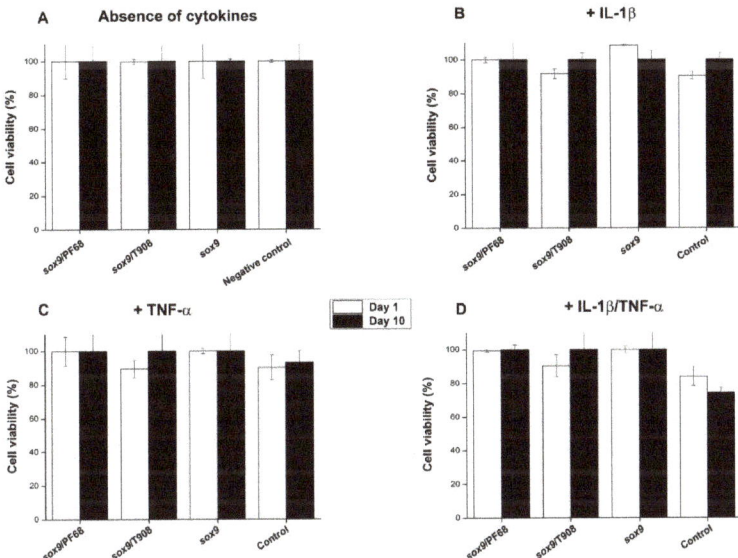

Figure 4. Cell viability in rAAV-FLAG-hsox9 modified human OA chondrocytes using micellar systems. Cell monolayer cultures were directly transduced with the rAAV/polymeric micelles (**A**) or after pre-incubation for 4 h with IL-1β (10 ng/mL) (**B**), TNF-α (100 ng/mL) (**C**), or IL-1β/TNF-α (10/100 ng/mL) (**D**), as described in Figures 1–3 and in the Materials and Methods.

4. Discussion

A potential means to counterbalance the disrupted cartilage homeostasis altered during OA disease is based on the correction of specific chondrocyte gene expression patterns [19]. Herein, transcription factors are critical mediators of cartilage metabolism prompting chondrogenesis in both physiologic and pathologic conditions [19]. Among them, SOX9 plays vital roles in the settlement of skeletal and cartilage formation [36] and the differentiation of chondrocytes [37]. Several studies have reported a decline in SOX9 expression in OA pathology [38,39]. Therefore, genetic adjustment of the levels of SOX9 expression may constitute a valuable strategy for re-equilibrating the disturbed balance characteristic of OA cartilage towards the synthesis of ECM compounds, affording the rescue of a native articular cartilage surface [19]. rAAV vectors are convenient carriers for efficiently and steadily targeting human OA chondrocytes [11,19] and avoiding the shortcomings and/or risks inherent to other types of vectors (short-term nonviral vectors, immunogenic adenoviral vectors, potentially tumorigenic retro-/lentiviral vectors) [40,41]. However, clinical administration of rAAV for OA treatments in patients may be hindered by the prevalence of circulating anti-AAV capsid antibodies in the subjects [42], especially in the synovial fluid from patients affected with joint disorders [20]. To overcome this hurdle, we evidenced the capability of PEO-PPO-PEO-based polymeric micelles (PF68 and T908) to efficiently and durably deliver rAAV vectors with increased stability and bioactivity to chondrocytes and mesenchymal stem cells (MSCs), affording protection against neutralizing antibodies [21,31]. Equally important, rAAV-mediated gene transfer of *sox9* via polymeric micelle delivery resulted in the remodeling of OA cartilage, with increased proteoglycan accumulation and cell proliferation in OA chondrocytes relative to free vector administration [23].

In light of these observations, the goal of the present study was to test the potentiality of these micellar nanocarriers to deliver the rAAV-FLAG-hsox9 vector to human OA chondrocytes in an environment similar to that in OA, i.e., in the presence of pro-inflammatory IL-1β and TNF-α cytokines [4,5,24]. First, and in good concordance with our previous findings [23], the data indicate that the transfer of rAAV-FLAG-h*sox9* to human OA chondrocytes via polymeric micelles led to enhanced levels of SOX9 expression over time relative to free vector treatment. Of note, rAAV-FLAG-h*sox9* transduction of chondrocytes prompted elevated and sustained levels of SOX9 expression in cells treated with IL-1β, especially when the vectors were carried by the polymeric micelles. A similar trend was observed in the presence of TNF-α alone or combined with IL-1β (IL-β/TNF-α condition), showing that delivery of the vectors via micellar systems to the highest levels of SOX9 expression. Likewise, rAAV-FLAG-h*sox9*-mediated treatment in the presence of IL-β/TNF-α increased the levels of SOX9 expression. These results are in agreement with previous work reporting an increased rAAV-mediated modification of fibroblast-like synoviocytes in conditions of inflammation [43].

The results next indicate that rAAV *sox9* treatment led to significantly higher levels of type-II collagen deposition compared with untransduced controls, most particularly when the vectors were delivered via polymeric micelles, concordant with our previous work when providing rAAV-FLAG-h*sox9* to experimental human osteochondral defects [23] and with the pro-anabolic properties of this transcription factor [44,45]. Of further note, while administration of IL-1β to chondrocyte cultures decreased the levels of type-II collagen deposition, in agreement with previous findings [7], transduction with rAAV-FLAG-h*sox9* reversed such undesirable effects by increasing type-II collagen deposition in IL-1β-treated chondrocytes especially when providing the construct via polymeric micelles, expanding earlier work using lentiviral delivery of *sox9* [8]. In this regard, the use of rAAV provides strong advantages for clinical translation, as they do not carry the risk of insertional mutagenesis inherent to lentiviruses [9]. Similar observations were made following TNF-α treatment (alone or combined with IL-1β) and genetic modification via rAAV-FLAG-h*sox9*, with increased type-II collagen deposition especially using polymeric micelle-guided rAAV gene transfer. Also remarkably, SOX9 overexpression via rAAV was capable of reverting the inhibitory effects of the cytokines upon the deposition of proteoglycans and the proliferation index [7], especially when delivering the therapeutic construct in polymeric micelles, again expanding work with lentiviral gene delivery of *sox9* [8], and concordant with the pro-anabolic activities of the transcription factor [45]. Moreover, no detrimental effects were noted, regardless of the gene transfer method adopted, as previously described with rAAV [23], and SOX9 overexpression was again capable to counteract the cytotoxic effects of the cytokines by preserving the viability of the OA chondrocytes, in agreement with work highlighting the role of SOX9 to preserve chondrocyte survival [8].

5. Conclusions

The present study shows the potentiality of polymeric micelles as powerful rAAV controlled delivery systems to counteract the specific contribution of major OA-associated inflammatory cytokines in chondrocyte cultures. Here, we provide concrete evidence that encapsulation of an rAAV vector carrying a *sox9* sequence in such systems promotes significant SOX9 expression levels capable of increasing the deposition of major ECM components (type-II collagen, proteoglycans) and the cell survival processes in human OA chondrocytes while reversing their downregulation afforded by OA cytokines. While this work evidence the utility of such micellar systems to tackle the OA phenotype in chondrocytes in a 2D environment, work is currently ongoing to broaden this investigation at longer time points and to support the present findings when cells are embedded in their own pericellular matrix using an experimental model of osteochondral defect in situ [22,23] where the chondrocytes may also be influenced by interplay with subchondral bone cells that have key roles in OA development and progression. Overall, such observations show the effectiveness of polymeric micelles as rAAV controlled delivery systems in an inflammatory environment, making them attractive tools for the treatment for chronic inflammatory diseases like OA.

Author Contributions: Conceptualization, A.R.-R. and M.C.; methodology, A.R.-R. and M.C.; software, J.U. and A.R.-R.; validation, A.R.-R. and M.C.; formal analysis, J.U., A.R.-R. and M.C.; investigation, J.U., A.R.-R. and M.C.; resources, A.R.-R. and M.C.; data curation, J.U. and A.R.-R.; writing—original draft preparation, A.R.-R. and M.C. writing—review and editing, A.R.-R. and M.C.; visualization, A.R.-R. and M.C.; supervision, A.R.-R. and M.C.;

project administration, A.R.-R. and M.C.; funding acquisition, A.R.-R. and M.C. All authors have read and agreed to the published version of the manuscript.

Funding: This research was funded by the DEUTSCHE FORSCHUNGSGEMEINSCHAFT (DFG RE 328/2-1 to A.R.R., M.C.).

Acknowledgments: The authors acknowledge R.J. Samulski (The Gene Therapy Center, University of North Carolina, Chapel Hill, NC, USA), X. Xiao (The Gene Therapy Center, University of Pittsburgh, Pittsburgh, PA, USA), and E.F. Terwilliger (Division of Experimental Medicine, Harvard Institutes of Medicine and Beth Israel Deaconess Medical Center, Boston, MA, USA) for providing the genomic AAV-2 plasmid clones, the pXX2 and pXX6 plasmids, and the 293 cell line. The authors also thank G. Scherer (Institute for Human Genetics and Anthropology, Albert-Ludwig University, Freiburg, Germany) for providing the human *sox9* cDNA. A.R.R. thanks the InTalent program from UDC-Inditex for the research grant.

Conflicts of Interest: The authors declare no conflict of interest.

References

1. Hermann, W.; Lambova, S.; Muller-Ladner, U. Current treatment options for osteoarthritis. *Curr. Rheumatol. Rev.* **2018**, *14*, 108–116. [CrossRef] [PubMed]
2. Loeser, R.F.; Goldring, S.R.; Scanzello, C.R.; Goldring, M.B. Osteoarthritis: A disease of the joint as an organ. *Arthritis Rheum.* **2012**, *64*, 1697–1707. [CrossRef] [PubMed]
3. Poole, A.R. Osteoarthritis as a whole joint disease. *HSS J.* **2012**, *8*, 4–6. [CrossRef]
4. Kapoor, M.; Martel-Pelletier, J.; Lajeunesse, D.; Pelletier, J.P.; Fahmi, H. Role of proinflammatory cytokines in the pathophysiology of osteoarthritis. *Nat. Rev. Rheumatol.* **2011**, *7*, 33–42. [CrossRef]
5. Goldring, M.B.; Otero, M. Inflammation in osteoarthritis. *Curr. Opin. Rheumatol.* **2011**, *23*, 471–478. [CrossRef]
6. Fernandes, J.C.; Martel-Pelletier, J.; Pelletier, J.P. The role of cytokines in osteoarthritis pathophysiology. *Biorheology* **2002**, *39*, 237–246.
7. Hwang, S.G.; Yu, S.S.; Poo, H.; Chun, J.S. C-jun/activator protein-1 mediates interleukin-1beta-induced dedifferentiation but not cyclooxygenase-2 expression in articular chondrocytes. *J. Biol. Chem.* **2005**, *280*, 29780–29787. [CrossRef]
8. Lu, H.; Zeng, C.; Chen, M.; Lian, L.; Dai, Y.; Zhao, H. Lentiviral vector-mediated over-expression of sox9 protected chondrocytes from il-1beta induced degeneration and apoptosis. *Int. J. Clin. Exp. Pathol.* **2015**, *8*, 10038–10049.
9. Schlimgen, R.; Howard, J.; Wooley, D.; Thompson, M.; Baden, L.R.; Yang, O.O.; Christiani, D.C.; Mostoslavsky, G.; Diamond, D.V.; Duane, E.G.; et al. Risks associated with lentiviral vector exposures and prevention strategies. *J. Occup. Environ. Med.* **2016**, *58*, 1159–1166. [CrossRef]
10. Smith, R.H. Adeno-associated virus integration: Virus versus vector. *Gene Ther.* **2008**, *15*, 817–822. [CrossRef]
11. Madry, H.; Cucchiarini, M.; Terwilliger, E.F.; Trippel, S.B. Recombinant adeno-associated virus vectors efficiently and persistently transduce chondrocytes in normal and osteoarthritic human articular cartilage. *Hum. Gene Ther.* **2003**, *14*, 393–402. [CrossRef]
12. Cucchiarini, M.; Madry, H.; Ma, C.; Thurn, T.; Zurakowski, D.; Menger, M.D.; Kohn, D.; Trippel, S.B.; Terwilliger, E.F. Improved tissue repair in articular cartilage defects in vivo by rAAV-mediated overexpression of human fibroblast growth factor 2. *Mol. Ther.* **2005**, *12*, 229–238. [CrossRef] [PubMed]
13. Hiraide, A.; Yokoo, N.; Xin, K.Q.; Okuda, K.; Mizukami, H.; Ozawa, K.; Saito, T. Repair of articular cartilage defect by intraarticular administration of basic fibroblast growth factor gene, using adeno-associated virus vector. *Hum. Gene Ther.* **2005**, *16*, 1413–1421. [CrossRef] [PubMed]
14. Cucchiarini, M.; Orth, P.; Madry, H. Direct rAAV sox9 administration for durable articular cartilage repair with delayed terminal differentiation and hypertrophy in vivo. *J. Mol. Med.* **2013**, *91*, 625–636. [CrossRef] [PubMed]
15. Cucchiarini, M.; Madry, H. Overexpression of human IGF-I via direct rAAV-mediated gene transfer improves the early repair of articular cartilage defects in vivo. *Gene Ther.* **2014**, *21*, 811–819. [CrossRef]
16. Ortved, K.F.; Begum, L.; Mohammed, H.O.; Nixon, A.J. Implantation of rAAV5-IGF-I transduced autologous chondrocytes improves cartilage repair in full-thickness defects in the equine model. *Mol. Ther.* **2015**, *23*, 363–373. [CrossRef] [PubMed]

17. Ulrich-Vinther, M.; Stengaard, C.; Schwarz, E.M.; Goldring, M.B.; Soballe, K. Adeno-associated vector mediated gene transfer of transforming growth factor-beta1 to normal and osteoarthritic human chondrocytes stimulates cartilage anabolism. *Eur. Cell Mater.* **2005**, *10*, 40–50. [CrossRef]
18. Venkatesan, J.K.; Rey-Rico, A.; Schmitt, G.; Wezel, A.; Madry, H.; Cucchiarini, M. rAAV-mediated overexpression of TGF-beta stably restructures human osteoarthritic articular cartilage in situ. *J. Transl. Med.* **2013**, *11*, 211. [CrossRef]
19. Cucchiarini, M.; Thurn, T.; Weimer, A.; Kohn, D.; Terwilliger, E.F.; Madry, H. Restoration of the extracellular matrix in human osteoarthritic articular cartilage by overexpression of the transcription factor sox9. *Arthritis Rheum.* **2007**, *56*, 158–167. [CrossRef]
20. Cottard, V.; Valvason, C.; Falgarone, G.; Lutomski, D.; Boissier, M.C.; Bessis, N. Immune response against gene therapy vectors: Influence of synovial fluid on adeno-associated virus mediated gene transfer to chondrocytes. *J. Clin. Immunol.* **2004**, *24*, 162–169. [CrossRef]
21. Rey-Rico, A.; Frisch, J.; Venkatesan, J.K.; Schmitt, G.; Rial-Hermida, I.; Taboada, P.; Concheiro, A.; Madry, H.; Alvarez-Lorenzo, C.; Cucchiarini, M. PEO-PPO-PEO carriers for rAAV-mediated transduction of human articular chondrocytes in vitro and in a human osteochondral defect model. *ACS Appl. Mater. Interfaces* **2016**, *8*, 20600–20613. [CrossRef] [PubMed]
22. Rey-Rico, A.; Venkatesan, J.K.; Schmitt, G.; Concheiro, A.; Madry, H.; Alvarez-Lorenzo, C.; Cucchiarini, M. rAAV-mediated overexpression of TGF-beta via vector delivery in polymeric micelles stimulates the biological and reparative activities of human articular chondrocytes in vitro and in a human osteochondral defect model. *Int. J. Nanomed.* **2017**, *12*, 6985–6996. [CrossRef] [PubMed]
23. Rey-Rico, A.; Venkatesan, J.K.; Schmitt, G.; Speicher-Mentges, S.; Madry, H.; Cucchiarini, M. Effective remodelling of human osteoarthritic cartilage by sox9 gene transfer and overexpression upon delivery of rAAV vectors in polymeric micelles. *Mol. Pharm.* **2018**, *15*, 2816–2826. [CrossRef] [PubMed]
24. Berenbaum, F. Osteoarthritis as an inflammatory disease (osteoarthritis is not osteoarthrosis!). *Osteoarthr. Cartil.* **2013**, *21*, 16–21. [CrossRef] [PubMed]
25. Samulski, R.J.; Chang, L.S.; Shenk, T. Helper-free stocks of recombinant adeno-associated viruses: Normal integration does not require viral gene expression. *J. Virol.* **1989**, *63*, 3822–3828. [CrossRef]
26. Samulski, R.J.; Chang, L.S.; Shenk, T. A recombinant plasmid from which an infectious adeno-associated virus genome can be excised in vitro and its use to study viral replication. *J. Virol.* **1987**, *61*, 3096–3101. [CrossRef]
27. Venkatesan, J.K.; Ekici, M.; Madry, H.; Schmitt, G.; Kohn, D.; Cucchiarini, M. Sox9 gene transfer via safe, stable, replication-defective recombinant adeno-associated virus vectors as a novel, powerful tool to enhance the chondrogenic potential of human mesenchymal stem cells. *Stem Cell Res. Ther.* **2012**, *3*, 22. [CrossRef]
28. Tao, K.; Rey-Rico, A.; Frisch, J.; Venkatesan, J.K.; Schmitt, G.; Madry, H.; Lin, J.; Cucchiarini, M. rAAV-mediated combined gene transfer and overexpression of tgf-beta and sox9 remodels human osteoarthritic articular cartilage. *J. Orthop. Res.* **2016**, *34*, 2181–2190. [CrossRef]
29. Venkatesan, J.K.; Frisch, J.; Rey-Rico, A.; Schmitt, G.; Madry, H.; Cucchiarini, M. Impact of mechanical stimulation on the chondrogenic processes in human bone marrow aspirates modified to overexpress sox9 via rAAV vectors. *J. Exp. Orthop.* **2017**, *4*, 22. [CrossRef]
30. Frisch, J.; Venkatesan, J.K.; Rey-Rico, A.; Schmitt, G.; Madry, H.; Cucchiarini, M. Determination of the chondrogenic differentiation processes in human bone marrow-derived mesenchymal stem cells genetically modified to overexpress transforming growth factor-beta via recombinant adeno-associated viral vectors. *Hum. Gene Ther.* **2014**, *25*, 1050–1060. [CrossRef]
31. Rey-Rico, A.; Venkatesan, J.K.; Frisch, J.; Rial-Hermida, I.; Schmitt, G.; Concheiro, A.; Madry, H.; Alvarez-Lorenzo, C.; Cucchiarini, M. Peo-ppo-peo micelles as effective rAAV-mediated gene delivery systems to target human mesenchymal stem cells without altering their differentiation potency. *Acta Biomater.* **2015**, *27*, 42–52. [CrossRef] [PubMed]
32. Vincenti, M.P.; Brinckerhoff, C.E. Early response genes induced in chondrocytes stimulated with the inflammatory cytokine interleukin-1beta. *Arthritis Res.* **2001**, *3*, 381–388. [CrossRef] [PubMed]
33. Schuerwegh, A.J.; Dombrecht, E.J.; Stevens, W.J.; Van Offel, J.F.; Bridts, C.H.; De Clerck, L.S. Influence of pro-inflammatory (IL-1 alpha, IL-6, TNF-alpha, IFN-gamma) and anti-inflammatory (il-4) cytokines on chondrocyte function. *Osteoarthr. Cartil.* **2003**, *11*, 681–687. [CrossRef]

34. Stanton, L.A.; Sabari, S.; Sampaio, A.V.; Underhill, T.M.; Beier, F. P38 map kinase signalling is required for hypertrophic chondrocyte differentiation. *Biochem. J.* **2004**, *378*, 53–62. [CrossRef] [PubMed]
35. Woods, A.; Wang, G.; Beier, F. Rhoa/rock signaling regulates sox9 expression and actin organization during chondrogenesis. *J. Biol. Chem.* **2005**, *280*, 11626–11634. [CrossRef] [PubMed]
36. Bi, W.; Deng, J.M.; Zhang, Z.; Behringer, R.R.; de Crombrugghe, B. Sox9 is required for cartilage formation. *Nat. Genet.* **1999**, *22*, 85–89. [CrossRef]
37. Ikeda, T.; Kamekura, S.; Mabuchi, A.; Kou, I.; Seki, S.; Takato, T.; Nakamura, K.; Kawaguchi, H.; Ikegawa, S.; Chung, U.I. The combination of sox5, sox6, and sox9 (the sox trio) provides signals sufficient for induction of permanent cartilage. *Arthritis Rheum.* **2004**, *50*, 3561–3573. [CrossRef]
38. Salminen, H.; Vuorio, E.; Saamanen, A.M. Expression of sox9 and type IIa procollagen during attempted repair of articular cartilage damage in a transgenic mouse model of osteoarthritis. *Arthritis Rheum.* **2001**, *44*, 947–955. [CrossRef]
39. Aigner, T.; Gebhard, P.M.; Schmid, E.; Bau, B.; Harley, V.; Poschl, E. Sox9 expression does not correlate with type II collagen expression in adult articular chondrocytes. *Matrix Biol.* **2003**, *22*, 363–372. [CrossRef]
40. Madry, H.; Cucchiarini, M. Advances and challenges in gene-based approaches for osteoarthritis. *J. Gene Med.* **2013**, *15*, 343–355. [CrossRef]
41. Evans, C.H.; Huard, J. Gene therapy approaches to regenerating the musculoskeletal system. *Nat. Rev. Rheumatol.* **2015**, *11*, 234–242. [CrossRef] [PubMed]
42. Calcedo, R.; Wilson, J.M. Humoral immune response to AAV. *Front. Immunol.* **2013**, *4*, 341. [CrossRef] [PubMed]
43. Traister, R.S.; Fabre, S.; Wang, Z.; Xiao, X.; Hirsch, R. Inflammatory cytokine regulation of transgene expression in human fibroblast-like synoviocytes infected with adeno-associated virus. *Arthritis Rheum.* **2006**, *54*, 2119–2126. [CrossRef] [PubMed]
44. Xie, W.F.; Zhang, X.; Sakano, S.; Lefebvre, V.; Sandell, L.J. Trans-activation of the mouse cartilage-derived retinoic acid-sensitive protein gene by sox9. *J. Bone Miner. Res.* **1999**, *14*, 757–763. [CrossRef] [PubMed]
45. Furumatsu, T.; Matsumoto-Ogawa, E.; Tanaka, T.; Lu, Z.; Ozaki, T. Rock inhibition enhances aggrecan deposition and suppresses matrix metalloproteinase-3 production in human articular chondrocytes. *Connect. Tissue Res.* **2014**, *55*, 89–95. [CrossRef] [PubMed]

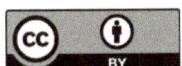 © 2020 by the authors. Licensee MDPI, Basel, Switzerland. This article is an open access article distributed under the terms and conditions of the Creative Commons Attribution (CC BY) license (http://creativecommons.org/licenses/by/4.0/).

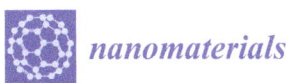

Article

Amphiphilic "Like-A-Brush" Oligonucleotide Conjugates with Three Dodecyl Chains: Self-Assembly Features of Novel Scaffold Compounds for Nucleic Acids Delivery

Anna S. Pavlova, Ilya S. Dovydenko, Maxim S. Kupryushkin, Alina E. Grigor'eva, Inna A. Pyshnaya and Dmitrii V. Pyshnyi *

Institute of Chemical Biology and Fundamental Medicine SB RAS, 630090 Novosibirsk, Russia; pavlova@niboch.nsc.ru (A.S.P.); dovydenko_il@niboch.nsc.ru (I.S.D.); kuprummax@niboch.nsc.ru (M.S.K.); grigoryeva@niboch.nsc.ru (A.E.G.); pyshnaya@niboch.nsc.ru (I.A.P.)
* Correspondence: pyshnyi@niboch.nsc.ru; Tel.: +7-383-363-5151

Received: 31 August 2020; Accepted: 25 September 2020; Published: 29 September 2020

Abstract: The conjugation of lipophilic groups to oligonucleotides is a promising approach for improving nucleic acid-based therapeutics' intracellular delivery. Lipid oligonucleotide conjugates can self-aggregate in aqueous solution, which gains much attention due to the formation of micellar particles suitable for cell endocytosis. Here, we describe self-association features of novel "like-a-brush" oligonucleotide conjugates bearing three dodecyl chains. The self-assembly of the conjugates into 30–170 nm micellar particles with a high tendency to aggregate was shown using dynamic light scattering (DLS), atomic force (AFM), and transmission electron (TEM) microscopies. Fluorescently labeled conjugates demonstrated significant quenching of fluorescence intensity (up to 90%) under micelle formation conditions. The conjugates possess increased binding affinity to serum albumin as compared with free oligonucleotides. The dodecyl oligonucleotide conjugate and its duplex efficiently internalized and accumulated into HepG2 cells' cytoplasm without any transfection agent. It was shown that the addition of serum albumin or fetal bovine serum to the medium decreased oligonucleotide uptake efficacy (by 22.5–36%) but did not completely inhibit cell penetration. The obtained results allow considering dodecyl-containing oligonucleotides as scaffold compounds for engineering nucleic acid delivery vehicles.

Keywords: lipid conjugates; amphiphilic oligonucleotides; self-assembly; phosphoryl guanidines; nucleic acid delivery

1. Introduction

Synthetic oligonucleotide conjugates with lipophilic groups are in the focus of considerable attention as nucleic acid (NA)-based biological tools in a wide range of fields of biotechnology and biomedicine [1,2]. Lipid-oligonucleotide conjugates (LOCs) are particularly interesting as delivery vehicles, which bring therapeutic oligonucleotides (e.g., antisense oligomers or siRNA) to their intracellular targets [3–6]. Negatively charged native oligonucleotides show poor cell penetration [5,6]. Their conjugation with lipophilic moieties can improve cellular uptake by providing an additional anchor for membrane binding [7–11].

Due to their amphipathic nature, oligonucleotide conjugates with lipophilic groups can self-assemble in aqueous solutions and form micelles [10,12–18] and their aggregates [10,11,14], vesicular assemblies [19,20], and more complex self-aggregation structures [2,11,21]. Generally, these structures are nearly spherical in shape [10,15,16,20,22,23]. The size and the shape of self-assembling structures may greatly depend on experimental conditions: ionic strength, pH, and temperature; the type of lipophilic group; the length and nucleotide sequence of an oligomer in the LOC [2,17].

Cargo systems can be based as well on the attachment of lipophilic groups directly to a specific antisense oligonucleotide [10,24,25], to one of the siRNA strands [11,21,26,27] or more complex delivery formulations [13,23,28,29]. Furthermore, LOCs suit for the construction of oligonucleotide delivery system based on the liposomal-type spherical nucleic acids (SNA) [30–32]. The hydrophobic micellar core of LOC particles also serves as a carrier for extremely poor soluble pharmaceuticals [14,23,29] and fluorescent dyes [13,19].

Substantial characteristics of lipid-oligonucleotide conjugates include good biocompatibility and low toxicity [10,11,33]. LOCs improve pharmacokinetics and biodistribution of antisense oligomers (ASO) compared with native unconjugated oligonucleotides [4]. This advance is generally attributed to enhanced LOC binding to serum proteins. The association of the LOCs with one or more serum proteins (albumin, etc.) is also believed to participate in their cellular uptake mechanisms [4]. Albumin is the major blood protein that binds and transports numerous endogenous and exogenous substances, including fatty acids and other poor water-soluble compounds [34]. Lipid-oligonucleotide conjugates can easily bind as well to hydrophobic sites of the albumin [5,22]. It appears to affect their circulation half-life and bioavailability, e.g., for intravenous administration of LOC-based pharmaceuticals. Modifications of the oligonucleotide backbone (phosphorothioate (PS), morpholino, peptide nucleic acids, 2'-O-methyl, 2'-fluoro, and others) combined with lipophilic group enhance nuclease resistance of oligonucleotides, thus increasing their in vivo circulation lifetime [4–6].

So far, cholesterol is one of the most investigated lipophilic groups conjugated with oligonucleotides to improve cellular uptake [4,5,8]. Other promising modifications of this kind are fatty acids and lipid chains [6]. For example, Imetelstat (GRN163L), a palmitoyl-tethered thio-phosphoramidate oligomer, provides telomerase inhibition in the treatment of myeloproliferative disorders or neoplasms [6,24]. An interesting type of conjugates is represented by LOCs with "like-a-brush" lipid moieties attached to the oligonucleotide backbone [10,14,20,35]. Conjugation in such a manner gives the rise of hydrophobicity of the LOC lipophilic segment, in contrast to the consecutive linear combination. Earlier, we designed a non-nucleoside monomer to incorporate dodecyl groups into the oligonucleotides and synthesized dodecyl-containing conjugates with hydrophobicity comparable to that of corresponding cholesterol derivatives [36]. It was recently demonstrated that three dodecyl oligonucleotide conjugates (DOCs) are efficient and non-toxic transport molecules for ASO delivery into the A549 and HEK293 cells, which provide the transfection efficacy comparable to that of Lipofectamine 2000 [33].

In the present work, we report on self-assembly features of amphiphilic "like-a-brush" oligonucleotide conjugates functionalized at 5' and 3'-ends with three dodecyl groups [36]. These DOCs were studied for their abilities to form micellar structures and to penetrate the HepG2 tumor cells. In vitro investigation of self-assembling features of DOCs by dynamic light scattering (DLS), electrophoretic mobility shift assay (EMSA), fluorescence spectroscopy, transmission electron (TEM) and atomic force (AFM) microscopies, flow cytometry, and confocal microscopy substantially extended current knowledge on micelle-like structures of "like-a-brush" lipophilic oligonucleotide conjugates. The obtained results establish the potential of DOCs as nucleic acid delivery tools.

2. Materials and Methods

2.1. General Remarks

Buffers composition: TA—50 mM Tris-Acetate, pH 7.5; TAM—50 mM Tris-Acetate, pH 7.5, 15 mM $MgCl_2$; TAN—50 Tris-Acetate, pH 7.5, 100 mM NaCl. All buffers were filtered through 0.22 μm Millipore Syringe Filter units (Merck, KGaA, Darmstadt, Germany, and/or its affiliates). Oligonucleotides and DOCs were incubated in 1.5 mL DNA LoBind tubes (Eppendorf AG, Hamburg, Germany).

2.2. Materials

Nile Red (9-diethylamino-5H-benzo[alpha]phenoxazine-5-one ($C_{20}H_{18}N_2O_2$), Merck, KGaA, Darmstadt, Germany, and/or its affiliates), bovine serum albumin (BSA) (Sigma-Aldrich Chemie Gmbh, Munich, Germany), Stains-All (Acros Organics, Fair Lawn, NJ, USA). Unless otherwise stated, all commercial reagents and solvents were used without additional purification. All chemicals used in this work were molecular biology grade or higher. Water was 18 MΩ grade (purified by a Simplicity 185 water system (Millipore, Burlington, MA, USA).

2.3. Oligonucleotides and Conjugates Synthesis

Standard phosphoramidite solid-phase synthesis of all modified/unmodified and conjugated/unconjugated oligonucleotides was carried out on the ASM-800 DNA/RNA synthesizer (Biosset, Novosibirsk, Russia). Oligonucleotides were synthesized at 0.2 µmol scale, using standard commercial 2-cyanoethyl deoxynucleoside phosphoramidites and CPG solid supports (Glen Research, Sterling, VA, USA). The phosphoramidite for introducing non-nucleosidic dodecyl-containing units was obtained as described [36] and used as a 0.1 M solution in anhydrous acetonitrile with the extension of the coupling time from 1 to 10 min. Oligonucleotides with internucleoside uncharged phosphoryl 1,3-dimethylimidazolidine-2-imino groups (phosphoryl guanidines, PG) were synthetized by NooGen LLC as described earlier [37–39]. 6-carboxyfluorescein (FAM) labeling of the oligonucleotides was performed using commercially available 5′- and 3′-modifiers (2-Dimethoxytrityloxymethyl-6-(3′,6′-dipivaloylfluorescein-6-yl-carboxamido)-hexyl-1-O-[(2-cyanoethyl)-(N,N-diisopropyl)]-phosphoramidite from Glen Research, Sterling, VA, USA and 3′-FAM-CPG (Figure S1) from Primetech ALC, Minsk, Belarus) according to the manufacturer's protocols. All oligomers after cleavage and deblocking from CPG were purified by RP-HPLC and their structures (for examples see Figures S3–S5) were confirmed by MALDI TOF or ESI mass spectrometry (for additional information see Supp. Inf., Section S1, Table S1, Figure S6).

2.4. Critical Aggregation Concentration (CAC) Determination by Nile Red Encapsulation Assay

Formation of the DOC micelles was characterized as described in the literature [23], using Nile Red as a fluorescent probe. A 10 mM stock solution of the Nile Red in ethanol was used for all experiments. Briefly, 0.7 µM, 1 µM, 3 µM, 10 µM, 30 µM, and 50 µM of the DOC or control oligonucleotide were incubated in eppendorfs with 100 µM Nile Red in TA or TAM buffer at 25 °C for 3 h. After incubation, time samples were transferred in TPP® tissue culture plates (Sigma-Aldrich Chemie GmbH, Buchs, Switzerland). The fluorescence intensity spectra of the Nile Red were obtained at room temperature using a CLARIOStar® Microplate reader (BMG LABTECH GmbH, Ortenberg, Germany). Fluorescent measurements were taken at the excitation wavelength of 550 nm and the emission was monitored from 570 to 740 nm. The oligonucleotide without dodecyl chains was used as a control. The critical aggregation concentration (CAC) could be calculated by tracking the fluorescence intensity of Nile Red as a function of the sample concentration. CAC values were calculated from the plot of the emission intensity at 645 nm (in TA buffer) or 630 nm (in TAM) versus the log of concentrations (M) of dodecyl oligonucleotide conjugates. The CAC was obtained from the intersection of two straight tangents to these regions' lines.

2.5. Characterization of Assembled DOCs Micellar Structures by DLS

The size distributions of micellar particles of pre-assembled DOCs were determined by dynamic light scattering technique using a Zetasizer Nano-ZS (Malvern Panalytical Ltd., Malvern, UK) at 25 °C. The DOCs (5 µM) were prepared in TAM buffer and after 3 h of incubation measurements of the size were conducted.

2.6. Characterization of Assembled DOCs Micellar Structures by AFM

Atomic force microscopy was performed using a MultiMode 8™ scanning probe microscope (Bruker, Santa Barbara, CA, USA) connected to a NanoScope® V controller (Veeco, Plainview, NY, USA). The images were obtained using tapping mode in air with NSG10_DLC cantilevers (typical curvature radius 1 nm, resonant frequency 255 kHz, force constant 11.5 N/m) from NT-MDT Spectrum Instruments (Zelenograd, Moscow, Russia). Oligonucleotides containing dodecyl groups were diluted to 1.5 µM in TAM buffer. The reactions were equilibrated for 3 h at 25 °C before 6 µL of this solution was deposited onto a freshly cleaved mica surface (7 × 7 mm, NT-MDT Spectrum Instruments, Zelenograd, Moscow, Russia) and allowed to adsorb for 5 min. The surface was then washed thrice with 200 µL of 18 MΩ grade water and dried by strong argon flow. Samples were dried for 10 min prior to imaging.

2.7. Characterization of Assembled DOCs Micellar Structures by TEM

Dodecyl oligonucleotide conjugates were diluted to 5 µM in TAM buffer. The reactions were equilibrated for 3 h at 25 °C before a drop of this sample was adsorbed for 1 min on the copper grid covered with formvar film which was stabilized using carbon evaporation. Then excess of liquid was removed with filter paper, and a grid was placed for 5–10 s on a drop of 1% uranyl acetate, excess liquid was collected with filter paper. All grids were examined using a transmission electron microscope JEM-1400 (JEOL, Tokyo, Japan), and images were obtained using a Veleta (EM SIS, Münster, Germany) digital camera. All measurements were made using program package iTEM (EM SIS, Münster, Germany).

2.8. EMSA and BSA Binding Experiments

Electrophoretic mobility shift assay was carried out using Thermo Scientific™ Owl™ Dual-Gel Vertical Electrophoresis System (P8DS-2, Owl, Thermo Fisher Scientific Inc., Waltham, MA, USA) at 25, 35, or 37 °C, 7–8 W for 3–4 h. Briefly, control oligonucleotides and DOCs were diluted to the required concentration in 20 µl of corresponding buffer solution (TA, TAM, or TAN) and incubated for 2 h prior to loading onto the native PAAG. In BSA binding experiments, the protein was added to the oligonucleotides after 2 h of incubation and then the probes were additionally incubated for 1 h prior to loading onto the gel. After electrophoretic separation, the DNA and BSA bands were visualized by Stains-All staining and in the case of FAM-labeled oligonucleotides by scanning and recording the image using VersaDoc™ MP 4000 Molecular Imager® System (Bio-Rad, Hercules, CA, USA) after excitation at 488 nm. For Stains-All staining (0.05% (w/v) Stains-All in 50% (v/v) formamide), the gel after the run was stained in the dark chamber for 10 min. Destaining was accomplished by removing the gel from the staining solution and exposing it to the light until sufficient destaining had occurred. The gel was then immediately scanned using an Epson Perfection 4990 Photo scanner (Epson, Los Alamitos, CA, USA).

2.9. Fluorescence Quenching Experiments

1.5 µM FAM-labeled oligonucleotides and DOCs were prepared in 18 MΩ grade water, TA, or TAM buffer solutions. The samples were equilibrated for 3 h at 25 °C before transferring into the flat bottom 96-well microplates (TPP®, Sigma-Aldrich Chemie GmbH, Buchs, Switzerland) and measured through reading fluorescence intensity spectra on a CLARIOstar® plate reader (BMG LABTECH GmbH, Ortenberg, Germany) in top-read mode, with excitation at 488 nm (16 nm bandpass) and emission scanning from 503 nm to 619 nm (10 nm bandpass). Wells for background subtraction contained all components except FAM-labeled nucleic acids. Reactions were set up in triplicate in each experiment. To check the fluorescence quenching, the values of the fluorescence intensities at 520 nm, representative of fluorescence emission maximums for this dye, were compared for each of the solution conditions. Quenching efficiency (QE) was defined as QE = $(F_{TAM} \times 100)/F_{TA}$, where F_{TA} is the fluorescence intensity value of the oligomer in TA buffer, and F_{TAM}—in TAM buffer, respectively.

2.10. Cell Culture

For all experiments, we used the hepatocellular carcinoma (HepG2) cell line obtained from Russian Cell Culture Collection, Institute of Cytology of the Russian Academy of Science (St. Petersburg, Russia). Cells were cultivated at 37 °C and 5% CO_2 in DMEM medium with GlutaMAX™ containing 4.5 g/L glucose, supplemented with 10% fetal bovine serum (FBS), 100 U/mL penicillin, 100 µg/mL streptomycin (all from Gibco™ by Life Technologies® Corporation, Paisley, UK).

2.11. Cells Transfection

One day before the carrier-free transfection procedure, cells were seeded in 24-well plates at a density of 1.2×10^5 cells/well. Then cells were washed with PBS and treated for 4 h with a medium containing fluorescently labeled dodecyl oligonucleotide conjugate FAM-D-17^{PG} or duplex D-17^{PG}/FAM-17′ (250 µL/well). We used six versions of the medium composition for cell transfection procedure: (a,d) fresh DMEM (245 µL) and FAM-D-17^{PG} or D-17^{PG}/FAM-17′ (5 µL, 250 µM); (b,e) fresh DMEM with 10% FBS (245 µL) and FAM-D-17^{PG} or D-17^{PG}/FAM-17′ (5 µL, 250 µM); (c,f) fresh DMEM (240 µL), filtered through 0.45 µm bovine serum albumin (5 µL, 1.5 mM) and FAM-D-17^{PG} or D-17^{PG}/FAM-17′ (5 µL, 250 µM). For each condition, three independent transfections were prepared.

2.12. Cellular Accumulation Assay

For cellular accumulation assay, 4 h post-transfection cells were washed with PBS to eliminate fluorescently labeled unbound oligonucleotides. Next 24 h, cells were cultivated in full medium. Then, the cells were washed with PBS, trypsinized and suspended in PBS. The accumulation of oligomers was evaluated using NovoCyte (ACEA Biosciences, San Diego, CA, USA) flow cytometer. More than 5000 cells from each sample were analyzed using NovoExpress software (ACEA Biosciences).

2.13. Confocal Fluorescence Microscopy

For confocal microscopy, HepG2 cells cultivated in 1 cm^2 chambers slide (Lab-Tek, Thermo Fisher Scientific Inc., Waltham, MA, USA) were transfected with conjugate FAM-D-17^{PG} or duplex D-17^{PG}/FAM-17′ to the final concentration of 5 µM in the media with various composition (see Section 2.11). Right after transfection, cells were washed twice with PBS to eliminate fluorescently labeled unbound oligonucleotides. Washed cell were fixed with 4% paraformaldehyde in DMEM for 30 min and washed twice with PBS. After removing the chamber, the microscopic slide containing cells was mounted with the cover slip glass using ProLong Gold antifade reagent with DAPI (Life Technologies, Eugene, OR, USA), then the slide was kept 24 h in the dark at room temperature. LSM 710 confocal microscope (Carl Zeiss Microscopy GmbH, Jena, Germany) was used in conjunction with Zen imaging software, and images were acquired with a Zeiss 63×/1.40 oil immersion objective. The excitation/emission laser wavelengths were 405 nm (to detect cell nuclei stained with DAPI), 488 nm (to detect FAM).

2.14. Statistical Analysis

Each variant of conditions was tested in three or more independent experiments for all investigations. The values reported are expressed as mean ± standard deviation (SD) for at least three independent experiments.

3. Results

3.1. Oligonucleotides and DOCs in this Study

In the first step, we designed and synthesized 13-, 17-, and 22-mer oligonucleotide conjugates with three dodecyl chains (Figure 1a). The structures and nucleotide sequences of the oligomers used in this study are given in Figure 1. While planning the synthesis of oligonucleotides with non-nucleoside units bearing dodecyl chains, we considered that the free terminal hydroxyethyl group of this unit can cause degradation of the modified oligonucleotide during the deprotection step in basic aqueous solutions [40,41]. Therefore, we added an extra thymidylate unit at 3′- (FAM-17-D (Figure S3)) or 5′-end (D-13, D-13^{PG}, D-17, D-17^{PG}, D-17-FAM (Figure S4), D-22^{PG}) of corresponding oligomers to overcome this problem. Two phosphoryl guanidine [37,39] (PG) modifications were introduced at 3′-ends of D-13^{PG}, D-17^{PG} (Figure S5), and D-22^{PG} oligomers to enhance their stability in serum (Figure 1a,c).

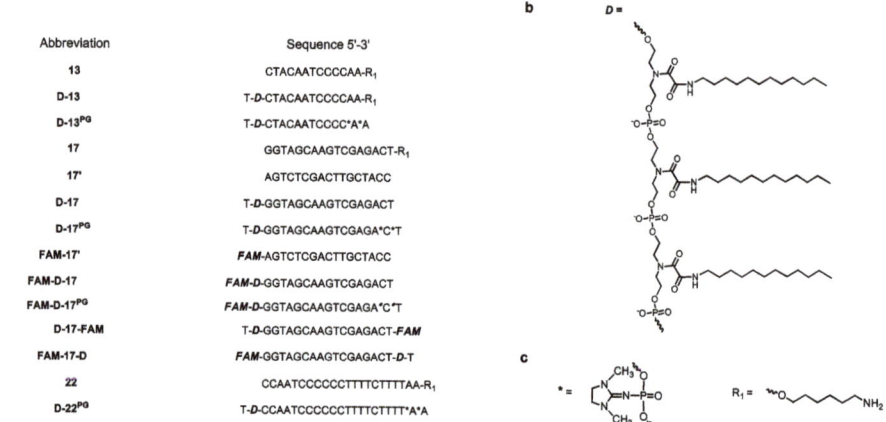

Figure 1. The sequences of oligonucleotides and their conjugates studied in this work (**a**), the structure of "like-a-brush" dodecyl-containing non-nucleoside backbone part of dodecyl oligonucleotide conjugates (DOC) (**b**). All oligonucleotides are deoxy. D-13^{PG}, D-17^{PG}, FAM-D-17^{PG}, D-22^{PG} are oligodeoxynucleotides partially substituted with phosphoryl guanidine groups (PG); * indicated a position of PG modification, R$_1$ is the linker with the terminal amino group protecting 3′-end of indicated oligomers from nuclease degradation (**c**). Here, 6-carboxyfluorescein (FAM) is represented 6-carboxyfluorescein residue (See Section 2.3). During post-chromatographic purification, dodecyl-containing oligonucleotides (especially D-17, D-17^{PG}, and FAM-D-17^{PG}) tended to aggregate, which resulted in significant salting-out of the conjugates at millimolar range concentrations used in the experiments.

3.2. CAC Determination by Nile Red Encapsulation Assay

Further testing by Nile Red encapsulation assay to determine the critical concentration of aggregation for D-17^{PG} partially explained our observations. The Nile Red dye fluoresces intensively in the hydrophobic lipid environment but shows negligible fluorescence in an aqueous medium. Due to these properties, it is applied to determine the LOC's critical aggregation concentration (CAC) value [42]. The incubation of a certain amount of the dye with D-17^{PG} at varying concentrations revealed an increase in the fluorescence intensity of Nile Red (Figure S7), which evidenced for its encapsulation in a non-polar microenvironment of micellar structure. Control oligonucleotide without dodecyl chains gave no significant increase in Nile Red fluorescence intensity (Figure S7). The CAC value of the DOC micellar particles was extremely sensitive to the presence of magnesium ions. In our work, the CAC of D-17^{PG} conjugate in 15 mM MgCl$_2$ (in TAM buffer) was above 1.2 µM (Figure S8a), while without magnesium ions, the CAC value (in TA buffer) was above 25 µM (Figure S8b).

We supposed that the self-assembly of the DOCs occurs with the formation of micellar particles composed of hydrophobic dodecyl inner core and hydrophilic oligonucleotide in the exterior shell corona. Considering this, Mg^{2+} ions can impact the CAC value of DOC micelles by reducing electrostatic repulsion between the oligonucleotides' charged phosphate groups, stabilizing the micelle structure, and facilitating its formation.

3.3. DLS Experiments

The size of DOC micellar structures was characterized by DLS measurements. After preincubation in TAM buffer, the average hydrodynamic diameter (D_h) of D-13 particles was found to be 45.77 ± 13.03 nm (Table 1, Figure 2b), as compared to 5.43 ± 1.60 nm for 13-mer control oligonucleotide without dodecyl groups (Figure 2a). As shown in Figure 2, the assemblies of the DOCs have one peak of populations, which is shifted relative to the control oligonucleotide, and fairly low values of polydispersity indexes (PDI) (Table 1). The intensity distribution also showed one peak of populations with an increase in particle diameter compared to the number mean, which is usually typical for DLS results (Figure S9). Similar results were obtained for longer 17-mer DOC (D-17, Table 1, Figure 2d,e), with the addition of the fact that the D_h value of D-17 particles was less than that of D-13 (Table 1).

Table 1. The average hydrodynamic diameter (D_h) of the DOC micellar particles.

DOC Type	D_h [1], nm	PDI
D-13	45.77 ± 13.03	0.109
D-13^{PG}	65.30 ± 33.66	0.241
D-17	32.67 ± 9.07	0.214
D-17^{PG}	169.63 ± 96.40	0.225
D-22^{PG}	80.76 ± 31.33	0.148

[1] as calculated by dynamic light scattering (DLS) measurements after 3 h incubation of 5 µM DOC in TAM buffer.

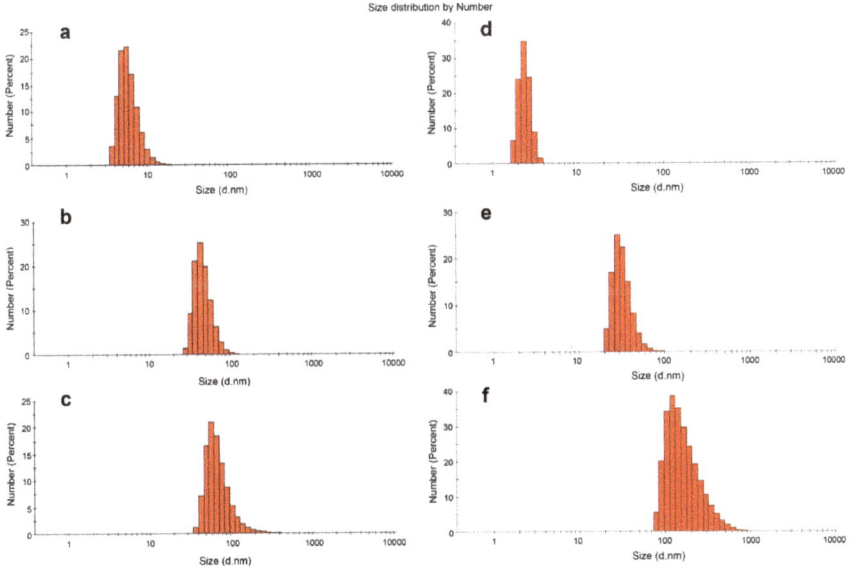

Figure 2. Size distributions of the control oligonucleotides 13 (**a**), 17 (**d**) compared with D-13 (**b**), D-13^{PG} (**c**), D-17^{PG} (**e**) and D-17^{PG} (**f**) conjugates (after 3 h incubation at 5 µM in TAM buffer) as measured by DLS. The D-13^{PG} dodecyl oligonucleotide conjugate with two uncharged PG groups assembled into slightly enlarged micellar particles compared to its DNA analog D-13 (Table 1, Figure 2c). Interestingly, we observed a considerable increase in the size of D-17^{PG} self-assemblies (Table 1, Figure 2f). We attributed these results to the multiple micellar complexes that appeared in a short time in this case, or to more complex micellar structures. Such micellar aggregates of 129.96 ± 73.36 (PDI 0.216) nm in diameter were detected after 24 h incubation for D-17 conjugate.

The average hydrodynamic diameter of D-22^{PG} particles was similar to that of D-13^{PG} assemblies (Table 1). DOC particles formed in solution appear to be much larger than typical NA micelles (up to

10 nm), and their size lies in the range characteristic for vesicle or lamellar structures (up to 500 nm). The non-polar, uncharged PG modification in D-13^{PG} and D-17^{PG} may contribute to forming a more densely packed corona of the oligonucleotide chains around the larger micelle core compared to their deoxy counterparts D-13 and D-17. The results demonstrate no direct correlation between the size of micellar particles and the oligomer length of the DOCs due to the additional impact of the nucleotide sequence, which well correlates with our preliminary DLS studies. We measured hydrodynamic diameters of two additional 22-mer dodecyl conjugates with different heteronucleotide sequences. Micellar particles formed by 5′ D-CTTGACTTTGGGGATTGTAG*G*G 3′ (here D is a three-dodecyl unit and * marks a phosphoryl guanidine modification) and 5′ D-AATACTGCCATTTGTACTG*C*T 3′ conjugates were of 12.15 ± 0.10 and 11.82 ± 1.66 nm correspondingly, while D-22^{PG} formed the particles of increased diameter. The reason for these rather contradictory results remains unclear. We can hypothesize that two additionally studied conjugates can form secondary structures: the sequence of 5′ D-CTTGACTTTGGGGATTGTAG*G*G 3′ contains two G-tracts of 3 and 4 consecutive guanines, which suggests the ability of quadruplex formation, and the sequence of 5′ D-AATACTGCCATTTGTACTG*C*T 3′ may form hairpin and partial self-dimer (Figure S10a). Interestingly, the nucleotide sequence of D-17^{PG} and D-17 also enables a formation of self-dimer of eight nucleotide bases (Figure S10b), which may contribute to the formation of larger particles and/or to accelerate their aggregation. Here, we only briefly discussed the effects of the oligonucleotide length and sequence of the LOC on the micelle size. This issue requires further studies on a wider series of oligonucleotides.

3.4. Atomic Force Microscopy

The morphology, dispersity, and relative size of the DOC micelles were investigated by AFM. As shown in Figure 3a, the D-17 sample contains spherical structures with a diameter of 30.5 ± 5.2 nm. The average height of 1.4 ± 0.6 nm for these particles corresponds to those obtained for nucleic acid samples [16,22,23,43]. The average diameter value is in line with our DLS results and correlates with the results of some previous AFM studies of the LOC-formed micellar structures [16,22].

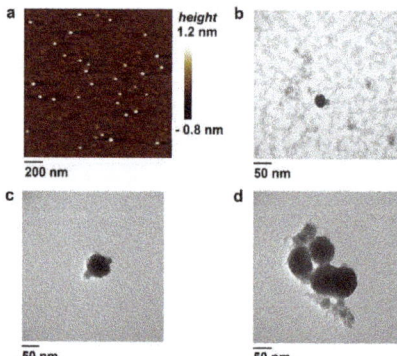

Figure 3. Characterization of D-17 (**a,b**) and D-17^{PG} (**c,d**) micelles in TAM buffer by atomic force (AFM) (**a**) and transmission electron (TEM) (**b–d**), contrasting using uranyl acetate) microscopies. Scale bars are indicated. Each sample contained 1.5 µM (AFM) or 5 µM (TEM) of the corresponding oligomer.

TEM visualization of the D-17 conjugate revealed discrete spherical particles and aggregates (Figure S17) with a size of about 30 nm (Figure 3b). The aggregates represent clusters of individual particles (<10) (Figure S17f). D-17^{PG} particles varied in size from 25 to 50 nm (Figure 3c) and contained more aggregates than the D-17 sample (Figure 3d, Figure S18). This result can also be partly associated with the influence of two uncharged phosphoryl guanidine groups in the sugar-phosphate backbone of D-17^{PG} conjugate, probably facilitating particle aggregation.

In concordance with DLS results, AFM and TEM data indicated that the self-association of DOCs in aqueous solutions leads to the formation of micellar particles with a high tendency to aggregate.

3.5. Electrophoretic Mobility Shift Assay

The investigation of DOCs self-assembly by EMSA also showed results well-consistent with the DLS data. As shown in Figure 4a, the D-17^{PG} sample forms extremely large structures (or aggregates), which cannot move along the gel and remain close to wells' bottoms (Figure 4a, Lanes 2–5). At the same time, micellar D-13^{PG} particles demonstrated higher electrophoretic mobility than D-22^{PG} (Figure 4a, Lanes 7 and 9 correspondingly). Analysis of the electrophoretic mobility of D-17^{PG} at the indicated time of incubation demonstrated that low-mobility structures form in as little as 30 min (Figure 4a, Lane 2). All control oligonucleotides without dodecyl chains were characterized by significantly higher electrophoretic mobilities as compared to the conjugates (Figure 4a, Lanes 1, 6, 8).

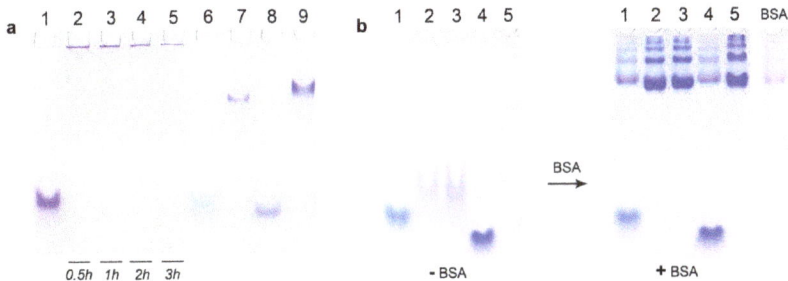

Figure 4. Comparative electrophoretic mobilities of control oligonucleotides and dodecyl oligonucleotide conjugates. (**a**) 17 (Lane 1), D-17^{PG}* (Lanes 2–5), 13 (Lane 6), D-13^{PG} (Lane 7), 22 (Lane 8), D-22^{PG} (Lane 9) investigated by electrophoretic mobility shift assay (EMSA) in non-denaturing 6.5% PAAG after 3 h* incubation in TAM buffer, at 25 °C; each sample contained 20 µM of the oligomer. (**b**) 13 (Lane 1), D-13 (Lane 2), D-13^{PG} (Lane 3), 17 (Lane 4), D-17^{PG} (Lane 5) investigated by non-denaturing 8% PAGE after 3 h incubation at 35 °C and additional no (−BSA) or adding (+BSA) of 45 µM bovine serum albumin (BSA without oligomers control lane is depicted on the right); each sample contained 25 µM of the oligomer in TAN buffer. Bands were visualized by Stains-All staining. * This conjugate was loaded into the wells after the indicated time of incubation.

Next, we compared the affinity of DOCs and dodecyl-free oligonucleotides to serum albumin. Having confirmed the formation of DOC micelles by D-13, D-13^{PG}, and D-17^{PG} conjugates in conditions similar to physiologic (Figure 4b, (−BSA), Lanes 2,3,5), we added the bovine serum albumin (BSA) and allowed the reaction mixture to equilibrate for 30 min. After incubation with BSA (1.8 molar excess relative to the oligomer), the dodecyl-containing conjugates completely bound to albumin in contrast to the parent control oligonucleotides 13, 17 (Figure 4b, ((+BSA), Lanes 2,3,5).

Albumin possesses seven major binding sites for fatty acids with high and moderate affinity [44]. Interestingly, we have demonstrated that D-13^{PG} DOC is highly associated with BSA even at the 0.1–0.15 molar excess (that is, the lack) of the protein (Figure S19). This corresponds to the interaction of one albumin molecule with approximately ten DOC molecules. These results point that in blood serum with high levels of albumin (about 0.5–0.6 mM), DOCs would be most probably entirely bound by this protein.

As expected, the EMSA (Figure 5) proved the complete association with the proteins either for FAM-17'/D-17^{PG} duplex (Lanes 6,7) or FAM-D-17^{PG} conjugate (Lanes 10,11) in the medium supplemented with BSA, as well as with 10% FBS. The FAM-17′/17 control duplex remained unbound in this assay (Lanes 2–3).

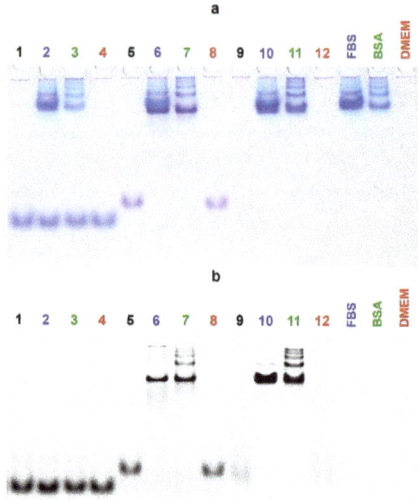

Figure 5. Comparative electrophoretic mobilities of 5 µM control duplex FAM-17′/17 (Lanes 1–4), dodecyl-containing duplex FAM-17′/D-17^{PG} (Lanes 5–8) and the FAM-D-17^{PG} conjugate (Lanes 9–12) investigated by EMSA in non-denaturing 8% PAAG after 2 h incubation at 37 °C in DMEM medium (depicted in red), DMEM supplemented with 30 µM BSA (depicted in green), DMEM supplemented with 10% fetal bovine serum (FBS) (depicted in blue). All medium conditions without oligomers control lanes are depicted on the right in corresponding colors. Indicated oligomers after incubation in PBS are depicted in black for additional controls. Bands were visualized after electrophoresis by Stains-All staining (**a**) and by recording the image after scanning with laser excitation at 488 nm (**b**). It is interesting to note that during the electrophoretic analysis of micellar assemblies of FAM-labeled DOCs, we observed significant fluorescence quenching of their bands, in contrast with the bands of non-conjugated control oligomers (Figure 5, Lanes 9, 12, Figure S20).

3.6. Fluorescence Quenching Experiments

The dyes in the vicinity of micellar arrangements can displace a complex physicochemical and photophysical behavior. Some studies evidenced that the fluorescence intensity of fluorescein derivatives may depend not only on the pH value [45], but also on the complicated intermolecular, hydrophobic/electrostatic interactions between the fluorophore, and the lipids in the microenvironment. It is important to gain insights into these non-specific interactions of the LOCs with the dyes that are widely used to detect intracellular localization of NA-based constructs. The fluorescence quenching of some dyes can be induced by dynamic (or collisional), static, or combined dynamic and static complex mechanisms. Self-quenching and fluorescence resonance energy transfer (FRET) can often occur, due to molecular interactions between the molecules of fluorophores themselves in proximity to each other [46].

To explore if self-assembly affects the fluorescence of 6-carboxyfluorescein (FAM) residue combined with DOCs, we investigated fluorescence intensities (FI) and absorption spectra of FAM-labeled oligomers with dodecyl groups. Dodecyl-free oligonucleotide FAM-17′ served as a control. The obtained results evidence for 86–87% fluorescence quenching of FAM-D-17 under the conditions of micelle formation in TAM buffer, in comparison with FI value in TA buffer lacking Mg^{2+}, where 17-mer DOC did not reach CAC at the used concentration (Figure 6). At the same time, in the case of dye-labeled control oligonucleotide FAM-17′, the addition of Mg^{2+} did not affect the fluorescence intensity (Figure 6).

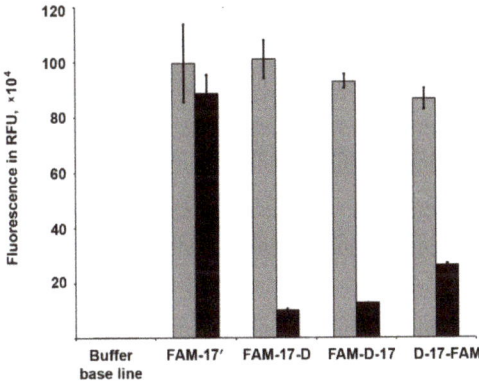

Figure 6. Fluorescence intensity values of 1.5 μM fluorescently labeled FAM-17′, FAM-17-D, FAM-D-17, and D-17-FAM oligomers in TAM (black columns) or TA (grey columns) buffer conditions. For excitation and emission scanning parameters, see Section 2.9. We hypothesized that during the FAM-D-17 self-assembly, FAM residues are encapsulated into the micelle core, thereby interacting with each other in close proximity and providing significant fluorescence quenching. For instance, fluorescence from Oregon green residues in dye-conjugated titin molecules quenched in the native folded state of the protein due to the proximity of dye residues [47].

Further, we compared the FI values of FAM-17-D and D-17-FAM conjugates in the presence/absence of magnesium ions. These DOCs bear dodecyl chains and the FAM residue at the opposite ends of the 17-mer oligonucleotide, which is assumed to exclude dye encapsulation in the micellar inner core. We supposed that if interactions inside the core cause the fluorescence decrease, these conjugates will demonstrate the smaller quenching degree. Interestingly, the fluorescence intensity of the D-17-FAM, as expected, was quenched less (by 67–72%), while the FI value of the other conjugate FAM-17-D with 5′-terminal dye residue surprisingly decreased by 89–91%. We attribute this difference to the existence of multiple mechanisms of molecular interactions involved in fluorescence quenching. Fluorescence of fluorescein and its derivatives are extremely sensitive for the quenching, even to the type of the binding linker [48]. An earlier finding of fluorescence quenching of 6-carboxyfluorescein in liposomes was reported decades ago [49]. The authors concluded that dimerization of the dye and energy transfer to nonfluorescent dimers made a major contribution to the mechanisms of this concentration quenching phenomenon. The absorbance spectra of FAM-D-17, FAM-17-D, and D-17-FAM DOCs also contain shoulders at about 468 nm (Figure S21). Furthermore, these spectra show differences in absorbance of the conjugates in solutions with or without Mg^{2+} (Figure S21), so a possibility of ground-state complex formation also cannot be excluded. It has been reported that Mg^{2+} ions up to 15 mM do not cause appreciable fluorescence quenching of 5′-fluorescein-labeled DNA oligonucleotides [50]. On the other hand, 5-FAM and TAMRA-modified oligonucleotides significant fluorescence quenching during hybridization with a complementary strand is caused by photoinduced electron transfer between the fluorophore and nucleotide base [51]. It has been revealed that guanine bases can strongly quench the fluorescence of the dyes mentioned above. The presence of two guanines at 5′-end of the FAM-D-17 and FAM-17-D DOCs can add one more step to complex molecular interactions of quenching mechanisms. These underlying diverse and probe-dependent mechanisms are still exactly unknown and require careful use of fluorophores in LOC-based systems.

3.7. Cellular Uptake of Three Dodecyl-Containing Conjugates

We also examined the cellular accumulation of FAM-labeled lipophilic oligonucleotide conjugates bearing three dodecyl groups (FAM-D-17^{PG}) or their duplex (D-17^{PG}/FAM-17′). The concentration of oligonucleotides was determined by CAC to ensure that oligonucleotide derivatives present in an aggregated state in the transfection solution. As shown above, the addition of BSA or FBS to the DOC aggregates leads to the protein binding of the lipophilic conjugate (Figure 5). To define the influence of BSA or other serum proteins on cellular internalization of DOCs, the transfection of HepG2 cells was performed with 5 µM concentrations of conjugated oligonucleotide in DMEM, either alone or supplemented with 10% FBS or 30 µM BSA. Prior to transfection procedure, we verified the stability of FAM-D-17^{PG} conjugate and D-17^{PG}/FAM-17′ duplex in 10% FBS (Figure S22). The efficacy of transfection was evaluated using flow cytofluorometry. The results demonstrated that DOCs penetrate the human cells with different efficacy, depending on the medium (Figure 7).

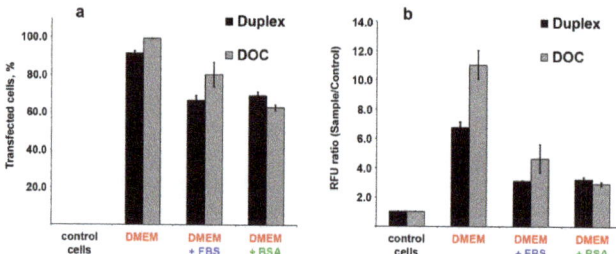

Figure 7. Cellular uptake of fluorescently labelled DOC (FAM-D-17^{PG}) and its duplex (D-17^{PG}/FAM-17′) estimated by flow cytometry after 4 h incubation of HepG2 cells with conjugates and additional followed 14 h without it: (**a**) percentage of FAM-positive HepG2 cells in the population; (**b**) normalized median value of the cell fluorescence to the autofluorescence of control cells. The highest transfection efficacy was achieved for cells treated with FAM-D-17^{PG} in DMEM (Figure 7a,b). All cells were transfected (Figure 7a), and the median value of their fluorescence intensity exceeded that of cells' auto-fluorescence 11 ± 1 times (Figure 7b). High efficacy of transfection was also reached for cells transfected with duplex D-17^{PG}/FAM-17′ in DMEM (Figure 7a). Surprisingly, the median value of cells' fluorescence was almost two times lower than for cells treated with a single stranded dodecyl-containing oligonucleotide (Figure 7b).

We attributed the difference in cells' fluorescence intensity to the different numbers of fluorescent groups in the aggregates. The formation of micellar structures of similar size with oligonucleotides exposed on surface and dodecyl groups forming a hydrophobic core requires a comparable number of oligonucleotide molecules. This comes from the fact that the size of oligonucleotide or duplex determines the curvature of the particle's surface and, therefore, its diameter. However, in the duplex, only one strand bears a fluorescent group, so the aggregate formed by a duplex with a diameter of 85.4 ± 17.0 nm (DLS data in PBS) contain twice less FAM groups than the aggregate formed by single strand conjugate with a diameter of 96.9 ± 47.8 nm.

The presence of BSA or BSA-containing FBS in the transfection media decreases the transfection efficacy (Figure 7a) and the accumulation of the oligonucleotide cargo in the cell (Figure 7b). We explain this result by the fact that aggregates formed by both oligonucleotides conjugated with three dodecyl groups and their duplexes appear in the BSA/DOCs associates (Figure 5, Lanes 7,11). The obtained data suggest that binding to albumin inhibits DOC's cell penetration since accumulation rates of oligonucleotide-albumin complexes are lower than those for aggregates or linear nucleic acids. Surprisingly, the efficacy of FAM-D-17^{PG} accumulation in cells in the presence of FBS is higher than in the presence of BSA only (Figure 7a). This difference can be explained by the presence of other lipids in FBS, including fatty acids, which can compete with conjugate's dodecyl groups for interaction with albumin [34,44,52]. In this case, the fraction of unbound FAM-D-17^{PG} released from protein/DOCs associates can penetrate cells. At the same time, D-17^{PG}/FAM-17' duplex in the presence of FBS demonstrated results comparable to those for BSA containing transfection. The reason for the difference between single stranded molecules of FAM-D-17^{PG} and D-17^{PG}/FAM-17' duplexes in this context is a larger negative net charge of the duplex [33].

The most intensive fluorescence was registered for the cells treated with DMEM-diluted FAM-D-17^{PG} or D-17^{PG}/FAM-17' (Figure 8a,d). Fluorescent signals of the medium intensity were found in cells transfected with FAM-D-17^{PG} dissolved in DMEM supplemented with 10% FBS (Figure 8b); for other samples, FAM signals were too low (Figure 8c,e,f). In FAM-positive cells, a fluorescent signal was evenly distributed throughout the cytoplasm, and no co-localization with nuclei was revealed.

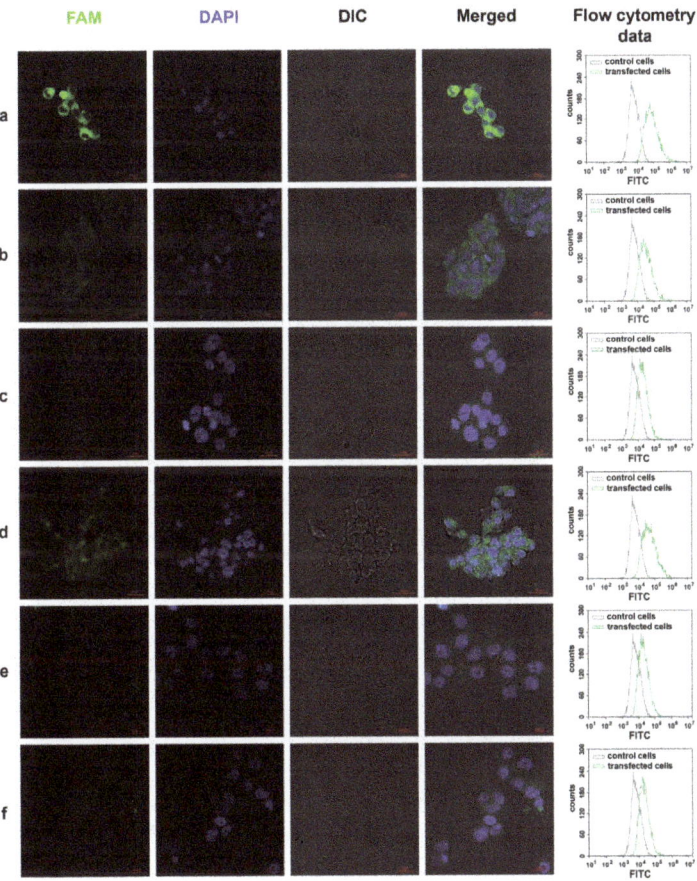

Figure 8. Qualitative (confocal fluorescent microscopy imaging) and quantitative (flow cytometry data) characterizations of HepG2 cells treated with 5 μM fluorescently labeled either FAM-D-17^{PG} (**a–c**) DOC or D-17^{PG}/FAM-17' (**d–f**) duplex in DMEM medium (**a,d**); in DMEM supplemented with 10% FBS (**b,e**); in DMEM supplemented with 30 μM BSA (**c,f**). The red bar in confocal fluorescent images corresponds to 20 μm. Our experiments are consistent with a previous study reporting micelle formation for other DNA-based amphiphilic conjugates depended on the presence of Mg^{2+} [15,16]. In another study, the authors also suggested that Mg^{2+} stabilizes all the lipid-oligonucleotides micellar assemblies, probably due to the Mg^{2+}-mediated neutralization of the oligonucleotide negative charges [53].

These results indicate that oligonucleotides conjugated with three dodecyl groups can penetrate cultured human cells both as disassembled molecules and in aggregated form.

4. Discussion

In recent years, several approaches have been proposed to employ "like-a-brush" LOCs as useful tools in the field of NA-based formulations [10,14,18,22,33,35,53–56]. Most of them rely on the conjugates bearing the diacyl lipid group. A few data have been reported on the features of triple lipophilic chains-tethered oligonucleotides [14,33]. Their investigations are generally limited by high hydrophobicity, fast self-aggregation, and salting out in aqueous solution. So far, only one paper reports two 15-mer oligoadenylate and oligothymidylate LOCs containing three "like-a-brush" hydrophobic chains [14]. The particle size and shape for the latter conjugate were characterized by DLS, TEM, and scanning electron microscopy, while highly hydrophobic oligoadenylate LOC irreversibly self-aggregated immediately after the deblocking procedure [14].

The present research aimed to investigate 13-, 17-, and 22-mer "like-a-brush" triple chains- contained DOCs for their self-assembly features and the ability to enter the cells. We have chosen heteronucleotide sequences for these oligomers and inserted two phosphoryl guanidine modifications at 3'-end of some conjugates during standard phosphoramidite solid-phase synthesis to provide additional nuclease stability [37,39]. Due to high hydrophobicity, DOCs form micellar particles in micromolar concentrations and require extreme caution to avoid their salting out during the work.

We observed a larger size of D-13 and D-17 DOC particles as compared with another 15-mer oligothymidylate LOC, also containing "like-a-brush" hydrophobic moiety with three aliphatic tails [14]. In turn, the conjugates containing phosphoryl guanidine modifications D-13^{PG}, D-17^{PG}, D-22^{PG} formed larger micellar assemblies than their DNA counterparts. There is a little discussion in the literature that tends to focus on the oligonucleotide length, sequence, and modified sugar-phosphate backbone of the LOC regarding the size of a micelle formed. The research also reported various sizes of LOC self-assemblies, which demonstrated the required biological effect. The impact of nucleotide sequence on LOC micellar assemblies' size was described for two 19-mer PS conjugates bearing identical diacyl lipid groups at their 5'-ends. While the oligomer 5'-AACTTGTTTCCTGCAGGTGA-3' formed small particles of ~11 nm, 5'-CGTGTAGGTACGGCAGATC-3' yielded micellar structures with the size of more than 100 nm [10]. Recently it was shown [11] that BODIPY-conjugated 10- and 25-mer oligodeoxythymidylates self-aggregate with a formation of the same assemblies of 94.1 ± 20.4 and 75.5 ± 4.4 nm, correspondingly. Self-association of siRNA with one BODIPY-attached strand into nanosized aggregates of ~140 nm in aqueous solution was shown to be indispensable for the high cellular uptake of these duplexes and efficient gene regulation by RNA interference [11]. The siRNA-squalene conjugates also demonstrated self-organizing in water with the formation of ~165 nm particles, and after intravenous injections, inhibited tumor growth in a mice xenograft model of papillary thyroid carcinoma [21]. Most reports deal with the development of LOC-based constructions for anticancer therapy [10,13,21,23,24,29,35]. Passive targeting via enhanced permeability and retention (EPR) effect requires a 5–200 nm hydrodynamic size range for the formulations [57,58]. Therefore, the ability of DOCs to self-assembly into micellar particles and their aggregates of 30–170 nm in size seems to open the way for further in vitro and in vivo studies to examine their cell penetration efficacy.

Given the high plasma concentration of albumin in vivo, we evaluated the affinity of DOCs for association with BSA. Other findings confirm our BSA binding experiments. It was reported that approximately 93% of LOC micelles dissociated into a non-micellar state when incubated in vitro with 0.1 mM BSA [22]. Size exclusion chromatography method has shown that diacyl lipid conjugated PS oligonucleotide in aqueous solution elutes as micelles, but after the following incubation with FBS, nearly 50% of this conjugate co-migrate with the albumin fraction [54]. In another work, siRNA bearing short-chain fatty acid residues such as lauroyl did not bind to lipoproteins in vivo, either associated with serum albumin or remained unbound [26]. Interestingly, monododecyl-containing siRNA bound to albumin with the highest affinity (K_d ~200 µM) among other investigated lipophilic residues, and the protein was saturated with these conjugates at 1:3.6 molar ratio [26].

The readily occurred interaction of DOCs with albumin can increase their overall in vivo lifetime [5]. An analogy can be drawn with recent reviews regarding more extensively studied interaction of PS modified therapeutics with proteins [59,60]. Oligonucleotides modified in PS backbone bind to a number of plasma proteins, including albumin. Plasma proteins binding increase the circulation half-life of PS oligomers which is crucial to maintain their distribution to peripheral tissues [60].

On the other hand, a well-known criticism of increased affinity of LOCs for binding by albumin refers to observations of subsequent conjugates accumulation in the liver and lymph nodes than in other organs [54,61]. To find a possible solution to this challenge, an interesting experiment was carried out with stable G-quadruplex-locked DNA micelles, which could not associate with serum albumin [22]. Cellular uptake of these conjugates was negligible in comparison with DNA micelles without intermolecular G-quadruplexes, which retain the ability to albumin bind [22].

In contrast to this limitation, other studies established albumin as a drug carrier [62]. Of particular interest are several features of albumin, which are responsible for the accumulation of this plasma protein in solid tumors [34,63]. The Paclitaxel albumin-bound particles known as Abraxane® are used in cancer therapy [62]. Recent research [35] suggested using in situ albumin targeting for development of carrier-free RNAi-based cancer therapies. The synthesized siRNA conjugated to a diacyl lipid moiety, which rapidly binds albumin in situ, was shown to achieve 19-fold greater tumor accumulation and 46-fold increase in per-tumor-cell uptake in a mouse orthotopic model of human triple-negative breast cancer as well as elicits sustained silencing in an in vivo tumor model [35]. The tumor:liver accumulation ratio of more than 40:1 achieved by this diacyl lipid-tethered siRNA is a promising result for LOC-based formulations. Future studies in this area are therefore required more attention to design of the research. Although most LOCs bind to albumin with high affinity, studies reporting the effect on intracellular uptake during the transfection are scarce. Recently it was found that BSA treatment reduces cell penetration of PS ASOs and their lipid conjugates in a protein concentration-dependent manner [25]. Interestingly, the cellular uptake efficacy of the lipid-conjugated PS ASO was reduced much stronger than that of the parental unconjugated oligonucleotide. Almost all other articles describe cells in vitro transfection in the absence of serum and/or albumin in the media [10,11,21,22,25], although understanding the features of interactions between LOCs and proteins is crucial for their use in vivo.

Taken together, in this study, we obtained key results proving that DOCs represent the attractive objects for further design of transport systems in oligonucleotide-based therapeutics. For future in vivo research of the DOCs, a principal issue is to evaluate the importance of the ability to form spherical micellar particles in aqueous media in front of their high protein binding affinity.

5. Conclusions

To summarize, we designed and conveniently synthesized DOCs containing three "like-a-brush" lipophilic chains. Phosphoryl guanidine modifications were introduced at the 3' end of some DOCs to prolong the plasma exposure. In the current work, we present the investigation of self-assembling and cell-penetrating features of these conjugates. DLS, AFM, and TEM techniques showed self-association of dodecyl oligonucleotide conjugates into spherical micellar particles and their nanosized aggregates (<200 nm). These structures are highly bound by serum albumin, which can increase their circulation half-life and bioavailability. It was found that DOCs and their duplexes can penetrate HepG2 cells by mimicking the spherical architecture or anchoring nonspecifically to the membranes both in the absence (with high efficacy) and in the presence of serum albumin (with reduced efficacy). These results, along with recently obtained data [33] indicate a strong potential to consider these conjugates as essential nanomaterials to develop nucleic acid delivery tools for biomedical applications.

Supplementary Materials: The following are available online at http://www.mdpi.com/2079-4991/10/10/1948/s1, Figure S1: The structure of 3′-FAM CPG used in this work, Figure S2: Comparative electrophoretic mobilities of oligonucleotides and DOCs, Figures S3–S5: The structures of FAM-17-D, D-17-FAM and FAM-D-17^{PG} conjugates, Figure S6: Typical MALDI TOF and ESI mass spectra of the conjugates, Figure S7,S8: Self-assembly of 17-mer DOC by Nile Red binding assay, Figure S9: Dynamic light scattering measurements, Figure S10: Possible structures of DOCs self-dimers, Figures S11–S16: AFM additional images, Figures S17,S18: TEM additional images, Figure S19: BSA binding with D-13^{PG} conjugate, Figure S20: Fluorescence quenching additional image, Figure S21: Absorbance spectra of FAM-D-17, FAM-17-D, D-17-FAM, Figure S22: The stability of FAM-D-17^{PG} conjugate and FAM-17′/D-17^{PG} duplex used for transfection in 10% FBS, Table S1: Experimental and theoretical molecular masses of the DOCs.

Author Contributions: Methodology, resources, investigation, formal analysis, visualization, validation, data curation, writing—original draft preparation, funding acquisition, A.S.P.; investigation, formal analysis, visualization, writing—original draft preparation (flow cytometry and confocal microscopy imaging), funding acquisition, I.S.D.; resources, formal analysis, visualization, M.S.K.; investigation, formal analysis, visualization, A.E.G.; data validation, project administration, funding acquisition, I.A.P.; conceptualization, methodology, data validation, supervision, writing—review and editing, D.V.P. All authors have read and agreed to the published version of the manuscript.

Funding: This research and APC was funded by the Russian Science Foundation (Project #19-15-00217). Fluorescence quenching experiments and AFM were carried out by A.S.P. and supported by Russian State funded budget project of ICBFM SB RAS # 0245-2019-0002.

Acknowledgments: The authors acknowledge Marat F. Kasakin, leading engineer of the Core Facility of Mass Spectrometric Analysis (ICBFM SB RAS) for recording of the MALDI TOF and ESI mass spectra. Authors thank Georgiy Yu. Shevelev (Laboratory of Synthetic Biology, ICBFM SB RAS) for useful technical assistance during AFM investigations followed by helpful discussions.

Conflicts of Interest: The authors declare no conflict of interest.

References

1. Gissot, A.; Camplo, M.; Grinstaff, M.W.; Barthélémy, P. Nucleoside, nucleotide and oligonucleotide based amphiphiles: A successful marriage of nucleic acids with lipids. *Org. Biomol. Chem.* **2008**, *6*, 1324–1333. [CrossRef]
2. Patwa, A.; Gissot, A.; Bestel, I.; Barthélémy, P. Hybrid lipid oligonucleotide conjugates: Synthesis, self-assemblies and biomedical applications. *Chem. Soc. Rev.* **2011**, *40*, 5844–5854. [CrossRef]
3. Raouane, M.; Desmaële, D.; Urbinati, G.; Massaad-Massade, L.; Couvreur, P. Lipid Conjugated Oligonucleotides: A Useful Strategy for Delivery. *Bioconjugate Chem.* **2012**, *23*, 1091–1104. [CrossRef]
4. Craig, K.; Abrams, M.; Amiji, M. Recent preclinical and clinical advances in oligonucleotide conjugates. *Expert Opin. Drug Deliv.* **2018**, *15*, 629–640. [CrossRef]
5. Osborn, M.F.; Khvorova, A. Improving Small Interfering RNA Delivery In Vivo Through Lipid Conjugation. *Nucleic Acid Ther.* **2018**, *28*, 128–136. [CrossRef]
6. Benizri, S.; Gissot, A.; Martin, A.; Vialet, B.; Grinstaff, M.W.; Barthélémy, P. Bioconjugated Oligonucleotides: Recent Developments and Therapeutic Applications. *Bioconjugate Chem.* **2019**, *30*, 366–383. [CrossRef]
7. Boutorin, A.S.; Gus'kova, L.V.; Ivanova, E.M.; Kobetz, N.D.; Zarytova, V.F.; Ryte, A.S.; Yurchenko, L.V.; Vlassov, V.V. Synthesis of alkylating oligonucleotide derivatives containing cholesterol or phenazinium residues at their 3′-terminus and their interaction with DNA within mammalian cells. *FEBS Lett.* **1989**, *254*, 129–132. [CrossRef]
8. Dovydenko, I.; Tarassov, I.; Venyaminova, A.; Entelis, N. Method of carrier-free delivery of therapeutic RNA importable into human mitochondria: Lipophilic conjugates with cleavable bonds. *Biomaterials* **2016**, *76*, 408–417. [CrossRef]
9. Borisenko, G.G.; Zaitseva, M.A.; Chuvilin, A.N.; Pozmogova, G.E. DNA modification of live cell surface. *Nucleic Acids Res.* **2009**, *37*, e28. [CrossRef]
10. Karaki, S.; Benizri, S.; Mejías, R.; Baylot, V.; Branger, N.; Nguyen, T.; Vialet, B.; Oumzil, K.; Barthélémy, P.; Rocchi, P. Lipid-oligonucleotide conjugates improve cellular uptake and efficacy of TCTP-antisense in castration-resistant prostate cancer. *J. Control. Release* **2017**, *258*, 1–9. [CrossRef]
11. Asahi, W.; Kurihara, R.; Takeyama, K.; Umehara, Y.; Kimura, Y.; Kondo, T.; Tanabe, K. Aggregate Formation of BODIPY-Tethered Oligonucleotides That Led to Efficient Intracellular Penetration and Gene Regulation. *ACS Appl. Bio Mater.* **2019**, *2*, 4456–4463. [CrossRef]
12. Liu, H.; Zhu, Z.; Kang, H.; Wu, Y.; Sefan, K.; Tan, W. DNA Based Micelles: Synthesis, Micellar Properties and Size-dependent Cell Permeability. *Chemistry* **2010**, *16*, 3791–3797. [CrossRef] [PubMed]

13. Chen, T.; Wu, C.S.; Jimenez, E.; Zhu, Z.; Dajac, J.G.; You, M.; Han, D.; Zhang, X.; Tan, W. DNA Micelle Flares for Intracellular mRNA Imaging and Gene Therapy. *Angew. Chem. Int. Ed.* **2013**, *52*, 2012–2016. [CrossRef]
14. Pokholenko, O.; Gissot, A.; Vialet, B.; Bathany, K.; Thiéry, A.; Barthélémy, P. Lipid oligonucleotide conjugates as responsive nanomaterials for drug delivery. *J. Mater. Chem. B* **2013**, *1*, 5329–5334. [CrossRef] [PubMed]
15. Edwardson, T.G.W.; Carneiro, K.M.M.; Serpel, C.J.; Sleiman, H.F. An Efficient and Modular Route to Sequence-Defined Polymers Appended to DNA. *Angew. Chem. Int. Ed.* **2014**, *53*, 1–6. [CrossRef]
16. Trinh, T.; Chidchob, P.; Bazzi, H.S.; Sleiman, H.F. DNA micelles as nanoreactors: Efficient DNA functionalization with hydrophobic organic molecules. *Chem. Commun.* **2016**, *52*, 10914–10917. [CrossRef]
17. Cozzoli, L.; Gjonaj, L.; Stuart, M.C.A.; Poolman, B.; Roelfes, G. Responsive DNA G-quadruplex micelles. *Chem. Commun.* **2018**, *54*, 260–263. [CrossRef]
18. Kauss, T.; Arpin, C.; Bientz, L.; Nguyen, P.V.; Vialet, B.; Benizri, S.; Barthélémy, P. Lipid oligonucleotides as a new strategy for tackling the antibiotic resistance. *Sci. Rep.* **2020**, *10*, 1054. [CrossRef]
19. Dentinger, P.M.; Simmons, B.A.; Cruz, E.; Sprague, M. DNA-Mediated Delivery of Lipophilic Molecules via Hybridization to DNA-Based Vesicular Aggregates. *Langmuir* **2006**, *22*, 2935–2937. [CrossRef]
20. Thompson, M.P.; Chien, M.-P.; Ku, T.-H.; Rush, A.-M.; Gianneschi, N.C. Smart Lipids for Programmable Nanomaterials. *Nano Lett.* **2010**, *10*, 2690–2693. [CrossRef]
21. Raouane, M.; Desmaele, D.; Gilbert-Sirieix, M.; Gueutin, C.; Zouhiri, F.; Bourgaux, C.; Lepeltier, E.; Gref, R.; Ben Salah, R.; Clayman, G.; et al. Synthesis, Characterization, and in Vivo Delivery of siRNA-Squalene Nanoparticles Targeting Fusion Oncogene in Papillary Thyroid Carcinoma. *J. Med. Chem.* **2011**, *54*, 4067–4076. [CrossRef] [PubMed]
22. Jin, C.; Liu, X.; Bai, H.; Wang, R.; Tan, J.; Peng, X.; Tan, W. Engineering Stability-Tunable DNA Micelles Using Photocontrollable Dissociation of an Intermolecular G-Quadruplex. *ACS Nano* **2017**, *11*, 12087–12093. [CrossRef] [PubMed]
23. Shu, Y.; Yin, H.; Rajabi, M.; Li, H.; Vieweger, M.; Guo, S.; Shu, D.; Guo, P. RNA-based micelles: A novel platform for paclitaxel loading and delivery. *J. Control. Release* **2018**, *276*, 17–29. [CrossRef] [PubMed]
24. Herbert, B.-S.; Gellert, G.C.; Hochreiter, A.; Pongracz, K.; Wright, W.E.; Zielinska, D.; Chin, A.C.; Harley, C.B.; Shay, J.W.; Gryaznov, S.M. Lipid modification of GRN163, an N3′→P5′ thio-phosphoramidate oligonucleotide, enhances the potency of telomerase inhibition. *Oncogene* **2005**, *24*, 5262–5268. [CrossRef] [PubMed]
25. Wang, S.; Allen, N.; Prakash, T.P.; Liang, X.; Crooke, S.T. Lipid Conjugates Enhance Endosomal Release of Antisense Oligonucleotides Into Cells. *Nucleic Acids Ther.* **2019**, *29*, 245–255. [CrossRef]
26. Wolfrum, C.; Shi, S.; Jayaprakash, K.N.; Jayaraman, M.; Wang, G.; Pandey, R.K.; Rajeev, K.G.; Nakayama, T.; Charrise, K.; Ndungo, E.M.; et al. Mechanisms and optimization of in vivo delivery of lipophilic siRNAs. *Nat. Biotechnol.* **2007**, *25*, 1149–1157. [CrossRef]
27. Roloff, A.; Nelles, D.A.; Thompson, M.P.; Yeo, G.W.; Gianneschi, N.C. Self-Transfecting Micellar RNA: Modulating Nanoparticle Cell Interactions via High Density Display of Small Molecule Ligands on Micelle Coronas. *Bioconjugate Chem.* **2018**, *29*, 126–135. [CrossRef]
28. Simonova, O.N.G.; Pishnyi, D.V.; Vlassov, V.V.; Zenkova, M.A. Modified Concatemeric Oligonucleotide Complexes: New System for Efficient Oligonucleotide Transfer into Mammalian Cells. *Hum. Gene Ther.* **2008**, *19*, 532–546. [CrossRef]
29. Charbgoo, F.; Alibolandi, M.; Taghdisi, S.M.; Abnous, K.; Soltani, F.; Ramezani, M. MUC1 aptamer-targeted DNA micelles for dual tumor therapy using doxorubicin and KLA peptide. *Nanomedicine* **2018**, *14*, 685–697. [CrossRef]
30. Banga, R.G.; Chernyak, N.; Narayan, S.P.; Nguyen, S.T.; Mirkin, C.A. Liposomal Spherical Nucleic Acids. *J. Am. Chem. Soc.* **2014**, *136*, 9866–9869. [CrossRef]
31. Banga, R.G.; Meckes, B.; Narayan, S.P.; Sprangers, A.J.; Nguyen, S.T.; Mirkin, C.A. Cross-Linked Micellar Spherical Nucleic Acids from Thermoresponsive Templates. *J. Am. Chem. Soc.* **2017**, *139*, 4278–4281. [CrossRef] [PubMed]
32. Meckes, B.; Banga, R.G.; Nguyen, S.T.; Mirkin, C.A. Enhancing the Stability and Immunomodulatory Activity of Liposomal Spherical Nucleic Acids through Lipid-Tail DNA Modifications. *Small* **2018**, *14*, 1702909. [CrossRef] [PubMed]
33. Markov, O.V.; Filatov, A.V.; Kupryushkin, M.S.; Chernikov, I.V.; Patutina, O.A.; Strunov, A.A.; Chernolovskaya, E.L.; Vlassov, V.V.; Pyshnyi, D.V.; Zenkova, M.A. Transport Oligonucleotides—A Novel System for Intracellular Delivery of Antisense Therapeutics. *Molecules* **2020**, *25*, 3663. [CrossRef] [PubMed]

34. Frei, E. Albumin binding ligands and albumin conjugate uptake by cancer cells. *Diabetol. Metab. Syndr.* **2011**, *3*, 11. [CrossRef] [PubMed]
35. Sarett, S.M.; Werfel, T.A.; Lee, L.; Jackson, M.A.; Kilchrist, K.V.; Brantley-Sieders, D.; Duvall, C.L. Lipophilic siRNA targets albumin in situ and promotes bioavailability, tumor penetration, and carrier-free gene silencing. *Proc. Natl. Acad. Sci. USA* **2017**, *114*, E6490–E6497. [CrossRef]
36. Kupryushkin, M.S.; Nekrasov, M.D.; Stetsenko, D.A.; Pyshnyi, D.V. Efficient Functionalization of Oligonucleotides by New Achiral Nonnucleosidic Monomers. *Org. Lett.* **2014**, *16*, 2842–2845. [CrossRef]
37. Kupryushkin, M.S.; Pyshnyi, D.V.; Stetsenko, D.A. Phosphoryl guanidines: A new type of nucleic acid analogues. *Acta Nat.* **2014**, *6*, 116–118. [CrossRef]
38. Stetsenko, D.A.; Kupryushkin, M.S.; Pyshnyi, D.V. Modified Oligonucleotides and Methods for Their Synthesis. International Patent No. WO2,016,028,187A1, 22 June 2014.
39. Lomzov, A.A.; Kupryushkin, M.S.; Shernyukov, A.V.; Nekrasov, M.D.; Dovydenko, I.S.; Stetsenko, D.A.; Pyshnyi, D.V. Diastereomers of a mono-substituted phosphoryl guanidine trideoxyribonucleotide: Isolation and properties. *Biochem. Biophys. Res. Commun.* **2019**, *513*, 807–811. [CrossRef]
40. Poulsen, C.S.; Pedersen, E.B.; Nielsen, C. DNA conjugated phenoxyaniline intercalators synthesis of diethanolaminoacetamide-type linkers. *Acta Chem. Scand.* **1999**, *53*, 425–431. [CrossRef]
41. Hébert, N.; Davis, P.W.; DeBaets, E.L.; Acevedo, O.L. Synthesis of N-substituted hydroxyprolinol phosphoramidites for preparation of combinatorial libraries. *Tetrahedron Lett.* **1994**, *35*, 9509–9512. [CrossRef]
42. Greenspan, P.; Mayer, E.P.; Fowler, S.D. Nile Red: A Selective Fluorescent Stain for Intracellular Lipid Droplets. *J. Cell Biol.* **1985**, *100*, 965–973. [CrossRef] [PubMed]
43. Bustamante, C.; Vesenka, J.; Tang, C.L.; Rees, W.; Guthold, M.; Keller, R. Circular DNA Molecules Imaged in Air by Scanning Force Microscopy. *Biochemistry* **1992**, *31*, 22–26. [CrossRef]
44. Van der Vusse, G.J. Albumin as Fatty Acid Transporter. *Drug Metab. Pharmacokinet.* **2009**, *24*, 300–307. [CrossRef] [PubMed]
45. Sjöback, R.; Nygren, J.; Kubista, M. Absorption and fluorescence properties of fluorescein. *Spectrochim. Acta A* **1995**, *51*, L7–L21. [CrossRef]
46. Zhegalova, N.G.; He, S.; Zhou, H.; Kim, D.M.; Berezin, M.Y. Minimization of self-quenching fluorescence on dyes conjugated to biomolecules with multiple labeling sites via asymmetrically charged NIR fluorophores. *Contrast Media Mol. Imaging* **2014**, *9*, 355–362. [CrossRef] [PubMed]
47. Zhuang, X.; Ha, T.; Kim, H.D.; Centner, T.; Labeit, S.; Chu, S. Fluorescence quenching: A tool for single-molecule protein-folding study. *Proc. Natl. Acad. Sci. USA* **2000**, *97*, 14241–14244. [CrossRef]
48. Kim, T.W.; Park, J.-H.; Hong, J.-I. Self-quenching Mechanism: The Influence of Quencher and Spacer on Quencher-fluorescein Probes. *Bull. Korean Chem. Soc.* **2007**, *28*, 1221–1223. [CrossRef]
49. Chen, R.F.; Knutson, J.R. Mechanism of Fluorescence Concentration Quenching of Carboxyfluorescein in Liposomes: Energy Transfer to Nonfluorescent Dimers. *Anal. Biochem.* **1988**, *172*, 61–77. [CrossRef]
50. Rupich, N.; Chiuman, W.; Nutiu, R.; Mei, S.; Flora, K.K.; Li, Y.; Brennan, J.D. Quenching of Fluorophore-Labeled DNA Oligonucleotides by Divalent Metal Ions: Implications for Selection, Design, and Applications of Signaling Aptamers and Signaling Deoxyribozymes. *J. Am. Chem. Soc.* **2006**, *128*, 780–790. [CrossRef]
51. Torimura, M.; Kurata, S.; Yamada, K.; Yokomaku, T.; Kamagata, Y.; Kanagawa, T.; Kurane, R. Fluorescence-Quenching Phenomenon by Photoinduced Electron Transfer between a Fluorescent Dye and a Nucleotide Base. *Anal. Sci.* **2001**, *17*, 155–160. [CrossRef]
52. Villard, P.-H.; Barlesi, F.; Armand, M.; Dao, T.-M.-A.; Pascussi, G.-M.; Fouchier, F.; Champion, S.; Dufour, C.; Giniès, C.; Khalil, A.; et al. CYP1A1 Induction in the Colon by Serum: Involvement of the PPARα Pathway and Evidence for a New Specific Human PPREα Site. *PLoS ONE* **2011**, *6*, e14629. [CrossRef] [PubMed]
53. Vialet, B.; Gissot, A.; Delzor, R.; Barthélémy, P. Controlling G-quadruplex formation via lipid modification of oligonucleotide sequences. *Chem. Commun.* **2017**, *53*, 11560–11563. [CrossRef] [PubMed]
54. Liu, H.; Moynihan, K.D.; Zheng, Y.; Szeto, G.L.; Li, A.V.; Huang, B.; Van Egeren, D.S.; Park, C.; Irvine, D.G. Structure-based Programming of Lymph Node Targeting in Molecular Vaccines. *Nature* **2014**, *507*, 519–522. [CrossRef] [PubMed]
55. Wu, C.; Chen, T.; Han, D.; You, M.; Peng, L.; Cansiz, S.; Zhu, G.; Li, C.; Xiong, X.; Jimenez, E.; et al. Engineering of Switchable Aptamer Micelle Flares for Molecular Imaging in Living Cells. *ACS Nano* **2013**, *7*, 5724–5731. [CrossRef] [PubMed]

56. Wilner, S.E.; Sparks, S.E.; Cowburn, D.; Girvin, M.E.; Levy, M. Controlling lipid micelle stability using oligonucleotide headgroups. *J. Am. Chem. Soc.* **2015**, *137*, 2171–2174. [CrossRef]
57. Golombek, S.K.; May, J.-N.; Theek, B.; Appold, L.; Drude, N.; Kiessling, F.; Lammers, T. Tumor Targeting via EPR: Strategies to Enhance Patient Responses. *Adv. Drug Deliv. Rev.* **2018**, *130*, 17–38. [CrossRef]
58. Danhier, F. To exploit the tumor microenvironment: Since the EPR effect fails in the clinic, what is the future of nanomedicine? *J. Control. Release* **2016**, *244*, 108–121. [CrossRef]
59. Crooke, S.T.; Vickers, T.A.; Liang, X.-H. Phosphorothioate modified oligonucleotide—protein interactions. *Nucleic Acids Res.* **2020**, *48*, 5235–5253. [CrossRef]
60. Crooke, S.T.; Seth, P.P.; Vickers, T.A.; Liang, X.-H. The Interaction of Phosphorothioate-Containing RNA Targeted Drugs with Proteins Is a Critical Determinant of the Therapeutic Effects of These Agents. *J. Am. Chem. Soc.* **2020**, *142*, 14754–14771. [CrossRef]
61. Akinc, A.; Zumbuehl, A.; Goldberg, M.; Leshchiner, E.S.; Busini, V.; Hossain, N.; Bacallado, S.A.; Nguyen, D.N.; Fuller, J.; Alvarez, R.; et al. A Combinatorial Library of Lipid-Like Materials for Delivery of RNAi Therapeutics. *Nat. Biotechnol.* **2008**, *26*, 561–569. [CrossRef]
62. Zhang, Y.; Sun, T.; Jiang, C. Biomacromolecules as carriers in drug delivery and tissue engineering. *Acta Pharm. Sin. B* **2017**, *8*, 34–50. [CrossRef] [PubMed]
63. Kratz, F. A clinical update of using albumin as a drug vehicle—A commentary. *J. Control. Release* **2014**, *190*, 331–336. [CrossRef] [PubMed]

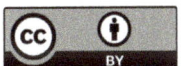

© 2020 by the authors. Licensee MDPI, Basel, Switzerland. This article is an open access article distributed under the terms and conditions of the Creative Commons Attribution (CC BY) license (http://creativecommons.org/licenses/by/4.0/).

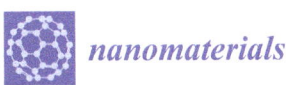

Article

Tyrosine-Modification of Polypropylenimine (PPI) and Polyethylenimine (PEI) Strongly Improves Efficacy of siRNA-Mediated Gene Knockdown

Sandra Noske, Michael Karimov, Achim Aigner * and Alexander Ewe *

Rudolf-Boehm-Institute for Pharmacology and Toxicology, Clinical Pharmacology, Leipzig University, Faculty of Medicine, 04107 Leipzig, Germany; Sandra.noske@medizin.uni-leipzig.de (S.N.); michael.karimov@medizin.uni-leipzig.de (M.K.)
* Correspondence: achim.aigner@medizin.uni-leipzig.de (A.A.); alexander.ewe@medizin.uni-leipzig.de (A.E.); Tel.: +49-(0)341-9724660 (A.A.)

Received: 12 August 2020; Accepted: 7 September 2020; Published: 10 September 2020

Abstract: The delivery of small interfering RNAs (siRNA) is an efficient method for gene silencing through the induction of RNA interference (RNAi). It critically relies, however, on efficient vehicles for siRNA formulation, for transfection in vitro as well as for their potential use in vivo. While polyethylenimines (PEIs) are among the most studied cationic polymers for nucleic acid delivery including small RNA molecules, polypropylenimines (PPIs) have been explored to a lesser extent. Previous studies have shown the benefit of the modification of small PEIs by tyrosine grafting which are featured in this paper. Additionally, we have now extended this approach towards PPIs, presenting tyrosine-modified PPIs (named PPI-Y) for the first time. In this study, we describe the marked improvement of PPI upon its tyrosine modification, leading to enhanced siRNA complexation, complex stability, siRNA delivery, knockdown efficacy and biocompatibility. Results of PPI-Y/siRNA complexes are also compared with data based on tyrosine-modified linear or branched PEIs (LPxY or PxY). Taken together, this establishes tyrosine-modified PPIs or PEIs as particularly promising polymeric systems for siRNA formulation and delivery.

Keywords: polypropylenimine dendrimers; polyethylenimines; tyrosine-modified polypropylene-imines; tyrosine-modified polyethlyenimines; PPI-Y; siRNA transfection; polymeric nanoparticles

---

1. Introduction

Severe diseases including cancer are often associated with the aberrant or uncontrolled expression of pathologically relevant genes. The use of small interfering RNAs (siRNAs) for inducing gene knockdown through RNA interference (RNAi) has become a powerful and promising technology to specifically downregulate target genes by harnessing a highly conserved cellular protein machinery called RNA-induced silencing complex (RISC) [1,2]. Today, siRNAs for any target RNA sequence of interest can be easily designed and synthetically generated [3]. They are thus also able to target proteins which are otherwise undruggable by small molecules and offer new therapeutic strategies. This also includes the knockdown of non-protein encoding mRNAs such as "long noncoding RNAs" (lncRNA) which are crucial biological regulators [4]. However, siRNAs are large and negatively charged molecules, which impair their cellular delivery and uptake, and are very susceptible to nuclease degradation. To address these issues, siRNAs can be chemically modified, e.g., by introducing non-natural nucleotide analogues or the covalent coupling targeting moieties [5,6], and/or it is often required to formulate them into nanoparticles.

In the recent years, several lipid molecules [7–9], cationic polymers [10,11], inorganic nanoparticles and other systems have been investigated for nucleic acid delivery [12–14]. Cationic materials are able to form nano-sized complexes through electrostatic interactions and efficiently protect their payload. For liver-related diseases, suitable siRNA carriers have already been established and, more recently, the first siRNA-based therapeutics have been translated into the clinic. In 2018, Patisiran (ONPATTRO®) was approved by the FDA. Relying on a liposomal siRNA formulation, Patisiran downregulates transthyretin in the liver for the treatment of hereditary transthyretin-mediated amyloidosis (hATTR) [15]. The second siRNA therapeutic, Givosiran (GIVLAARI®), was approved one year later for targeting aminolevulinic acid synthase 1 (ALAS1) in the treatment of acute hepatic porphyrias (AHPs). Givosiran is an siRNA bearing extensive chemical modifications and it is coupled to GalNAc for the targeted delivery to hepatocytes [16,17]. Despite these impressive advances, most siRNA delivery systems are unable to efficiently deliver siRNAs into target sites other than the liver, thus showing serious limitations, for example, in anti-tumor therapies [18,19]. In this context, polymeric nanoparticles may be particularly promising due to their versatility based on the implementation of chemical modifications.

There are several rate-limiting steps which need to be addressed when using nanosized carriers for systemic application. On the extracellular level, nanocarriers bind serum-components which may lead to aggregation, decomposition and/or opsonization by phagocytic cells. Poor tissue penetration and low internalization rates, followed by insufficient endo-/lysosomal release and intracellular siRNA release into the correct compartment are further limiting steps on the cellular/intracellular level [20,21].

Cationic polymers are promising candidates for addressing these issues, and in particular polyethylenimines (PEIs) are widely explored in this regard. PEIs are commercially available in branched and linear structures over a wide range of molecular weights (0.8–100 kDa). Branched PEIs comprise of amines in every third position, at a 1:2:1 ratio of 1°:2°:3° amines. The linear form consists of only secondary and a very few primary amines [22–25]. Polypropylenimine dendrimers (PPI) are another class of commercially available cationic polymers. PPIs are highly branched molecules with well-defined structure and size. They are composed of a diaminobutane core molecule and propylene imine repeating units. PPI dendrimers contain only tertiary amines in the interior and primary amines at the surface (see Figure 1); the number of repeating units determines the so-called 'generation' of the dendrimer and the number of surface functionalities [26]. However, in contrast to (larger) pDNA molecules, PPI dendrimers have not been explored so extensively for delivering siRNAs [27]. Marked differences have been observed between the delivery of siRNA and pDNA when choosing the optimal PPI generation. The smaller G3 PPI dendrimer (1687 Da, 16 1° amines) has been identified as most efficient for pDNA complexation and gene expression [28]. For the delivery of the smaller and more rigid siRNA molecules or small oligonucleotides, the G4 PPI (3514 Da, 32 1° amines) showed the highest uptake rates and gene knockdown efficiencies, when compared G3 and G5 PPI dendrimers [29]. Still, another study used the PPI G3 for the siRNA mediated knockdown of the ubiquitin ligase ITCH in various pancreatic cancer cell lines, showing an ~ 50% downregulation only at high siRNA concentrations (5 µg/200 µL) [30].

When considering PEIs or PPIs for therapeutic nucleic acid delivery, there are major concerns impeding their clinical translation. While it is well known that the transfection efficacy of these polymers increases with the molecular weight or number of generations, this is usually associated in parallel with higher cytotoxicity. Furthermore, PEI and PPI complexes tend to aggregate over time in physiological buffers or upon contact with biological fluids, e.g., serum [28,31–33].

Due to the large content of reactive amines in PEIs and PPIs, their chemical modification has been extensively explored, for further improvement of PEI- and PPI-based delivery systems. A general approach towards reducing cytotoxicity of cationic polymers is the shielding of the strong cationic charge by PEGylation. Although this strategy improved the biocompatibility and colloidal stability of the complexes, their cellular uptake and transfection efficacies were decreased [34,35]. To address this issue, targeting moieties have been introduced for cell specific internalization of pDNA- and siRNA complexes. This was shown for the coupling of the luteinizing hormone-releasing hormone (LHRH) peptide or folate onto the distal end of G4 or G5 PPI dendrimers [36,37]. In another approach, G4 PPI was modified with maltose for improved biocompatibility, and the loss of cellular uptake was compensated by coupling of an anti-EGFRvIII single chain antibody [38]. Other chemical modifications focused only on pDNA delivery. Another widely explored method for modifying cationic polymers is the introduction of lipophilic molecules. Here, biological activities were improved; for example after alkylcarboxylation of G4 PPI with 10-bromodeconoic acid or fluorination of G3-G5 PPIs with heptafluorobutyric acid [39,40]. Other studies explored PPI copolymers like PPI-poly-L-lysine, PPI-oligoethylenimine or PPI-Pluronic® P123 [33,41,42]. Smaller molecules were found to be efficient as well. The coupling of amino acids arginine, leucine or lysine strongly enhanced gene expression efficiencies of G3 PPI-based complexes and even of the very small G2 PPI [43,44]. Similarly, the modification of the larger G4/G5 PPIs with heterocyclic amines (histidine, piperazine-2-carboxyilic acid and 3-pyridyl acetic acid) reduced cytotoxicity, while leading to higher gene expression levels [45].

In stark contrast, chemical modifications of PPI-based systems with the aim of improving siRNA delivery have been barely explored at all. For creating a library, G1 PPI was modified with various alkyl epoxides, prior to formulation with PEG-lipids and siRNA to form nanoparticles. The most efficient derivative was a C16-modified G1 PPI that was able to downregulate Tie2 in endothelial cells in vitro and in vivo [46]. Another approach anchored G3 PPI onto gold nanoparticles. The Au-G3/siRNA complexes achieved a 70% knockdown of the target gene BCl-2, with negligible nonspecific toxicity [47]. Alternatively, an optimized formulation rather than a covalent modification employed the polyphenol epigallocatechin-3-O-gallate (EGCG) for pre-mixing with siRNA, prior to complexation with a G2 PPI. This ternary complex reduced luciferase reporter gene activity by 70% [48]. These findings identify PPI dendrimers as attractive candidates for further improvement. Moreover, PPI dendrimers are available at large scales and more defined structures compared to "normal" polymers, which is of particular importance when it comes to medical applications [49].

Recently, we selected a range of branched low molecular weight PEIs (2, 5, and 10 kDa) which were modified with tyrosine at the primary amines, yielding the tyrosine-grafted PEIs P2Y, P5Y and P10Y, respectively. This modification strongly enhanced siRNA-mediated knockdown efficiencies of different target genes in various cell lines at very low polymer/siRNA ratios, with a 70–90% target gene downregulation. Notably, even in the case of the smallest 2 kDa PEI, which is otherwise biologically inactive, tyrosine modification achieved knockdown efficacies of 50%. In addition, the colloidal stability of the tyrosine-modified PEI complexes upon incubation with serum was markedly improved [50–52]. More recently, we extended this strategy towards the modification of linear PEIs. Linear PEIs are more biocompatible than their branched counterparts and they can be produced with narrow polydispersities [53]. However, in their unmodified form, linear PEIs cannot sufficiently deliver siRNA into cells. We selected 2.5, 5, 10 and 25 kDa linear PEIs for tyrosine modification. Again, all new polymer derivatives, called LP2.5Y, LP5Y, LP10Y and LP25Y, showed excellent knockdown efficacies of 80–90% in various cell lines, including hard-to-transfect cells. The most active candidates, the linear LP10Y as well as the branched P5Y and P10Y, have also been successfully evaluated in tumor xenograft mouse models for siRNA-mediated oncogene targeting [54].

Thus, as shown previously, and in this paper, the tyrosine modification of branched or linear, small PEIs markedly improves their efficacy and biocompatibility. Based on these findings, we have now extended this approach for the first time towards a PPI dendrimer and present the superior properties of a tyrosine-modified fourth generation PPI ("PPI-G4-Y"). This covers the physicochemical characterization of the PPI-G4-Y/siRNA complexes which show high complexation efficacy and complex stability, and little surface charge. High biological activity and low cytotoxicity were found and compared to various tyrosine-modified branched and linear PEI complexes in different cell lines. In combination with first in vivo biocompatibility studies, our data identify PPI-G4-Y dendrimers as versatile and particularly promising siRNA delivery platform.

2. Materials and Methods

2.1. Materials

All chemicals and reagents were of analytical grade. Unmodified polymers used here were as follows: 10 kDa branched PEI (Polysciences, Eppelheim, Germany), 5 kDa branched PEI (a kind gift from BASF, Ludwigshafen, Germany), 5 kDa and 10 kDa linear PEIs (Sigma-Aldrich, Taufkirchen, Germany) and PPI dendrimer generation 4 (SyMO-Chem, Eindhoven, The Netherlands). N-Boc-tyrosine-OH, N-hydroxysuccinimide, EDC·HCl and benzotriazole-1-yl-oxy-tris-pyrrolidino-phosphonium hexafluorophosphate (PyBOP) were from Carbolution Chemicals (Saarbrücken, Germany). Dry N,N-Dimethylformamide (DMF) and dimethylsulfoxide (DMSO) was from VWR (Darmstadt, Germany), Trifluoroacetic acid (TFA) and diisopropylamine (DIPEA) were from Carl Roth (Karlsruhe, Germany). Dialysis tubes (MWCO 1 kDa and 3.5 kDa) were Spectra/Por, from Serva (Heidelberg, Germany).

Cell culture plastics and consumables were purchased from Sarstedt (Nümbrecht, Germany). Cell culture media were from Sigma-Aldrich (Taufkirchen, Germany) and fetal calf serum was from Biochrom (Berlin, Germany). The cell lines HT29 (colorectal carcinoma), PC3 (prostate carcinoma), MV4-11 (biphenotypic B-myelomonocytic leukemia) were obtained from ATCC/LGC Promochem (Wesel, Germany). The cells were routinely tested for Mycoplasma using the Venor$^{(R)}$ GeM Classic kit (Minerva Biolabs, Berlin, Germany) and determined to be free of any contamination. All cell lines were cultivated in a humid atmosphere at 37 °C and 5% CO_2. HT29 and PC3 cells were grown in Iscove's Modified Dulbecco Medium (IMDM), and MV-4-11 cells were cultured in RPMI 1640 medium. All media were supplemented with 10% FCS and 2 mM alanyl-glutamine. Cell culture and all transfection experiments were conducted in the absence of antibiotics. Stably dual expressing EGFP/Luciferase-expressing reporter cell lines were prepared by lentiviral transduction as previously described [52].

SiRNA sequences and RT-qPCR primer sequences are given in Table S1.

2.2. Chemical Synthesis of Tyrosine-Modified PPI

For the tyrosine-modification of the PPI G4 dendrimer, Boc (*tert*-butyloxycarbonyl) protected tyrosine (0.282 g, 1.0 mmol) was dissolved in 3 mL dry DMSO in a glass vial and PyBOP (0.616 g, 1.18 mmol) was slowly added and stirred for 15 min. In a separate glass vial, the PPI G4 dendrimer (0.1 g, 0.9 mmol in primary amines) was dissolved in dry DMSO and DIPEA (200 µL, 0.151 mol) was added. Next, the pre-activated tyrosine mixture was slowly added to the PPI solution and stirred for 48 h at room temperature. Thereafter, DMSO and other low molecular weight impurities were removed by dialysis (MWCO 1 kDa) against methanol for 6 h. The methanol was removed *in vacuo* and the modified dendrimer was dissolved in 5 mL TFA and left stirring overnight to remove the Boc group. Excess TFA was then removed by co-evaporation with methanol. Finally, the crude polymer was dissolved in 0.1 M HCl and excessively purified by dialysis against 0.05 M HCl for 24 h, then against water for 48 h with intermediate water exchange. Lyophilization yielded the tyrosine-modified PPI as white/yellowish fluffy powder. The degree of substitution was confirmed by ^{1}H-NMR (Avance III, 400 MHz, Bruker BioSpin, Rheinstetten, Germany) and calculated as described in [35], indicating an almost complete tyrosine functionalization of the outer primary amines. ^{1}H-NMR (400 MHz, D_2O) δ 1.47–2.17 (m, PPI, 4.023 H), 2.45–3.37 (m, PPI +CH_2 tyrosine, 9.38 H), 3.93 (m, CH tyrosine, 1 H), 6.86–6.88 (d, H_{Ar} tyrosine, 2H), 7.11–7.13 (d, H_{Ar} tyrosine, 2H).

The tyrosine-modified 5 kDa and 10 kDa branched PEIs (P5Y, P10Y) and linear PEIs (LP5Y, LP10Y) were prepared as described previously according to similar protocols [50,54].

2.3. Complex Preparation and Characterization

For standard transfection studies, the cells were seeded at a density of 35,000 cells per well of a 24 well plate in 0.5 mL fully supplemented medium. The following day, the cells were transfected with the polyplexes. The polyplexes were prepared at a polymer/siRNA mass ratio of 2.5 unless indicated otherwise. For a 24 well plate format, 0.4 µg siRNA in 12.5 µL HN buffer (150 mM NaCl, 10 mM HEPES, pH 7.4) and 1 µg tyrosine-modified polymer in 12.5 µL HN buffer were diluted in two separate tubes. The polymer dilution was added to the siRNA dilution, thoroughly mixed and incubated at room temperature for 30 min. After adding the polyplexes to the cells, no further medium change was performed.

The hydrodynamic diameters and zeta potentials of the PPI-G4-Y/siRNA complexes were measured by dynamic light scattering (DLS) and phase analysis light scattering (PALS), using the Brookhaven ZetaPALS system (Brookhaven Instruments, Holtsville, NY, USA). Polyplexes containing 5 µg siRNA in 250 µL total volume were prepared as described above and diluted to 1.7 mL in ultrapure water. The data were analyzed using the manufacturer's software, applying the viscosity and refractive index of pure water at 25 °C. For size determination, polyplexes were measured in five runs, with a run duration of 1 min per experiment. Zeta potentials were analyzed in ten runs, with each run containing ten cycles using the Smoluchowski model.

To study the complexation efficacy, agarose gel electrophoresis was used. Briefly, 0.2 µg siRNA was complexed in a total volume of 25 µL as described above at the different polymer/siRNA mass ratios indicated in the figure. The polyplexes were mixed with 10× loading dye and run on a 2% (w/v) agarose gel containing ethidium bromide at 80 V in TAE running buffer (20 mM EDTA, 40 mM Tris, 20 mM acetic acid). Unbound siRNA bands were visualized under UV illumination.

For assessing the complex stability of PPI-G4-Y/siRNA complexes, mass ratio of 3.75 was used. Complexes containing 0.2 µg siRNA in 25 µL were incubated with increasing amounts of heparin, incubated for 30 min at room temperature and subjected to agarose gel electrophoresis as described above.

To analyze the influence of FCS on the knockdown efficacies, PPI-G4-Y/siRNA complexes were further incubated in the presence of various FCS concentrations and storage conditions (fresh: 1 h at RT, 3 d at RT or 3 d at 37 °C).

2.4. Luciferase Assay and Flow Cytometry

Knockdown efficiencies were analyzed by measuring reporter gene activities (luciferase or enhanced green fluorescent protein, EGFP) 72 h after transfection. For the determination of luciferase activity, the medium was aspirated and the cells were lysed with 300 µL Luciferase Cell Culture Lysis Reagent (Promega, Mannheim, Germany) for 30 min at room temperature. In a test tube 10 µL cell lysate was mixed with 25 µL luciferin reagent (Beetle-Juice Kit, PJK, Kleinblittersdorf, Germany) and immediately measured in a luminometer (Berthold, Bad Wildbad, Germany).

EGFP expression levels were determined by flow cytometry. The cells were harvested by trypsinization and centrifuged for 3 min at 3,000 rpm, prior to resuspension of the cell pellets in FACS buffer (0.5 mL PBS, 1% FCS, 0.1% NaN$_3$). 20,000 cells in the vital gate were measured in an Attune® Acoustic Focusing Cytometer (Applied Biosystems, Foster City, CA, USA).

2.5. RT-qPCR

Knockdown efficiencies on the mRNA level were analyzed by RT-qPCR. Seventy-two hours after transfection, the total RNA was isolated using a combined TRI reagent (TRIfast, VWR, Darmstadt, Germany) and silica column protocol as previously described [52]. One microgram of total RNA was reverse transcribed using the RevertAid™ H Minus First Strand cDNA Synthesis Kit (Thermo Fisher Scientific; Schwerte, Germany). The cDNA synthesis mixture was incubated at 25 °C for 10 min, 42 °C for 60 min, and heat denatured at 70 °C for 10 min.

For quantitative real time PCR, the cDNA was diluted 1:10 with diethyl pyrocarbonate (DEPC)-water and 4 µL were mixed with 5 µL PerfeCTa SYBR Green FastMix (Quantabio, Beverly, MA) and 1 µL 5 µM primer mix. The RT-qPCR was performed using a Real-Time PCR System (Applied Biosystems) with the following instrument settings: pre-incubation at 95 °C for 2 min, followed by 45 amplification cycles (95 °C for 15 s, 55 °C for 15 s, 72 °C for 15 s). Levels were normalized for RPLP0. Primer sequences are given in Table S2.

2.6. Proliferation and LDH Release

Acute cell damage upon transfection was determined by measuring the lactate dehydrogenase (LDH) release, using the Cytotoxicity Detection Kit from Roche (Mannheim, Germany) according to the manufacturer's protocol. In brief, 35,000 cells were seeded in a 24 well plate. One hour prior to transfection, the medium was replaced with fresh medium and the cells were transfected with the polyplexes as described above containing 0.4 µg siRNA. After 24 h, the medium was harvested. Medium from untreated cells served as negative control and medium of cells treated with Triton X-100 (2% final concentration) was used as positive control (= 100% value) and fresh medium was included for the background value. In a 96 well plate, 50 µL medium was mixed with 50 µL reagent mix and incubated for 30 min in the dark at room temperature. The absorbance was measured at 490 nm and 620 nm as a reference filter in a plate reader (Thermo Fisher, Schwerte, Germany). Acute cytotoxicity values are presented as a percentage of the positive control after subtracting the background.

For the determination of the cell viability/metabolic activity 10,000 cells in 100 µL medium were seeded per well of a 96 well plate. The following day, the cells were transfected with polyplexes at different amounts as indicated in the figure. Numbers of viable/metabolically active cells were measured 72 h after transfection by using the colorimetric WST-8 Cell Counting Kit (Dojindo Molecular Technologies EU, Munich, Germany). Briefly, after replacing the medium with 50 µL of a 1:10 dilution of WST-8 in serum-free medium, the cells were incubated for 1 h at 37 °C. The absorbance was measured at 450 nm and 620 nm as a reference wavelength in a plate reader.

2.7. Erythrocyte Aggregation and Hemolysis

Erythrocyte aggregation and hemolysis assays were performed for analyzing possible damaging effects of the polyplexes after incubation. Red blood cells from healthy mice were isolated by repeated washing steps with Ringer's solution and centrifugation for 5 min at 5,000 rpm until the solution became clear. After the last centrifugation step, the red blood cells were resuspended in 0.9% NaCl solution. For the determination of erythrocyte aggregation, 1×10^6 cells were diluted in 150 µL 0.9% NaCl solution and incubated with the PPI-G4-Y/siRNA polyplexes or with 750 kDa branched PEI as positive control for 2 h at 37 °C. The cells were mounted onto coverslips and examined by bright field microscopy.

The hemolytic activity of the polyplexes was determined by incubating 50 µL polyplex solution with 50 µL cell suspension containing 1.5×10^7 cells in saline for 1 h at 37 °C. Erythrocytes incubated with pure HN buffer served as negative control while cells lysed with 2% Triton X-100 were used as positive control (= 100% value).

2.8. Blood Serum Markers and Immunostimulation

Animal studies were performed according to the national regulations and approved by the local authorities (Landesdirektion Sachsen). The mice were kept in cages with rodent chow (ssniff, Soest, Germany) and water available *ad libitum*. Immunocompromised nude mice were maintained and worked with under sterile aseptic conditions.

For analyzing the immunostimulating cytokines TNF-α and INF-γ, PPI-G4-Y/siCtrl complexes containing 10 µg siRNA in 150 µL were intravenous (i.v.) injected twice within 24 h into healthy C57BL/6 mice. The blood was collected four hours after the last injection. Untreated mice served as negative control and mice treated with a single dose of 50 µg lipopolysaccharide (LPS from E.coli O111:B4; Sigma-Aldrich) were used as positive control. The serum levels of TNF-α and INF-γ were measured using ELISA kits (PreproTech, Hamburg, Germany) according the manufacturer's instructions.

For measuring the blood serum markers alanine-aminotransferase (ALAT), creatinine and urea, healthy nude mice were intraperitoneal (i.p.) and i.v. injected with complexes containing 10 µg siRNA as detailed in the figure. The mice were treated twice within 24 h and the blood was collected 72 h after the first injection. Untreated mice served as negative control. The serum was diluted 1:1 and analyzed using an AU480 (Beckman Coulter, Krefeld Germany).

2.9. Statistics

Statistical analyses were performed by Student's t-test or One-way ANOVA, and significance levels are * = $p < 0.03$, ** = $p < 0.01$, *** = $p < 0.001$ and # = not significant. Unless indicated otherwise, differences between specific and non-specific treatment were analysed, with at least n = 3.

3. Results

3.1. Generation and Analysis of Tyrosine-Modified PPI-G4 and (L)PEIs, and Their Corresponding siRNA Complexes

Tyrosine-modified ("Y") fourth generation ("G4") polypropylenimine ("PPI") dendrimers (PPI-G4-Y; Figure 1A) were generated according to the synthesis scheme shown in Figure S1A. Based on our previous studies for the tyrosine-modified branched PEIs, all 32 primary amines of the PPI dendrimer were subjected to tyrosine modification. More specifically, the primary amines of the PPI dendrimer were coupled with tyrosine by using PyBOP and DMSO as solvent. The Boc deprotection with TFA and extensive purification by dialysis finally yielded the modified PPI dendrimer as white, fluffy powders. 1H-NMR analysis confirmed the structure of PPI-G4-Y (Figure S1B) and the average number of tyrosine per dendrimer was calculated to be 30. Tyrosine-modified branched and linear PEIs (Figure 1A, lower panels) were prepared as described previously [50,54].

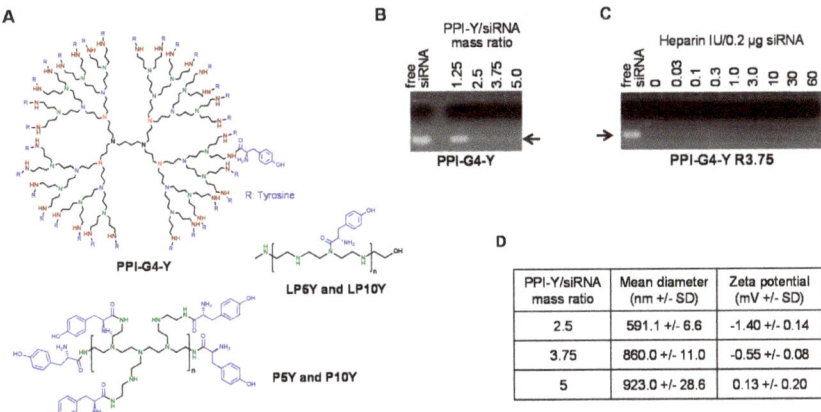

Figure 1. (**A**) Structures of tyrosine-modified PPI-G4 ("PPI-G4-Y"; upper panel) as well as tyrosine-grafted branched or linear polyethylenimines (PEIs) (lower panels; numbers indicate molecular weights of PEI). (**B**) Analysis of PPI-G4-Y-mediated siRNA complexation efficacy, dependent on polymer/siRNA mass ratios. (**C**) Determination of PPI-G4-Y/siRNA complex stability by heparin displacement assay. (**D**) Size and zeta potential of PPI-G4-Y/siRNA complexes at different mass ratios.

The analysis of complexation efficacies at various polymer/siRNA stoichiometries by agarose gel electrophoresis revealed complete siRNA complexation already at a PPI-G4-Y/siRNA mass ratio of 2.5, as indicated by the absence of the free siRNA band (Figure 1B). Thus, mass ratio 2.5 was used in the further experiments, unless indicated otherwise. The finding of a particularly high complexation efficacy of the tyrosine-modified PPI dendrimer was comparable to previous results on linear or branched low molecular weight PEIs upon their tyrosine-modification, with similarly low mass ratios being sufficient even for the complexation of small RNA molecules like siRNAs.

Likewise, PPI-G4-Y/siRNA complexes showed very high stability against heparin displacement, with no siRNA release even at heparin concentrations as high as 60 IU/0.2 µg siRNA (Figure 1C). While similar increases in complex stability had been obtained previously upon tyrosine-modification of PEIs, the complete absence of siRNA release upon heparin treatment as seen here for PPI-G4-Y/siRNA complexes was reminiscent to LP10Y/siRNA complexes [54]. Considering, however, that LP10Y/siRNA- as well as PPI-G4-Y/siRNA complexes display biological activity which must be based on the release of intact siRNA molecules, this demonstrates that heparin displacement seems to somewhat over-estimate complex stabilities and thus only poorly reflect the situation in biological media. Still, it should be noted that PPI-G4-Y/siRNA complexes, comparable to LP10Y/siRNA complexes, show particularly high stabilities even when prepared at very low polymer/siRNA ratios.

Zetasizer measurements revealed rather large PPI-G4-Y/siRNA complex sizes with diameters of almost 600 nm already at mass ratio 2.5. They increased even further when using more polymer for complexation and were then in the range of ~ 800–900 nm (Figure 1D). Thus, despite essentially complete siRNA complexation already at mass ratio 2.5 (see above), the addition of more PPI-G4-Y dendrimer still contributed to the complex formation. This was also associated with alterations in the zeta potential. More specifically, while PPI-G4-Y/siRNA complexes were slightly negative at mass ratio 2.5 and, to a lesser extent, at mass ratio 3.75, they turned even slightly positive at the higher mass ratio 5 (Figure 1D). In conclusion, comparably large complexes with very little surface charge were obtained when using PPI-G4-Y.

3.2. Biological Efficacies of siRNA Complexes Based on PPI-G4-Y- or Various Tyrosine-Modified PEIs

The beneficial effects of tyrosine-modification also became evident when analyzing knockdown efficacies. The use of PPI-G4 dendrimers for siRNA transfection into stably luciferase expressing PC3-EGFP/Luc reporter cells yielded no reduction of luciferase at all, independent of complex stoichiometries up to mass ratio 5 (Figure 2A, left).

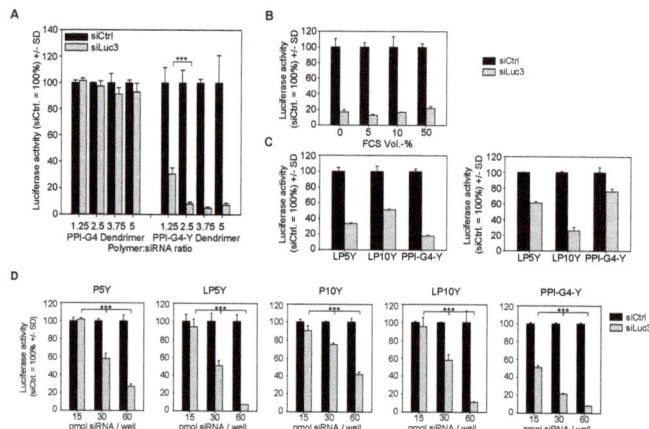

Figure 2. (**A**) Knockdown efficacies of PPI-G4 dendrimer-based siRNA complexes with (right) or without (left) tyrosine modification, as determined by luciferase knockdown in PC3-EGFP/Luc reporter cells. Bars show results upon transfection with complexes containing negative control siRNA (black) or luciferase-specific siRNA (grey), respectively, with black bars normalized to 100%. UT: untreated. (**B**) Knockdown efficacies upon pre-incubation of the complexes in the presence of FCS at various concentrations. (**C**) Knockdown efficacies of tyrosine-modified PPI- or PEI-based siRNA complexes in HT29-EGFP/Luc (upper panel) or MV4-11-EGFP/Luc cells (lower panel). (**D**) Dose-dependent knockdown efficacies of various tyrosine-modified PPI- or PEI-based siRNA complexes in HT29-EGFP/Luc cells.

In stark contrast, > 90% reduction of luciferase activity was observed upon incubation of cells with PPI-G4-Y/siRNA complexes. In agreement with the above results, ratio 2.5 proved to be sufficient for reaching maximum knockdown efficacy (Figure 2A, right).

When analyzing luciferase activity values normalized to untreated control cells, rather than those normalized to the respective PPI-G4-Y/negative control siRNA complexes as in Figure 2A, it was also seen that PPI-G4-Y/siRNA complexes prepared at ratios 1.25 or 2.5 exerted very few non-specific effects, with luciferase activity upon PPI-G4-Y/siCtrl transfection remaining comparable with untreated (Figure S2A, right). In contrast, at least in this cell line, non-specific reduction of luciferase activity was observed at ratios 3.75 or higher. Knockdown efficacies were not impaired by high protein content, i.e., no decrease in siRNA activity was seen in the presence of FCS at a concentration as high as 50% (Figure 2B). In fact, higher protein concentrations rather protected knockdown activity upon storage at various temperatures for three days (Figure S3). Gene targeting on the protein level, as determined by reduced luciferase activity, was also paralleled by decreased mRNA levels (Figure S2B), further substantiating the specificity of the siRNA-mediated knockdown. Results were comparable to previously described tyrosine-modified PEIs, e.g., to P5Y/siRNA complexes.

Knockdown efficacies and the definition of optimal complexes, however, were also found to be dependent on the cell line. In HT29-EGFP/Luc colon carcinoma cells, PPI-G4-Y/siRNA complexes showed better knockdown activity than their counterparts based on tyrosine-modified linear 5 kDa or 10 kDa PEI (LP5Y/siRNA or LP10Y/siRNA complexes; Figure 2C). In particular the LP10Y/siRNA complexes which had previously been found to efficiently mediate gene knockdown showed only moderate ~ 50% reduction of their target gene (Figure 2C, upper panel). In contrast, in MV4-11-EGFP/Luc B-myelomonocytic leukemia cells the same complexes were particularly efficient while little knockdown was achieved when using PPI-G4-Y (Figure 2C, lower panel). Maximum achievable knockdown efficacies, however, also proved to be dose-dependent. The lesser activity of LP10Y/siRNA complexes in HT29-EGFP/Luc cells observed above was not seen any more when doubling complex amounts: while at 15 and 30 pmol/well major differences between both polymers were seen, 60 pmol led to a very profound > 90% reduction of luciferase also in the case of LP10Y-based complexes (Figure 2D, right). This was comparable with LP5Y/siRNA complexes, whereas their counterparts based on branched 5 or 10 kDa PEI (P5Y, P10Y) showed somewhat lesser efficacy in HT29 cells (Figure 2D, left and center). In other cell lines, knockdown efficacies were rather comparable and were also seen when targeting other genes. In PC3-EGFP/Luc cells, the transfection of siRNAs specific for EGFP led to profound reduction of EGFP fluorescence, as determined by flow cytometry (Figure 3A, Figure S2C).

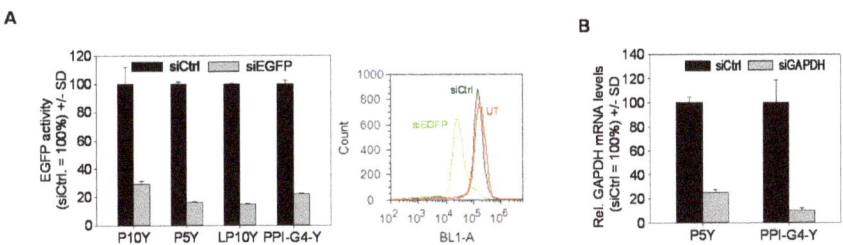

Figure 3. (**A**) Knockdown efficacies of various tyrosine-modified PPI- or PEI-based siRNA complexes targeting EGFP in PC3-EGFP/Luc cells (left). EGFP levels were determined by flow cytometry (see right panel and Figure S2C for original data). (**B**) Reduction of GAPDH mRNA levels in PC3 cells.

In the case of all polymers, the direct comparison between untreated and negative control siRNA transfected cells revealed no differences, indicating the absence of non-specific effects. Finally, when switching to an endogenous gene rather than stably, but ectopically expressed reporter genes, similar results were obtained. As shown for glyceraldehyde 3-phosphate dehydrogenase (GAPDH), PPI-G4-Y/siRNA complexes led to an ~ 90% reduction of the target gene (Figure 3B).

Taken together, this identifies complexes based on PPI-G4-Y, as alternative to tyrosine-modified linear or branched PEIs, as very efficient for siRNA-mediated knockdown in various cell lines, with some differences seen dependent on the cell line and the complex amounts used for transfection.

3.3. Biocompatibility of siRNA Complexes Based on PPI-G4-Y- or Various Tyrosine-Modified PEIs

Beyond knockdown efficacy, biocompatibility is a major variable determining optimal complexes for transfection. Complexes based on PPI-G4-Y as well as those based on tyrosine-modified linear or branched PEIs proved to be highly biocompatible, as seen in cell viability assays in PC3 cells (Figure 4A). Notably, in particular transfection with PPI-G4-Y/siRNA complexes preserved cell viability by 100%. The absence of acute toxicity was also confirmed by LDH release assays, indicating no acute cell damage upon transfection with any of the tested complexes (Figure 4B). In line with this, no adverse effects on erythrocytes were observed, as shown here for PPI-G4-Y/ siRNA complexes. Erythrocytes incubated with PPI-G4-Y/siRNA complexes revealed no signs of aggregation, leaving them indistinguishable from their untreated counterparts (Figure 4C). Likewise, independent of complex amounts, no hemoglobine release from erythrocytes was detected (Figure 4D).

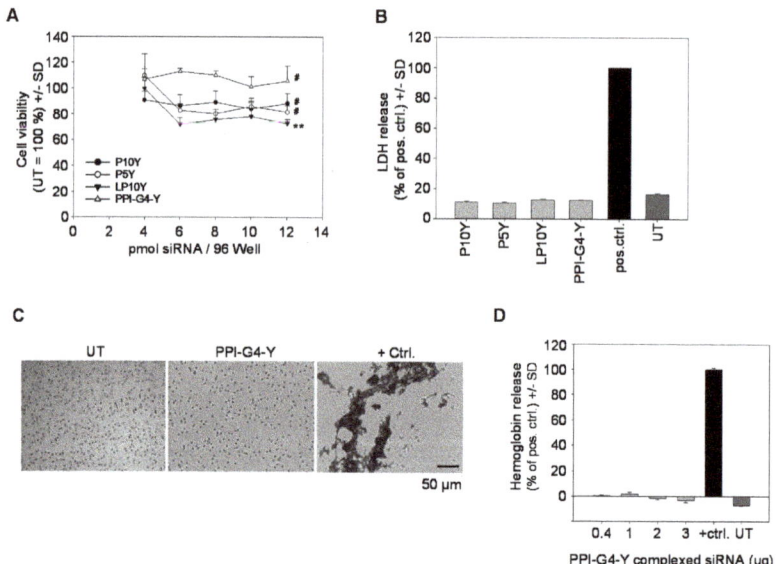

Figure 4. (**A**) Analysis of PC3 cell viability by WST-8 based measurement of viable cells upon transfection with various tyrosine-modified PPI- or PEI-based siRNA complexes at different amounts (indicated by siRNA amounts on the x-axis). Statistics analyze differences of the highest siRNA amounts (12 pmol) to untreated. (**B**) Assessment of acute cytotoxicity in PC3 cells by lactate dehydrogenase (LDH) into the medium. (**C**) Analysis of hemoglobin aggregation and (**D**) of hemoglobin release upon incubation of erythrocytes with PPI-G4-Y/siRNA complexes.

3.4. In Vivo Biocompatibility of siRNA Complexes Based on PPI-G4-Y- or Various Tyrosine-Modified PEIs

Studies on the biocompatibility of nanoparticles based on tyrosine-modified PPI or PEIs were also extended towards their application in vivo. Administration routes were intravenous (i.v.) or, considering the previously observed high efficacy and systemic availability of PEI-based nanoparticles, intraperitoneal (i.p.) injection [50,55]. In the case of PEI/siRNA complexes, these two modes of administration had previously shown marked differences in biodistribution and bioavailability, and thus both were included. After two injections, blood samples were taken and analyzed for serum markers. Levels of urea (Figure 5A) and creatinine (Figure 5B) after treatment were found identical to the untreated negative control, indicating the absence of nephrotoxic effects. For the assessment of hepatotoxicity, alanine-aminotransferase levels were determined. In some cases, minor increases in alanine-aminotransferase (ALAT) levels were detected, but did not reach statistical significance (Figure 5C). Finally, immune stimulation was measured as well. In this case, studies were restricted to i.v. administration since cytokine activation occurs in a narrow time window and thus requires immediate bioavailability of the whole sample. To cover a very short as well as a somewhat longer time range, two injections of PPI-G4-Y/siRNA complexes within 24 h were performed, prior to the determination of TNFα and IFNγ levels. While a profound increase in the levels of both cytokines was observed in the lipopolysaccharide (LPS) positive control group, treatment with PPI-G4-Y/siRNA complexes led to no (TNFα) and or a slight, statistically not significant (IFNγ) alteration in serum levels (Figure 5D). In line with this, no alterations in animal appearance or behavior were observed throughout the experiments.

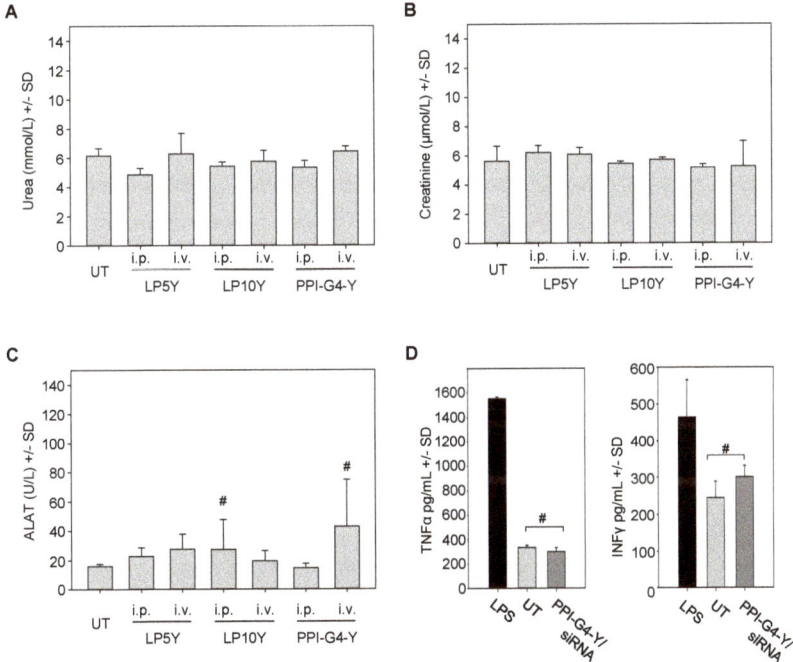

Figure 5. Determination of serum levels of (**A**) urea, (**B**) creatinine and (**C**) alanine-aminotransferase (ALAT) levels upon intraperitoneal (i.p.) or intravenous (i.v.) injection of mice with the tyrosine-modified PPI- or PEI-based siRNA complexes indicated on the x-axis. (**D**) Measurement of TNFα (left) and INFγ serum levels (right) upon i.v. injection of PPI-G4-Y/siRNA complexes.

4. Discussion

Tyrosine-modified polymers based on linear or branched PEIs have been identified as highly efficient for siRNA delivery in this and previous studies [50–52,54,56–58]. In this paper, we introduce for the first time the extension of this approach towards PPI dendrimers. In contrast to their non-modified counterparts, the tyrosine-grafted polymers show substantially increased complexation efficacy and complex stability, which is particularly critical for small oligonucleotides like siRNAs and also allows for using smaller polymers at lower mass ratios. The latter aspect may also provide a difference with regard to previous studies on unmodified PPI, where, when using higher siRNA concentrations than in our experiments, considerable knockdown was observed [29,30]. The positive effect of tyrosine grafting may rely on the contribution of others than electrostatic interactions, including π–π and cation–π interactions as suggested previously [59–61]. Notably, however, even the markedly enhanced complex stabilities still allow for efficient intracellular siRNA release, as seen from the high knockdown efficacies. In this context, it should be noted that the analysis of complex decomposition by heparin displacement has repeatedly proven to be insufficient since its results, falsely, suggested no siRNA release at all. Rather, studies in the presence of biological media like protein-containing cell or tissue lysates seem to be more appropriate in this regard [54].

Another major bottleneck for nanoparticle activity is their efficient cellular delivery and uptake. Notably, despite their large sizes, especially in the case of the PPI-G4-Y/siRNA complexes, and their very low (if at all) surface charge, cellular internalization of tyrosine-modified PEI- or PPI-based nanoparticles proved to be high. This indicates that surface charge is not a major determinant of nanoparticle activity. Still, the larger sizes may come with issues in vivo, e.g., regarding the penetration into intact tissue. In the case of P10Y/siRNA [50] or LP10Y/siRNA complexes [54], however, high biological activities in xenograft tumors were observed, arguing against major problems related to size. While it remains to be seen if this is also true for the even larger PPI-G4-Y/ siRNA complexes, it can already be noted that even sizes of almost 600 nm did not lead to issues regarding biocompatibility after i.v. injection. Also, limited tissue penetration and thus altered biodistribution may prove beneficial with regard to specificities for certain compartments and cell types. In this context, it could be of interest that we found PPI-G4-Y/siRNA complexes to be particularly efficient for macrophage transfection in vitro (data not shown). Thus, they may well represent candidates for preferentially transfecting these cells also in vivo, without the introduction of targeting moieties for targeted delivery. Taken together, these aspects provide the basis and clearly call for future in vivo experiments, covering biodistribution upon different modes of administration, gene knockdown in various target cells including tumor cells, stroma cells as well as hematopoietic cells, and therapeutic effects in relevant tumor models. While beyond the scope of this paper, we have already selected a relevant siRNA dosage (10 µg) for our toxicity studies presented here, based on previous results on PEI/siRNA or P10Y/siRNA complexes [50,55]. Thus, the combination of these and previous data, i.e., (i) the absence of toxicity at (ii) dosages previously identified in PEI-based systems as relevant for therapy, and (iii) in the light of the even enhanced transfection efficacy seen here, provides a strong basis for extensive in vivo and therapy studies.

The very high biocompatibilities in vitro and in vivo described here for PPI-G4-Y/siRNA complexes as well as in our previous studies for tyrosine-modified PEIs may be readily explained by the low nanoparticle zeta potentials, considering that positive surface charges have been associated with cytotoxicity [62], and the comparably little polymer amounts required for siRNA complexation. Still, more detailed studies will be required for comprehensively analyzing their toxicological profile. As reported previously, G4 PPI induced DNA damages in a COMET assay but no effects were observed in the case of a maltose-modified G4 PPI derivative. Likewise, G4 PPI, but not the maltose-modified G4 PPI, showed toxic effects in vivo, e.g., changes in serum parameters, body weight and behavior. These studies indicate that PPI dendrimers, when chemically modified, are interesting starting materials for synthesizing new effective and biocompatible polymers for nucleic acid delivery. In this regard, the approach of combining tyrosine-grafting with the introduction of biodegradable linkers at defined branching points in the polymer will be of particular interest. It should be noted, however, that the systems reviewed and described here rely on a comparably minor chemical modification, thus increasing the likeliness of their possible translation into the clinics. It must be kept in mind that successful systems for therapeutic siRNA delivery will have to combine maximum efficacy and biocompatibility with favorable properties with regard to manufacturing, upscaling, charge variability and GMP production.

5. Conclusions

This paper, as well as previous studies, establish tyrosine-modified PPIs or PEIs as particularly promising polymeric systems for siRNA formulation and delivery. Low chemical complexity, as in the case of tyrosine modifications, and particularly defined structure and size, as in the case of PPI dendrimers, in combination with the optimal molecular weight (G4) may leave PPI-G4-Y as particularly promising for siRNA formulation.

Supplementary Materials: The following are available online at http://www.mdpi.com/2079-4991/10/9/1809/s1, Figure S1: Synthesis scheme and 1H-NMR analysis of PPI-G4-Y. Figure S2: Knockdown efficacies of various tyrosine-modified PPI- or PEI-based siRNA complexes. Figure S3: Knockdown efficacies upon storage of PPI-G4-Y/siRNA complexes at various temperatures for three days, in the presence of different FCS concentrations.

Author Contributions: Conceptualization, A.E. and A.A.; investigation, S.N., M.K., A.E.; resources, A.A.; writing—original draft preparation, S.N., M.K., A.A. and A.E.; writing—review and editing, A.E. and A.A.; supervision, A.E. and A.A.; funding acquisition, A.A. All authors have read and agreed to the published version of the manuscript.

Funding: This research was funded by grants from the Deutsche Forschungsgemeinschaft (DFG; AI 24/21-1; AI 24/24-1) and the Deutsche Krebshilfe (70111616) to A.A.

Acknowledgments: The authors are grateful to Markus Böhlmann and Anne-Kathrin Krause for expert mouse maintenance, to Gabriele Oehme for help in cell culture experiments, the core unit "fluorescence technologies" (Kathrin Jäger) for cell sorting; Tamara Haustein (Institute for Organic Chemistry) for recording the NMR spectra.

Conflicts of Interest: The authors declare no conflict of interest. The funders had no role in the design of the study; in the collection, analyses, or interpretation of data; in the writing of the manuscript, or in the decision to publish the results.

References

1. Chakraborty, C.; Sharma, A.R.; Sharma, G.; Doss, C.G.P.; Lee, S.-S. Therapeutic miRNA and siRNA: Moving from Bench to Clinic as Next Generation Medicine. *Mol. Ther. Nucleic Acids* **2017**, *8*, 132–143. [CrossRef] [PubMed]
2. Setten, R.L.; Rossi, J.J.; Han, S.-P. The current state and future directions of RNAi-based therapeutics. *Nat. Rev. Drug Discov.* **2019**, *18*, 421–446. [CrossRef] [PubMed]
3. Fakhr, E.; Zare, F.; Teimoori-Toolabi, L. Precise and efficient siRNA design: A key point in competent gene silencing. *Cancer Gene Ther.* **2016**, *23*, 73–82. [CrossRef] [PubMed]
4. Friedrich, M.; Wiedemann, K.; Reiche, K.; Puppel, S.-H.; Pfeifer, G.; Zipfel, I.; Binder, S.; Köhl, U.; Müller, G.A.; Engeland, K.; et al. The Role of lncRNAs TAPIR-1 and -2 as Diagnostic Markers and Potential Therapeutic Targets in Prostate Cancer. *Cancers* **2020**, *12*, 1122. [CrossRef]
5. Benizri, S.; Gissot, A.; Martin, A.; Vialet, B.; Grinstaff, M.W.; Barthélémy, P. Bioconjugated Oligonucleotides: Recent Developments and Therapeutic Applications. *Bioconjug. Chem.* **2019**, *30*, 366–383. [CrossRef]
6. Gooding, M.; Malhotra, M.; Evans, J.C.; Darcy, R.; O'Driscoll, C.M. Oligonucleotide conjugates—Candidates for gene silencing therapeutics. *Eur. J. Pharm. Biopharm.* **2016**, *107*, 321–340. [CrossRef]
7. Kuboyama, T.; Yagi, K.; Naoi, T.; Era, T.; Yagi, N.; Nakasato, Y.; Yabuuchi, H.; Takahashi, S.; Shinohara, F.; Iwai, H.; et al. Simplifying the Chemical Structure of Cationic Lipids for siRNA-Lipid Nanoparticles. *ACS Med. Chem. Lett.* **2019**, *10*, 749–753. [CrossRef]
8. Kulkarni, J.A.; Darjuan, M.M.; Mercer, J.E.; Chen, S.; van der Meel, R.; Thewalt, J.L.; Tam, Y.Y.C.; Cullis, P.R. On the Formation and Morphology of Lipid Nanoparticles Containing Ionizable Cationic Lipids and siRNA. *ACS Nano* **2018**, *12*, 4787–4795. [CrossRef]
9. Lin, Z.; Bao, M.; Yu, Z.; Xue, L.; Ju, C.; Zhang, C. The development of tertiary amine cationic lipids for safe and efficient siRNA delivery. *Biomater. Sci.* **2019**, *7*, 2777–2792. [CrossRef]
10. Peng, L.; Wagner, E. Polymeric Carriers for Nucleic Acid Delivery: Current Designs and Future Directions. *Biomacromolecules* **2019**, *20*, 3613–3626. [CrossRef]
11. Ulkoski, D.; Bak, A.; Wilson, J.T.; Krishnamurthy, V.R. Recent advances in polymeric materials for the delivery of RNA therapeutics. *Expert Opin. Drug Deliv.* **2019**, *16*, 1149–1167. [CrossRef] [PubMed]

12. Conde, J.; Ambrosone, A.; Hernandez, Y.; Tian, F.; McCully, M.; Berry, C.C.; Baptista, P.V.; Tortiglione, C.; de La Fuente, J.M. 15 years on siRNA delivery: Beyond the State-of-the-Art on inorganic nanoparticles for RNAi therapeutics. *Nano Today* **2015**, *10*, 421–450. [CrossRef]
13. Steinbacher, J.L.; Landry, C.C. Adsorption and release of siRNA from porous silica. *Langmuir* **2014**, *30*, 4396–4405. [CrossRef] [PubMed]
14. Krasheninina, O.A.; Apartsin, E.K.; Fuentes, E.; Szulc, A.; Ionov, M.; Venyaminova, A.G.; Shcharbin, D.; de La Mata, F.J.; Bryszewska, M.; Gómez, R. Complexes of Pro-Apoptotic siRNAs and Carbosilane Dendrimers: Formation and Effect on Cancer Cells. *Pharmaceutics* **2019**, *11*, 25. [CrossRef] [PubMed]
15. Adams, D.; Gonzalez-Duarte, A.; O'Riordan, W.D.; Yang, C.-C.; Ueda, M.; Kristen, A.V.; Tournev, I.; Schmidt, H.H.; Coelho, T.; Berk, J.L.; et al. Patisiran, an RNAi Therapeutic, for Hereditary Transthyretin Amyloidosis. *N. Engl. J. Med.* **2018**, *379*, 11–21. [CrossRef] [PubMed]
16. Gonzalez-Aseguinolaza, G. Givosiran—Running RNA Interference to Fight Porphyria Attacks. *N. Engl. J. Med.* **2020**, *382*, 2366–2367. [CrossRef]
17. Balwani, M.; Sardh, E.; Ventura, P.; Aguilera Peiró, P.; Rees, D.C.; Stölzel, U.; Bissell, M.D.; Bonkovsky, H.; Windyga, J.; Anderson, K.E.; et al. Phase 3 Trial of RNAi Therapeutic Givosiran for Acute Intermittent Porphyria. *N. Engl. J. Med.* **2020**, *382*, 2289–2301. [CrossRef]
18. Lorenzer, C.; Dirin, M.; Winkler, A.-M.; Baumann, V.; Winkler, J. Going beyond the liver: Progress and challenges of targeted delivery of siRNA therapeutics. *J. Control. Release* **2015**, *203*, 1–15. [CrossRef]
19. Zuckerman, J.E.; Davis, M.E. Clinical experiences with systemically administered siRNA-based therapeutics in cancer. *Nat. Rev. Drug Discov.* **2015**, *14*, 843–856. [CrossRef]
20. Dominska, M.; Dykxhoorn, D.M. Breaking down the barriers: siRNA delivery and endosome escape. *J. Cell Sci.* **2010**, *123*, 1183–1189. [CrossRef]
21. Whitehead, K.A.; Langer, R.; Anderson, D.G. Knocking down barriers: Advances in siRNA delivery. *Nat. Rev. Drug Discov.* **2009**, *8*, 129–138. [CrossRef] [PubMed]
22. Boussif, O.; Lezoualc'h, F.; Zanta, M.A.; Mergny, M.D.; Schermann, D.; Demeneix, B.; Behr, J.-P. A versatile vector for gene and oligo transfer into cells in culture and in vivo: Polyethylenimine. *Proc. Natl. Acad. Sci. USA* **1995**, *92*, 7297–7301. [CrossRef] [PubMed]
23. Höbel, S.; Aigner, A. Polyethylenimines for siRNA and miRNA delivery in vivo. *Wiley Interdiscip. Rev. Nanomed. Nanobiotechnol.* **2013**, *5*, 484–501. [CrossRef] [PubMed]
24. Jiang, C.; Chen, J.; Li, Z.; Wang, Z.; Zhang, W.; Liu, J. Recent advances in the development of polyethylenimine-based gene vectors for safe and efficient gene delivery. *Expert Opin. Drug Deliv.* **2019**, *16*, 363–376. [CrossRef]
25. Neu, M.; Fischer, D.; Kissel, T. Recent advances in rational gene transfer vector design based on poly(ethylene imine) and its derivatives. *J. Gene Med.* **2005**, *7*, 992–1009. [CrossRef]
26. Palmerston Mendes, L.; Pan, J.; Torchilin, V.P. Dendrimers as Nanocarriers for Nucleic Acid and Drug Delivery in Cancer Therapy. *Molecules* **2017**, *22*, 1401. [CrossRef]
27. Dzmitruk, V.; Apartsin, E.; Ihnatsyeu-Kachan, A.; Abashkin, V.; Shcharbin, D.; Bryszewska, M. Dendrimers Show Promise for siRNA and microRNA Therapeutics. *Pharmaceutics* **2018**, *10*, 126. [CrossRef]
28. Zinselmeyer, B.H.; Mackay, S.P.; Schätzlein, A.; Uchegbu, I. The Lower-Generation Polypropylenimine Dendrimers Are Effective Gene-Transfer Agents. *Pharm. Res.* **2002**, *19*, 960–967. [CrossRef]
29. Taratula, O.; Savla, R.; He, H.; Minko, T. Poly(propyleneimine) dendrimers as potential siRNA delivery nanocarrier: From structure to function. *IJNT* **2011**, *8*, 36. [CrossRef]
30. De La Fuente, M.; Jones, M.-C.; Santander-Ortega, M.J.; Mirenska, A.; Marimuthu, P.; Uchegbu, I.; Schätzlein, A. A nano-enabled cancer-specific ITCH RNAi chemotherapy booster for pancreatic cancer. *Nanomedicine* **2015**, *11*, 369–377. [CrossRef]
31. Malloggi, C.; Pezzoli, D.; Magagnin, L.; de Nardo, L.; Mantovani, D.; Tallarita, E.; Candiani, G. Comparative evaluation and optimization of off-the-shelf cationic polymers for gene delivery purposes. *Polym. Chem.* **2015**, *6*, 6325–6339. [CrossRef]
32. Kafil, V.; Omidi, Y. Cytotoxic impacts of linear and branched polyethylenimine nanostructures in A431 cells. *BioImpacts* **2011**, *1*, 23–30. [CrossRef] [PubMed]
33. Russ, V.; Günther, M.; Halama, A.; Ogris, M.; Wagner, E. Oligoethylenimine-grafted polypropylenimine dendrimers as degradable and biocompatible synthetic vectors for gene delivery. *J. Control. Release* **2008**, *132*, 131–140. [CrossRef] [PubMed]

34. Somani, S.; Laskar, P.; Altwaijry, N.; Kewcharoenvong, P.; Irving, C.; Robb, G.; Pickard, B.S.; Dufès, C. PEGylation of polypropylenimine dendrimers: Effects on cytotoxicity, DNA condensation, gene delivery and expression in cancer cells. *Sci. Rep.* **2018**, *8*, 9410. [CrossRef] [PubMed]
35. Stasko, N.A.; Johnson, C.B.; Schoenfisch, M.H.; Johnson, T.A.; Holmuhamedov, E.L. Cytotoxicity of polypropylenimine dendrimer conjugates on cultured endothelial cells. *Biomacromolecules* **2007**, *8*, 3853–3859. [CrossRef]
36. Taratula, O.; Garbuzenko, O.B.; Kirkpatrick, P.; Pandya, I.; Savla, R.; Pozharov, V.P.; He, H.; Minko, T. Surface-engineered targeted PPI dendrimer for efficient intracellular and intratumoral siRNA delivery. *J. Control. Release* **2009**, *140*, 284–293. [CrossRef]
37. Sideratou, Z.; Kontoyianni, C.; Drossopoulou, G.I.; Paleos, C.M. Synthesis of a folate functionalized PEGylated poly(propylene imine) dendrimer as prospective targeted drug delivery system. *Bioorg. Med. Chem. Lett.* **2010**, *20*, 6513–6517. [CrossRef]
38. Tietze, S.; Schau, I.; Michen, S.; Ennen, F.; Janke, A.; Schackert, G.; Aigner, A.; Appelhans, D.; Temme, A. A Poly(Propyleneimine) Dendrimer-Based Polyplex-System for Single-Chain Antibody-Mediated Targeted Delivery and Cellular Uptake of SiRNA. *Small* **2017**, *13*. [CrossRef]
39. Hashemi, M.; Fard, H.S.; Farzad, S.A.; Parhiz, H.; Ramezani, M. Gene transfer enhancement by alkylcarboxylation of poly(propylenimine). *Nanomed. J.* **2013**, *1*, 55–62.
40. Liu, H.; Wang, Y.; Wang, M.; Xiao, J.; Cheng, Y. Fluorinated poly(propylenimine) dendrimers as gene vectors. *Biomaterials* **2014**, *35*, 5407–5413. [CrossRef]
41. Byrne, M.; Victory, D.; Hibbitts, A.; Lanigan, M.; Heise, A.; Cryan, S.-A. Molecular weight and architectural dependence of well-defined star-shaped poly(lysine) as a gene delivery vector. *Biomater. Sci.* **2013**, *1*, 1223–1234. [CrossRef] [PubMed]
42. Gu, J.; Hao, J.; Fang, X.; Sha, X. Factors influencing the transfection efficiency and cellular uptake mechanisms of Pluronic P123-modified polypropyleneimine/pDNA polyplexes in multidrug resistant breast cancer cells. *Colloid Surface B* **2016**, *140*, 83–93. [CrossRef] [PubMed]
43. Aldawsari, H.; Edrada-Ebel, R.; Blatchford, D.R.; Tate, R.J.; Tetley, L.; Dufès, C. Enhanced gene expression in tumors after intravenous administration of arginine-, lysine- and leucine-bearing polypropylenimine polyplex. *Biomaterials* **2011**, *32*, 5889–5899. [CrossRef] [PubMed]
44. Kim, T.-I.; Baek, J.-U.; Zhe Bai, C.; Park, J.-S. Arginine-conjugated polypropylenimine dendrimer as a non-toxic and efficient gene delivery carrier. *Biomaterials* **2007**, *28*, 2061–2067. [CrossRef] [PubMed]
45. Hashemi, M.; Tabatabai, S.M.; Parhiz, H.; Milanizadeh, S.; Amel Farzad, S.; Abnous, K.; Ramezani, M. Gene delivery efficiency and cytotoxicity of heterocyclic amine-modified PAMAM and PPI dendrimers. *Mater. Sci. Eng. C* **2016**, *61*, 791–800. [CrossRef]
46. Khan, O.F.; Zaia, E.W.; Jhunjhunwala, S.; Xue, W.; Cai, W.; Yun, D.S.; Barnes, C.M.; Dahlman, J.E.; Dong, Y.; Pelet, J.M.; et al. Dendrimer-Inspired Nanomaterials for the in Vivo Delivery of siRNA to Lung Vasculature. *Nano Lett.* **2015**, *15*, 3008–3016. [CrossRef]
47. Chen, A.M.; Taratula, O.; Wei, D.; Yen, H.-I.; Thomas, T.; Thomas, T.J.; Minko, T.; He, H. Labile catalytic packaging of DNA/siRNA: Control of gold nanoparticles "out" of DNA/siRNA complexes. *ACS Nano* **2010**, *4*, 3679–3688. [CrossRef]
48. Shen, W.; Wang, Q.; Shen, Y.; Gao, X.; Li, L.; Yan, Y.; Wang, H.; Cheng, Y. Green Tea Catechin Dramatically Promotes RNAi Mediated by Low-Molecular-Weight Polymers. *ACS Cent. Sci.* **2018**, *4*, 1326–1333. [CrossRef]
49. Maitz, M.F. Applications of synthetic polymers in clinical medicine. *Biosurf. Biotribol.* **2015**, *1*, 161–176. [CrossRef]
50. Ewe, A.; Przybylski, S.; Burkhardt, J.; Janke, A.; Appelhans, D.; Aigner, A. A novel tyrosine-modified low molecular weight polyethylenimine (P10Y) for efficient siRNA delivery in vitro and in vivo. *J. Control. Release* **2016**, *230*, 13–25. [CrossRef]
51. Ewe, A.; Höbel, S.; Heine, C.; Merz, L.; Kallendrusch, S.; Bechmann, I.; Merz, F.; Franke, H.; Aigner, A. Optimized polyethylenimine (PEI)-based nanoparticles for siRNA delivery, analyzed in vitro and in an ex vivo tumor tissue slice culture model. *Drug Deliv. Transl. Res.* **2017**, *7*, 206–216. [CrossRef] [PubMed]
52. Ewe, A.; Noske, S.; Karimov, M.; Aigner, A. Polymeric Nanoparticles Based on Tyrosine-Modified, Low Molecular Weight Polyethylenimines for siRNA Delivery. *Pharmaceutics* **2019**, *11*, 600. [CrossRef]

53. Tauhardt, L.; Kempe, K.; Knop, K.; Altuntaş, E.; Jäger, M.; Schubert, S.; Fischer, D.; Schubert, U.S. Linear Polyethyleneimine: Optimized Synthesis and Characterization—On the Way to "Pharmagrade" Batches. *Macromol. Chem. Phys.* **2011**, *212*, 1918–1924. [CrossRef]
54. Karimov, M.; Schulz, M.; Kahl, T.; Noske, S.; Kubczak, M.; Gockel, I.; Thieme, R.; Büch, T.; Reinert, A.; Ionov, M.; et al. Tyrosine-modified linear PEIs for highly efficacious and biocompatible siRNA delivery in vitro and in vivo. *Nano Res.* **2020**, Submitted.
55. Höbel, S.; Koburger, I.; John, M.; Czubayko, F.; Hadwiger, P.; Vornlocher, H.-P.; Aigner, A. Polyethylenimine/small interfering RNA-mediated knockdown of vascular endothelial growth factor in vivo exerts anti-tumor effects synergistically with Bevacizumab. *J. Gene Med.* **2010**, *12*, 287–300. [CrossRef]
56. Troiber, C.; Edinger, D.; Kos, P.; Schreiner, L.; Kläger, R.; Herrmann, A.; Wagner, E. Stabilizing effect of tyrosine trimers on pDNA and siRNA polyplexes. *Biomaterials* **2013**, *34*, 1624–1633. [CrossRef]
57. Creusat, G.; Thomann, J.-S.; Maglott, A.; Pons, B.; Dontenwill, M.; Guérin, E.; Frisch, B.; Zuber, G. Pyridylthiourea-grafted polyethylenimine offers an effective assistance to siRNA-mediated gene silencing in vitro and in vivo. *J. Control. Release* **2012**, *157*, 418–426. [CrossRef]
58. Creusat, G.; Rinaldi, A.-S.; Weiss, E.; Elbaghdadi, R.; Remy, J.-S.; Mulherkar, R.; Zuber, G. Proton sponge trick for pH-sensitive disassembly of polyethylenimine-based siRNA delivery systems. *Bioconjug. Chem.* **2010**, *21*, 994–1002. [CrossRef]
59. Dougherty, D.A. Cation-π Interactions in Chemistry and Biology- A New View of Benzene, Phe, Tyr, and Trp. *Science* **1996**, *271*, 163–168. [CrossRef]
60. Edwards-Gayle, C.J.C.; Greco, F.; Hamley, I.W.; Rambo, R.P.; Reza, M.; Ruokolainen, J.; Skoulas, D.; Iatrou, H. Self-Assembly of Telechelic Tyrosine End-Capped PEO Star Polymers in Aqueous Solution. *Biomacromolecules* **2018**, *19*, 167–177. [CrossRef]
61. Roviello, G.N.; Roviello, V.; Autiero, I.; Saviano, M. Solid phase synthesis of TyrT, a thymine-tyrosine conjugate with poly(A) RNA-binding ability. *RSC Adv.* **2016**, *6*, 27607–27613. [CrossRef] [PubMed]
62. Fröhlich, E. The role of surface charge in cellular uptake and cytotoxicity of medical nanoparticles. *Int. J. Nanomed.* **2012**, *7*, 5577–5591. [CrossRef] [PubMed]

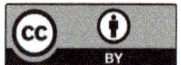

© 2020 by the authors. Licensee MDPI, Basel, Switzerland. This article is an open access article distributed under the terms and conditions of the Creative Commons Attribution (CC BY) license (http://creativecommons.org/licenses/by/4.0/).

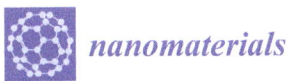

Article

pH-Sensitive Dendrimersomes of Hybrid Triazine-Carbosilane Dendritic Amphiphiles-Smart Vehicles for Drug Delivery

Evgeny Apartsin [1,2,3,*], Nadezhda Knauer [1,4], Valeria Arkhipova [1,2], Ekaterina Pashkina [1,4], Alina Aktanova [1,4], Julia Poletaeva [1], Javier Sánchez-Nieves [5,6], Francisco Javier de la Mata [5,6,7] and Rafael Gómez [5,6,7,*]

1. Institute of Chemical Biology and Fundamental Medicine SB RAS, 8, Lavrentiev ave., 630090 Novosibirsk, Russia; knauern@gmail.com (N.K.); v.arkhipova@g.nsu.ru (V.A.); pashkina.e.a@yandex.ru (E.P.); aktanova_al@mail.ru (A.A.); fabaceae@yandex.ru (J.P.)
2. Department of Natural Sciences, Novosibirsk State University, 630090 Novosibirsk, Russia
3. Laboratoire de Chimie de Coordination, CNRS, 31077 Toulouse, France
4. Research Institute of Fundamental and Clinical Immunology, 630099 Novosibirsk, Russia
5. Departamento de Química Orgánica y Química Inorgánica, UAH-IQAR, Universidad de Alcalá, 28805 Alcalá de Henares, Spain; javier.sancheznieves@uah.es (J.S.-N.); javier.delamata@uah.es (F.J.d.l.M.)
6. Networking Research Center on Bioengineering, Biomaterials and Nanomedicine (CIBER-BBN), 28029 Madrid, Spain
7. Instituto Ramón y Cajal de Investigación Sanitaria, IRYCIS, 28034 Madrid, Spain
* Correspondence: eka@niboch.nsc.ru (E.A.); rafael.gomez@uah.es (R.G.)

Received: 7 August 2020; Accepted: 22 September 2020; Published: 23 September 2020

Abstract: Supramolecular constructions of amphiphilic dendritic molecules are promising vehicles for anti-cancer drug delivery due to the flexibility of their architecture, high drug loading capacity and avoiding off-target effects of a drug. Herein, we report a new class of amphiphilic dendritic species—triazine-carbosilane dendrons readily self-assembling into pH-sensitive dendrimersomes. The dendrimersomes efficiently encapsulate anticancer drugs doxorubicin and methotrexate. Chemodrug-loaded dendrimersomes have dose-related cytotoxic activity against leukaemia cell lines 1301 and K562. Our findings suggest that triazine-carbosilane dendrimersomes are prospective drug carriers for anti-cancer therapy.

Keywords: carbosilane; dendron; triazine; amphiphile; self-assembly; vesicles; pH-sensitive; doxorubicin; methotrexate; leukaemia

---

1. Introduction

The use of engineered nanosized constructions as drug delivery systems has become an emerging area of attention in recent years due to their ability to improve pharmacological properties of cargo compounds, i.e., improving selectivity and efficiency of drug delivery into target cells/tissues, reducing off-target effects of drugs, and protecting drugs from the biological environment amid the delivery [1]. Furthermore, nanoconstructions are expected to release a cargo in a controllable manner upon the action of external stimuli (changes of ambient pH or temperature, enzymatic digestion etc.) [2]. In light of this, the use of supramolecular assemblies for drug delivery seems to be very promising [3].

Dendritic molecules, dendrimers and dendrons, are versatile platforms to design supramolecular nanoconstructions for robust drug delivery [4–8]. In particular, carbosilane dendrimers are efficient tools for antibacterial [9] and antiviral therapy [10], nucleic acid delivery [11], cancer treatment [12], imaging [13], functional nanomaterials [14,15], and so on. It should be noted that dendritic architectures give room to design various types of supramolecular constructions based on the molecular topology of building blocks. Systematic studies conducted using amphiphilic dendrons revealed the effect of both the structure of the hydrophobic part and the dendron generation as amphiphilic part on their assembly into supramolecular constructions of given topology: micelles, unilamellar or multilamellar vesicles [16–18]. These regularities are implemented in the development of dendron-based nanoconstructions for biomedical applications [19–23].

To increase the loading capacity, the formation of vesicle-like assemblies (dendrimersomes) is preferred over micelle-like ones. This can be achieved by branching the hydrophobic part in the focal point of dendron. In this work, we suggest the use of a triazine moiety as a branching point. Triazine-based synthons can be easily prepared by the controllable substitution in cyanuric chloride [24]; they have already been shown to be versatile building blocks both for building dendrimer scaffolds [25] and for the functionalisation of dendrimer surface [26]. Furthermore, triazine cycle gets protonated in slightly acidic medium (pH~5.5) [27], which can be useful for the design of pH-sensitive constructions [28].

Herein, we report the synthesis of a new class of functional dendritic species—amphiphilic triazine-carbosilane dendrons. We aim to study the self-assembly of dendrons in physiological conditions as well as to explore the potential of dendrons' self-assemblies for drug delivery. As a representative and emerging model, leukaemia cell lines have been chosen. Leukaemia is a severe cancer of frequent occurrence. At present, despite advances of chemotherapy, the survival rate in adult patients with acute lymphoblastic leukaemia does not exceed 50% [29]. The prognosis for chronic leukaemia is more favorable; however, some aggravations, so-called blast crises that require special treatment may occur [30]. In view of this, the development of novel approaches to increase the efficacy of chemotherapy, in particular, nanomedicine-based ones, is highly important.

2. Materials and Methods

2.1. General Information

Organic solvents were dried and freshly distilled under argon prior to use. Reagents were obtained from commercial sources and used as received. Dendron precursor BrG_2V_4 was obtained as described elsewhere [31].

Water solutions of chemicals, amphilhiles, and chemodrugs as well as buffer solutions were prepared using milliQ® deionized water. Sonication of amphiphile solutions was done in a Sonorex Super RK 31 H ultrasonic bath (Bandelin Electronic, Berlin, Germany). Dialysis was done using SnakeSkin dialysis membranes MWCO 3500 (Thermo Fisher, Waltham, MA, USA).

2.2. Analytical and Spectroscopic Techniques

^1H and ^{13}C and spectra were recorded on Varian Unity VXR-300 (Varian Inc., Palo Alto, CA) and Bruker AV400 (Bruker, Karlsruhe, Germany) instruments. Chemical shifts (δ, ppm) were measured relative to residual ^1H and ^{13}C resonances for $CDCl_3$ used as solvent. ESI-TOF analysis was carried out in an Agilent 6210 TOF LC/MS mass spectrometer (Agilent, Santa Clara, CA, USA).

UV-vis spectra were recorded using an Eppendorf Biospectrophotometer (Eppendorf, Hamburg, Germany). Measurements were done at 25 °C using 1 mm thick quartz cells. Fluorescence spectra were recorded using a CLARIOstar microplate reader (BMG LABTECH, Ortenberg, Germany).

Hydrodynamic diameter of the supramolecular aggregates obtained was determined in plastic disposable microvolume cells using a Zetasizer Nano ZS particle analyzer (Malvern Instruments, Manchester, UK), equipped with NBS. The measurements were made at 25 °C. Zeta potential values were measured in plastic disposable cells DTS 1061 using Malvern Instruments Nanosizer ZS particle analyser. 10 mM of Na phosphate buffer was used to prepare solutions.

Transmission electron microscopy (TEM) images were obtained using a Veleta digital camera (EM SIS, Muenster, Germany) mounted on a JEM 1400 transmission electron microscope (JEOL, Tokyo, Japan) at the accelerating voltage of 80 kV. Samples were stained with 0.1% uranyl acetate.

2.3. Cell Experiments

Human T-cell leukemia cell line 1301 and human chronic myelogenous leukemia cell line K562 (European collection of authenticated cell cultures, Sigma Aldrich, Merck KGaA, Germany) were used. Cells were cultivated in the RPMI-1640 cell medium containing 10% foetal calf serum (HyClone Laboratories, South Logan, UT, USA), 0.3 mg/mL L-glutamine (Vector, Russia), 50 µg/mL gentamicin (DalChimPharm, Khabarovsk, Russia), and 25 µg/mL tienam (Merck Sharp & Dohme, Kenilworth, NJ, USA) in a humidified atmosphere containing 5% CO_2 at 37 °C.

2.4. Statistical Analysis

We used GraphPad Prism software and Statistica 7.0 software for data analysis and visualization. The Mann–Whitney criterion was used; the differences were considered to be significant if $p < 0.05$.

2.5. Synthesis of Dendron Amphiphiles

2.5.1. 2,4-dodecylamino-6-chloro-1,3,5-triazine

Cyanuric chloride (970 mg, 5.26 mmol) and dodecylamine (2.0 g, 10.8 mmol) were mixed in 150 mL $CHCl_3$. The mixture was cooled with an ice bath, then 10% aqueous KOH was added up to the pH~10. The reaction mixture was stirred overnight at room temperature, then organic phase was separated, the solvent was evaporated under vacuum, and the solid residue was recrystallized from the mixture $CHCl_3$:CH_3OH (5:1) to yield the desired product as white solid (2.28 g, 90%).

^1H NMR (400 MHz, $CDCl_3$) δ 0.86 (t, J = 6.8 Hz, 6H, H_a), 1.18–1.37 (m, 32H, H_b), 1.52–1.64 (m, 8H, H_c, H_d), 3.45 (q, J = 6.8 Hz, 4H, H_e), 6.03 (s, 2H, H_f). ^{13}C NMR (101 MHz, $CDCl_3$) δ 14.1, 22.6, 26.6, 28.5–29.9 (m), 31.9, 41.5, 165.8, 169.7, 171.0. MS: $[M + H]^+$ 482.40 amu (calcd 481.39 amu).

2.5.2. 2,4-dodecylamino-6-piperazino-1,3,5-triazine

2,4-didodecylamino-6-chloro-1,3,5-triazine (600 mg, 1.2 mmol) and piperazine (645 mg, 7.5 mmol) were mixed in 15 mL $CHCl_3$; the reaction mixture was stirred at room temperature. When the starting triazine derivative was fully consumed, as shown by TLC (5% CH_3OH in CH_2Cl_2), the solution was washed several times with 1M NaOH, then with water. The organic phase was separated, dried over Na_2SO_4, and the solvent was removed under vacuum to yield the desired product as yellowish solid (600 mg, 92%).

^1H NMR (400 MHz, $CDCl_3$) δ 0.87 (t, J = 6.5 Hz, 6H, H_a), 1.20–1.37 (m, 36H, H_b, H_c), 1.52 (t, 4H_d), 1.81 (s, 1H, H_i), 2.85 (s, 4H, H_h), 3.33 (d, 4H, H_g), 3.72 (s, 4H, H_e), 4.75 (s, 2H, H_f). ^{13}C NMR (101 MHz, $CDCl_3$) δ 14.1, 22.7, 27.0, 28.6–30.3 (m), 31.9, 40.7, 44.2, 46.1, 165.2, 166.3. MS: $[M + H]^+$ 532.51 amu (calcd 531.50 amu).

2.5.3. Vinyl-Terminated Dendron G2

2,4-didodecylamino-6-piperazino-1,3,5-triazine (220 mg, 0.41 mmol) and vinyl-terminated carbosilane dendron BrG$_2$V$_4$ (140 mg, 0.3 mmol), K$_2$CO$_3$ (70 mg, 0.5 mmol) were mixed in 30 mL acetone in a sealed ampule with catalytic amounts of 18-crown-6 and KI added. The reaction mixture was stirred for 24 h at 90 °C. The reaction completion was monitored by TOCSY ^{1}H NMR following the disappearance of BrCH$_2$ protons. When the reaction was over, the solvent was removed under vacuum, the residue was dissolved in ethyl acetate and washed with brine. The organic phase was dried over Na$_2$SO$_4$, and the solvent was removed. The crude product was purified by silica gel column chromatography (eluent: ethyl acetate:hexane 1:1) to yield functionalized dendron as light-yellow oil (245 mg, 90%).

^{1}H NMR (400 MHz, CDCl$_3$) δ −0.12 (s, 3H, H$_m$), 0.10 (s, 6H, H$_q$), 0.46 (m, 2H, H$_l$), 0.53 (m, 4H, H$_n$), 0.67 (m, 4H, H$_p$), 0.84 (t, J = 6.5 Hz, 6H, H$_a$), 1.19–1.35 (m, 42H, H$_b$, H$_c$, H$_k$, H$_o$), 1.50 (t, J = 7.3 Hz, 6H, H$_d$, H$_j$), 2.32 (t, J = 7.8 Hz, 2H, H$_i$), 2.42 (t, J = 5.1 Hz, 4H, H$_h$), 3.30 (d, J = 6.6 Hz, 4H, H$_g$), 3.76 (s, 4H, H$_e$), 4.88 (s, 2H, H$_f$), 5.59–6.21 (m, 12H, H$_r$). ^{13}C NMR (101 MHz, CDCl$_3$) δ -5.2, -5.1, 13.9, 14.1, 18.3, 18.5, 18.7, 22.0, 22.7, 26.9, 28.7–30.1 (m), 30.7, 30.9, 31.9, 40.6, 42.9, 53.2, 58.6, 132.6, 137.1, 164.7, 166.1.

2.5.4. Amphiphilic Dendron G2

Functionalized vinyl-terminated dendron (400 mg, 0.44 mmol), 2-(dimethylamino)ethanethiol hydrochloride (275 mg, 1.76 mmol) and dimethoxyphenylacetophenone (DMPA) (12 mg, 0.044 mmol) were dissolved in 5 mL of mixture THF:CH$_3$OH (1:2). The reaction mixture was deoxygenated by bubbling argon and irradiated by UV for 2 h (365 nm, 120W). Then, another 12 mg (0.044 mmol) of DMPA was added, and the reaction mixture was irradiated for another 2 h. The reaction completion was monitored by ^{1}H NMR. After the reaction was completed, the solvents were removed under vacuum and then the residue was dissolved in methanol. Afterward, it was precipitated in diethyl ether, and after the solvent was separated, the solid was dried under vacuum to afford the desired dendron as light-yellow solid (495 mg, 75%). For characterization, the dendron was deprotonated with K$_2$CO$_3$.

^{1}H NMR (400 MHz, CDCl$_3$) δ −0.10 (s, 3H, H$_m$), −0.01 (s, 6H, H$_q$), 0.46 (m, 2H, H$_l$), 0.52 (m, 4H, H$_n$), 0.59 (m, 4H, H$_p$), 0.85 (s, 6H, H$_a$), 1.25 (m, 42H, H$_b$, H$_c$, H$_k$, H$_o$), 1.49 (m, 6H, H$_d$, H$_j$), 2.23 (s, 24H, H$_v$), 2.32 (m, 2H, H$_i$), 2.40 (m, 4H, H$_h$), 2.47 (m, 8H, H$_u$), 2.53 (m, 8H, H$_s$), 2.61 (m, 8H, H$_t$), 3.31 (s, 4H,

H$_g$), 3.75 (s, 4H, H$_e$), 4.71 (s, 2H, H$_f$). ^{13}C NMR (101 MHz, CDCl$_3$) δ -5.3, -5.1, 14.1, 14.6, 18.3, 18.7, 22.1, 22.7, 27.0, 27.7, 29.0–30.1 (m), 31.9, 37.0, 40.6, 42.9, 45.4, 53.3, 59.3, 127.7, 128.5, 165.0, 166.2. MS: [M + H]$^+$ 1329.00 amu (calcd 1327.99 amu).

2.6. CMC Measurements

Association of dendron molecules into supramolecular constructions was studied by fluorescence spectroscopy using pyrene as a marker [32]. Aliquots of pyrene solution in acetone (5 μL, 20 μM) were dispensed in 200 μL glass vials and the solvent was removed under vacuum. Then, solutions of the amphiphilic dendron (100 μL, 0.3 to 100 μM) in 10 mM sodium phosphate buffer, pH 7.0 (PB) or 10 mM phosphate-buffered saline, pH 7.0–7.4 (PBS) were added. Samples were sonicated for 30 min and then incubated for 2 days at room temperature. After the incubation, the samples were transferred into the wells of 96-well black microplate COSTAR 96 half-area, and pyrene fluorescence spectra were recorded in the range 360–500 nm upon excitation at 345 ± 5 nm. The ratio of fluorescence intensities I_{373}/I_{383} was plotted against $-lgC$, fitted with Boltzmann sigmoidal curve ($r^2 > 0.95$), and the $-lg(CMC)$ values were estimated from the fitting data.

2.7. Study of the pH-Dependence of the Particle Size

The water solution of amphiphilic dendron in a glass vial (1 mL, 100 μM) was sonicated for 30 min and then incubated overnight at room temperature. 100 μL aliquots of the solution were taken into plastic Eppendorf-type test tubes, and 5 μL of 200 mM sodium phosphate buffer (pH 7.0; 6.5; 6.0; 5.5; 5.0) was added. The samples were incubated at room temperature for 2 h, then DLS profiles of the samples were recorded.

2.8. Drug Encapsulation

A drop of water solution of amphiphilic dendron (10 μL, 10 mM) and a drop of water solution (10 μL, 10 mM) of a doxorubicin hydrochloride (DOX), sodium methotrexate (MTX) or 5-fluorouracil (5FU) were rapidly mixed in 1 mL of deionized water; an UV-vis spectrum of the sample [As-mixed] was recorded. The solution was sonicated for 30 min and then incubated for 2 days at room temperature; an UV-vis spectrum of the sample [After treatment] was recorded. Non-encapsulated chemodrug was removed by dialysis against deionized water (4 × 200 mL, 6 h); an UV-vis spectrum of the sample [After dialysis] was recorded. The degree of chemodrug encapsulation was estimated from UV-vis spectra as a ratio of a chemodrug absorption at λ_{max} before and after dialysis. Drug loading capacity was estimated as a ratio of the weight of encapsulated drug to the total weight of nanoparticles neglecting the weight of the dendron washed off during the dialysis. The real loading capacity values are thus higher than estimated.

The UV-vis spectra of chemodrugs at different stages of encapsulation into dendrimersomes are shown in the Figure 1. DLS and zeta potential distribution profiles of drug-loaded dendrimersomes were recorded.

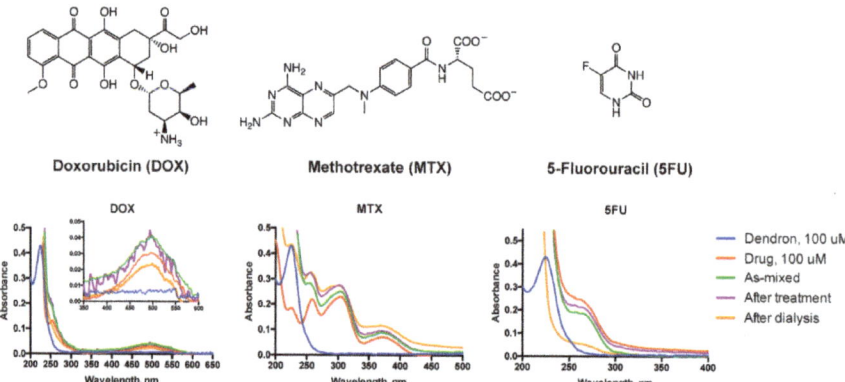

Figure 1. Structures of the chemodrugs used in the work: doxorubicin (DOX), methotrexate (MTX) and 5-fluorouracil (5FU) (**top**). UV-vis spectra of chemodrugs upon encapsulation into dendrimersomes (**bottom**).

2.9. Drug Release from Dendrimersomes

Doxorubicin-loaded dendrimersomes solution (65 µM DOX) was placed in a 200 µL Eppendorf-type plastic tube, sealed with a dialysis membrane and incubated in 5 mL of 10 mM Na phosphate buffer pH 7.0; 6.5; 6.0 for 24 h upon gentle stirring. At given time points, 50 µL aliquots of dialysis buffer were taken, and their fluorescence was read at 590 nm. Fluorescence intensity was plotted vs. incubation time and fitted with a first order kinetic curve ($r^2 > 0.95$).

2.10. WST Assay

10^4 1301 cells were cultivated in total volume 100 µL in flat-bottomed 96-well cell culture plates (TPP, Switzerland) for 72 h in the presence of blank chemodrug-loaded dendrimersomes as well as free drugs. Non-treated cells were cultivated in parallel as a control.

After cultivation, 10 µL of the WST-1 reagent (Takara Bio Inc, Kusatsu, Japan) per well was added, and the plates were incubated for 4 h. To evaluate the cell viability, optical absorbance at 450 nm was directly read against the background control, the reference was read at 620 nm (TriStar LB 941 Multimode Microplate Reader, Berthold Technologies GmbH&Co., Bad Wildbad, Germany). Cell viability was calculated as a ratio of absorbance of treated cells samples to that of non-treated control, then converted into percentage. Cell viability values were plotted against lgC, fitted with Boltzmann sigmoidal curve ($r^2 > 0.95$), and the $-\lg(IC_{50})$ values were estimated from the fitting data.

2.11. Drug Internalization Studies

0.5×10^6 1301 cells were cultivated in total volume 100 µL in flat-bottomed 48-well cell culture plates (TPP, Switzerland) for 4 h. Then, water solutions of amphiphilic dendron (5 µM), doxorubicin (3 µM) or doxorubicin-loaded dendrimersomes (doxorubicin content 3 µM) were added. The equal volume of PBS was added to control cells. After cultivation, cells were collected, washed once with PBS, then 50 µL of acidic glycine solution were added, gently pipetted for 30 s and washed again with PBS. Flow cytometric analysis was performed on a FACSCanto II cytometer (BD Biosciences, San Jose, CA, USA). The analysis was made in FITC and PE channels. 15,000 to 50,000 events per sample were acquired and analysed using FACSDiva 6.1.2 software.

1301 cells were incubated with blank dendrimersomes, doxorubicin and doxorubicin-loaded dendrimersomes (6.6 µM DOX) in complete cell culture media for 4 h in humidified atmosphere containing 5% CO_2 at 37 °C, then fixed in ethanol and glacial acetic acid. Samples were stained with

DAPI solution (1.5 µg/mL) with the addition of antifade solution (10 µL) for 20 min, protected from light. The cells were visualized under fluorescence microscopy (Axiopscop 40, Zeiss, Oberkochen, Germany).

2.12. Apoptosis Induction Studies

0.5×10^6 1301 cells were cultivated in total volume 250 µL for 72 h with amphiphilic dendron (5 µM), doxorubicin (3 µM) or doxorubicin-loaded dendrimersomes (doxorubicin content 3 µM). Non-treated cells were cultivated in parallel as a control. After cultivation, cells were collected, washed twice in cold Cell Staining Buffer (Biolegend, San Diego, CA, USA) and resuspended in Annexin V Binding Buffer (Biolegend, CA, USA). Ice-cold 70% ethanol solution was used for the necrosis induction control; and doxorubicin-treated cells were taken as the apoptosis induction control. For cell staining, the solutions of FITC Annexin V (5 µL per probe with $0.25–1.0 \times 10^7$ cells) and 7-AAD (5 µL per probe with $0.25–1.0 \times 10^7$ cells) were added. Cells were gently pipetted and incubated for 15 min at room temperature in the dark. Then, 400 µL of Annexin V Binding Buffer were added to each tube. Flow cytometric analysis was performed on a FACSCanto II cytometer (BD Biosciences, San Jose, CA, USA). 40,000 to 100,000 events per sample were acquired and analyzed using FACSDiva software. All experiments were run in triplicates.

3. Results and Discussion

3.1. Synthesis of the Amphiphilic Dendron

The novel dendritic amphiphile designed herein consists of a branched hydrophobic moiety (substituted triazine) and a cationic carbosilane dendron conjugated through a piperazine moiety, a convenient linker allowing further dendron grafting in relatively mild conditions.

We have synthesized the amphiphile in a convergent way (Scheme 1). The hydrophobic triazine unit has been obtained by the substitution of two chlorides in cyanuric chloride with dodecylamino-residues followed by the subsequent grafting of piperazine. The vinyl-terminated carbosilane dendron G2 having bromine in the focal point has been obtained starting from 4-bromobutylmethyldichlorosilane by iterative hydrosilylation and Grignard reaction steps as described earlier [33]. Two units, namely triazine and dendron ones, were conjugated by simple nucleophilic substitution, and vinyl residues at the periphery of the dendron have been modified via thiol-ene reaction. The resulting amphiphilic molecule contains two hydrophobic tails long enough to form a bilayer, a stimuli-sensitive triazine unit, and a branched polycationic dendron unit.

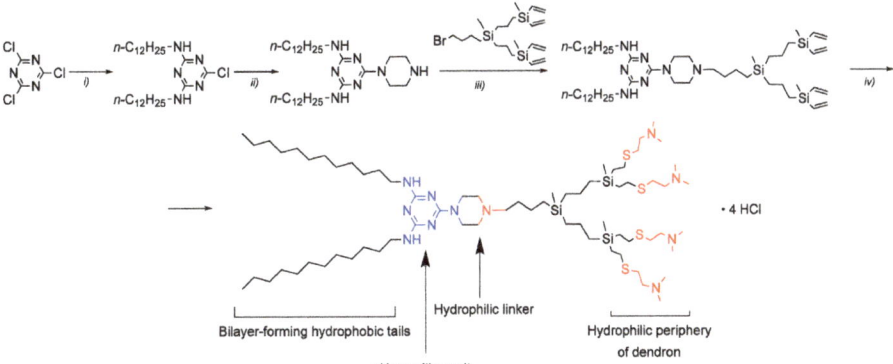

Scheme 1. Synthesis of the amphiphilic dendron: (**i**) n-C$_{12}$H$_{25}$NH$_2$, CHCl$_3$, NaOH (aq.), 90%; (**ii**) piperazine, CHCl$_3$, 92%; (**iii**) K$_2$CO$_3$, 18-crown-6, KI, acetone, 90%; (**iv**) HS(CH$_2$)$_2$N(CH$_3$)$_2$·HCl, DMPA, 365 nm UV, THF:CH$_3$OH, 75%.

3.2. Self-Assembly of Dendrimersomes

Dendritic amphiphile molecules are efficiently self-organised into supramolecular associates in water medium. The CMC determination plots in PB and PBS are given in the Figure 2. Comparing two plots, a clear difference is observed. In a low-salt solution (PB), there is only one association stage, quite broad in terms of concentration range, with CMC of 9.5 ± 1.2 µM. In contrast, at physiological salt concentration (PBS), there are two association stages with CMC of 2.1 ± 1.0 µM and 21 ± 1.1 µM. Apparently, the high salt concentration fosters the association of dendron molecules at low concentrations, with these aggregates further rearranging into vesicle-like dendrimersomes at higher concentrations.

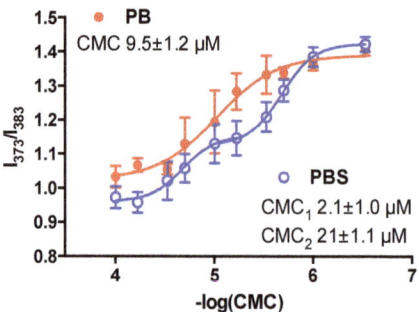

Figure 2. I_{373}/I_{383} plots corresponding to the amphiphilic dendron association in PB and PBS.

Vesicle-like nanoconstructions, dendrimersomes, are readily assembled upon quite simple treatment (short sonication and relaxation). High uniformity of nanoconstructions' topology and size, likely defined by the molecular structure of the dendron precursor, is achieved without specific post-treatment (e.g., extrusion). Having been formed at neutral pH, dendrimersomes have mean diameter of 20–30 nm; however, when put into acidic medium (pH below 6.5), they reorganize into larger particles 100–150 nm diameter (Figure 3). TEM shows that the vesicle-like structure of dendrimersomes is maintained upon reorganization.

Based on the findings above, we suggest a provisional scheme of the bilayer behaviour (Figure 3D). The main driving force of self-assembly is the interaction of hydrophobic tails of amphiphilic dendron molecules additionally stabilized by stacking interactions of triazine moieties [34]. On the other hand, the bilayer structure is destabilized by the steric and electrostatic repulsion of dendron fragments. Such a balance of factors favouring and unfavouring the bilayer stability likely gives the supramolecular flexibility to the whole dendrimersome. In acidic medium, triazine moieties get protonated, and the stacking is distorted. Thus, the stabilizing factor turns into the destabilizing one; this causes loosening of the bilayer followed by fusion with other vesicles.

It is worth noting that the effects of pH-sensitivity are observed at slightly acidic pH (below 6.5), which corresponds to early stages of endosome maturation. Thus, once delivered into a cell by endocytosis, an encapsulated biologically active cargo can be released into the cytosol in the most favourable moment to escape endosomes. Fusing dendrimersomes can contribute to the endosomal escape release by assisting the endosome membrane disruption.

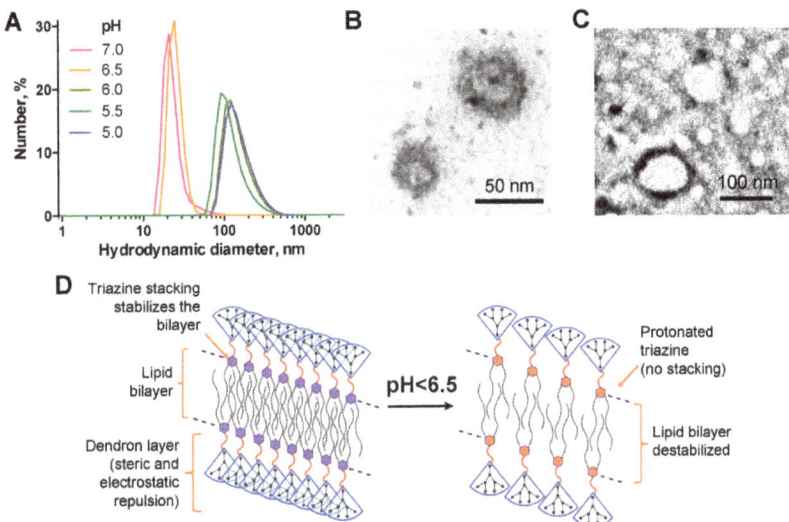

Figure 3. Self-assembly of dendritic amphiphiles. DLS profiles for supramolecular associates of dendron (100 μM) exposed to different pH in 10 mM Na-phosphate buffer (**A**); representative TEM images of dendrons' supramolecular associates at pH 7.0 (**B**) and pH 5.0 (**C**); tentative scheme of the pH-dependent behaviour of a dendron bilayer (**D**).

3.3. Drug Loading into Dendrimersomes

To explore the potential of dendrimersomes as drug carriers, we encapsulated three anti-tumor drugs—doxorubicin, methotrexate and 5-fluorouracil into dendrimersomes. Concentrated solutions of a drug and a dendron were rapidly mixed in water, sonicated and incubated for 48 h, followed by removal of non-encapsulated drug by dialysis. This procedure yields drug-loaded dendrimersomes with low size dispersion (PDI < 0.3) with a high degree of drug encapsulation (ca. 65% for doxorubicin and 75% for methotrexate) (Table 1). On the contrary, 5-fluorouracil encapsulated much less efficiently: for ca. 25%. The differences in the drug encapsulation efficiency resulted in 10-fold variation of the drug loading capacity: ~20% for doxorubicin and methotrexate vs. ~2% for 5-fluorouracil (Table 1). Such a dissimilarity is likely explained by the hydrophobicity of the encapsulated compound: doxorubicin and methotrexate can not only be entrapped into the inner cavity of a dendrimersomes but also incorporated into a bilayer (that can be observed in the TEM images (Figure 4) by the thickening of dendrimersomes' membranes), whereas for 5-fluorouracil, the entrapment likely prevails. Thus, the efficiency of 5-fluorouracil encapsulation can give an idea of the efficiency of the physical entrapment of compounds into the hydrophilic interior of dendrimersomes. It should be noted that methotrexate appeared to be additionally retained on the dendrimersomes' surface due to electrostatic interactions, as suggested by zeta potential values and TEM images. Drug-loaded dendrimersomes have mean diameter less than 100 nm that makes them suitable for drug delivery studies (Table 1).

Table 1. Properties of drug-loaded dendrimersomes.

Sample [1]	Particle Size [2], nm	PDI	Zeta Potential [2], mV	Drug Encapsulation [2], %	Drug Loading Capacity [3], %
DOX@DS	92 ± 38	0.213	41.3 ± 7.3	65 ± 10	>20.0
MTX@DS	46 ± 17	0.292	1.2 ± 4.5	75 ± 10	>20.0
5FU@DS	75 ± 30	0.216	11.0 ± 5.7	25 ± 5	>2.1

[1] DS-dendrimersomes; [2] Mean ± S.D.; [3] rough estimation, see Section 2.8.

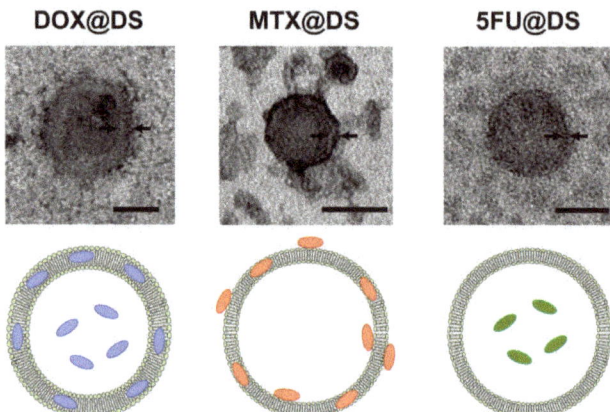

Figure 4. Representative TEM images of doxorubicin-loaded (DOX@DS), methotrexate-loaded (MTX@DS) and 5-fluorouracil-loaded (5FU@DS) dendrimersomes (top) and cartoons showing tentative drug distribution in dendrimersomes (bottom). Scale bar represents 50 nm. Black arrows show the thickness of a bilayer.

We have studied the pH dependence of the drug release from dendrimersomes using doxorubicin-loaded constructions as a model. The release was followed by measuring fluorescence intensity of dialysate (see Section 2.9). The rate of the drug release from dendrimersomes has not been found to increase significantly in slightly acidic medium (Figure S1): The half-release time being 6.3 ± 1.4 h at the pH 7.0 decreased to 6.0 ± 1.5 h (pH 6.5) and 5.4 ± 1.4 h (pH 6.0). However, overall fluorescence intensity of dialysate was higher with the decrease of the pH. The completeness of the doxorubicin release from dendrimersomes after 24 h was >80%. Thus, the pH-dependent behaviour shown for blank dendrimersomes (Figure 3) likely takes place in drug-loaded constructions as well, triggering the release of a drug in slightly acidic media frequently occurring in endocytic vesicles at early stages of endosome maturation [35].

3.4. Cytotoxic Activity of Drug-Loaded Dendrimersomes Towards Cancer Cells

We have tested the performance of triazine-carbosilane dendrimersomes as drug carriers by doing a comparative study of cytotoxic effects of nanoconstructions loaded with doxorubicin and methotrexate towards two leukaemia cell lines, 1301 and K562. 5-Fluorouracil-loaded dendrimersomes were excluded from the study due to the insufficient encapsulation efficiency resulting in the low concentration of the drug in the nanoparticle preparations.

Cell lines 1301 and K562 have been chosen as targets, for they represent leukaemia variants related to different types of progenitor cells: 1301 is the acute T-cell leukaemia cell line; K562 is chronic myelogenous leukaemia cell line derived from the cells of a patient having blast crises [36]. Thus, the use of these cell lines permits to estimate the efficiency of drug-loaded nanoconstructions in the haemoblastosis therapy.

The ability of drug-loaded dendrimersomes to suppress the viability of target cell lines was studied using WST-1 assay. Dose-response cytotoxic effects of nanoconstructions were observed. Doxorubicin-loaded dendrimersomes have been found to be less cytotoxic in comparison with free drug at low concentrations (below 1 µM) and exhibit similar activity at higher concentrations (Figure 5A,B). These differences are likely connected with the slow release of doxorubicin from dendrimersomes, so, being taken at low concentrations, they do not cause a commeasurable cytotoxic effect, which results in higher cell viability after treatment. In the case of methotrexate, free drug and drug-loaded dendrimersomes possess similar cytotoxicity (Figure 5C,D): In most cases, there were no statistically significant differences found between two groups. In general, the cytotoxic effects have been observed at dendron concentrations below the IC_{50} (Table 2, Figure S2), which permits to assign them to the encapsulated chemodrugs.

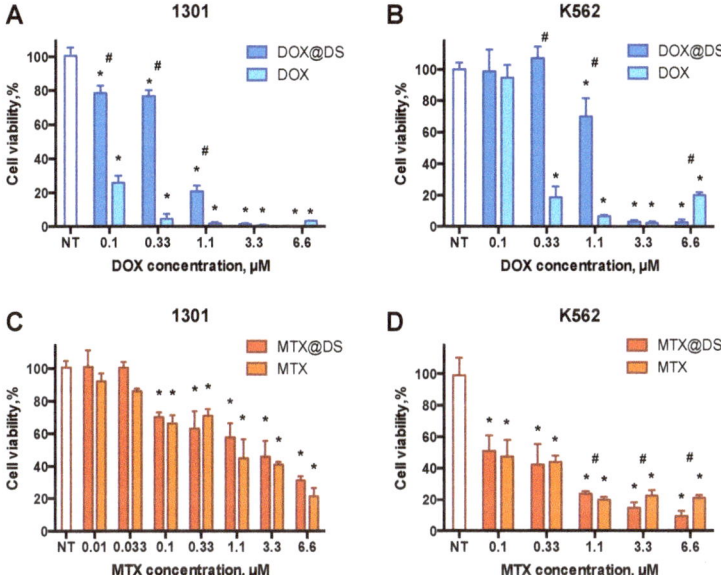

Figure 5. Viability profiles of 1301 (**A,C**) and K562 (**B,D**) cells after incubation with free chemodrugs and drug-loaded dendrimersomes. NT—non-treated cells. Incubation for 72 h, then WST-1 assay, data are presented as Mean ± S.D. (n = 5). * $p < 0.05$ vs. NT; # $p < 0.05$ free drug vs. drug@DS.

Table 2. IC_{50} values of blank dendrimersomes, chemodrugs and drug-loaded dendrimersomes towards 1301 and K562 cells.

Sample [1]	1301	K562
DS	5.4 ± 1.4 µM	4.6 ± 2.6 µM
DOX	0.059 ± 0.021 µM [2]	0.20 ± 0.08 µM
DOX@DS	0.71 ± 0.13 µM	1.2 ± 0.6 µM
MTX	0.99 ± 0.34 µM	0.046 ± 0.03 µM [2]
MTX@DS	0.99 ± 0.40 µM	0.15 ± 0.08 µM

[1] DS-dendrimersomes; [2] value predicted from data fitting

The differences observed between effects of doxorubicin- and methotrexate-loaded dendrimersomes on the viability of target cells are likely explained by the distribution of drugs in dendrimersomes. Since doxorubicin is mostly retained in the hydrophobic part of a vesicle, it is released as a result of reorganization (or even dissociation) of the carrier nanoparticle. Meanwhile, methotrexate is retained mostly at the surface of dendrimersomes, so it can be released relatively easier.

To understand the effects of drug-loaded dendrimersomes better, we have quantified cell subpopulations at different stages of cell death after the treatment with blank dendrimersomes, free drug and drug-loaded nanoconstructions. As a model system, we have taken doxorubicin-loaded dendrimersomes and 1301 cells as a cell model.

Both free doxorubicin and doxorubicin-loaded dendrimersomes have been shown to be efficiently accumulated in 1301 cells (Figures S3 and S4). However, treating cells with free doxorubicin (3 µM) resulted in slight increasing of early and late apoptosis cell fractions in comparison with control (ca. 10% each), whereas doxorubicin-loaded dendrimersomes (3 µM doxorubicin) caused a sharp increase of late apoptosis and necrosis cell fractions (50% and 20%, respectively) (Figure 6 and Figure S5). Blank dendrimersomes do not cause any significant effect on the 1301 cells in comparison to control at the concentration used (5 µM dendron). Certain differences with WST data likely occurred due to methodological features of the techniques.

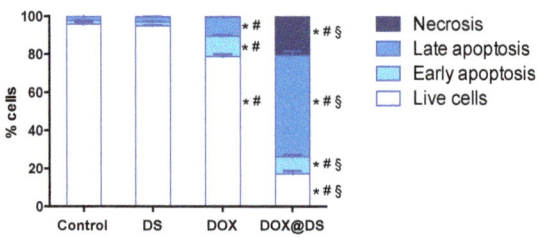

Figure 6. Induction of cell death in 1301 cells by blank dendrimersomes (DS), free doxorubicin (DOX) and doxorubicin-loaded dendrimersomes (DOX@DS). Incubation for 72 h, then FITC-Annexin V/7AAD staining, flow cytometry. Data are presented as mean ± S.D. (n = 3). * $p < 0.05$ vs. control group; # $p < 0.05$ vs. DS group; § $p < 0.05$ vs. DOX group.

Our findings show that the encapsulation does not improve the rate of accumulation of doxorubicin into tumour cells, however, the cytotoxic effect of the doxorubicin-containing nanoconstruction is visibly higher. This likely occurs due to the switch of the mechanism of drug penetration into a cell. Remarkably, the presence of serum, an important component of the cell culture medium, does not suppress the dendrimersomes' penetration into cells nor their cytostatic activity. The interaction of nanoconstructions with serum components is known to imminently take place during co-incubation with cells. We suppose that the encapsulation of anti-cancer chemodrugs into dendrimersomes can prolongate their persistence in the organism as well as reduce side effects. Such a phenomenon has been reported while using supramolecular associates [37] and macromolecules, in particular, dendrimers [38,39], as carriers for chemodrugs. In respect of novel amphiphilic triazine-carbosilane dendrimersomes reported herein, this hypothesis deserves further validation in animal experiments.

4. Conclusions

In summary, we have designed a new class of dendritic amphiphiles self-assembling into vesicle-like nanosized supramolecular associates (dendrimersomes). Rationally designed molecular topology of dendrons permits to use simple procedures to yield monodisperse nanoparticles. Because the reorganization is driven by subtle changes of ambient pH, triazine-carbosilane dendrimersomes can be useful as carriers for the delivery of sensitive, poorly soluble or highly toxic compounds into cells. As a proof-of-concept study, we attempted to encapsulate anti-cancer drugs doxorubicin and methotrexate and to deliver them into human leukaemia cells. The encapsulation, though efficient, does not change the vesicular topology of nanoconstructions. Drug-loaded dendrimersomes efficiently penetrate into cells and induce cell death. Our findings suggest that triazine-carbosilane dendrimersomes hold considerable potential for nanomedicine as stimuli-sensitive drug carriers.

Supplementary Materials: The following are available online at http://www.mdpi.com/2079-4991/10/10/1899/s1, Figure S1: Kinetic profiles of the doxorubicin release; Figure S2: Dendron biocompatibility; Figure S3: Flow cytometry plots; Figure S4: Fluorescence microscopy images; Figure S5: Flow cytometry plots.

Author Contributions: Conceptualization, N.K., E.P., E.A.; methodology, N.K., E.P., J.P., J.S.-N., E.A.; investigation, N.K., V.A., E.P., A.A., J.P., E.A.; data curation, N.K., V.A., J.P., E.P., E.A.; writing—original draft preparation, N.K., E.P., E.A.; writing—review and editing, F.J.d.l.M., R.G., E.A.; visualization, N.K., J.P., E.A.; supervision, F.J.d.l.M., R.G., E.A.; funding acquisition, F.J.d.l.M., R.G., E.A. All authors have read and agreed to the published version of the manuscript.

Funding: This study was supported by RFBR grant No. 18-33-20109, grant of the President of the Russian Federation No. MK-2278.2019.4, by MINECO grant CTQ-2017-85224-P, Consortium NANODENDMED-II-CM

(B2017/BMD-3703) and IMMUNOTHERCAN-CM (B2017/BMD3733). The project has received funding from the European Union's Horizon 2020 research and innovation programme under the Marie Skłodowska-Curie grant agreement No 844217. This article is based upon work from COST Action CA 17140 "Cancer Nanomedicine from the Bench to the Bedside" supported by COST (European Cooperation in Science and Technology). CIBER-BBN is an initiative funded by the VI National R&D&i Plan 2008–2011, Iniciativa Ingenio 2010, Consolider Program, CIBER Actions and financed by the Instituto de Salud Carlos III with assistance from the European Regional Development Fund. E.A. appreciates the financial support through the Gíner de los Ríos scholarship from the University of Alcalá.

Acknowledgments: The authors thank Margarita Barkovskaya (RIFCI) for fluorescence microscopy images as well as Alya Venyaminova (ICBFM) and Vladimir Kozlov (RIFCI) for the management support.

Conflicts of Interest: The authors declare no conflict of interest. The funders had no role in the design of the study; in the collection, analyses, or interpretation of data; in the writing of the manuscript, or in the decision to publish the results.

References

1. Jain, K.; Mehra, N.K.; Jain, N.K. Potentials and emerging trends in nanopharmacology. *Curr. Opin. Pharmacol.* **2014**, *15*, 97–106. [CrossRef]
2. Li, Z.; Ye, E.; David; Lakshminarayanan, R.; Loh, X.J. Recent Advances of using hybrid nanocarriers in remotely controlled therapeutic delivery. *Small* **2016**, *12*, 4782–4806. [CrossRef]
3. Movassaghian, S.; Merkel, O.M.; Torchilin, V.P. Applications of polymer micelles for imaging and drug delivery. *Wiley Interdiscip. Rev. Nanomed. Nanobiotechnol.* **2015**, *7*, 691–707. [CrossRef]
4. Dzmitruk, V.; Apartsin, E.; Ihnatsyeu-Kachan, A.; Abashkin, V.; Shcharbin, D.; Bryszewska, M. Dendrimers show promise for sirna and microrna therapeutics. *Pharmaceutics* **2018**, *10*, 126. [CrossRef]
5. Knauer, N.; Pashkina, E.; Apartsin, E. Topological aspects of the design of nanocarriers for therapeutic peptides and proteins. *Pharmaceutics* **2019**, *11*, 91. [CrossRef]
6. Palmerston Mendes, L.; Pan, J.; Torchilin, V. Dendrimers as nanocarriers for nucleic acid and drug delivery in cancer therapy. *Molecules* **2017**, *22*, 1401. [CrossRef]
7. Bolu, B.; Sanyal, R.; Sanyal, A. Drug delivery systems from self-assembly of dendron-polymer conjugates. *Molecules* **2018**, *23*, 1570. [CrossRef]
8. Sandoval-Yañez, C.; Castro Rodriguez, C. Dendrimers: Amazing Platforms for Bioactive Molecule Delivery Systems. *Materials* **2020**, *13*, 570. [CrossRef]
9. Fernandez, J.; Acosta, G.; Pulido, D.; Malý, M.; Copa-Patiño, J.L.; Soliveri, J.; Royo, M.; Gómez, R.; Albericio, F.; Ortega, P.; et al. Carbosilane dendron–peptide nanoconjugates as antimicrobial agents. *Mol. Pharm.* **2019**, *16*, 2661–2674. [CrossRef]
10. Sepúlveda-Crespo, D.; de la Mata, F.J.; Gómez, R.; Muñoz-Fernández, M.A. Sulfonate-ended carbosilane dendrimers with a flexible scaffold cause inactivation of HIV-1 virions and gp120 shedding. *Nanoscale* **2018**, *10*, 8998–9011. [CrossRef]
11. Krasheninina, O.; Apartsin, E.; Fuentes, E.; Szulc, A.; Ionov, M.; Venyaminova, A.; Shcharbin, D.; De la Mata, F.; Bryszewska, M.; Gómez, R. Complexes of pro-apoptotic siRNAs and carbosilane dendrimers: Formation and effect on cancer cells. *Pharmaceutics* **2019**, *11*, 25. [CrossRef]
12. Sánchez-Milla, M.; Muñoz-Moreno, L.; Sánchez-Nieves, J.; Malý, M.; Gómez, R.; Carmena, M.J.; de la Mata, F.J. Anticancer activity of dendriplexes against advanced prostate cancer from protumoral peptides and cationic carbosilane dendrimers. *Biomacromolecules* **2019**, *20*, 1224–1234. [CrossRef]
13. Carloni, R.; Sanz del Olmo, N.; Ortega, P.; Fattori, A.; Gómez, R.; Ottaviani, M.F.; García-Gallego, S.; Cangiotti, M.; de la Mata, F.J. Exploring the interactions of ruthenium (ii) carbosilane metallodendrimers and precursors with model cell membranes through a dual spin-label spin-probe technique using EPR. *Biomolecules* **2019**, *9*, 540. [CrossRef]
14. Gutierrez-Ulloa, C.E.; Buyanova, M.Y.; Apartsin, E.K.; Venyaminova, A.G.; de la Mata, F.J.; Gómez, R. Carbon nanotubes decorated with cationic carbosilane dendrons and their hybrids with nucleic acids. *ChemNanoMat* **2018**, *4*, 220–230. [CrossRef]
15. Pędziwiatr-Werbicka, E.; Gorzkiewicz, M.; Horodecka, K.; Abashkin, V.; Klajnert-Maculewicz, B.; Peña-González, C.E.; Sánchez-Nieves, J.; Gómez, R.; de la Mata, F.J.; Bryszewska, M. Silver nanoparticles surface-modified with carbosilane dendrons as carriers of anticancer siRNA. *Int. J. Mol. Sci.* **2020**, *21*, 4647. [CrossRef]

16. Percec, V.; Wilson, D.A.; Leowanawat, P.; Wilson, C.J.; Hughes, A.D.; Kaucher, M.S.; Hammer, D.A.; Levine, D.H.; Kim, A.J.; Bates, F.S.; et al. Self-Assembly of janus dendrimers into uniform dendrimersomes and other complex architectures. *Science* **2010**, *328*, 1009–1014. [CrossRef]
17. Peterca, M.; Percec, V.; Leowanawat, P.; Bertin, A. Predicting the size and properties of dendrimersomes from the lamellar structure of their amphiphilic janus dendrimers. *J. Am. Chem. Soc.* **2011**, *133*, 20507–20520. [CrossRef]
18. Thota, B.N.S.; Berlepsch, H.v.; Böttcher, C.; Haag, R. Towards engineering of self-assembled nanostructures using non-ionic dendritic amphiphiles. *Chem. Commun.* **2015**, *51*, 8648–8651. [CrossRef]
19. Wei, T.; Chen, C.; Liu, J.; Liu, C.; Posocco, P.; Liu, X.; Cheng, Q.; Huo, S.; Liang, Z.; Fermeglia, M.; et al. Anticancer drug nanomicelles formed by self-assembling amphiphilic dendrimer to combat cancer drug resistance. *Proc. Natl. Acad. Sci. USA* **2015**, *112*, 2978–2983. [CrossRef] [PubMed]
20. Liu, X.; Zhou, J.; Yu, T.; Chen, C.; Cheng, Q.; Sengupta, K.; Huang, Y.; Li, H.; Liu, C.; Wang, Y.; et al. Adaptive amphiphilic dendrimer-based nanoassemblies as robust and versatile siRNA delivery systems. *Angew. Chem. Int. Ed.* **2014**, *53*, 11822–11827. [CrossRef]
21. Gutierrez-Ulloa, C.E.; Buyanova, M.Y.; Apartsin, E.K.; Venyaminova, A.G.; de la Mata, F.J.; Valiente, M.; Gómez, R. Amphiphilic carbosilane dendrons as a novel synthetic platform toward micelle formation. *Org. Biomol. Chem* **2017**, *15*, 7352–7364. [CrossRef] [PubMed]
22. Mencia, G.; Lozano-Cruz, T.; Valiente, M.; de la Mata, J.; Cano, J.; Gómez, R. New ionic carbosilane dendrons possessing fluorinated tails at different locations on the skeleton. *Molecules* **2020**, *25*, 807. [CrossRef] [PubMed]
23. Gutierrez-Ulloa, C.E.; Sepúlveda-Crespo, D.; García-Broncano, P.; Malý, M.; Muñoz-Fernández, M.A.; de la Mata, F.J.; Gómez, R. Synthesis of bow-tie carbosilane dendrimers and their HIV antiviral capacity: A comparison of the dendritic topology on the biological process. *Eur. Polym. J.* **2019**, *119*, 200–212. [CrossRef]
24. Moreno, K.X.; Simanek, E.E. Identification of diamine linkers with differing reactivity and their application in the synthesis of melamine dendrimers. *Tetrahedron Lett.* **2008**, *49*, 1152–1154. [CrossRef]
25. Lim, J.; Simanek, E.E. Triazine dendrimers as drug delivery systems: From synthesis to therapy. *Adv. Drug Deliv. Rev.* **2012**, *64*, 826–835. [CrossRef]
26. Bagul, R.S.; Hosseini, M.M.; Shiao, T.C.; Roy, R. "Onion peel" glycodendrimer syntheses using mixed triazine and cyclotriphosphazene scaffolds. *Can. J. Chem.* **2017**, *95*, 975–983. [CrossRef]
27. Ji, K.; Lee, C.; Janesko, B.G.; Simanek, E.E. Triazine-Substituted and acyl hydrazones: Experiment and computation reveal a stability inversion at low pH. *Mol. Pharm.* **2015**, *12*, 2924–2927. [CrossRef]
28. Poletaeva, J.; Dovydenko, I.; Epanchintseva, A.; Korchagina, K.; Pyshnyi, D.; Apartsin, E.; Ryabchikova, E.; Pyshnaya, I. Non-Covalent associates of siRNAs and AuNPs enveloped with lipid layer and doped with amphiphilic peptide for efficient siRNA delivery. *Int. J. Mol. Sci.* **2018**, *19*, 2096. [CrossRef] [PubMed]
29. Onciu, M. Acute lymphoblastic leukemia. *Hematol. Oncol. Clin. N. Am.* **2009**, *23*, 655–674. [CrossRef] [PubMed]
30. Saußele, S.; Silver, R.T. Management of chronic myeloid leukemia in blast crisis. *Ann. Hematol.* **2015**, *94*, 159–165. [CrossRef]
31. Fuentes-Paniagua, E.; Peña-González, C.E.; Galán, M.; Gómez, R.; De La Mata, F.J.; Sánchez-Nieves, J. Thiol-ene synthesis of cationic carbosilane dendrons: A new family of synthons. *Organometallics* **2013**, *32*, 1789–1796. [CrossRef]
32. Aguiar, J.; Carpena, P.; Molina-Bolívar, J.A.; Carnero Ruiz, C. On the determination of the critical micelle concentration by the pyrene 1:3 ratio method. *J. Colloid Interface Sci.* **2003**, *258*, 116–122. [CrossRef]
33. Sánchez-Nieves, J.; Ortega, P.; Muñoz-Fernández, M.Á.; Gómez, R.; de la Mata, F.J. Synthesis of carbosilane dendrons and dendrimers derived from 1,3,5-trihydroxybenzene. *Tetrahedron* **2010**, *66*, 9203–9213. [CrossRef]
34. Mooibroek, T.J.; Gamez, P. The s-triazine ring, a remarkable unit to generate supramolecular interactions. *Inorganica Chim. Acta* **2007**, *360*, 381–404. [CrossRef]
35. Parkar, N.S.; Akpa, B.S.; Nitsche, L.C.; Wedgewood, L.E.; Place, A.T.; Sverdlov, M.S.; Chaga, O.; Minshall, R.D. Vesicle formation and endocytosis: Function, machinery, mechanisms, and modeling. *Antioxid. Redox Signal.* **2009**, *11*, 1301–1312. [CrossRef]
36. Klein, E.; Vánky, F.; Ben-Bassat, H.; Neumann, H.; Ralph, P.; Zeuthen, J.; Polliack, A. Properties of the K562 cell line, derived from a patient with chronic myeloid leukemia. *Int. J. Cancer* **1976**, *18*, 421–431. [CrossRef]
37. Fahmy, S.A.; Brüßler, J.; Alawak, M.; El-Sayed, M.M.H.; Bakowsky, U.; Shoeib, T. Chemotherapy based on supramolecular chemistry: A promising strategy in cancer therapy. *Pharmaceutics* **2019**, *11*, 292. [CrossRef]

38. Abedi-Gaballu, F.; Dehghan, G.; Ghaffari, M.; Yekta, R.; Abbaspour-Ravasjani, S.; Baradaran, B.; Ezzati Nazhad Dolatabadi, J.; Hamblin, M.R. PAMAM dendrimers as efficient drug and gene delivery nanosystems for cancer therapy. *Appl. Mater. Today* **2018**, *12*, 177–190. [CrossRef]
39. Hossain Sk, U.; Kojima, C. Dendrimers for Drug Delivery of Anticancer Drugs. In *Frontiers in Clinical Drug Research-Anti-Cancer Agents*; Rahman, A., Ed.; Bentham Science Publishers: Shardjah, UAE, 2015; pp. 3–25. ISBN 978-1-68108-073-4.

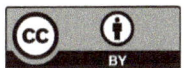

© 2020 by the authors. Licensee MDPI, Basel, Switzerland. This article is an open access article distributed under the terms and conditions of the Creative Commons Attribution (CC BY) license (http://creativecommons.org/licenses/by/4.0/).

MDPI
St. Alban-Anlage 66
4052 Basel
Switzerland
Tel. +41 61 683 77 34
Fax +41 61 302 89 18
www.mdpi.com

Nanomaterials Editorial Office
E-mail: nanomaterials@mdpi.com
www.mdpi.com/journal/nanomaterials

www.ingramcontent.com/pod-product-compliance
Lightning Source LLC
LaVergne TN
LVHW070127100526
838202LV00016B/2241